Image-Guided Interventions

Terry Peters • Kevin Cleary
Editors

Image-Guided Interventions

Technology and Applications

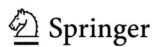 Springer

Editors

Terry Peters
Imaging Research Laboratories
Robarts Research Institute
University of Western Ontario
100 Perth Drive
London, ON N6A 5K8
Canada

Kevin Cleary
Radiology Department
Imaging Science and Information
  Systems (ISIS) Center
2115 Wisconsin Ave. NW, Suite 603
Washington, DC 20057
USA

ISBN: 978-0-387-73856-7   e-ISBN: 978-0-387-73858-1

Library of Congress Control Number: 2007943573

We would like to express our deepest gratitude to our colleague Jackie C. Williams, MA, for taking on the burden of Executive Editor of this book, for haranguing the authors, ensuring the manuscripts were delivered in time, editing them to perfection, and moulding them into the consistent format of the book. Without Jackie's dedicated involvement and professional skills, the production of this book could not have moved forward!

Foreword

Technical and clinical developments in the field of image-guided interventions have reached a stage **which makes the appearance of this book particularly timely. The chapters are by leading researchers, many of whom have been important contributors to the International Conference series Medical Image Computing and Computer Assisted Interventions (MICCAI).

The chapters provide excellent reviews that will be useful to a range of readers. While the material will generally be most accessible to those with a technical background (engineers, computer scientists, and physicists), books like this are increasingly important for clinical practitioners (surgeons and other interventionists) as well as clinical researchers and students with a background in medicine or biology. The field is emphatically cross-disciplinary, and close cooperation between the medical and the technical experts is critical. Constant preoccupation with high-volume patient throughput often inhibits the participation of highly trained clinicians in technically challenging research and well-written sources such as this volume, which can be used by clinicians as well as scientists, make a real contribution.

During interventions where images provide guidance, the effector may of course be the hand of the surgeon, but there are many exciting developments involving remote effectors where the surgeon is distanced from the final actions. Partially autonomous robotic systems, for example, in orthopaedic surgery (Chap. 12), allow much improved reliability for certain procedures. Micromanipulators potentially allow finer-scale interventions that are increasing in importance, particularly when the effector is at the end of an endoscope. In the future, we will also see the use of effectors with no mechanical link to the outside world, and such devices have the potential to function at a microscopic scale. The strength of this book is to include radiation therapy as one of the effectors (Chaps. 16 and 17).

The engineers involved in the design of all types of effectors including robots and remotely controlled devices need to remain fully engaged with image computing and clinical research in this cross-disciplinary field: whole-system integration is the key to future success. This remains a strong part of the philosophy of the MICCAI conferences.

What are the key areas which determine progress and future directions? This book provides several pointers. An important limitation of image guidance arises when images acquired earlier become out-of-date before a procedure is completed, because of physiological or pathological changes in the tissue and especially because of changes brought about by the intervention itself. Some *developments in intra-operative imaging* that provide regularly updated imaging are covered in the book (including MRI in Chaps. 10 and 14, and ultrasound in Chap. 15), and we look forward to further significant advances in these and other modalities. Developments in modelling of tissue deformations and in *non-rigid registration* (Chap. 7) continue to be important. This has particular relevance for thoraco-abdominal interventions (Chap. 13).

Evaluating the benefits and risks of image-guided interventions is of central importance (Chap. 18 and *passim*). Benefits for certain procedures has now been demonstrated in many clinical specialities. However, making the procedures available to patients in routine practice faces the huge hurdle of persuading healthcare funders of the *cost-effectiveness* of procedures. As healthcare costs generally increase, demonstrating improvements in the quality of care is not enough to secure support for clinical use, but quantifying benefit in economic terms, beloved by many health economists, is a very inexact process and often open to a wide range of interpretations. It is likely that in the short term image-guided systems will continue to make inroads into clinical practice only for isolated applications. Researchers need to continue to work very hard to generate quantitative and qualitative validation data. In some countries and clinical specialties, there is at present often great reluctance of funders and managers to support the introduction of new technology. But as patients and the public perception of the nature of the improvements provided by image-guided interventions continues to rise, demand will increase to a level which will greatly facilitate subsequent developments.

Alan Colchester

Professor of Clinical Neuroscience and Medical Image Computing,
University of Kent, Canterbury, England

Consultant Neurologist, Guy's & St. Thomas's Hospitals,
London and East Kent Hospitals Trust

Medical Image Computing and Computer-Assisted Intervention Board
Chairman 1999–2007 and Society President 2004–2007

Preface

This book had its genesis in 2003, when Dr. Lixu Gu of Shanghai Jiatong University asked whether we would consider organizing a workshop on image-guided interventions at the 2005 International Symposium on Engineering in Medicine and Biology in Shanghai, China. We agreed and our subsequent workshop included five individual speakers and covered neurological, orthopedic, and abdominal applications of image-guided interventions, with the inclusion of issues on visualization and image processing. After the symposium, Springer-Verlag approached us about editing a book on the basis of the workshop, and we decided that such a book would indeed fill a niche in the literature, but to do its justice, it would need to cover more than the original five topics.

We asked Jackie Williams to take on the role of Executive Editor, and over the next six months, we received agreement from the authors represented in this book, which includes 18 chapters divided between principles and applications. The title, "Image-Guided Interventions" was deliberately chosen over "Image-Guided Surgery" or "Minimally-Invasive Surgery and Therapy," as it covers the widest range of both therapeutic and surgical procedures, and reflects the recognition that the basic principles covered in the first part of the book are applicable to all such procedures. In addition, the inclusion of two chapters dealing with radiation-based therapies recognizes the convergence between surgery and radiation therapy in terms of the guidance technologies.

This book is aimed at both the graduate student embarking on a career in medical imaging, and the practicing researcher or clinician who needs a snapshot of the state-of-the-art in both the principles and practice of this discipline. Accordingly, the book begins with a historical overview of the development of image guidance for medical procedures, and follows with discussions of the critical components of tracking technologies, visualization, augmented reality, image registration (both rigid and nonrigid) image segmentation, and image acquisition. A chapter on the important issue of software development for image-guided systems is also included, as is one on the equally important issue of validation.

In the application section, examples are presented on the use of image guidance for focused ultrasound therapy, neurosurgery, orthopedics, abdominal surgery, prostate therapy, and cardiac applications. Finally, the linkages between image-guided surgery and radiation therapy are highlighted in chapters on the clinical application of radiosurgery and radiation oncology.

We sincerely thank our colleagues for agreeing to assist us in this endeavor, and for putting up with our incessant demands over the past year.

Terry Peters
London, ON, Canada

Kevin Cleary
Washington, DC, USA

November 2007

Contents

Contributors

Dean Barratt
University College London, London, United Kingdom

Filip Banovac
Georgetown University, Washington, DC, USA

Wolfgang Birkfellner
Medical University, Vienna, Austria

Jill Bruno
Georgetown University Medical Center, Washington, DC, USA

Tim Carter
University College London, London, United Kingdom

Rosanna Chan
Washington Hospital Center, Washington, DC

Kevin Cleary
Georgetown University, Washington, DC, USA

Greg Clement
Brigham & Women's Hospital, Boston, MA, USA

Bill Crum
Centre for Medical Image Computing, University College London,
London, United Kingdom

Sonja Dieterich
Radiation Physics Division, Stanford University Medical Center,
Stanford, CA, USA

Donal B. Downey
Royal Inland Hospital, Kamloops, British Columbia, Canada

Chandima Edirisinghe
Robarts Research Institute, London, Ontario, Canada

Fiona Fennessy
Brigham & Women's Hospital, Boston, MA, USA

Aaron Fenster
Robarts Research Institute and University of Western Ontario,
London, Ontario, Canada

Kirk Finnis
Medtronic Inc

RL Galloway
Dept of Biomedical Engineering, Vanderbilt University, Nashville, TN

Lori Gardi
Robarts Research Institute, London, Ontario, Canada

Mary Gospodarowicz
Princess Margaret Hospital/University Health Network, Toronto,
Ontario, Canada

Michael A. Guttman
National Institutes of Health, National Heart, Lung and Blood
Institute, Department of Health and Human Services, Bethesda, MD

Ting Guo
Robarts Research Institute and University of Western Ontario,
London, Ontario, Canada

David Hawkes
University College London, London, United Kingdom

Anthony Hodgson
University of British Columbia, Centre for Hip Health, Vancouver
Hospital, Vancouver, British Columbia, Canada

D.R. Holmes III
Mayo Clinic College of Medicine, Rochester, MN, USA

Keith A. Horvath
National Institutes of Health, Bethesda, MD

Johann Hummel
Medical University, Vienna, Austria

Luis Ibanez
Kitware Inc., Clifton Park, NY, USA

Jonathan Irish
Princess Margaret Hospital/University Health Network, Toronto,
Ontario, Canada

David Jaffray
University of Toronto, Ontario, Canada

Pierre Jannin
INSERM, Faculté de Médecine CS, Rennes Cedex, France
INRIA, Rennes, France

Ferenc Jolesz
Brigham & Women's Hospital, Boston, MA, USA

Ali Khamene
Siemens Corporate Research, USA

Manabu Kinoshita
Brigham & Women's Hospital, MA, USA

Werner Korb
University Leipzig, Leipzig, Germany

Robert J. Lederman
National Institutes of Health, Bethesda, MD

Jamie McClelland
University College London, London, United Kingdom

Nathan McDannold
Brigham & Women's Hospital, Boston, MA, USA

Elliot R. McVeigh
Johns Hopkins University, Baltimore, MD, USA

W. J. Niessen
Erasmus MC, Rotterdam, The Netherlands and Delft University
of Technology, The Netherlands

Brian O'Sullivan
Princess Margaret Hospital/University Health Network, Toronto,
Ontario, Canada

Andrew Parrent
London Health Sciences Centre and University of Western Ontario,
London, Ontario, Canada

Terry Peters
Robarts Research Institute and University of Western Ontario,
London, Ontario, Canada

M.E. Rettmann
Mayo Clinic College of Medicine, Rochester, MN, USA

R.A. Robb
Mayo Clinic College of Medicine, Rochester, MN, USA

James Rodgers
Director of Radiation Physics, Georgetown University Hospital,
Washington, DC, USA

Frank Sauer
Siemens Corporate Research, USA

Jeffrey Siewerdsen
Department of Medical Biophysics, University of Toronto, Ontario,
Canada

Clare Tempany
Brigham & Women's Hospital, Boston, MA, USA

Sebastian Vogt
Siemens Corporate Research, USA

Zhouping Wei
Philips Healthcare, Cleveland, Ohio, USA

Emmanuel Wilson
Georgetown University, Washington, DC, USA

Kenneth H. Wong
Georgetown University, Washington, DC, USA

Jason Wright
Georgetown University Medical Center, Washington, DC, USA

Ziv Yaniv
Georgetown University, Washington, DC, USA

List of Abbreviations

AAM	Active appearance models
ABS	American brachytherapy society
AC	Alternating current
AC-PC	Anterior commissural-posterior commissural
AP	Anterior-posterior
API	Application programming interface
API	Application user interface
AR	Augmented reality
AVS	Advanced visualization systems
BBB	Blood brain barrier
BPH	Benign prostatic hyperplasia
CABG	Coronary artery bypass graft
CAMC	Computer augmented mobile C-arm
CAOS	Computer-assisted orthopedic surgery
CAS	Computer-assisted surgery
CCD	Charge-coupled device
CFR	Code of federal regulations
CT	Computed tomography
CTV	Clinical target volume
DBS	Deep brain stimulation
DC	Direct current
DICOM	Digital imaging and communications
DOF	Degrees of freedom
DRR	Digitally reconstructed radiograph
DSA	Digital subtraction angiography
DTI	Diffusion tensor imaging
EBRT	External beam radiation therapy
EMTS	Electromagnet tracking systems
ENT	Ear, nose, and throat
EP	Electrophysiological
FFD	Free form deformation
FLE	Fiducial localization error
FMEA	Failure mode and effect analysis
fMRI	Functional magnetic resonance imaging
FOV	Field of view

FRACAS	FRActure computer assisted surgery
FRE	Fiducial registration error
FTA	Fault tree analysis
FUS	Focused ultrasound
GHTF	Global harmonization task force
GPU	Graphics processing unit
GRADE	The grading of recommendations assessment, development and evaluation
GTV	Gross tumor volume
GUI	Graphical user interface
HCTA	Health care technology assessment
HDR	High dose rate
HIFU	High intensity focused ultrasound
HKA	Hip–knee–ankle
HMD	Head-mounted display
HMM	Hidden Markov model
ICP	Iterative closest point
ICRU	The International Commission of Radiological Units
iCT	Intraoperative computed tomography
IEC	International electrotechnical commission
IGI	Image-guided intervention
IGS	Image-guided surgery
IGSTK	Image-guided surgical toolkit
iMRI	Intraoperative magnetic resonance imaging
IMRT	Intensity modulated radiation therapy
IR	Infrared
ISRCTN	The International Standard Randomized Controlled Trial Number
ITK	Insight segmentation and registration toolkit
IV	Integral videography
kNN	k nearest neighbors
kVCT	Kilovoltage computed tomography
kVp	Peak kilovoltage
LCD	Liquid crystal display
LED	Light-emitting diodes
Linac/LINAC	Linear accelerator
LPS	Left posterior superior
MEG/EEG	Magneto- and electro-encephalography
MER	Microelectrode recording
MI	Mutual information
MLC	Multi-leaf collimator
MRgFUS	MRI-guided focused ultrasound
MRI	Magnetic resonance imaging

MV	Megavoltage
MVCT	Megavoltage computed tomography
NCC	Normalized cross correlation
NHLBI	The National Heart, Lung, and Blood Institute of the National Institute of Health
NMI	Normalized mutual information
NURBS	Non-uniform rational B-splines
OAR	Organs at risk
OR	Operating room
OTS	Optical tracking systems
PACS	Picture archiving and communications systems
PAI	Pubic arch interference
PCA	Principal components analysis
PD	Parkinson's disease
PDE	Partial differential equation
pdf	probability density functions
PET	Positron emission tomography
PID	Proportional integral and derivative
PMMA	Polyethyl methacrylate
PRA	Probabilistic risk analysis
PRCT	Prospective randomized clinical trial
PRF	Proton resonant frequency
PRV	Planning risk volume
PTV	Planning target volume
RAS	Remote access service
RCT	Randomized clinical trials
RMS	Root mean square
RP	Radical prostatectomy
rtMRI	Real time magnetic resonance imaging
SAD	Sum of absolute differences
SBRT	Stereotactic body radiation therapy
SDM	Statistical deformation model
SISCOM	Subtraction interictal SPECT co-registered to MRI
SPECT	Single photon emission computed tomography
SPET	Single photon emission tomography
SRS	Stereotactic radiosurgery
SSD	Sum of squared differences
SSM	Statistical shape model
STARD	Standard for reporting of diagnostic accuracy
STN	Subthalamic nucleus
STS	Soft tissue sarcoma

SVD	Singular value decomposition
THA	Total hip arthroplasty
THR	Total hip replacement
TKA	Total knee arthroplasty
TKR	Total knee replacement
TRE	Target registration error
TRUS	Transrectal ultrasound
TUUS	Transurethral ultrasound
UML	Unified modeling language
UNC	University of North Carolina
US	Ultrasound
Vc	Ventralis caudalis
VF	Virtual fluoroscopy
VGA	Video graphics adaptor
Vim	Ventralis intermedius
VTK	Visualization toolkit

Chapter 1

Overview and History of Image-Guided Interventions

Robert Galloway and Terry Peters

Abstract

Although the routine use of image-guided intervention (IGI) is only about 20 years old, it grew out of stereotactic neurosurgical techniques that have a much longer history. This chapter introduces stereotactic techniques and discusses the evolution of image-guided surgical techniques enabled by the introduction of modern imaging modalities, computers, and tracking devices. Equally important in the evolution of this discipline were developments in three-dimensional (3D) image reconstruction, visualization, segmentation, and registration. This chapter discusses the role that each has played in the development of systems designed for IGI. Finally, a number of challenges are identified that currently are preventing IGI to progress.

1.1 Introduction

At the time of writing, the modern embodiment of the field of image-guided intervention (IGI) is approximately 20 years old. Currently, the general task of IGI can be subdivided into five smaller processes and a handful of general concepts. The subprocesses are to

1. gather preoperative data, generally in the form of tomographic images;
2. localize and track the position of the surgical tool or therapeutic device;
3. register the localizer volume with the preoperative data;
4. display the position of the tool with regard to medically important structures visible in the preoperative data; and
5. account for differences between the preoperative data and the intraoperative reality.

T. Peters and K. Cleary (eds.), *Image-Guided Interventions.*
© Springer Science + Business Media, LLC 2008

Underlying IGI are two fundamental concepts:

1. three-dimensional position data can be used to guide a physiological or medical procedure and
2. path, pose, and orientation make the problem at least six dimensional.

Although IGI is only 20 years old, the concepts and subprocesses have been developed, tested, and refined for over a hundred years. It also is interesting to note that the first known medical application of x-ray imaging was taken with therapeutic, not diagnostic, intent. A mere 8 days after the publication of Roentgen's first paper on x-ray imaging in 1895, J. H. Clayton, a casualty surgeon in Birmingham, England, used a bromide print of an x-ray to remove an industrial sewing needle from a woman's hand [Burrows 1986]. Barely a month later, John Cox, Professor of Physics at McGill University in Montreal [Cox and Kirkpatrick 1896], successfully removed a bullet from the leg of a victim based upon the radiograph that had been made of the limb. Not only was the projectile successfully removed on the basis of the radiograph, it was later used as evidence during a suit against the man who had shot the victim.

1.2   Stereotaxy

Horsley and Clark [1908] published a paper on a device that embodied several concepts and methods central to IGI 12 years after Clayton's landmark procedure. This device was a frame (Fig. 1.1) affixed to a subject's head (in this case, a monkey), and aligned using external anatomic landmarks, such as the auditory canals and the orbital rims. Using that alignment, the device allowed electrodes to be introduced into the skull and moved to locations within a Cartesian space defined by the frame. Horsley and Clark called their device a stereotaxic frame and brought several ideas to the forefront, notably the use of an external device to define a space within an anatomical structure, and the guidance of a tool or sensor to a point within that space. Horsley and Clark also used serial sections and illustrations derived from the sections to map where they wanted to move their instruments. This idea presaged tomographic imaging by more than 50 years. Horsley and Clark also introduced the concept of a spatial brain atlas. In an atlas, the user assumes that certain structures or functions can be found at particular spatial settings on the frame. The fundamental flaw in their system was that they assumed the monkey brains possessed a constant structure; that is, that one monkey's brain is the same as another. This led them to believe that external structures (auditory canals and orbital rims) could be used to accurately predict the location of internal structures.

To resolve these issues, and for stereotaxy to progress from physiological experiments on monkeys to medical procedures on humans, a methodology for obtaining patient specific information about internal structures

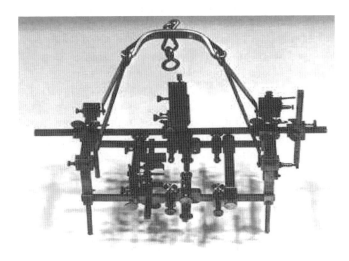

Fig. 1.1. The Horsley–Clarke stereotactic frame

had to be developed. Development of that methodology for the human head would take several decades.

It is curious as to why stereotaxy, and later, image guidance, arose in the field of neurosurgery but not in other therapeutic fields, although there are two probable reasons. The first is that the brain is the only organ encased entirely in bone. This allows the rigid attachment of an external guidance device to the skull, providing a platform for guidance. The second reason is that the brain tissue is largely non-redundant and non-regenerative, so the tissue in the path of the surgical target may be more crucial than the targeted tissue. The advantage of a guidance technology able to limit damage to healthy tissue was sufficient to overcome the usual inertia and resistance toward the adaptation of a new, complex technology.

Further development was hampered by the need for patient-specific information and target localization within the brain. The only realistic way to gather patient-specific information is to image it, and in the early years of medical imaging, plane-film x-ray was the only real choice. Given the high x-ray absorption of the surrounding skull and the relatively subtle changes in x-ray absorption between soft tissues, the soft tissue compartments of the head provided little contrast in a plane-film x-ray, which only displayed differences in the line-integral absorption of the x-ray beams. It was Dandy's [1918, 1919] invention of pneumoencephalography and ventriculography that allowed for some contrast between soft tissue compartments of the brain, providing patient-specific measurements of brain anatomy.

The availability of this imaging capability led Spiegel et al. [1947] to develop the first human stereotactic frame. Their device, while mechanically echoing the Horsley and Clark [1908] frame of almost 40 years earlier, was designed so that two orthogonal images, one anterior-posterior (AP) and the other side-to-side (lateral), could be made. The frame was constructed in such a way that it appeared in the images together with information about the patient's anatomy. Again, the images are projections of interior structures, so finding a three-dimensional point in the anatomy required it being precisely identified in both the AP and lateral images to resolve the third dimension. Although the Spiegel frame opened the door to human stereotaxy, its major weakness was how the frame was attached to the head. They used a plaster cast that swathed the patient's head and held struts attached to the frame. The plaster cast was held to the skin by friction and if the skin moved under the weight of the frame, it changed the relationship between the frame position and the anatomic structures.

Whether inspired by Spiegel and his colleagues or by independent creation, a number of surgeons developed their own stereotactic frames in the late 1940s and early 1950, the details of which can be found in Gildenberg and Tasker [1998] and Galloway [2001]. Four systems, in particular, deserve some additional mention. Tailarach [Talairach 1957; Talairach and Tourneau 1988, 1993] revisited the idea of a spatial atlas. His approach was to assume that all brains were not the same, but varied by a series of proportions. This meant that if certain anatomical structures could be visualized and measured, they could be used as scaling terms to an atlas, thus allowing a general atlas to be "fit" to a specific patient. Such a technique presaged the automatic rigid [Collins et al. 1994] and non-rigid [Collins and Evans 1997] registration methods used for intra-patient comparisons today. In addition, Chapter 6: Rigid Registration, and Chapter 7: Nonrigid Registration, give more detailed descriptions of these topics.

In Germany, Traugott Riechert and Wolff [1951] and later Fritz Mundinger [1982] developed a device that differed from all the preceding frames. This frame dealt with the head, not in a Cartesian format, but in spherical coordinates. This allowed access to structures within the head by moving along the cortical surface. This process also reduced the maximum distance from the frame to the head, thus reducing the effect of inaccurate angular positioning.

Leksell [Leksell 1951; Leksell and Jernberg 1980] also realized the advantage of breaking from Cartesian coordinates, but his system was structured on polar coordinates and introduced the idea of moving the device (a moveable arc mounted on the frame), such that its isocenter could be aligned with the target position (Fig. 1.2). By moving the arc so that the target was always at its center, all probes, electrodes, or other surgical instruments could be the same length. When at their fullest extent, the target was reached. Leksell [1968, 1983] also realized that other forms of therapy, such as radiation treatment, would be enhanced by improved guidance and he later developed the "Gamma Knife" system for radiation delivery (also see Chapter 16: Radiosurgery, for more discussion).

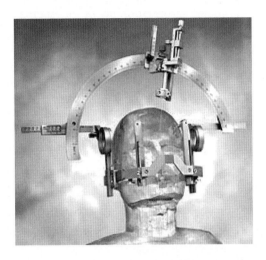

Fig. 1.2. Modern Leksell Frame equipped with isocentric targeting device

Of the stereotactic frames developed in the 1960s, the Todd–Wells [Todd 1967] is notable, not so much for its design, but for the fact that it served as the foundation for a number of other stereotactic systems. These include the Brown–Roberts–Wells (BRW) frame, the Cosman-Roberts–Wells (CRW) frame, and the Compass System.

For most of its history, the role of stereotaxy was to allow the surgeon close access to the target. Most stereotactic cases were for treatment of seizures or movement disorders, and consisted of ablation of erratically firing cells. Since such cells are radiographically indistinguishable from the surrounding healthy tissue, the surgeon had to determine the area of the brain to approach based on physical examination, and then use images to capture patient-specific information to locate the zone. The targeting was then refined by moving an electrode through the area until pathologic electrical signals were detected, or a desired patient response was elicited through stimulation.

In a 1987 article in Neurosurgery entitled, "Whatever Happened to Stereotactic Surgery?" Gildenberg [1987] documented the steep reduction in the number of stereotactic procedures after the introduction of L-Dopa in 1967. This was a good example of a medical treatment supplanting a surgical approach. At the time of writing, it is rather interesting to see the rise in deep brain stimulation, a surgical procedure that deals with the failure in the long-term use of L-Dopa and its pharmacological descendents.

1.3   The Arrival of Computed Tomography

In 1973, Hounsfield and EMI [Hounsfield 1973] announced the invention of the computed tomography (CT) scanner, which allowed the direct acquisition of three-dimensional image information about the internal structures of the brain. With CT, the voxels were highly non-isotropic due to the thickness of the slice (typically 13 mm in 1973). Although Hounsfield and EMI had had a difficult time finding commercial backers for the technology, it was quickly embraced by the diagnostic radiology community [Davis and Pressman 1974]. In the early 1970s, EMI's main activity was the recording and marketing of popular music and it is probable that the success of the Beatles in the 1960s was directly responsible for funding EMI's development of the CT scanner.

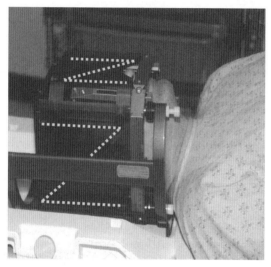

Fig. 1.3. "N"-bar system (embedded in acrylic frame but highlighted as *dashed lines*) attached to a stereotactic frame prior to imaging, as a means of registering the image to the patient

During this period of development, the therapeutic side was not lagging behind. Bergstrom and Greitz [1976] described their early experience of CT using stereotactic frames, and this was followed by many other reports describing the adaptation of CT in stereotactic surgery. In 1979, Brown published a methodology for determining the three-dimensional stereotactic position of any target point visible in a tomographic image. His method required placing radio-opaque bars that formed a letter "N" on the sides and the front of the frame worn by the patient. There were several important consequences of this technology. First, it made each voxel in the image independently addressable in both image space and physical space, removing the need to match target points on two plain-film x-rays. By removing the requirement that a target be unambiguously determined in two images, the choice of targets and therefore the targeting precision increased dramatically. The second consequence of the Brown "N" bar system is that it allowed the integration of the localization system and the registration process (Fig. 1.3). A frame with an N-bar system could serve both as a rigid tool platform and as a means of registration. One clever technique developed by Gildenberg and Kaufman [1982] allowed for the transfer of target points from a CT image into pseudo AP and lateral images, allowing pre- N-bar systems to make use of the new imaging modality.

In spite of the success of CT, the use of radiographs for stereotactic surgery did not entirely disappear. When vascular structures were involved, it was often necessary to use angiography alongside the CT images to ensure vascular-free pathways to the target. When using angiographic images, an alternative fiducial marker configuration comprising two sets of point objects on frame-mounted plates perpendicular to the central rays of lateral and AP x-ray beams were employed [Peters et al. 1994]. This configuration is similar to that described earlier, except that locations of points determined using the angiograms could now be directly related to the three-dimensional coordinate system defined by the CT image volume. Each of these points appears clearly in the projection images, and their positions can be used to precisely determine the imaging geometry. Using this approach, three-dimensional localization of structures within the brain could be achieved using orthogonal (or even stereoscopic) image pairs [Henri et al. 1991a,b] while superimposing them on the appropriate CT image.

Beyond the mechanics of using an old technology with new data, the presence of volumetric imaging allowed surgeons to consider new applications. Led by Kelly, then of the Mayo Clinic [Kall et al. 1985; Kelly 1986], surgeons began to use CT-based stereotaxy for surgeries beyond the classic cell ablations for movement and seizure disorders. Tumor, vascular, and functional surgeries were all facilitated using the information from tomographic images, a process that gained even more momentum with the release of the first magnetic resonance imaging systems in the late 1970s.

1.3.1 Computer Systems Come of Age

One development crucial to image-guided procedures that should not be overlooked is the August 1981 release of the IBM personal computer (PC). Although a number of neurosurgery systems had used computing systems (most notably the work by Shelden et al. [1980]), they required either specialty computer systems or massive amounts of data reduction, usually performed at the console of the tomographic imaging system. One of the first PC-based systems, with capabilities to plan stereotactic procedures from CT, MRI, or digital subtraction angiography (DSA), was that of Peters et al. [1987, 1989]. This increase in computing power triggered one of the most important changes in thinking, which was crucial to the advent of IGI. Prior to CT, for all types of medical images, the message was embedded in the medium. The images were formed on the method of display, for example, photographic film, whether the procedure involved plane-film x-ray, angiograms, or ultrasound. Using CT, the images existed as numbers *first* and then became converted to either film or cathode-ray displays. It should be noted that a large number of small computers existed prior to the IBM PC, but the legitimizing effect that the support of such a prominent company lent to this new technology cannot be ignored.

Stereotaxis can be grossly simplified as a process in which one "locates the target in the images, then moves to the target in physical space." In the mid- to late 1980s, at least four groups realized that the workflow of that process could be reversed. The new idea became to "determine present surgical position and display that position on the images." This made trajectory decisions an active process in the Operating Room ("how do I get from here to my target?"), but it allowed all the image information to be used actively as that decision was made or modified. It also provided multiple landmarks, so that there was no need to designate tumor margins as a surface of targets, or blood vessels as targets to be avoided. Such systems generally dispensed with the frame, performing image-to-patient registration using homologous landmarks instead. Thus the term "frameless stereotaxy" was born.

All the first four systems used tomographic images, a three-dimensional localizer/tracker, and a registration methodology. Initially, all four systems used anatomic landmarks as fiducials, generally the nasion of the nose and the tragi of the ears, so the difference was in the localization systems and in the methodology of display. We identify these four as simultaneous discovery/invention, because it is clear that work was proceeding on all four before the first public disclosure was made. They will be discussed here in the order of publications of first manuscripts.

1.4   Image-Guided Surgery

The first of the "frameless stereotactic" systems came from Roberts' lab at Dartmouth [Friets et al. 1989; Roberts et al. 1986]. They used a spark gap sonic system (there is further discussion on this in Section 1.5.1 of this chapter) affixed to the operating microscope with a single, dynamically updated tomographic image. The second published system was from the group at the Tokyo Police Hospital [Kosugi et al. 1988; Watanabe et al. 1987]. Here, an off-the-shelf articulated arm was used as a localizer, and the display consisted of a scanned sheet of tomographic images. In the 3 years between the first Roberts' paper and the first from the Vanderbilt group [Galloway et al. 1989], there had been a significant increase in the available computing power and display capabilities of small computers. Based on this technology boost, the Vanderbilt group [Galloway et al. 1993; Maciunas et al. 1992] developed an articulated arm designed exclusively for neurosurgery and for simultaneously displaying the surgical position on three dynamically updated orthogonal cut planes. The last of the four pioneering systems was also a custom articulated arm and perpendicular display [Adams et al. 1990a]. This system was noteworthy for two reasons. First, it addressed one of the major problems in articulated arms, which is the weight of the system, by suspending the arm from a fixed stand. The second reason was that this system was proposed for otolaryngology as well as neurosurgical procedures.

From these beginnings, articulated arms of various configurations were developed by research labs [Guthrie and Adler 1992; Koivukangas et al. 1993] and used in early commercial systems. However, articulated arms represented conflicting requirements. To be accurate, the arms could not flex appreciably over their length, requiring short, thick, arm segments. For ease of use, however, the arms needed low mass (and thus low inertia), but the base of the arm had to be mounted well away from the patient. These requirements forced the design of long, slender segments. It was the conflict between these requirements that prompted the development of free-hand localizers.

1.5   Three-Dimensional Localization

Three-dimensional localization can be achieved by means of geometric, triangulation, and inertial guidance. Articulated arms are a subclass of geometric localizers, and determine the position and angulation of the tip by measuring changes in arm angle and/or length from an initial zero point. All articulated arms used to date for surgery have been revolute arms, that is, they have fixed-length arms and they determine position by sensing the angles between the arms. The new (2006) da Vinci "S" surgical robot from Intuitive Surgical Inc. (Sunnyvale, CA), and some of the robotic biopsy work by Cleary et al. [2003] can be seen as the first step toward localizers that sense length change.

Considerable work has been performed on inertial guidance systems in aircraft and ships, and miniaturization of the component parts has made the creation of a handheld device possible. However, even in air and water craft, inertial systems are being supplanted by global positioning systems, a method of triangulation.

If geometric systems have conflicting requirements, and inertial systems are impractical for handheld tracking, the method of choice for localization and tracking must be some form of triangulation. There are two distinct methods of creating a triangulation system: fixed receiver and fixed emitter. In a fixed receiver system, three or more one-dimensional receivers (or two or more two-dimensional receivers) are placed in a known space in a known geometry to define a relative Cartesian space. An emitter placed in that space produces an energy pulse of some type. This pulse propagates to the receivers, and either the distances (generally through a time-of-flight

(TOF) calculation) or the angles between the emitter and the receivers are determined, allowing the location of the emitter to be calculated relative to the sensors. If one wishes to track and localize an object and determine its location and orientation, then three or more emitters must be placed on the object. Although three is the minimum required mathematically, all triangulation measurements contain noise that leads to spatial uncertainty. This uncertainty can be mitigated by placing additional transmitters on the object, converting the solution from a deterministic to a least-squares error minimization with concomitant noise reduction.

The other form of triangulation, fixed emitter, turns the geometry around. For fixed emitter, the tracked object holds the sensor and the transmitter defines the Cartesian space. Because it is easier to make small magnetic or radio frequency receivers than it is to make effective transmitters, most magnetic tracking systems are of the fixed emitter type.

There is one special case of localizer that is a hybrid fixed receiver, fixed emitter. The Beacon System (Calypso Medical Technologies Inc. Seattle, WA) uses a passive, implanted device that receives an energizing radio-frequency pulse and then emits a frequency-shifted response to fixed receivers [Balter et al. 2005]. An array of receivers permits the received signals to be decoded in terms of the position of the transponders.

1.5.1 Handheld Localizers

As was the case with the creation of what we now call image-guided surgery, it is difficult to sort out the beginning of devices that provide freehand localization and tracking. Clearly, three-dimensional localizers other than articulated arms had been available for decades prior to their use in surgery. However, at least three groups in the early 1990s proposed the use of sonic, TOF triangulation systems for tracking surgical tools in neuro-surgery. These three groups were those of Barnett at the Cleveland Clinic [Barnett et al. 1993], Bucholz at St. Louis University [Bucholz and Smith 1993], and Reinhardt et al. [1993] in Basel. In all of these systems, as in the Roberts' tracked microscope, receivers were placed in a fixed geometry at known locations. A source of sound beyond the human audible frequency range is transmitted as a pulse, and the time taken for the sound to reach each of the receivers is measured. The distances between the receivers and the emitters are calculated by measuring the TOF and dividing by the speed of sound. From these distances the emitter location can be determined.

Sonic systems suffer from two major problems, both of which are related to the speed of sound. The first problem is that while the speed of sound at standard temperature and pressure (STP) in air is nominally 330 m/s; humidity and temperature can cause variations sufficient to cause significant localization errors. Speed of sound induced errors can be overcome by using a surfeit of emitters that free the speed of sound from being a single constant, but the second problem limits the number of transmitters.

The second problem is that the receivers must be placed at least a meter from the patient to allow for measurable differences in TOF. This means it takes 3 ms for the pulse to reach the receiver. To prevent confounding echoes being detected as new source firing, the source activations must be spread out by at least 9 ms for a 1 m source/receiver distance. To resolve a three-dimensional device in space and attitude, at least three independent, non-collinear emitters are required. From the argument above, it is clear that more than four would be preferable. Using five as an arbitrary number, then five independent transmissions would be needed, each of 9 ms or 45 ms in total. During that time, the tracked object cannot move. If the receivers are moved further away from the patient, this problem becomes worse. In the case of the Roberts' tracked microscope, the inertia of the microscope prevented rapid motion, mitigating this effect. However, in a handheld tracking system for surgery, such a requirement puts an unreasonable burden on the surgeon to pay attention to the requirements of the tool. If the tool moves when the emitters are firing, then the solution to the equation degenerates and the answer becomes invalid. This was addressed by some developers by inserting a switch, which was to be pressed when the tool had settled into a desired position. While the switch addresses (to some extent) the motion-induced error, the system is no longer a localizer/tracker, but has become merely a localizer.

If the problem with sonic localizers is the speed of sound, then why not use light? Strobe-based, three-dimensional video position tracking had been known for a number of years, and the development in the 1980s of increasingly more efficient infrared light-emitting diodes (IREDs) made lightweight moving emitter configurations possible. There were initially two fundamental approaches, which were supplemented by a third approach that arrived later. The first approach used active IREDs as emitters. This made use of the sensitivity of charge-coupled device (CCD) light sensors sensitivity to near infrared light. By placing a visible light filter in front of the sensor, it became relatively easy to distinguish the IREDs from other light sources in the room. Two distinct systems emerged from this approach: the Optotrak 3020 (Northern Digital Inc, Waterloo, ON, Canada) [Maciunas et al. 1992; Zamorano et al. 1994] and the Flashpoint 3D localizer and Dynamic Reference Frame head tracker (Pixsys, Boulder, Colorado) [Tebo et al. 1996]. Both systems were adapted into surgical guidance systems. To address the price disparity between the Optotrak 3020 and the Flashpoint, Northern Digital developed a smaller system known as the Polaris, which has become the most commonly used localizer in image-guided systems.

The second optical approach was the direct offspring of video techniques used in biomechanics, automotive destructive testing, and other active deformation applications. Here the target was a passive reflector, often a pattern of lines and bars that can be extracted from two video images. In some ways this is a throwback to stereotactic frames and the need to locate points in AP and lateral x-rays; however, there is greater control in target geometry. One of the most successful approaches was the VISLAN project [Thomas et al. 1996; Colchester et al. 1996] from Guy's Hospital. A slightly different approach came from Brigham and Women's' Hospital, where a single camera was used, but a laser stripe was passed over the object [Grimson et al. 1998]. This technique cannot provide real-time tracking, but has found new applications in shape identification using laser range scanners [Sinha et al. 2005].

The major advantage of reflective systems is the low cost of the "emitter." These are merely reflective structures that can be as simple as patterns printed on a laser printer [Balanchandran et al. 2006]. The major problem with visible-light reflective techniques is that ambient light can confound the system. In an attempt to retain the advantages of passive systems, but to mitigate this weakness, Northern Digital developed a version of the Polaris that used infrared reflective balls mounted on their tracked probes [Wiles et al. 2004]. Such a technique retains the wireless nature and light weight of reflective systems, but filters the reflected light to allow clear identification of the reflectors.

All optical systems, whether active or passive, require that a line-of-sight be maintained between the emitter and the receiver. In some applications, such as when a flexible tool is desired, optical techniques are not optimal. A number of researchers, beginning with Manwaring et al. [1994], have used electromagnetic systems (See footnote in Chapter 2 Tracking Devices, page 26) for their tracking. The major advantage of these fixed-emitter systems is that as the EM signal can pass through the body, the sensor can be placed on the tip of the tool that enters the body. This spares the device from the errors caused by calculating the tool tip from the device trajectory, and allows the tool to be as flexible as desired. The use of flexible tools opens the way for tomogram-guided interventional radiology [Banovac et al. 2002]. Electromagnetic tracking has not yet attained the accuracy of optical tracking, and the presence of large metal structures in medical procedures and operating rooms can cause significant localization errors [Birkfellner et al. 1998a,b]. Chapter 2 discusses tracking in more detail.

1.6   Registration Techniques

The development of tomographic image sets providing three-dimensional information about the patient anatomy, location, and extent of disease, and the advent of three-dimensional spatial localizer/trackers has prompted the development of techniques to determine the relationship between these distinct spaces. This process is known as registration. When the mathematical relationship between a point in one space and the homologous point in another space is known, the spaces are considered registered. If that relationship can be reduced to a single common translation and rotation, the registration is considered rigid. In the field of stereotaxy, as the frame was visible in the image, registration was automatic. Once the frames were removed with the rise of image-guided surgery, then techniques had to be developed to map one space to another.

The obvious method to register these spaces was to identify homologous points in both the image space and the physical space. Use of these intrinsic points coupled with least square error transformation techniques, such as that of Arun et al. [1987] or Horn [1987], allows for the rapid registration of spaces. However, there are two problems with such methods. The first is that distinct points on the human body are not easily identified. Most shapes are rounded and it is difficult to pick out points either in image space or in physical space. The second problem is that the spatial uncertainty in a tomographic image in the thickness of the slice makes it impossible to determine precisely where the point lies within the slice.

Given the dearth of good intrinsic points to serve as reference points or fiducials, researchers have tried placing extrinsic objects with desirable characteristics on the patient for use in registration. These fiducial markers have been designed to stick to the skin [Zinreich et al. 1994] or be implanted into the bone [Maurer et al. 1997]. Because the markers were of a known size and geometry, and were designed to appear in more than one image slice, the spatial uncertainty of localization was greatly reduced. The mathematics of marker registration and marker design are discussed in detail in Fitzpatrick and Galloway [2001].

The field of registration has been dominated by the techniques of image-to-image registration, whether across modalities for the same patient, time series for the same patient, or across subjects for the creation of image atlases. In image-to-image registration, point-based registration has the advantage of having the most easily quantified outcomes, but for the reasons discussed above, the need for prospective placement of fiducial markers limits the usefulness of point-based techniques. Retrospective techniques that do not rely on point identification are clearly preferable, given a few qualifications. One of the first techniques was from Pelizzari et al. [1989] where surfaces were extracted from image sets and fitted together like a hat on a head. The greatest advantage of the surface registration was its ability to be used retrospectively; the greatest disadvantage was that it was difficult to quantify the quality of the registration.

In a landmark paper by West et al. [1997], a controlled experiment of image-to-image registration techniques was performed. Image sets with hidden point-based information were made available to researchers in the field, so they could use their own techniques for registration of the image sets. After they were satisfied with the registration their algorithms created, the hidden information was unveiled and the registration quality was then quantified. This study showed that point-based and volume-based [Hill et al. 1994] image-to-image registration techniques performed significantly better than surface-based registrations, after which the surface-based techniques fell rather into disfavor.

IGI requires image-to-physical space registration, and volumetric techniques are impractical, if not impossible. This has led to a slow reappearance of surface-based techniques for image space to physical registration. The problem of quantification of the registration quality remains, although there are glimmers of new techniques that allow the determination of which surfaces will provide good surface registration [Benincasa et al. 2006].

Physical space surfaces can be obtained by tracked intraoperative imaging such as ultrasound [Lavallee et al. 2004] by moving a tracked probe over a surface, or by the use of a laser range scanner [Herring et al. 1998]. The physical space surface is generally a cloud of three space points, which then can be matched to an extracted surface from image space via a number of iterative mathematical approaches. Most of the mathematical approaches are related to the iterative closest point algorithm developed by Besl and McKay [1992]. Further details on registration can be found in Chapter 6: Rigid Registration, and Chapter 7: Nonrigid Registration.

1.7   Display

The last component of early IGI systems is the display of surgical position and trajectory. The display task is often overlooked as being less important than the localizer or registration step, but it is the step where the data can most easily be misrepresented.

With the advent of modern tomography, good localizers, and functioning registration methodologies, the IGI task is inherently at least a four-dimensional task (three spatial dimensions plus time). Yet, even the most modern of displays can only display two spatial dimensions at once and even holographic displays only display the surfaces of the objects that were imaged with the hologram. So the challenge is to display four dimensions (three space + time) of information on a three-dimensional (two space + time) display. In addition, such a display must be as intuitive as possible, so the surgeon does not spend time and effort understanding the display instead of considering the surgery.

As discussed earlier, the four-quadrant, cardinal plane display common to most guidance systems was independently invented by Galloway et al. [1993] and Adams et al. [1990]. By presenting slices in standard orientations with perpendicular information, such displays allow for the transmission of multidimensional information in a relatively easy-to-grasp presentation. However, at any given point in time, the presented information is only the slices congruent with the estimated surgical position. If the surgeon wishes to consider moving obliquely to those planes, the anatomy to be traversed by such a move is not shown on the display.

In the 1990s, a new class of computer called a workstation began to become available to IGI system designers. One of the principles discerning features of workstations compared with other computers was the concern with the graphical performance of the machine. Workstations typically provide a great ability to perform sophisticated rendering and other graphics functions. Developers began to consider image pixels as textures that could be applied to shapes, allowing for display of transverse, sagittal, and coronal information on the same rendering [Barillot et al. 1991]. However, those systems still were hampered by the dimensional problem of the display. What surgeons needed to see was not their location, but the structures that were immediately beneath their location.

A group at Brigham and Women's Hospital attempted to address this problem with a methodology they called "enhanced reality" [Grimson et al. 1996]. Here, the tomographic data was reduced to important structures, such as the tumor and nearby blood vessels. These structures were then rendered and mixed into a perspective display according to the surgeon's viewpoint. By placing internal objects within such a display, the aim was to display the head as being transparent, allowing the surgeon to understand the location and orientation of internal structures.

One of the challenges of designers of IGI systems in dealing with three-dimensional data is that the human visual system is really only 2.5 dimensional in space. Binocular vision allows a viewer to understand the relative position of structures, but not to see within. The Montreal Neurological Institute has a long history [Henri et al. 1990; Peters et al. 1990a,b] of obtaining stereo pair angiograms that allow the viewer to determine the relative positions of vessels and vascular abnormalities. Angiograms do this well, because only by visualizing the vessels can you reduce the information density. There is no pressing reason to see inside the vessel for the guidance of therapy.

In addition, to accomplish true binocular vision, there must be an image presented to the right eye, and a distinct image presented to the left eye. If either eye perceives the image presented to the other, the binocular effect is lost. The need for complete separation has led to the development of various forms of head-up displays. Clearly, the operating microscope is a logical place for insertion of data; however, inserting information into the visual stream without disturbing the light microscopy function presents some challenges to the designers [Edwards et al. 1995]. Other designers do not employ the microscope at all [Birkfellner et al. 2000], but use small monitors to display information separately to each eye. Surgeon acceptance remains a challenge for this approach.

1.8   The Next Generation of Systems

Currently, what are the remaining challenges? Although advancements have been made in imaging, localizers, registration, and display, no one can claim that the ideal has been found for any of them. In addition, one of the fundamental concepts of the whole field, which is that the images represent the present state of the physiology, is only a first approximation. Attempts to address this by decreasing the time between image and intervention led to the development of intraoperative tomography [Fichtinger et al. 2005]. However, there has not been a significant advancement in medical outcomes to justify the cost and complexity of such systems. Research is ongoing to see if the cost and complexity can be reduced.

A separate approach is to attempt to understand and model the deformations that occur both peri-procedurally and intra-procedurally. Again, the ongoing march of performance to price of computers is allowing for large, mathematically sophisticated models [Cash et al. 2005; Paulsen et al. 1999; Warfield et al. 2005] to calculate solutions in surgically appropriate time scales.

We are rapidly closing in on the twentieth anniversary of what is now called IGI, with new applications being developed almost monthly. A whole generation of neurosurgeons has completed their residencies, culminating in an expectation that operating rooms will come readily equipped with image guidance systems. It is a tribute to the designers that their systems have become commoditized, but acceptance should not breed complacency. As evidenced by the rest of this book, there is exciting work still to be done and problems yet to be solved.

References

Adams L, Krybus W, Meyerebrecht D, Rueger R, Gilsbach JM, Moesges R, and Schloendorff G. (1990). "Computer-assisted surgery." *IEEE Comput Graph Appl*, 10(3), 43–51.

Arun KS, Huang TS, and Blostein SD. (1987). "Least-squares fitting of 2 3-D point sets." *IEEE Trans Pattern Anal Mach Intell*, 9(5), 699–700.

Balanchandran R, Labadie R, and Fitzpatrick JM. (2006). "Validation of a Fiducial Frame System for Image-guided Otologic Surgery Utilizing Bahar Bone Screws." *ISBI 2006*, Arlington, VA.

Balter JM, Wright JN, Newell LJ, Friemel B, Dimmer S, Cheng Y, Wong J, Vertatschitsch E, and Mate TP. (2005). "Accuracy of a wireless localization system for radiotherapy." *Int J Radiat Oncol Biol Phys*, 61(3), 933–937.

Banovac F, Levy EB, Lindisch DJ, Pearce A, Onda S, and Clifford M. (2002). "Feasibility of percutaneous transabdominal portosystemic shunt creation." *Surg Radiol Anat*, 24(3–4), 217–221.

Barillot C, Lachmann F, Gibaud B, and JM S. (1991). "Three-dimensional display of MRI data in neurosurgery: segmentation and rendering aspects." *SPIE Medical* SPIE, Newport Beach, CA, 54–65.

Barnett GH, Kormos DW, Steiner CP, and Weisenberger J. (1993). "Intraoperative localization using an armless, frameless stereotactic wand. Technical note." *J Neurosurg*, 78(3), 510–514.

Benincasa A, Clements L, Herrell S, Chang S, Cookson M, and Galloway R. (2006). "Feasibility study for image guided kidney surgery: assessment of required intraoperative surface for accurate image to physical space registrations." *SPIE Medical Imaging* SPIE, San Diego, CA, 554–562.

Bergstrom M, and Greitz T. (1976). "Stereotaxic computed tomography." *AJR Am J Roentgenol*, 127(1), 167–170.

Besl PJ, and McKay ND. (1992). "A Method for Registration of 3-D Shapes." *IEEE Trans Pattern Anal Mach Intell*, 14(2), 239–256.

Birkfellner W, Figl M, Huber K, Watzinger F, Wanschitz F, Hanel R, Wagner A, Rafolt D, Ewers R, and Bergmann H. (2000). "The varioscope AR – A head-mounted operating microscope for augmented reality." *Med Image Comput Comput Assist Interv*, 1935, 869–877.

Birkfellner W, Watzinger F, Wanschitz F, Enislidis G, Kollmann C, Rafolt D, Nowotny R, Ewers R, and Bergmann H. (1998a). "Systematic distortions in magnetic position digitizers." *Med Phys*, 25(11), 2242–2248.

Birkfellner W, Watzinger F, Wanschitz F, Ewers R, and Bergmann H. (1998b). "Calibration of tracking systems in a surgical environment." *IEEE Trans Med Imaging*, 17(5), 737–742.

Brown RA. (1979). "A computerized tomography-computer graphics approach to stereotaxic localization." *J Neurosurg*, 50(6), 715–720.

Bucholz R, and Smith K. (1993). "A comparison of sonic digitizers versus light emitting diode-based localization." In: *Interactive Image-Guided Neurosurgery*, Maciunas RJ, ed., American Association of Neurological Surgeons, pp. 179–200.

Burrows E. (1986). *Pioneers and Early Years: A History of British Radiology*. Colophon Press, Alderney.

Cash DM, Miga MI, Sinha TK, Galloway RL, and Chapman WC. (2005). "Compensating for intraoperative soft-tissue deformations using incomplete surface data and finite elements." *IEEE Trans Med Imaging*, 24(11), 1479–1491.

Cleary K, Watson V, Lindisch D, Patriciu A, Mazilu D, and Stoianovici D. (2003). "Robotically assisted interventions: Clinical trial for spinal blocks." *Med Image Comput Comput Assist Interv*, 2879(Pt 2), 963–964.

Colchester ACF, Zhao J, Holton-Tainter KS, Henri CJ, Maitland N, Roberts PTE, Harris CG, and Evans RJ. (1996). "Development and preliminary evaluation of VISLAN, a surgical planning and guidance system using intra-operative video imaging." *Med Image Anal*, 1, 73–90.

Collins DL, and Evans AC. (1997). "ANIMAL: Validation and applications of non-linear registration based segmentation." *Int J Pattern Recog Art Intel*, 11(8), 1271–1294.

Collins DL, Neelin P, Peters TM, and Evans AC. (1994). "Automatic 3D inter-subject registration of MR volumetric data in standardized Talairach space." *J Comput Assist Tomogr*, 18(2), 192–205.

Cox J, and Kirkpatrick RC. (1896). "The new photography with report of a case in which a bullet was photographed in the leg." *Montreal Medical Journal*, 24, 661–665.

Dandy W. (1918). "Ventriculography of the brain after injection of air into the cerebral ventricles." *Ann Surg*, 68, 5–11.

Dandy W. (1919). "Roentgenography of the brain after injection of air into the spinal canal." *Ann Surg*, 70, 397–403.

Davis DO, and Pressman BD. (1974). "Computerized tomography of the brain." *Radiol Clin North Am*, 12(2), 297–313.

Edwards PJ, Hawkes DJ, Hill DL, Jewell D, Spink R, Strong A, and Gleeson M. (1995). "Augmentation of reality using an operating microscope for otolaryngology and neurosurgical guidance." *J Image Guid Surg*, 1(3), 172–178.

Fichtinger G, Deguet A, Fischer G, Iordachita I, Balogh E, Masamune K, Taylor RH, Fayad LM, de Oliveira M, and Zinreich SJ. (2005). "Image overlay for CT-guided needle insertions." *Comput Aided Surg*, 10(4), 241–255.

Fitzpatrick J, and Galloway R. (2001). "Fiducial-based 3D image- and patient-space matching." *Automedica*, 20(1–2), 36–47.

Friets EM, Strohbehn JW, Hatch JF, and Roberts DW. (1989). "A frameless stereotaxic operating microscope for neurosurgery." *IEEE Trans Biomed Eng*, 36(6), 608–617.

Galloway R, Edwards C, Haden G, and Maciunas R. (1989). "An interactive, image-guided articulated arm for laser surgery." *Strategic Defense Initiative Organization's Fourth Annual Meeting on Medical Free-Electron Lasers*, Dallas, TX.

Galloway R, Edwards C, Lewis J, and Maciunas R. (1993). "Image display and surgical visualization in interactive image-guided neurosurgery." *Optical Engineering.*, 32(8), 1955–1962.

Galloway RL, Jr. (2001). "The process and development of image-guided procedures." *Annu Rev Biomed Eng*, 3, 83–108.

Gildenberg P, and Tasker R, eds. (1998). *Textbook of Stereotactic and Functional Neurosurgery*, McGraw-Hill, New York.

Gildenberg PL. (1987). "Whatever happened to stereotactic surgery?" *Neurosurgery*, 20(6), 983–987.

Gildenberg PL, and Kaufman HH. (1982). "Direct calculation of stereotactic coordinates from CT scans." *Appl Neurophysiol*, 45(4–5), 347–351.

Grimson E, Leventon M, Ettinger G, Chabrerie A, Ozlen F, Nakajima S, Atsumi H, Kikinis R, and Black P. (1998). "Clinical experience with a high precision image-guided neurosurgery system." *MICCAI*, Springer (LNCS), Boston, MA.

Grimson WEL, Ettinger GJ, White SJ, LozanoPerez T, Wells WM, and Kikinis R. (1996). "An automatic registration method for frameless stereotaxy, image guided surgery, and enhanced reality visualization." *IEEE Trans Med Imaging*, 15(2), 129–140.

Guthrie BL, and Adler JR. (1992). "Computer-assisted preoperative planning, interactive surgery, and frameless stereotaxy." *Clinical Neurosurgery,* 38, 112–131.

Henri CJ, Collins DL, and Peters TM. (1991a). "Multimodality image integration for stereotactic surgical planning." *Med Phys*, 18(2), 167–177.

Henri CJ, Collins DL, Pike GB, Olivier A, and Peters TM. (1991b). "Clinical experience with a stereoscopic image workstation." *SPIE – The International Society for Optical Engineering*, Bellingham, WA, San Jose, CA, 306–317.

Henri CJ, Peters TM, Lemieux L, and Olivier A. (1990). "Experience with a computerized stereoscopic workstation for neurosurgical planning." *IEEE Visualization in Biomedical Computing*, IEEE Press, 450–457.

Herring JL, Dawant BM, Maurer CR, Jr., Muratore DM, Galloway RL, and Fitzpatrick JM. (1998). "Surface-based registration of CT images to physical space for image-guided surgery of the spine: a sensitivity study." *IEEE Trans Med Imaging*, 17(5), 743–752.

Hill D, Studholme C, and Hawkes D. (1994). "Voxel similarity measures for automated image registration." *SPIE Medical Imaging*, SPIE, Newport Beach, 205–216.

Horn BKP. (1987). "Closed-form solution of absolute orientation using unit quaternions." *J Opt Soc Am a-Opt Image Sci Vis*, 4(4), 629–642.

Horsley V, and Clark R. (1908). "The structure and functions of the cerebellum examined by a new method." *Brain* 31(45–124).

Hounsfield GN. (1973). "Computerized transverse axial scanning (tomography). 1. Description of system." *Br J Radiol*, 46(552), 1016–1022.

Kall BA, Kelly PJ, Goerss S, and Frieder G. (1985). "Methodology and clinical experience with computed tomography and a computer-resident stereotactic atlas." *Neurosurgery*, 17(3), 400–407.

Kelly PJ. (1986). "Applications and methodology for contemporary stereotactic surgery." *Neurol Res*, 8(1), 2–12.

Koivukangas J, Louhisalmi Y, Alakuijala J, and Oikarinen J. (1993). Neuronavigator-guided cerebral biopsy. *Acta Neurochir Suppl.*, 58, 71–74.

Kosugi Y, Watanabe E, Goto J, Watanabe T, Yoshimoto S, Takakura K, and Ikebe J. (1988). "An articulated neurosurgical navigation system using MRI and CT images." *IEEE Trans Biomed Eng*, 35(2), 147–152.

Lavallee S, Merloz P, Stindel E, Kilian P, Troccaz J, Cinquin P, Langlotz F, and Nolte L. (2004). "Echomorphing: introducing an intraoperative imaging modality to reconstruct 3D bone surfaces for minimally invasive surgery." *4th Annual Meeting of the International Society for Computer Assisted Orthopaedic Surgery (CAOS-International)*, Chicago, IL, 38–39.

Leksell L. (1951). "The stereotaxic method and radiosurgery of the brain." *Acta Chir Scand*, 102(4), 316–319.

Leksell L. (1968). "Cerebral radiosurgery. I. Gammathalanotomy in two cases of intractable pain." *Acta Chir Scand*, 134(8), 585–595.

Leksell L. (1983). "Stereotactic radiosurgery." *J Neurol Neurosurg Psychiatry*, 46(9), 797–803.

Leksell L, and Jernberg B. (1980). "Stereotaxis and tomography. A technical note." *Acta Neurochir (Wien)*, 52(1–2), 1–7.

Maciunas RJ, Galloway RL, Jr., Fitzpatrick JM, Mandava VR, Edwards CA, and Allen GS. (1992). "A universal system for interactive image-directed neurosurgery." *Stereotact Funct Neurosurg*, 58(1–4), 108–113.

Manwaring KH, Manwaring ML, and Moss SD. (1994). "Magnetic field guided endoscopic dissection through a burr hole may avoid more invasive craniotomies. A preliminary report." *Acta Neurochir Suppl*, 61, 34–39.

Maurer CR, Jr., Fitzpatrick JM, Wang MY, Galloway RL, Jr., Maciunas RJ, and Allen GS. (1997). "Registration of head volume images using implantable fiducial markers." *IEEE Trans Med Imaging*, 16(4), 447–462.

Mundinger F. (1982). "CT stereotactic biopsy of brain tumors." In: *Tumors of the Central Nervous System in Infancy and Childhood*, Voth D. Gutjahr P., and Langmaid C., eds., Springer, Berlin Heidelberg New York.

Paulsen KD, Miga MI, Kennedy FE, Hoopes PJ, Hartov A, and Roberts DW. (1999). "A computational model for tracking subsurface tissue deformation during stereotactic neurosurgery." *IEEE Trans Biomed Eng*, 46(2), 213–225.

Pelizzari CA, Chen GT, Spelbring DR, Weichselbaum RR, and Chen CT. (1989). "Accurate three-dimensional registration of CT, PET, and/or MR images of the brain." *J Comput Assist Tomogr*, 13(1), 20–26.

Peters TM, Clark J, Pike B, Drangova M, and Olivier A. (1987). "Stereotactic surgical planning with magnetic resonance imaging, digital subtraction angiography and computed tomography." *Appl Neurophysiol*, 50(1–6), 33–38.

Peters TM, Clark JA, Pike GB, Henri C, Collins L, Leksell D, and Jeppsson O. (1989). "Stereotactic neurosurgery planning on a personal-computer-based work station." *J Digit Imaging*, 2(2), 75–81.

Peters TM, Henri C, Collins L, Pike B, and Olivier A. (1990a). "Clinical applications of integrated 3-D stereoscopic imaging in neurosurgery." *Australas Phys Eng Sci Med*, 13(4), 166–176.

Peters TM, Henri C, Pike GB, Clark JA, Collins L, and Olivier A. (1990b). "Integration of stereoscopic DSA with three-dimensional image reconstruction for stereotactic planning." *Stereotact Funct Neurosurg*, 54–55, 471–476.

Peters TM, Henri CJ, Munger P, Takahashi AM, Evans AC, Davey B, and Olivier A. (1994). "Integration of stereoscopic DSA and 3D MRI for image-guided neurosurgery." *Comput Med Imaging Graph*, 18(4), 289–299.

Reinhardt HF, Horstmann GA, and Gratzl O. (1993). "Sonic stereometry in microsurgical procedures for deep-seated brain tumors and vascular malformations." *Neurosurgery*, 32(1), 51–57; discussion 57.

Riechert T, and Wolff M. (1951). "A new stereotactic instrument for intracranial placement of electrodes." *Arch Psychiatr Nervenkr Z Gesamte Neurol Psychiatr*, 186(2), 225–230.

Roberts DW, Strohbehn JW, Hatch JF, Murray W, and Kettenberger H. (1986). "A frameless stereotaxic integration of computerized tomographic imaging and the operating microscope." *J Neurosurg*, 65(4), 545–549.

Shelden CH, McCann G, Jacques S, Lutes HR, Frazier RE, Katz R, and Kuki R. (1980). "Development of a computerized microstereotaxic method for localization and removal of minute CNS lesions under direct 3-D vision. Technical report." *J Neurosurg*, 52(1), 21–27.

Sinha TK, Dawant BM, Duay V, Cash DM, Weil RJ, Thompson RC, Weaver KD, and Miga MI. (2005). "A method to track cortical surface deformations using a laser range scanner." *IEEE Trans Med Imaging*, 24(6), 767–781.

Spiegel E, Wycis H, Marks M, and Lee A. (1947). " Stereotactic apparatus for operations on the human brain." *Science*, 106, 349–350.

Talairach J. (1957). *Atlas d'anatomie stéréotaxique; repérage radiologique indirect des noyaux gris centraux des régions mésencéphalo-sous-optique et hypothalamique de l'homme,* Masson, Paris.

Talairach J, and Tourneau P. (1988). *Co-planar stereotaxic atlas of the human brain,* Georg Thieme Verlag, Stuttgart, Germany.

Talairach J, and Tourneau P. (1993). *Referentially oriented cerebral MRI anatomy,* Georg Thieme Verlag, Stuttgart, Germany.

Tebo SA, Leopold DA, Long DM, Zinreich SJ, and Kennedy DW. (1996). "An optical SD digitizer for frameless stereotactic surgery." *IEEE Comput Graph Appl*, 16(1), 55–64.

Thomas DG, Doshi P, Colchester A, Hawkes DJ, Hill DL, Zhao J, Maitland N, Strong AJ, and Evans RI. (1996). "Craniotomy guidance using a stereo-video-based tracking system." *Stereotact Funct Neurosurg*, 66(1–3), 81–83.

Todd E. (1967). *Todd-Wells Manual of Stereotaxic Procedures*, Codman & Shurtleff, Randolph, Mass.

Warfield SK, Haker SJ, Talos IF, Kemper CA, Weisenfeld N, Mewes AU, Goldberg-Zimring D, Zou KH, Westin CF, Wells WM, Tempany CM, Golby A, Black PM, Jolesz FA, and Kikinis R. (2005). "Capturing intraoperative deformations: research experience at Brigham and Women's Hospital." *Med Image Anal*, 9(2), 145–162.

Watanabe E, Watanabe T, Manaka S, Mayanagi Y, and Takakura K. (1987). "Three-dimensional digitizer (neuronavigator): new equipment for computed tomography-guided stereotaxic surgery." *Surg Neurol*, 27(6), 543–547.

West J, Fitzpatrick JM, Wang MY, Dawant BM, Maurer CR, Jr., Kessler RM, Maciunas RJ, Barillot C, Lemoine D, Collignon A, Maes F, Suetens P, Vandermeulen D, van den Elsen PA, Napel S, Sumanaweera TS, Harkness B, Hemler PF, Hill DL, Hawkes DJ, Studholme C, Maintz JB, Viergever MA, Malandain G, Woods RP, et al. (1997). "Comparison and evaluation of retrospective intermodality brain image registration techniques." *J Comput Assist Tomogr*, 21(4), 554–566.

Wiles AD, Thompson DG, and Frantz DD. (2004). "Accuracy assessment and interpretation for optical tracking systems." *SPIE Medical Imaging, Visualization, Image-Guided Procedures, and Display*, San Diego, CA, 421–432.

Zamorano LJ, Nolte L, Kadi AM, and Jiang Z. (1994). "Interactive intraoperative localization using an infrared-based system." *Stereotact Funct Neurosurg*, 63(1–4), 84–88.

Zinreich SJ, and Zinreich ES. US Patent 5368030. (1994). "*Non invasive Multi-Modality Radiographic Surface Markers*." USA.

Chapter 2

Tracking Devices

Wolfgang Birkfellner, Johann Hummel, Emmanuel Wilson,

and Kevin Cleary

Abstract

Tracking devices are an essential component of an image-guided surgery system. These devices are used to track the position of instruments relative to the patient anatomy. Although early tracking systems were essentially mechanical digitizers, the field quickly adopted optical tracking systems because of their high accuracy and relatively large workspace. However, optical tracking systems require that a line-of-sight be maintained between the tracking device and the instrument to be tracked, which is not always convenient and precludes tracking of flexible instruments inside the body. Therefore, electromagnetic tracking systems were developed that had no line-of-sight requirement and could track instruments such as catheters and the tips of needles inside the body. The choice of tracking system is highly application dependent and requires an understanding of the desired working volume and accuracy requirements. To meet these needs, a variety of tracking devices and techniques have been introduced as described in this chapter.

2.1 Introduction

The advent of x-rays as a medical imaging modality at the turn of the last century brought about clinical interest in the 3D localization of internal anatomical structures. This was first realized with the invention of the stereotactic frame in the late 1920s, and its first use in humans for neurosurgical applications in the early 1940s. Targets within the cranium are relatively easy to localize because of visible landmarks such as the exterior auditory canals and inferior orbital rims, onto which the early stereotactic frames were fixed. The improved accuracy and benefits of this technique to existing surgery techniques led to the emergence of framed stereotactic approaches as standard practice by the early 1960s, with devices such as the Leksell frame and Mayfield clamp being widely used.

Advances in computed tomography (CT) and magnetic resonance imaging (MRI) by the mid-1980s led to the development of frameless

T. Peters and K. Cleary (eds.), *Image-Guided Interventions.*

© Springer Science + Business Media, LLC 2008

stereotaxy. Neurosurgical applications pioneered the early advances with this technique, but its use quickly spread to ENT and spine procedures. Frameless stereotaxy allowed for smaller incisions, less patient discomfort, shorter patient preparation times, and fewer restrictions on surgical access. Perhaps the single most crucial benefit was the capability for real-time overlay of CT and MRI images that facilitated a more exact roadmap of the patient anatomy and thereby more accurate surgical outcome.

The emergence of frameless stereotaxy was facilitated by position trackers, which can track surgical tools and enable the physician to register external landmarks to pre-operative images of the patient anatomy. Over the past 20 years, frameless stereotaxy has become the predominant influence on image-guided interventions. Techniques that were pioneered for neuro-surgical applications have been used in orthopedic, endoscopic, and, more recently, abdominal surgical procedures. The wide-ranging applications of image-guided surgery place differing emphasis on requirements. In addition, novel position tracking techniques and devices have also been introduced.

2.2   Tracking: A Brief History

The introduction and successful outcome of computer-aided surgery (CAS), or frameless stereotaxy in neurosurgery in the 1980s, relied heavily on position tracking devices. A well-established technology at the time that could provide accurate position information was a mechanical digitizer, consisting of a robotic arm with rotary encoders at the various linkage nodes. Position and orientation information of the robotic end effector is resolved using forward kinematics.

The use of mechanical digitizers facilitated frameless stereotaxy by localizing either an operating microscope's focus, or a surgical probe inside the patient's cranium [Reinhardt and Landolt 1989; Watanabe et al. 1987]. Early CAS systems used mechanical digitizers to replace the need for the Mayfield clamp, a staple of framed stereotaxy procedures. Due to the cumbersome nature of mechanical digitizers of the time, interest in alternative tracking methods led to the introduction of ultrasonic transducers for localization [Hata et al. 1997; Reinhardt and Zweifel 1990; Roberts et al. 1986]. However, ultrasonic solutions rely on the speed of sound, which is dependent on relative air moisture and surrounding temperature and is prone to obstruction; thereby lacking the robustness of mechanical digitizers.

The reliability of mechanical digitizers, such as the Faro arm [Zamorano et al. 1994], helped spearhead the development of a commercial product, the ISG Viewing Wand [Doshi et al. 1995; Sandeman et al. 1994]. The ISG Viewing Wand was used for a number of non-neurosurgical interventions in cranio- and maxillofacial surgery [Dyer et al. 1995; Hassfeld et al. 1995] and in ENT surgery [Carney et al. 1996; Freysinger et al. 1997; Nishizaki et al. 1996]. During early trials, a localization accuracy of approximately 2–3 mm [Sipos et al. 1996] was reported. Although the system served the purpose of localizing a probe relative to the fixed coordinate system of the Mayfield clamp, this approach posed several limitations in a clinical setting. A primary limitation of this approach was the inability to track multiple devices. In addition, sterilization issues and relatively cumbersome handling in the operating theater led researchers to move toward alternate tracking techniques.

Optical trackers proved to be an early answer to clinically feasible tracking systems. Systems such as the Optotrak 3020 (Northern Digital Inc., Waterloo, Ontario, Canada) [Nolte et al. 1995; Rohling et al. 1995], the Flashpoint 5000 (Boulder Innovation Group Inc., Boulder, Colorado, USA) [Anon 1998; Eljamel 1997; Li et al. 1999; Smith et al. 1994; Watzinger et al. 1999], and the Polaris (Northern Digital) [Khadem et al. 2000; Schmerber and Chassat 2001] were adopted. Figure 2.1 shows some of the commonly used optical tracking systems (OTS). Optical trackers evolved into the most reliable and accurate tracking solution. The early systems usually consisted of charge-coupled device (CCD) cameras and sequentially illuminated infrared (IR) light-emitting diodes (LED), and were integrated into image-guided systems such as the Neurostation, which finally evolved into the well-known StealthStation (Medtronic, Minneapolis, Minnesota, USA).

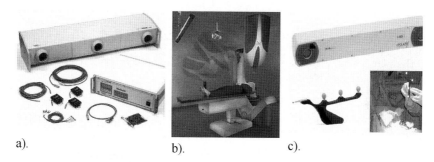

a).   b).   c).

Fig. 2.1. Examples of optical trackers: (**a**) Optotrak 3020 camera, control unit, and active markers (courtesy of Northern Digital), (**b**) Flashpoint active optical camera from Boulder Innovation Group used in the CyberKnife suite (courtesy of Accuray), (**c**) Polaris camera shown with passive marker tool and use in surgery (courtesy of Northern Digital)

Most OTS in use are wired devices that lead to increased clutter in the OR. A few wireless systems have been developed. VISLAN, an experimental system for neurosurgery [Colchester et al. 1996] shown in Fig. 2.2a, was one of the earliest efforts to use a videometric system to estimate patient pose and instrument orientation by identification of passive markers in video-image sequences. Another early effort was the use of the Qualisys tracking system [Gumprecht et al. 1999; Josefsson et al. 1996] in the VectorVision system by BrainLAB (Heimstetten, Germany) shown in Fig. 2.2b, now distributed by Advanced Realtime Tracking GmbH, Munich,

Germany. The de-facto standard at the time of writing is the Polaris tracking system with its variants, which provides both the option of wireless and wired tracking.

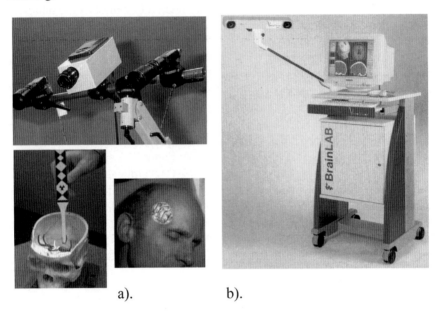

a).   b).

Fig. 2.2. Examples of IGS systems: (**a**) VISLAN system with pattern marked tool and image overlay (reprinted from Colchester 1996 with permission from Elsevier), (**b**) Brainlab VectorVision system (reprinted from Gumprecht 1999 with permission from the Congress of Neurological Surgeons)

The key limitation with the use of an OTS in a crowded operating theater is the line-of-sight requirement between the optical markers and the tracker camera, which led to the development of alternative tracking methods that avoided line-of-sight limitations. In particular, electromagnetic tracking systems (EMTS),[1] a technology well known from motion analysis [Meskers et al. 1999; Milne et al. 1996; van Ruijven et al. 2000; Wagner et al. 1996], helmet-mounted displays, and the animation industry, was proposed as a possible alternative. EMTS incorporating small coils or similar electromagnetic field sensors and multiple position measurement devices can easily be used in a clinical setting. Therefore, electromagnetic trackers

---

[1]The term "electromagnetic" tracking has historically been used to describe systems that are based on magnetic fields. Some researchers may argue that these systems should be called "magnetic" spatial measurement systems since they do not depend on the electric field component of the electromagnetic wave. However, we will use the term electromagnetic here to reflect common usage and the fact that a varying magnetic field has an associated electric component.

that were developed for military applications as well as motion capture solutions in general, were employed within CAS [Bottlang et al. 1998; Fried et al. 1997; Goerss et al. 1994, Javer et al. 2000; Reittner et al. 2002; Sagi et al. 2003; Suess et al. 2001; Wagner et al. 1995] motion detection in radiation oncology [Kirsch et al. 1997; Litzenberg et al. 2006; Seiler et al. 2000; Watanabe and Anderson 1997], image-guided radiological interventions [Wood et al. 2005; Khan et al. 2005; Zhang et al. 2006], endoscopic procedures [Deguchi et al. 2006; Hautmann et al. 2005; Solomon et al. 2000], and 3D B-mode ultrasound imaging [Barratt et al. 2001; Fristrup et al. 2004; Sumiyama et al. 2002].

2.3 Principles of Optical Tracking Systems

The broad use of OTS in industry has introduced many manufacturers and system variants with wide-ranging specifications. Clinical systems are a niche sector and the technology used for their operation has not changed significantly in recent years. Optical systems can be characterized as follows:

1. *Videometric tracking systems.* These systems identify marker patterns on video image sequences, usually taken using one or more calibrated video cameras. The well-known marker patterns on crash-test dummies as well as the videometric solutions implemented in the VISLAN system and the freely available AR Toolkit [Kato and Billinghurst 1999] fall into this category. Systems commercially available today, such as the Claron tracker (Claron Technology Inc., Toronto, Ontario, Canada), are provided in small form factors.

2. *IR-based tracking systems.* An optical band-pass filter eliminates all ambient light of other wavelengths, making the identification of optical markers a comparatively simple and reliable task. Two types of IR trackers exist, both used widely in clinical applications:

    1. *Active optical trackers.* Sterilizable LEDs operating in the near-IR range (approximately 900 nm wavelength) are used as markers, tracked by either two planar or three linear CCD units that form the camera module. The LEDs are fired sequentially and detected by each CCD unit. The central unit uses a process of triangulation based on the known geometric configuration and firing sequence of each LED and the known, fixed distance between the CCD elements. A minimum of three non-collinear LEDs are necessary for determining six degrees-of-freedom (DOF) pose information. Since the LEDs must be powered, traditionally active systems were also wired systems.

2. *Passive optical trackers.* These systems work in the near IR range. Instead of active markers, retroreflective spheres are illuminated by the camera in the near-IR spectrum. The pattern of the reflective markers, which has to be unique for each tracking probe so that unambiguous assignment of each probe is feasible, is identified on a 2D image. For this reason, these systems are always equipped with 2D CCD cameras. One big advantage of these systems is that no wires are needed between the tracking system and the tracked probes.

3. *Laser tracking systems.* Rather than localizing a set of LEDs, an array of photosensors is mounted to a rigid carrier. Two or three fans of coherent laser light emitted by conventional semiconductor lasers are reflected by rotating mirrors. The fan-shaped laser beam sweeps the digitizer volume. The position of the rigid body is estimated by simultaneously sampling the position of the sweep fan and the signal from the photosensor [Cash et al. 2007]. An example of such a tracker is the laserBIRD2 by Ascension Technology (Burlington, Vermont, USA). However, these systems have not found widespread use in medical applications.

A key reason for the success of optical tracking technology in the clinical environment has been its high accuracy and reliability. There have been a few scattered instances in clinical practice where the use of high-intensity IR from the emitter LEDs of passive IR trackers interferes with other IR devices in the operating room, but this is a rare occurrence. Despite their line-of-sight limitation, OTS are the standard in clinical applications at this time. Other examples of applications include high-precision radiation therapy of retinal diseases, where the beam is controlled by detection of eye motion [Petersch et al. 2004], or for motion correction in tomographic reconstruction [Buhler et al. 2004; Feng et al. 2006].

2.4   Principles of Electromagnetic Tracking

EMTS are a relatively new tracking technology in medical applications. Their main advantage is that they have no line-of-sight limitation, but their disadvantages include susceptibility to distortion from nearby metal sources and limited accuracy compared to optical tracking. These systems localize small electromagnetic field sensors in an electromagnetic field of known geometry. The EMTS used in medical imaging can be divided into three categories as described below. Figure 2.3 shows an example system from each category.

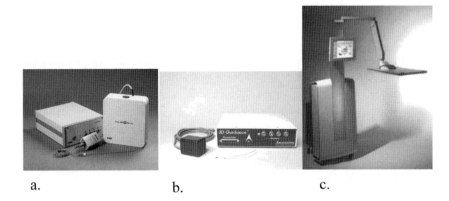

a.   b.   c.

Fig. 2.3. (**a**) Aurora AC-based system (courtesy of Northern Digital), (**b**) 3D Guidance pulsed-DC system (courtesy of Ascension), (**c**) transponder-based system (courtesy of Calypso Medical Systems)

1. *AC-driven tracking.* The earliest developed "classical" EMTS are driven by alternating current (AC). One of the earliest systems is from Polhemus Inc. (Colchester, Vermont, USA). This system consists of three coils arranged in a Cartesian coordinate system that emits an electromagnetic field composed of three dipole fields. Typical operating frequencies for the AC-driven magnetic trackers lie in the range of 8–14 kHz. Small search coils measure the induced voltage, which is proportional to the flux of the magnetic field. A thorough description of the principles of operation of AC-driven tracking systems can be found in Kuipers [1980]. As systems have evolved, manufacturers have employed different approaches to generate the electromagnetic field [Raab 1979]. An early iteration of the Northern Digital Aurora system used six coils in a tetrahedral arrangement [Seiler et al. 2000, 2007].

2. *DC-driven tracking.* As the name would suggest, rather than using an AC-driven magnetic field, these systems are driven by quasistatic direct current (DC). DC trackers are available from Ascension Technology. The magnetic induction within miniature active (fluxgate) sensors was originally measured after establishment of a stationary magnetic field, but current models employ passive microminiaturized sensors [Blood 1989].

3. *Passive or transponder systems.* These systems track position by localization of permanent magnets or implanted transponders. One such system in use for medical application is to assess the placement of nasogastric feeding tubes [Bercik et al. 2005]). Another system introduced recently for tumor position tracking during radiation therapy is the Calypso 4D system (Calypso Inc., Seattle, Washington, USA)

[Willoughby et al. 2006]. Since these systems are relatively new, they have not been widely used yet in image-guided interventions.

The main difference between AC and DC systems lies in their behavior when metallic objects are in close proximity to either the field emitter or the sensor. With an AC-based system, eddy currents are induced in conductive materials, which can then interfere with the continuously generated (i.e., never turned off) magnetic fields and distort the sensor readings. DC-based tracking systems can circumvent this problem by using static magnetic field measurements. With a DC-based system, the magnetic field is turned on and off at a certain frequency, allowing eddy currents to decay sufficiently to mitigate distortions caused by common conductive metals such as stainless steel (300 series), titanium, and aluminium.

A second issue is that ferromagnetic materials such as iron, nickel, cobalt, and some steels become strongly magnetic in the presence of an electromagnetic field. This phenomenon can also distort the reference magnetic field and thereby affect the measurement accuracy of the EMTS [Birkfellner et al. 1998a; Hastenteufel et al. 2006; King 2002; LaScalza et al. 2003; Milne et al. 1999; Poulin and Amiot 2002]. Another source of reference field distortion is magnetic stray fields from drives or other computer equipment and peripheral devices. Therefore, EMTS can be susceptible to measurement errors. To mitigate ferromagnetic errors, Ascension has recently introduced a planar (flat) transmitter with a built-in shield that negates metal distortions emanating from OR and procedural tables [Ashe 2003]. Both radio-translucent and radio-opaque models are available.

From the early days of application of EMTS in the virtual reality/augmented reality (AR) community to more recent applications in the medical field, methods to differentiate the systematic error or compensate for it have been studied extensively. For medical applications, methods to calibrate the work environment for changes in the magnetic field by interpolation or lookup table-based approaches have been proposed for EMTS [Birkfellner et al. 1998b; Meskers et al. 1999]. A more promising approach might lie in systems that can inherently detect field distortions.

The adoption of this technology for biomechanical applications has been slow, in part due to the aforementioned distortion factors. In fact, it was not until the introduction of miniature electromagnetic tracking sensors (small enough to embed in surgical instruments such as needles or catheters, as shown in Fig. 2.4) by companies such as Northern Digital in the last 5 years, and more recently by Ascension, that the use of EMTS provided a clear advantage not offered by any other existing tracking technology; the ability to track flexible instruments and to track instruments inside the body. Thus applications aimed at tracking inner organs using flexible instruments such as catheters and endoscopes were made possible, and more sophisticated algorithms capable of error detection have been developed recently [Ellsmere

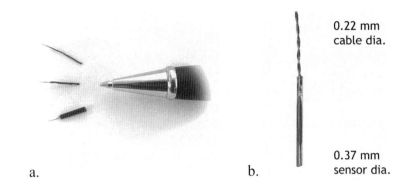

0.22 mm
cable dia.

0.37 mm
sensor dia.

a.   b.

Fig. 2.4 With growing interest in clinical applications of electromagnetic tracking, more companies have begun to produce miniaturized sensors: (**a**) 0.5 mm and 0.8 mm five DOF sensors and 1.8 mm six DOF sensor (courtesy of Northern Digital), (**b**) 0.37 mm five DOF sensor (courtesy of Ascension)

et al. 2004; Gepstein et al. 1997; Seiler et al. 2000; Solomon et al. 2000, 2003; Zaaroor et al. 2001].

Despite recent improvements in the technology, it should be noted that EMTS do not, in the general sense, compete with OTS in terms of tracking accuracy. From the application accuracy point of view, the difference between EMTS and OTS becomes smaller, since EMTS sensors tend to be closer to the point of interest. Therefore, extrapolation errors are less important. The lack of any line-of-sight limitation and the ability to track flexible endoscopes and catheters are the main advantage of EMTS. Several studies on the robustness and accuracy of the newer medical EMTS have been performed [Hummel et al. 2002, 2005, 2006; Schicho et al. 2005; Wagner et al. 2002] with reported accuracy in the range of a millimeter for a 0.5 m × 0.5 m × 0.5 m volume workspace. Due to the dependence of device accuracy on environment, which makes comparison of distortion effects a delicate matter, several groups have proposed standardized assessment protocols [Frantz et al. 2003; Hummel et al. 2005, 2006; Wilson et al. 2007].

2.5   Other Technologies

While this chapter has covered the most commonly used tracking systems in medical applications, other technologies exist that either have great potential for IGI applications in their current state, or which could be used for specific clinical procedures more efficiently than the present systems. An example of such a device is the "ShapeTape" (Measurand Inc, Fredericton, New Brunswick, Canada) [Koizumi et al. 2003] shown in Fig. 2.5. ShapeTape uses optical sensor linkages to measure torsion and flexion of fiber optic cables to determine position and pose along the entire length of the device.

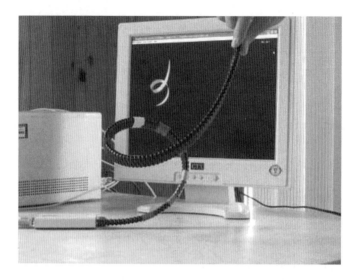

Fig. 2.5 Although the ShapeTape device shows potential, it has not yet seen any application in IGI systems (courtesy of Measurand)

This device has been used predominantly for reverse engineering and animation in the entertainment industry.

Another potential technology is the use of accelerometers and gyroscopes to measure acceleration and angular velocity, respectively, to determine tool pose. A sensor assembly with a pair of three such sensors aligned in the main coordinate axes is usually referred to as an inertial tracking system. Since acceleration is the second derivative of position with respect to time, and angular velocity is the first derivative, angular changes integrated over time from a known starting position yield translation and rotation. Inevitably, small measurement errors, either systematic or statistical (those caused by jitter), lead to increased error over time. Since error of this type is intrinsic, it cannot be tolerated for medical interventions. Despite these limitations, inertial sensors have found application in some biomechanical setups for measurement of joint motion [Zhou et al. 2006; Zhu and Zhou 2004] and as auxiliary sensing devices in hybrid motion tracking systems.

In both instances, the setup can be realized by a Kalman filtering algorithm [Kalman 1960] that uses a predictor-corrector structure to estimate the state of a dynamic system characterized by noisy or incomplete measurements. The expected position in the near future is predicted using the measurements from the inertial system. Such solutions were first presented in the AR community [Azuma and Bishop 1994], but they may not be applicable to image-guided surgery, as high update rates are not a necessity at present. The continuing efforts of the community of researchers to bring

AR to the operating theater [Birkfellner et al. 2002; Das et al. 2006; Edwards et al. 2000; Shahidi et al. 2002; Wacker et al. 2006] might render these approaches an important technology in the near future, especially since some of these visualization devices feature considerable optical magnification that complicates latency issues even further [Figl et al. 2005].

Another approach is to use hybrid navigation systems that combine two or more tracking technologies, such as EMTS and OTS, to provide continuous position data in case of obstruction or failure of any one tracking system. Hybrid systems of this nature have been proposed by several authors [Birkfellner et al. 1998b, Khan et al. 2006; Muench et al. 2004], sometimes in combination with calibration efforts for compensation of distortion in the EMTS. Since tracking systems are moderately expensive (in the $10,000 to $25,000 price range at the time of writing), using two tracking systems increases the cost of the image-guided system, while adding more equipment to an already congested clinical environment. For these reasons, interest in such systems to date has been largely academic.

Finally, medical imaging modalities can be used for tracking instruments during procedures. A simple example is tumor motion detection by identification of marker motion in electronic portal images (EPI) acquired during radiation therapy. In this case, the treatment beam is used as an imaging modality where the resulting absorption images resemble conventional x-ray imaging. One drawback of this technique is that the high-energy photons emitted by the accelerator provide rather poor image contrast. However, external or internal markers are easily detected in those perspective images [Aubin et al. 2003; Harada et al. 2002; Nederveen et al. 2001; Pang et al. 2002; Shimizu et al. 2000; Vetterli et al. 2006]. Another closely related technique is the tracking of guidewires or similar structures in fluoroscopic x-ray images during radiological interventions [Baert et al. 2003; van Walsum et al. 2005], and the localization of bronchoscopes from a comparison of virtual endoscopy images and actual bronchoscopy images [Mori et al. 2002], or angiography images and 3D rotational angiography data [van de Kraats et al. 2006]. A key methodology for these three examples is the use of 2D/3D registration techniques [Birkfellner et al. 2003; Hipwell et al. 2003; Lemieux et al. 1994; Livyatan et al. 2003; Penney et al. 1998; Skerl et al. 2006; Turgeon et al. 2005]. As these registration applications become faster with the advent of more rapid rendering techniques and computing capabilities [Birkfellner et al. 2005; Russakoff et al. 2005], improved image-based tracking may become the technology of choice for a variety of applications in interventional radiology and image-guided radiation therapy. Related work in this direction has been proposed that retrieves a starting point for an iterative registration process [Deguchi et al. 2006; Krueger et al. 2005].

2.6   Data Transmission and Representation

The protocol and interface used to transfer data from the tracker to the control computer and the representation of the transmitted data are important practical concerns for any researcher wishing to develop an IGS system. Historically, the most commonly used interface for tracking systems was the serial RS 232 interface and this is still the standard for many current systems. However, newer systems are transitioning to a USB interface as this is more standard with modern computers and can provide faster data rates. This interface is available for the newer Northern Digital systems such as the Polaris Spectra and Polaris Vicra as well as the 3D Guidance system from Ascension.

Equally relevant is the parameterization and representation of the data to be transmitted. It should be noted that some EMTS are ambiguous on data representation, as their digitizer volume is only defined as a hemisphere around the field emitter. The data representation is particularly confusing for rotations and orientation measures. From a mathematical perspective the rotation transformation forms a group named SO(3). These rotations are given as 3×3 matrices with two special properties:

1. the determinant of a rotation matrix is 1.
2. the inverse is formed by transposition of the matrix.

Providing a full rotation matrix would give an unambiguous representation of rigid body rotation, but suffers two drawbacks. First, transmission of nine matrix components requires bandwidth and takes time, especially when using slow serial communication lines. Second, interpolation and other non-trivial computations such as filtering algorithms are not easily accomplished using matrices.

The most straightforward parameterization of the rotation group is the use of three rotation angles around a Cartesian coordinate system, which are sometimes denoted as roll, pitch, and yaw. Unfortunately, this parameterization suffers from the non-commutativity of rotations given as rotation matrices. Providing three rotation angles, therefore, also requires directions on how to combine them to obtain a single rotation. As a result, the quaternion representation has become the generally accepted standard for parameterization of the rotation group. Quaternions are a quadruple of numbers consisting of a scalar component q_0 and a vector component $(q_1, q_2, q_3)^T$ associated to three complex units i, j, and k. They were first introduced to theoretical mechanics by Hamilton in the nineteenth century. Quaternions, while not commutative, provide a non-singular representation of the rotation group (thereby avoiding the so-called gimbal lock problem). Most modern tracking systems like the Northern Digital products and several trackers from Ascension use this representation. A compact description of quaternion kinematics can be found in Chou [1992]. The derivation of the quaternion representation from a conventional rotation matrix representation is given in Shepperd [1978].

2.7   Accuracy

Accuracy in image-guided surgery is a critical issue, and the aspect of validation in image-guided surgery systems is discussed in Chapter 18. There have been many papers describing accuracy evaluations of the tracker component on the overall outcome of image-guided surgery procedures. We can make the following general statements concerning accuracy:

1. Tracker accuracy is a crucial component of the overall target registration error (TRE) in image-guided surgery systems [Fitzpatrick et al. 1998].
2. Evaluation of image-guided surgery systems, including tracker performance, should take place with the specific intended clinical application in mind. The crucial questions are

   a. Can therapeutic outcome be improved by deploying an image-guided surgery system?
   b. Can this improvement be optimized by applying other (more accurate or more convenient) tracking technologies?

If trackers of different technologies or from different vendors are to be compared, one should aim at providing an experimental framework that makes comparison of measurements feasible for other groups. The principle of experiment repeatability is important and should be taken into account.

2.8   Conclusions

Position tracking is an essential component in image-guided surgery. Many different types and styles of tracking devices have been introduced and perhaps the ideal solution does not exist yet. The best choice of tracking device is highly application dependent.

Although the first image-guided system incorporated mechanical digitizers, these were replaced as more compact and less intrusive optical tracking devices emerged. In some sense, it would be appropriate to say that optical tracking is the standard benchmark with sufficient accuracy in applications where it is viable.

Over the last decade, companies have taken note of the growing prominence of image-guided interventions and developed systems targeted toward medical applications. This has resulted in EMTS with smaller profile sensors that facilitate the tracking of flexible instruments. Continual refinement and sophistication in measurement error detection and distortion correction could in time replace the use of optical trackers altogether in general surgery, interventional radiology, and image-guided radiation therapy. We also could expect to see optimized solutions for application groups (like miniature EMTS for endoscopy and catheterization and OTS for high-precision localization of rigid bodies). Simple-to-use interfaces and sufficient data update rates would greatly stimulate uptake of new devices for the development of image-guided intervention systems.

As intra-operative imaging becomes a more integral part of surgical and interventional routine, we assume that some applications for external tracking might be replaced by image processing methods rather than external position sensing. In addition, tracking does not need to be confined to instrument localization alone. Examples mentioned in this chapter on the use of tracking within biomechanics, radiation therapy, motion correction, and instrument position surveillance illustrate the myriad avenues in which tracking exhibits clear potential. To facilitate the research and development of interventional systems that serve the vast patient community is indeed a noble goal for researchers in the fields of clinical research, biomedical engineering, and medical physics.

References

Anon JB (1998). "Computer-aided endoscopic sinus surgery." *Laryngoscope*, 108(7), 949–61.

Ashe W (2003). "Magnetic position measurement system with field containment means." U.S. Patent 6,528,991.

Aubin S, Beaulieu L, Pouliot S, Pouliot J, Roy R, Girouard LM, Martel-Brisson N, Vigneault E, Laverdiere J (2003). "Robustness and precision of an automatic marker detection algorithm for online prostate daily targeting using a standard V-EPID." *Med Phys*, 30(7), 1825–32.

Azuma R, Bishop G (1994). Improving static and dynamic registration in an optical see-through HMD. *SIGGRAPH'04*, 197–204.

Baert SA, Viergever MA, Niessen WJ (2003). "Guide-wire tracking during endo vascular interventions." *IEEE Trans Med Imaging*, 22(8), 965–72.

Barratt DC, Davies AH, Hughes AD, Thom SA, Humphries KN (2001). "Accuracy of an electromagnetic three-dimensional ultrasound system for carotid artery imaging." *Ultrasound Med Biol*, 27(10), 1421–5.

Bercik P, Schlageter V, Mauro M, Rawlinson J, Kucera P, Armstrong D (2005). "Noninvasive verification of nasogastric tube placement using a magnet-tracking system: a pilot study in healthy subjects." *JPEN J Parenter Enteral Nutr*, 29(4), 305–10.

Birkfellner W, Figl M, Huber K, Watzinger F, Wanschitz F, Hummel J, Hanel R, Greimel W, Homolka P, Ewers R, Bergmann H (2002). "A head-mounted operating binocular for augmented reality visualization in medicine – design and initial evaluation." *IEEE Trans Med Imaging*, 21(8), 991–7.

Birkfellner W, Seemann R, Figl M, Hummel J, Ede C, Homolka P, Yang X, Niederer P, Bergmann H (2005). "Wobbled splatting-a fast perspective volume rendering method for simulation of x-ray images from CT." *Phys Med Biol*, 50(9), N73–N84.

Birkfellner W, Watzinger F, Wanschitz F, Enislidis G, Kollmann C, Rafolt D, Nowotny R, Ewers R, Bergmann H (1998a). "Systematic distortions in magnetic position digitizers." *Med Phys*, 25(11), 2242–8.

Birkfellner W, Watzinger F, Wanschitz F, Ewers R, Bergmann H (1998b). "Calibration of tracking systems in a surgical environment." *IEEE Trans Med Imaging*, 17(5), 737–42.

Birkfellner W, Wirth J, Burgstaller W, Baumann B, Staedele H, Hammer B, Gellrich NC, Jacob AL, Regazzoni P, Messmer P (2003). "A faster method for 3D/2D medical image registration-a simulation study." *Phys Med Biol*, 48(16), 2665–79.

Blood E (1989). "Device for quantitatively measuring the relative position and orientation of two bodies in the presence of metals utilizing direct current magnetic fields." U.S. Patent 4,849,692.

Bottlang M, Marsh JL, Brown TD (1998). "Factors influencing accuracy of screw displacement axis detection with a D.C.-based electromagnetic tracking system." *J Biomech Eng*, 120(3), 431–5.

Buhler P, Just U, Will E, Kotzerke J, van den Hoff J (2004). "An accurate method for correction of head movement in PET." *IEEE Trans Med Imaging*, 23(9), 1176–85.

Carney AS, Patel N, Baldwin DL, Coakham HB, Sandeman DR (1996). "Intra-operative image guidance in otolaryngology – the use of the ISG viewing wand." *J Laryngol Otol*, 110(4), 322–7.

Cash DM, Miga MI, Glasgow SC, Dawant BM, Clements LW, Cao Z, Galloway RL, Chapman WC (2007). Concepts and preliminary data toward the realization of image-guided liver surgery. *J Gastrointest Surg*, 11(7), 844–59.

Chou JCK (1992). "Quaternion kinematic and dynamic differential equations." *IEEE Trans Robotic Autom*, 8(1), 53–64.

Colchester AC, Zhao J, Holton-Tainter KS, Henri CJ, Maitland N, Roberts PT, Harris CG, Evans RJ (1996). "Development and preliminary evaluation of VISLAN, a surgical planning and guidance system using intra-operative video imaging." *Med Image Anal*, 1(1), 73–90.

Das M, Sauer F, Schoepf UJ, Khamene A, Vogt SK, Schaller S, Kikinis R, vanSonnenberg E, Silverman SG (2006). "Augmented reality visualization for CT-guided interventions: system description, feasibility, and initial evaluation in an abdominal phantom." *Radiology*, 240(1), 230–5.

Deguchi D, Akiyama K, Mori K, Kitasaka T, Suenaga Y, Maurer CR Jr, Takabatake H, Mori M, Natori H (2006). "A method for bronchoscope tracking by combining a position sensor and image registration." *Comput Aided Surg*, 11(3), 109–17.

Doshi PK, Lemieux L, Fish DR, Shorvon SD, Harkness WH, Thomas DG (1995). "Frameless stereotaxy and interactive neurosurgery with the ISG viewing wand." *Acta Neurochir Suppl*, 64, 49–53.

Dyer PV, Patel N, Pell GM, Cummins B, Sandeman DR (1995). "The ISG viewing wand: an application to atlanto-axial cervical surgery using the Le Fort I maxillary osteotomy." *Br J Oral Maxillofac Surg*, 33(6), 370–4.

Edwards PJ, King AP, Maurer CR Jr, de Cunha DA, Hawkes DJ, Hill DL, Gaston RP, Fenlon MR, Jusczyzck A, Strong AJ, Chandler CL, Gleeson MJ (2000). "Design and evaluation of a system for microscope-assisted guided interventions (MAGI)." *IEEE Trans Med Imaging*, 19(11), 1082–93.

Eljamel MS (1997). "Accuracy, efficacy, and clinical applications of the Radionics Operating Arm System." *Comput Aided Surg*, 2(5), 292–7.

Ellsmere J, Stoll J, Wells W 3rd, Kikinis R, Vosburgh K, Kane R, Brooks D, Rattner D (2004). "A new visualization technique for laparoscopic ultrasonography." *Surgery*, 136(1), 84–92.

Feng B, Gifford HC, Beach RD, Boening G, Gennert MA, King MA (2006). "Use of three-dimensional Gaussian interpolation in the projector/backprojector pair of iterative reconstruction for compensation of known rigid-body motion in SPECT." *IEEE Trans Med Imaging*, 25(7), 838–44.

Figl M, Ede C, Hummel J, Wanschitz F, Ewers R, Bergmann H, Birkfellner W (2005). "A fully automated calibration method for an optical see-through head-mounted operating microscope with variable zoom and focus." *IEEE Trans Med Imaging*, 24(11), 1492–9.

Fitzpatrick JM, West JB, Maurer CR Jr (1998). "Predicting error in rigid-body point-based registration." *IEEE Trans Med Imaging*, 17(5), 694–702.

Frantz DD, Wiles AD, Leis SE, Kirsch SR (2003). "Accuracy assessment protocols for electromagnetic tracking systems." *Phys Med Biol*, 48(14), 2241–51.

Freysinger W, Gunkel AR, Thumfart WF (1997). "Image guided endoscopic ENT surgery." *Eur Arch Otorhinolaryngol*, 254(7), 343–6.

Fried MP, Kleefield J, Gopal H, Reardon E, Ho BT, Kuhn FA (1997). "Image guided endoscopic surgery: results of accuracy and performance in a multicenter clinical study using an electromagnetic tracking system." *Laryngoscope*, 107(5), 594–601.

Fristrup CW, Pless T, Durup J, Mortensen MB, Nielsen HO, Hovendal CP (2004). "A new method for three-dimensional laparoscopic ultrasound model reconstruction." *Surg Endosc*, 18(11), 1601–4.

Gepstein L, Hayam G, Ben-Haim SA (1997). "A novel method for nonfluoroscopic catheter-based electroanatomical mapping of the heart. *In vitro* and *in vivo* accuracy results." *Circulation*, 95(6), 1611–22.

Goerss SJ, Kelly PJ, Kall B, Stiving S (1994). "A stereotactic magnetic field digitizer." *Stereotact Funct Neurosurg*, 63(1–4), 89–92.

Gumprecht HK, Widenka DC, Lumenta CB (1999). "BrainLab VectorVision Neuronavigation System: technology and clinical experiences in 131 cases." *Neurosurgery*, 44(1), 97–104.

Harada T, Shirato H, Ogura S, Oizumi S, Yamazaki K, Shimizu S, Onimaru R, Miyasaka K, Nishimura M, Dosaka-Akita H (2002). "Real-time tumor-tracking radiation therapy for lung carcinoma by the aid of insertion of a gold marker using bronchofiberscopy." *Cancer*, 95(8), 1720–7.

Hassfeld S, Muhling J, Zoller J (1995). "Intraoperative navigation in oral and maxillofacial surgery." *Int J Oral Maxillofac Surg*, 24(1 Pt 2), 111–9.

Hastenteufel M, Vetter M, Meinzer HP, Wolf I (2006). "Effect of 3D ultrasound probes on the accuracy of electromagnetic tracking systems." *Ultrasound Med Biol*, 32(9), 1359–68.

Hata N, Dohi T, Iseki H, Takakura K (1997). "Development of a frameless and armless stereotactic neuronavigation system with ultrasonographic registration." *Neurosurgery*, 41(3), 608–13.

Hautmann H, Schneider A, Pinkau T, Peltz F, Feussner H (2005). "Electromagnetic catheter navigation during bronchoscopy: validation of a novel method by conventional fluoroscopy." *Chest*, 128(1), 382–7.

Hipwell JH, Penney GP, McLaughlin RA, Rhode K, Summers P, Cox TC, Byrne JV, Noble JA, Hawkes DJ (2003). "Intensity-based 2-D-3-D registration of cerebral angiograms." *IEEE Trans Med Imaging*, 22(11), 1417–26.

Hummel J, Bax MR, Figl ML, Kang Y, Maurer C Jr, Birkfellner WW, Bergmann H, Shahidi R (2005). "Design and application of an assessment protocol for electromagnetic tracking systems." *Med Phys*, 32(7), 2371–9.

Hummel J, Figl M, Birkfellner W, Bax MR, Shahidi R, Maurer CR Jr, Bergmann H (2006). "Evaluation of a new electromagnetic tracking system using a standardized assessment protocol." *Phys Med Biol*, 51(10), N205–10.

Hummel J, Figl M, Kollmann C, Bergmann H, Birkfellner W (2002). "Evaluation of a miniature electromagnetic position tracker." *Med Phys*, 29(10), 2205–12.

Javer AR, Kuhn FA, Smith D (2000). "Stereotactic computer-assisted navigational sinus surgery: accuracy of an electromagnetic tracking system with the tissue debrider and when utilizing different headsets for the same patient." *Am J Rhinol*, 14(6), 361–5.

Josefsson T, Nordh E, Eriksson PO (1996). "A flexible high-precision video system for digital recording of motor acts through lightweight reflex markers." *Comput Methods Programs Biomed,* 49(2), 119–29.

Kalman RE (1960). "A new approach to linear filtering and prediction problems." *Trans ASME – J Basic Eng*, 82, 35–45.

Kato H, Billinghurst M (1999). "Marker Tracking and HMD Calibration for a video-based Augmented Reality Conferencing System." *Proceedings of the 2nd International Workshop on Augmented Reality (IWAR 99)*. October, San Francisco, CA.

Khadem R, Yeh CC, Sadeghi-Tehrani M, Bax MR, Johnson JA, Welch JN, Wilkinson EP, Shahidi R (2000). "Comparative tracking error analysis of five different optical tracking systems." *Comput Aided Surg*, 5(2), 98–107.

Khan MF, Dogan S, Maataoui A, Gurung J, Schiemann M, Ackermann H, Wesarg S, Sakas G, Vogl TJ (2005). "Accuracy of biopsy needle navigation using the Medarpa system – computed tomography reality superimposed on the site of intervention." *Eur Radiol*, 15(11), 2366–74.

Khan MF, Dogan S, Maataoui A, Wesarg S, Gurung J, Ackermann H, Schiemann M, Wimmer-Greinecker G, Vogl TJ (2006). "Navigation-based needle puncture of a cadaver using a hybrid tracking navigational system." *Invest Radiol*, 41(10), 713–20.

King DL (2002). "Errors as a result of metal in the near environment when using an electromagnetic locator with freehand three-dimensional echocardiography." *J Am Soc Echocardiogr*, 15(7), 731–5.

Kirsch S, Boksberger HU, Greuter U, Schilling C, Seiler PG (1997). "Real-time tracking of tumor positions for precision irradiation." In *Advances in Hadrontherapy*, Excerpta Medica International Congress Series 1144, Elsevier, 269–274.

Koizumi N, Sumiyama K, Suzuki N, Hattori A, Tajiri H, Uchiyama A (2003). "Development of a new three-dimensional endoscopic ultrasound system through endoscope shape monitoring." *Stud Health Technol Inform*, 94, 168–70.

Krueger S, Timinger H, Grewer R, Borgert J (2005). "Modality-integrated magnetic catheter tracking for x-ray vascular interventions." *Phys Med Biol*, 50(4), 581–97.

Kuipers JB (1980). "SPASYN – an electromagnetic relative position and orientation tracking system." *IEEE Trans Instrum Meas*, 29, 462–66.

LaScalza S, Arico J, Hughes R (2003). "Effect of metal and sampling rate on accuracy of Flock of Birds electromagnetic tracking system." *J Biomech*, 36(1), 141–4.

Lemieux L, Jagoe R, Fish DR, Kitchen ND, Thomas DG (1994). "A patient-to-computed-tomography image registration method based on digitally reconstructed radiographs." *Med Phys*, 21(11), 1749–60.

Li Q, Zamorano L, Jiang Z, Gong JX, Pandya A, Perez R, Diaz F (1999). "Effect of optical digitizer selection on the application accuracy of a surgical localization system-a quantitative comparison between the OPTOTRAK and flashpoint tracking systems." *Comput Aided Surg*, 4(6), 314–21.

Litzenberg DW, Balter JM, Hadley SW, Sandler HM, Willoughby TR, Kupelian PA, Levine L (2006). "Influence of intrafraction motion on margins for prostate radiotherapy." *Int J Radiat Oncol Biol Phys*, 65(2), 548–53.

Livyatan H, Yaniv Z, Joskowicz L (2003). "Gradient-based 2-D/3-D rigid registration of fluoroscopic X-ray to CT." *IEEE Trans Med Imaging*, 22(11), 1395–406.

Meskers CG, Fraterman H, van der Helm FC, Vermeulen HM, Rozing PM (1999). "Calibration of the "Flock of Birds" electromagnetic tracking device and its application in shoulder motion studies." *J Biomech*, 32(6), 629–33.

Milne AD, Chess DG, Johnson JA, King GJ (1996). "Accuracy of an electromagnetic tracking device: a study of the optimal range and metal interference." *J Biomech*, 29(6), 791–3.

Mori K, Deguchi D, Sugiyama J, Suenaga Y, Toriwaki J, Maurer CR Jr, Takabatake H, Natori H (2002). "Tracking of a bronchoscope using epipolar geometry analysis and intensity-based image registration of real and virtual endoscopic images." *Med Image Anal*, 6(3), 321–36.

Muench RK, Blattmann H, Kaser-Hotz B, Bley CR, Seiler PG, Sumova A, Verwey J (2004). "Combining magnetic and optical tracking for computer aided therapy." *Z Med Phys*, 14(3), 189–94.

Nederveen AJ, Lagendijk JJ, Hofman P (2001). "Feasibility of automatic marker detection with an a-Si flat-panel imager." *Phys Med Biol*, 46(4), 1219–30.

Nishizaki K, Masuda Y, Nishioka S, Akagi H, Takeda Y, Ohkawa Y (1996). "A computer-assisted operation for congenital aural malformations." *Int J Pediatr Otorhinolaryngol*, 36(1), 31–7.

Nolte LP, Zamorano L, Visarius H, Berlemann U, Langlotz F, Arm E, Schwarzenbach O (1995). "Clinical evaluation of a system for precision enhancement in spine surgery." *Clin Biomech*, 10(6), 293–303.

Pang G, Beachey DJ, O'Brien PF, Rowlands JA (2002). "Imaging of 1.0-mm-diameter radiopaque markers with megavoltage X-rays: an improved online imaging system." *Int J Radiat Oncol Biol Phys*, 52(2), 532–7.

Penney GP, Weese J, Little JA, Desmedt P, Hill DL, Hawkes DJ (1998). "A comparison of similarity measures for use in 2-D-3-D medical image registration." *IEEE Trans Med Imaging*, 17(4), 586–95.

Petersch B, Bogner J, Dieckmann K, Potter R, Georg D (2004). "Automatic real-time surveillance of eye position and gating for stereotactic radiotherapy of uveal melanoma." *Med Phys*, 31(12), 3521–7.

Poulin F, Amiot LP (2002). "Interference during the use of an electromagnetic tracking system under OR conditions." *J Biomech*, 35(6), 733–7.

Raab FH, Blood EB, Steiner TO, Jones HR (1979). "Magnetic position and orientation tracking system." *IEEE Trans Aerosp Electron Syst*, AES-15, 709–17.

Reinhardt HF, Landolt H (1989). "CT-guided "real time" stereotaxy." *Acta Neurochir Suppl (Wien)*, 46, 107–8.

Reinhardt HF, Zweifel HJ (1990). "Interactive sonar-operated device for stereotactic and open surgery." *Stereotact Funct Neurosurg*, 54–55, 93–7.

Reittner P, Tillich M, Luxenberger W, Weinke R, Preidler K, Kole W, Stammberger H, Szolar D. (2002). "Multislice CT-image guided endoscopic sinus surgery using an electromagnetic tracking system." *Eur Radiol*, 12(3), 592–6.

Roberts DW, Strohbehn JW, Hatch JF, Murray W, Kettenberger H (1986). "A frameless stereotaxic integration of computerized tomographic imaging and the operating microscope." *J Neurosurg*, 65(4), 545–9.

Rohling R, Munger P, Hollerbach JM, Peter T (1995). "Comparison of relative accuracy between a mechanical and an optical position tracker for image guided neurosurgery." *J Image Guid Surg*, 1(1), 30–4.

Russakoff DB, Rohlfing T, Mori K, Rueckert D, Ho A, Adler JR Jr, Maurer CR Jr (2005). "Fast generation of digitally reconstructed radiographs using attenuation fields with application to 2D-3D image registration." *IEEE Trans Med Imaging*, 24(11), 1441–54.

Sagi HC, Manos R, Benz R, Ordway NR, Connolly PJ (2003). "Electromagnetic field-based image guided spine surgery part I & II: results of a cadaveric study evaluating lumbar pedicle screw placement." *Spine*, 28(17), 2013–8 and E351–4.

Sandeman DR, Patel N, Chandler C, Nelson RJ, Coakham HB, Griffith HB (1994). "Advances in image-directed neurosurgery: preliminary experience with the ISG Viewing Wand compared with the Leksell G frame." *Br J Neurosurg*, 8(5), 529–44.

Schicho K, Figl M, Donat M, Birkfellner W, Seemann R, Wagner A, Bergmann H, Ewers R (2005). "Stability of miniature electromagnetic tracking systems." *Phys Med Biol*, 50(9), 2089–98.

Schmerber S, Chassat F (2001). "Accuracy evaluation of a CAS system: laboratory protocol and results with 6D localizers, and clinical experiences in otorhinolaryngology." *Comput Aided Surg*, 6(1), 1–13.

Seiler P (2007). "Device for determining the position of body parts and use of the same." U.S. Patent 7,204,796.

Seiler PG, Blattmann H, Kirsch S, Muench RK, Schilling C (2000). "A novel tracking technique for the continuous precise measurement of tumour positions in conformal radiotherapy." *Phys Med Biol*, 45(9), N103–10.

Shahidi R, Bax MR, Maurer CR Jr, Johnson JA, Wilkinson EP, Wang B, West JB, Citardi MJ, Manwaring KH, Khadem R (2002). "Implementation, calibration and accuracy testing of an image-enhanced endoscopy system." *IEEE Trans Med Imaging*, 21(12), 1524–35.

Shepperd SW (1978). "Quaternion from rotation matrix." *J Guid Control*, 1(3), 223–4.

Shimizu S, Shirato H, Kitamura K, Shinohara N, Harabayashi T, Tsukamoto T, Koyanagi T, Miyasaka K (2000). "Use of an implanted marker and real-time tracking of the marker for the positioning of prostate and bladder cancers." *Int J Radiat Oncol Biol Phys*, 48(5), 1591–7.

Sipos EP, Tebo SA, Zinreich SJ, Long DM, Brem H (1996). "In vivo accuracy testing and clinical experience with the ISG Viewing Wand." *Neurosurgery*, 39(1), 194–202.

Skerl D, Likar B, Pernus F (2006). "A protocol for evaluation of similarity measures for rigid registration." *IEEE Trans Med Imaging*, 25(6), 779–91.

Smith KR, Frank KJ, Bucholz RD (1994). "The NeuroStation-a highly accurate, minimally invasive solution to frameless stereotactic neurosurgery." *Comput Med Imaging Graph*, 18(4), 247–56.

Solomon SB, Dickfeld T, Calkins H (2003). "Real-time cardiac catheter navigation on three-dimensional CT images." *J Interv Card Electrophysiol*, 8(1), 27–36.

Solomon SB, White P Jr, Wiener CM, Orens JB, Wang KP (2000). "Three-dimensional CT-guided bronchoscopy with a real-time electromagnetic position sensor: a comparison of two image registration methods." *Chest*, 118(6), 1783–7.

Suess O, Kombos T, Kurth R, Suess S, Mularski S, Hammersen S, Brock M (2001). "Intracranial image guided neurosurgery: experience with a new electromagnetic navigation system." *Acta Neurochir (Wien)*, 143(9), 927–34.

Sumiyama K, Suzuki N, Kakutani H, Hino S, Tajiri H, Suzuki H, Aoki T (2002). "A novel 3-dimensional EUS technique for real-time visualization of the volume data reconstruction process." *Gastrointest Endosc,* 55(6), 723–8.

Talamini MA, Chapman S, Horgan S, Melvin WS (2003). "The Academic Robotics Group. A prospective analysis of 211 robotic-assisted surgical procedures." *Surg Endosc*, 17(10), 1521–4.

Turgeon GA, Lehmann G, Guiraudon G, Drangova M, Holdsworth D, Peters T (2005). "2D-3D registration of coronary angiograms for cardiac procedure planning and guidance." *Med Phys*, 32(12), 3737–49.

van de Kraats EB, van Walsum T, Kendrick L, Noordhoek NJ, Niessen WJ (2006). "Accuracy evaluation of direct navigation with an isocentric 3D rotational X-ray system." *Med Image Anal*, 10(2), 113–24.

van Ruijven LJ, Beek M, Donker E, van Eijden TM (2000). "The accuracy of joint surface models constructed from data obtained with an electromagnetic tracking device." *J Biomech*, 33(8), 1023–8.

van Walsum T, Baert SA, Niessen WJ (2005). "Guide wire reconstruction and visualization in 3DRA using monoplane fluoroscopic imaging." *IEEE Trans Med Imaging*, 24(5), 612–23.

Vetterli D, Thalmann S, Behrensmeier F, Kemmerling L, Born EJ, Mini R, Greiner RH, Aebersold DM (2006). "Daily organ tracking in intensity-modulated radiotherapy of prostate cancer using an electronic portal imaging device with a dose saving acquisition mode." *Radiother Oncol*, 79(1), 101–8.

Wacker FK, Vogt S, Khamene A, Jesberger JA, Nour SG, Elgort DR, Sauer F, Duerk JL, Lewin JS (2006). "An augmented reality system for MR image guided needle biopsy: initial results in a swine model." *Radiology*, 238(2), 497–504.

Wagner A, Ploder O, Enislidis G, Truppe M, Ewers R (1995). "Virtual image guided navigation in tumor surgery-technical innovation." *J Craniomaxillofac Surg*, 23(5), 217–3.

Wagner A, Ploder O, Zuniga J, Undt G, Ewers R (1996). "Augmented reality environment for temporomandibular joint motion analysis." *Int J Adult Orthodon Orthognath Surg*, 11(2), 127–36.

Wagner A, Schicho K, Birkfellner W, Figl M, Seemann R, Konig F, Kainberger F, Ewers R (2002). "Quantitative analysis of factors affecting intraoperative precision and stability of optoelectronic and electromagnetic tracking systems." *Med Phys*, 29(5), 905–12.

Wagner AA, Varkarakis IM, Link RE, Sullivan W, Su LM (2006). "Comparison of surgical performance during laparoscopic radical prostatectomy of two robotic camera holders, EndoAssist and AESOP: a pilot study." *Urology*, 68(1), 70–4.

Watanabe Y, Anderson LL (1997). "A system for nonradiographic source localization and real-time planning of intraoperative high dose rate brachytherapy." *Med Phys*, 24(12), 2014–23.

Watanabe E, Watanabe T, Manaka S, Mayanagi Y, Takakura K (1987). "Three-dimensional digitizer (neuronavigator): new equipment for computed tomography-guided stereotaxic surgery." *Surg Neurol*, 27(6), 543–7.

Watzinger F, Birkfellner W, Wanschitz F, Millesi W, Schopper C, Sinko K, Huber K, Bergmann H, Ewers R (1999). "Positioning of dental implants using computer-aided navigation and an optical tracking system: case report and presentation of a new method." *J Craniomaxillofac Surg*, 27(2), 77–81.

Willoughby TR, Kupelian PA, Pouliot J, Shinohara K, Aubin M, Roach M 3rd, Skrumeda LL, Balter JM, Litzenberg DW, Hadley SW, Wei JT, Sandler HM (2006). "Target localization and real-time tracking using the Calypso 4D localization system in patients with localized prostate cancer." *Int J Radiat Oncol Biol Phys*, 65(2), 528–34.

Wilson E, Yaniv Z, Zhang H, Nafis C, Shen E, Shechter G, Wiles A, Peters T, Lindisch D, Cleary K (2007). "A hardware and software protocol for the evaluation of electromagnetic tracker accuracy in the clinical environment: a multi-center study." *SPIE Medical Imaging*, 6509, 2T1–T11.

Wood BJ, Zhang H, Durrani A, Glossop N, Ranjan S, Lindisch D, Levy E, Banovac F, Borgert J, Krueger S, Kruecker J, Viswanathan A, Cleary K (2005). "Navigation with electromagnetic tracking for interventional radiology procedures: a feasibility study." *J Vasc Interv Radiol*, 16(4), 493–505.

Zaaroor M, Bejerano Y, Weinfeld Z, Ben-Haim S (2001). "Novel magnetic technology for intraoperative intracranial frameless navigation: *in vivo* and *in vitro* results." *Neurosurgery*, 48(5), 1100–7.

Zamorano L, Jiang Z, Kadi AM (1994). "Computer-assisted neurosurgery system: Wayne State University hardware and software configuration." *Comput Med Imaging Graph,* 18(4), 257–71.

Zhang H, Banovac F, Lin R, Glossop N, Wood BJ, Lindisch D, Levy E, Cleary K (2006). "Electromagnetic tracking for abdominal interventions in computer aided surgery." *Computer Aided Surgery*, 11(3), 127–36.

Zhou H, Hu H, Tao Y (2006). "Inertial measurements of upper limb motion." *Med Biol Eng Comput*, 44(6), 479–87.

Zhu R, Zhou Z (2004). "A real-time articulated human motion tracking using tri-axis inertial/magnetic sensors package." *IEEE Trans Neural Syst Rehabil Eng*, 12(2), 295–302.

Chapter 3

Visualization in Image-Guided Interventions

David Holmes III, Maryam Rettmann, and Richard Robb

Abstract

Visualization is one of the primary interfaces between an interventionalist and his patient. This interface is the final integration of several disparate data streams. To develop an appropriate image-guided interface, it is important to understand several aspects of the data acquisition, data processing, and visualization methodologies in the context of the interventional procedure. This chapter introduces the basics of data acquisition and processing for image guidance, including the benefits of both preoperative and intraoperative data streams. 2D and 3D visualization methodologies are described with examples. Several different systems for visualization are introduced, ranging from low-level hardware to software-only render engines. Several clinical examples of visualization for image guidance are described.

3.1 Introduction

The purpose of visualization in image-guided interventions (IGI) is to faithfully represent the patient and surgical environment, and to accurately guide the surgeon to navigate toward, and localize the treatment target during an intervention. This is a challenging task given the limited number and type of systems available for online, real-time imaging in the typical surgical suite. To address this challenge, IGI visualization software often incorporates both preoperative and intraoperative patient image data into the interventional situation. IGI visualizations may include other objects in the field of view (FOV), such as surgical instruments. Thus, visualization in IGI becomes an integration task that attempts to combine several disparate, but related, signals into a common framework and interface, with the goal of accurately guiding the interventionalist to the target during the procedure. Thus visualization in IGI ia an integration task that combines several disparate, but related signals into a common framework. The combined data are presented visually to accurately guide the interventionalist to the target during the procedure.

T. Peters and K. Cleary (eds.), *Image-Guided Interventions.*
© Springer Science + Business Media, LLC 2008

3.2   Coordinate Systems

Medical image data, together with tracking and other sensor data, are collected relative to a system-specific coordinate system. Different data streams may be collected in different frames of reference, so it is important to recognize and account for the different coordinate systems within a visualization system used in IGI applications. In the context of IGI, the term "coordinate system" can be used to describe either a general 3D spatial domain (which is usually a rectilinear frame of reference relative to a system specific origin) or an anatomical domain (which is a specialized frame of reference). Since the anatomical coordinate system is a particular form of a general 3D coordinate system, conversion between these two types of systems can be straightforward if each frame of reference is carefully defined and known.

The Cartesian coordinate system is convenient and common for use in IGI. Although other coordinate systems, such as cylindrical or polar, can be used during the acquisition of data, the Cartesian system is easy to understand and use. The 3D Cartesian coordinate system requires the definition of "handedness" (either right-handed or left-handed) to avoid ambiguity. Both hardware systems (i.e., graphics cards and trackers) and software systems (i.e., 3D visualization APIs) vary with regard to handedness. For example, OpenGL, a low-level application programming interface (API) for graphics hardware, uses a right-handed coordinate system [Segal and Akeley 2006], whereas Direct3D, another low-level graphics API, uses a left-handed coordinate system [Microsoft 2006].

There is a well-defined common coordinate system for anatomy, which can be found in most anatomy textbooks (e.g., [Gray 1918]). Anterior and posterior refer to front and back of the body, respectively. Superior is toward the head; inferior is toward the feet. Left and right refer to the subject's left side and right side. This anatomical coordinate system is also sometimes used to define the coordinate system for medical image storage. Coordinate systems for file formats are generally defined from low to high in each anatomical direction. For example, in the Analyze file format [Robb 2008a; Robb 2008b], the lowest dimension (e.g., the x dimension) spans from right to left, the y dimension spans from posterior to anterior, and the z dimension from inferior to superior. This coordinate system would be called an L(eft)–A(nterior)–S(uperior), or LAS, coordinate system. DICOM, the currently accepted standard for most medical image files and storage, is based on a Left Posterior Superior (LPS) system [DICOM 2006]. NIFTI, a neuroimaging file format, is stored as RAS [NIFTI].

The three orthogonal planes within a 3D medical image dataset are defined relative to an anatomical coordinate system. The transverse (or axial) plane is perpendicular to the inferior–superior line; the sagittal plane

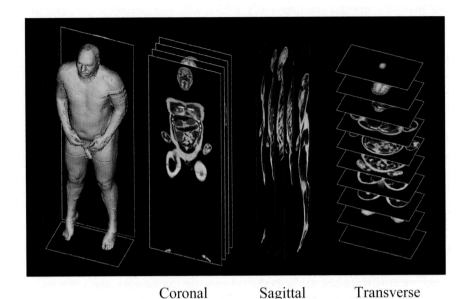

Coronal   Sagittal   Transverse

Fig. 3.1. Common anatomical orientation of 3D image data

is perpendicular to the left–right line; and the coronal plane is perpendicular to the anterior–posterior line. These three planes are used to define the orientation of a slice of data within a volume or 3D dataset. Figure 3.1 shows an example of the three orthogonal planes.

In designing a visualization paradigm for IGI, it is important to determine which coordinate system will serve as the primary reference, so that all other data can be transformed into a common spatial framework. It is convenient to use the coordinate system of the graphics subsystem or visualization API since the graphics must be as responsive as possible. Once the reference system is chosen, coordinate system transformations can be used to approximately align all system input and output data streams into a single frame of reference. Changing the handedness of a data stream requires a "flip" in the direction of one of the three axes. Changing the anatomical frame of reference requires more effort, because both the anatomical origin and handedness of the data must be addressed. To achieve this, a combination of rotations, translations, and flipping may be used.

3.3   Preoperative Images

Use of preoperative data is common in IGI and serves several purposes. Most importantly, it provides the necessary data to conduct pre-surgical planning and/or rehearsal. The pre-surgical plan is used to (1) understand the patient's normal anatomy, (2) understand the patient's disease, and (3) develop a treatment approach. Although it may not be intuitive that pre-surgical assessment is a consideration for IGI visualization, it is often an important component of the intervention, because it provides the patient-specific context for the interventionalist, even if it is not explicitly used during the procedure. In addition to pre-surgical planning, preoperative data can serve as a basic guidance tool during the procedure. The preoperative data must be in the form of high-quality images that provide excellent differentiation between normal and abnormal tissues (for planning) and an accurate representation of the patient (for guidance). In many cases, single modality imaging is insufficient for this task, and scans from multiple modalities may be required.

3.3.1 Computed Tomography

Computed tomography (CT) is an x-ray-based imaging method used to generate a 3D image volume of patient tissue densities [Hounsfield 1973]. Since most soft tissues in the body are of a similar density, the contrast resolution of CT may not be well suited for some clinical tasks, such as tumor visualization and/or delineation. By comparison, CT is excellent for imaging dense tissues and is therefore commonly used to visualize the skeletal anatomy and vascular structures (using injected x-ray opaque contrast material). There have been several developments in CT technology over the years including direct digital image acquisition, multiple detectors, and rapid scanning technologies (such as electron-beam CT and spiral CT) [Ritman 2003]. These developments have produced dramatic improvements in spatial and temporal resolution. Current CT technologies can acquire images with an isotropic voxel resolution 0.5 mm or less. In addition, using gating techniques, multi-detector CT scanners can acquire multiple image volumes every second.

For preoperative planning, CT scans are used in nearly all interventional disciplines, including cardiology [Budoff et al. 2006], neurology [Haydel et al. 2000], radiation oncology [Lattanzi et al. 2004; Spencer 2001], and orthopedic surgery [Lattanzi et al. 2004]. For orthopedic applications, CT scans are commonly used to estimate the size, shape, and location of bones to determine the optimal prosthesis for surgical implantation. In addition to selecting appropriate prosthetics, the CT scan can be used to virtually design and rehearse the approach for implantation, and again to guide the surgeon during the real procedure. Figure 3.2 shows a single sagittal image from a CT scan and a 3D rendering of the volume CT data. Such data used during surgical planning can be integrated with IGI hardware to provide intraoperative guidance.

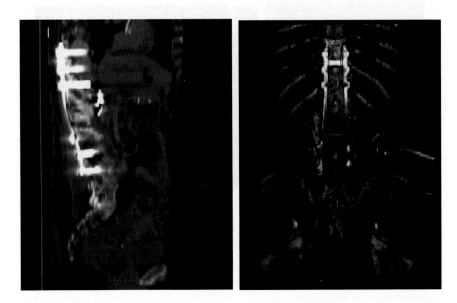

Fig. 3.2. CT image data provide excellent contrast between dense objects, such as bones and implants. On the *left*, a sagittal image of a patient after pedicle screw placement. The rendering on the *right* shows both the 3D anatomy and implanted screws

3.3.2 Magnetic Resonance Imaging

The principle of magnetic resonance imaging (MRI) is based on the phenomenon that atomic nuclei precess about an axis in the presence of a magnetic field [Bronskill and Sprawls 1993]. In MRI of biological tissues, the phenomenon is used to induce precession of hydrogen in water molecules. Due to the nuclear local interactions of water molecules within the body, contrast is generated by varying the local magnetic field and measuring the emission of RF energy. MRI provides excellent soft tissue differentiation and can be used to separately visualize normal and pathological tissue. An example is shown in Fig. 3.3, in which a large tumor is visible.

Both hardware and software engineering improvements over the last two decades have led to superior signal-to-noise, faster scans, and higher-resolution MR imaging. High-field strength MR scanners can now acquire sub-millimeter images of clinical quality [Pakin et al. 2006]. Parallel imaging methods can be used to dramatically reduce scan times [Blaimer et al. 2004]. In addition, special MR techniques such as functional MR (fMRI) [Baxendale 2002] and MR diffusion tensor imaging (DTI) [Le Bihan 2003]

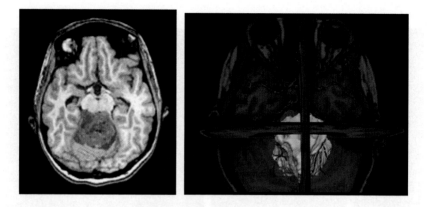

Fig. 3.3. MR imaging provides excellent soft tissue contrast. On the *left*, a single MR image slice of the head is shown. On the *right*, a 2D slice image is merged with the 3D segmented tumor and blood vessels

provide information on the biological function of tissue, which can be very useful in surgery planning.

3.3.3 Nuclear Image Scans and Other Functional Data

Nuclear image scans include both Positron Emission Tomography (PET) and Single Photon Emission Computed Tomography (SPECT) [Christian et al. 2003]. These scans require the injection of radionuclides that are differentially taken up into tissues based on the vascularity and patho-physiologic function of the organ of interest. PET imaging, for example, is commonly used for brain activity assessment, metastasized tumor identification, and myocardial viability testing (see Fig. 3.4). In general, these functional scans offer little anatomical differentiation; however, the functional information provides added value in detection and staging of disease. To compensate for poor anatomical differentiation, such images are often paired with an anatomical CT or MR image to provide correlated structure and function information [Hutton et al. 2002].

Often, pre-surgical planning includes one or more data streams other than standard medical images. Such functional signals can be useful in surgery planning, but lack anatomical detail. For example, in some neurosurgical procedures, electrodes are placed on the surface of the brain to record local functional activity (see Fig. 3.4). The electrode data, together with functional imaging data, can provide important feedback to a neurosurgeon during surgery [Zimmerman et al. 2004]. Visualization of these data can be achieved by mapping the signals into an anatomical image dataset.

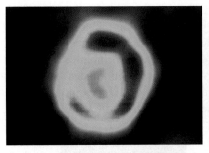 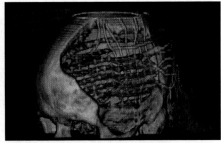

Fig. 3.4. Functional image data can be used to assess the physiology of a disease. For example, a PET scan of the heart (*left*) can be used to assess myocardial viability (regional perfusion). On the *right*, a CT scan is rendered to show placement of subdural electrodes that are used to evaluate brain function

3.4   Intraoperative Data

Image guidance may be used during both open and minimally invasive procedures. Although intraoperative imaging may be used for both types of procedures, minimally invasive procedures rely heavily on intraoperative imaging modalities, because the anatomical/pathological target cannot be observed directly by the interventionalist. Intraoperative imaging must be real time to provide adequate guidance while surgical instruments are manipulated by the operator. For this reason, intraoperative imaging may compromise spatial resolution and image fidelity in favor of improved temporal resolution.

3.4.1 X-Ray Fluoroscopy and Rotational Angiography

X-ray fluoroscopy has been the workhorse of intraoperative imaging for several decades. Despite concerns about radiation exposure, both acutely and chronically, x-ray fluoroscopy systems generate real-time images that can provide useful guidance during a procedure. An x-ray source and detector are used to rapidly (video rates of 30 Hz) collect 2D projection images through the body [Hendee and Ritenour 1992]. Even though the soft tissue contrast is generally poor, dense contrast agents and surgical instruments can be clearly identified within the images (see Fig. 3.5a).

Because x-ray fluoroscopy produces projection images, determining 3D anatomic morphology and/or the precise spatial position of surgical instruments can be difficult. Moreover, registration of the 2D fluoroscopy images to pre-acquired 3D image data is challenging. In some procedures, two x-ray fluoroscopy devices (biplane systems) are used to provide more useful 3D morphology and positional data.

Rotational angiography is an interventional scanning method in which an x-ray fluoroscopy system is iso-centrically rotated on a C-arm around the patient and multiple projection images are collected. The projection images can be reconstructed into a 3D volume using the same principles as used in CT reconstruction. Unlike monoplane x-ray fluoroscopic images, the resulting 3D dataset can provide an accurate description of 3D morphology of an object, and can help localize 3D instruments in the anatomic FOV.

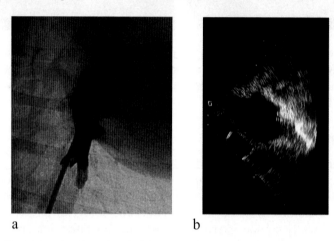

a   b

Fig. 3.5. Intraoperative imaging is important for guidance during minimally invasive procedures. X-ray fluoroscopy is the most common intraoperative imaging tool (a); however, for some procedures such as cardiac imaging, ultrasound may also be used because it can be used to collect real-time 2D and 3D data (b)

3.4.2 Intraoperative Ultrasound

Intraoperative ultrasound is used in many interventional procedures. Ultrasound scanners generate pulses of sound which propagate through tissue and reflect energy back when contacting overlapping tissue interfaces [Szabo 2004]. The reconstructed backscatter image often provides effective visualization of the anatomical morphology. Ultrasound imaging is also used to visualize other properties of tissue, including stiffness (through elastography) and flow (through Doppler imaging).

Ultrasound acquires true 2D images at real-time rates and does not use radiation. In addition, US scanners are compact, relatively inexpensive, and can be stored on mobile carts for use in multiple procedure rooms. Due to the advantages of ultrasound, it is commonly used for intraoperative imaging during cancer treatment [Guillonneau 2006], vascular atheterization [Nicholls et al. 2006], biopsy procedures [Gunneson et al. 2002], and several other interventions. To accommodate all these procedures, different ultrasound transducer configurations have been engineered to provide optimal imaging for specific anatomy. Figure 3.5b shows an ultrasound image of the left atrium obtained from an intracardiac ultrasound device.

3.4.3 Intraoperative CT and Intraoperative MR

Intraoperative CT (iCT) technology provides an alternative to standard fluoroscopy [Butler et al. 1998]. Like preoperative CT, iCT provides reliable x-ray imaging during a procedure; however, iCT data can be reconstructed as a 3D image volume. The ability to acquire CT quality images during a procedure facilitates more accurate placement of surgical instruments and implantable devices than that possible with fluoroscopy. Procedures that are conducted using iCT include prostate brachytherapy, tissue biopsy, and spine surgery.

Although expensive, intraoperative MR (iMR) is available and may be used during interventional procedures [Schenck et al. 1995]. Because MR imaging is used, the soft tissue contrast is more superior with iMR than other technologies. In order to use an iMR system, the room and surgical instruments must be designed and manufactured to be MR compatible. iMR has been used for guiding biopsies and neurosurgery, as well as other procedures.

3.5   Integration

Integration of image and sensor data often requires one or more processing steps. Of primary concern in integrating disparate data sources is addressing (a) what data streams or signals should be integrated? and (b) what is the relationship between the different data streams/signals? Addressing these two issues generally involves the process of segmentation and registration, respectively. Segmentation removes extraneous data so that the visualization can be focused on relevant anatomy and pathology. Registration aligns the separate data streams into a common coherent frame of reference.

3.5.1 Segmentation and Surface Extraction

Segmentation, as defined here, is the process of extracting relevant anatomy from medical images. For targeted interventions, segmented anatomy is important for visualization and quantification. Segmented anatomy is generally easier to display in real time and can provide an uncluttered visualization in which nonrelevant data have been removed. Segmented anatomy distinguishes boundaries among multiple anatomic structures, which makes measurement straightforward.

Methods for segmentation range from completely manual to fully auto-mated. The most accurate, but time-consuming method for segmentation is a manual approach, in which the anatomical regions of interest are traced by a human expert. Several data conditioning algorithms, including thres-holding and mathematical morphology, can help expedite manual segmen-tation, while advanced methods for segmentation of objects reduce the need for operator interaction. Some methods, such as seeded-region growing, active shape models, and level-set methods, require the placement of seed points within the image data to initialize an iterative algorithm. If initialized properly, these methods can be very effective for automatically segmenting anatomy. Another approach to segmentation is the use of statistical shape models and atlases. These methods are often very good for segmenting objects that have distinct anatomical characteristics and minor inter-subject variability.

Following segmentation, the surface of the segmented object is often parameterized into a compact polygonal model. In doing so, the amount of data necessary to represent the object can be reduced dramatically. Surface extraction can be challenging, however, because there is a trade-off between the accuracy of the surface and the amount of polygonal data required to faithfully represent the object surface. For example, one approach for surface extraction is to consider every voxel on the surface and create a polygon based on the local voxel neighborhood. One such method, called marching cubes, is very effective for extracting the surface at a high resolution [Lorensen and Cline 1987]. Unfortunately, a fully sampled surface can produce a large number of polygons, making it difficult to draw in three dimension. To address this issue, decimation (i.e., the reduction of polygons) is used to optimize the number and placement of polygons in the model. Decimation algorithms can identify surface regions with low curvature and replace several small polygons with one large polygon [Crouch and Robb 1997]. There are other methods for surface extraction including self-organizing maps [Aharon et al. 1997] and hybrid adapt/deform methods [Cameron et al. 1996]. Segmentation techniques are discussed in Chapter 8: Image Segmentation.

3.5.2 Registration

Registration is a process of spatial and temporal alignment of separate data streams. It is a critical component of IGIs because it brings together pre-procedural image data, intraoperative image data, the patient on the surgical table, and the surgical instruments. Registration methods also vary from completely manual to fully automated.

Manual registration is the most user-intensive method for registering data and is usually accomplished by the selection of spatially corresponding landmarks in multiple data volumes. Alternatively, a registration may be achieved by manual manipulation of the transformation matrix and visual feedback from a fused image. This method does not require the selection of corresponding landmarks; however, the process of manual refinement of the transformation matrix is tedious and may not yield an optimal solution.

Automated methods, which require little input from the user, are generally classified into two categories – feature based and intensity based. Feature-based methods generate a registration based on extracted features such as the surfaces of segmented objects, whereas intensity-based methods use similarity relationships among voxels of the multiple image data sets to find alignment. For some applications, an automated deformable registration may be used to align datasets that are very different. Due to the mathematical complexity of deformable registration, the algorithms may be computationally intensive and may have limited use during time-critical interventional procedures. Registration for IGI is discussed more fully in Chaps. 6 and 7.

3.6   Visualization

The principal goal for visualization during interventions is a clear, accurate representation of all relevant data with negligible latency. Basic 2D image display requires little computational overhead, and real-time update of the display can be achieved easily; 3D and 4D image display require substantial system resources and can significantly reduce the update frame rate of the system. However, 3D visualizations are generally more intuitive and useful. In practice, the use of visualization tools must be tailored to the particular application and will likely include a number of different techniques and approaches.

3.6.1   2D – Multi-Planar and Oblique

2D multi-planar displays represent an uncomplicated method for displaying medical image data, largely because the data have been collected and stored as a rectilinear volume, or at a minimum, a sequential collection of parallel 2D slices (a "stack" of images). Slices can be rapidly rendered on a computer monitor for review of the data and identification of anatomy or pathology. In addition to direct visualization of the image data, additional referential information can be added, including annotations, 2D contours, and patient demographics. In general, when presenting 2D image data, it is important to display each frame isotropically. In-plane imaging is generally acquired isotropically and is straightforward to display; however, displaying images that are orthogonal to the acquired orientation requires interpolation when the slice thickness and separation is larger than the in-plane resolution.

Presentation of multi-planar images often uses three separate panels – one for each orthogonal direction. Figure 3.6 shows a common screen layout for multi-planar image display. In a multi-panel display, all of the panels should generally be drawn at the same resolution, which may require interpolation of two frames of data when isotropic volume images are not provided. Because the amount of image data can range from several mega-bytes to several hundred megabytes, it is unrealistic to interpolate the data volumetrically. Instead, individual slices are interpolated when they are drawn on the screen. In some cases, it is beneficial to embed visual cues within a display process to provide context within and between images. Commonly used cues include the anatomical orientation, slice position, and linked cursors, as shown in Fig. 3.6.

Oblique image display is important for providing 2D slices of the data that are not orthogonal to the acquisition orientation. There are several methods for defining and computing oblique images. For example, selection of three points within a data volume can be used to uniquely define the oblique image plane. Alternatively, one point may be selected together with a vector that is normal to the oblique plane. The first approach is useful for creating images that cut along a dataset in a particular anatomical plane. For example, in Fig. 3.6, the oblique image shows sections of the aorta, left ven-tricle, and left atrium all within the same plane. The second approach is useful, for example, when a surgeon wants to generate an image plane per-pendicular to the tip of a surgical instrument. Oblique displays also may include visual cues to provide a context for the image plane.

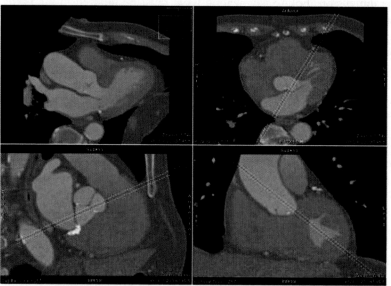

Fig. 3.6. A four-panel multiplanar display showing three mutually orthogonal images (*top right and bottom*) and an oblique image (*upper left*). Visual cues, such as the cursor link, provide feedback about the relationship between the images

3.6.2 3D Surface Rendering and 3D Volume Rendering

3D display on a 2D screen involves the mapping of a 3D object into a 2D image. To accomplish this, ray-tracing is used to rasterize the 3D object space into the 2D image. Ray-tracing algorithms project a line from a viewpoint into the 3D scene. In doing so, the ray passes through a plane that defines the 2D image to be drawn. Each ray cast into the scene interacts with the objects within the 3D FOV, either through transmission or reflection. When the ray interacts with an opaque object, the color of that object is then drawn into the corresponding pixel of the 2D image. By examining the local gradient about the intersecting point, the color can be adjusted to generate shadows. If the ray intersects with an object that has some transparency, then only a portion of the color of the object is drawn into the 2D image and the ray continues along the path. Ray-tracing can use parallel rays or diverging rays to generate orthographic renderings or perspective renderings, respectively. When creating a 3D visualization, it is important to consider several parameters, including the camera position, the look at point, the size of the 2D image, and the objects to be displayed. Once defined, manipulation of the scene is accomplished by applying a collection of transformations to the objects within the scene relative to the camera. A detailed description of rendering algorithms and implementations can be found in Foley et al. [1990].

3D visualizations are often generated using surface renderings because of the comparatively small amount of data necessary to render the object in three dimension. Following segmentation and surface extraction, the polygonal model that defines the surface of the object can be rapidly manipulated with graphics hardware to create dynamic visualizations. Using standard graphics hardware, surface renderings can be generated at up to 60 frames per second. To achieve high frame rates, however, it is important to reduce the number of polygons used to represent the objects. Conversely, by reducing the data, the model may not have sufficient resolution to accurately represent the underlying anatomy. Compromise must be achieved between desired update rate and image quality. An example of surface rendering is included in Fig. 3.7a.

Volume rendering involves projection of rays directly into a volume of data that has been placed within the 3D FOV. Although volume rendering offers great flexibility [Robb 2000a,b], there may be a penalty on performance due to the large amounts of data necessary to create an accurate visualization. Highly optimized rendering algorithms and high-performance computer hardware can significantly decrease computational latency. Volume rendering methods can be used to generate renderings based both on transmission and reflection. In transmission rendering, there is no consideration of object boundaries. Instead, each ray cast into the volume simply interacts with each voxel along its path until it exits the far end of the 3D FOV.

Voxel interaction is defined by a weighting function. Examples of transmission rendering include maximum intensity projection and summed voxel projection; however, the most common form of transmission volume rendering is volume compositing.

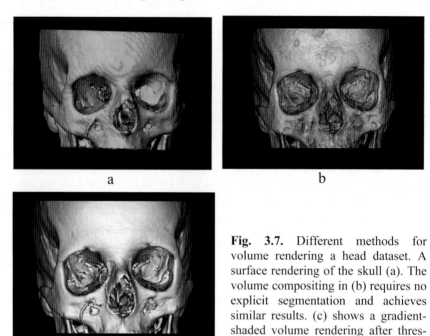

a   b

c

Fig. 3.7. Different methods for volume rendering a head dataset. A surface rendering of the skull (a). The volume compositing in (b) requires no explicit segmentation and achieves similar results. (c) shows a gradient-shaded volume rendering after thresholding for the skull

In compositing, rays are projected into the volume. For each voxel that the ray encounters, a lookup table is used to extract optical properties based on the value at that voxel (e.g., color and transparency information). The ray continues to traverse a line through the volume until it meets a stopping criterion, such as a predefined barrier or simply exiting the volume. All of the voxels traversed by the ray are incorporated to generate the final value for display of the 2D image pixel corresponding to that ray. The optical property lookup table is referred to as the transfer function, and can be manipulated to generate several different visual effects. An example of a volume compositing image, in which the voxel value is mapped to a gray-scale color and transparency, can be seen in Fig. 3.7b. Because a lookup table is used to map the voxel values into the resulting object properties, simple color/transparency volume compositing is well suited to medical image data in which different gray levels distinctly describe different anatomy. Accordingly, volume compositing is often used with CT data calibrated to

Hounsfield units for intensity, but not often used with MR or US data, which have no similar calibrated intensity scale. There are alternatively models for compositing transfer functions that have been proposed. In many cases, these approaches attempt to integrate either prior knowledge or advanced data processing in order to best delineate anatomical regions that are appropriate for visualization. An overview of transfer function methods can be found in Pfister et al. [2001].

Alternatively, a medical image dataset can be rendered using a reflectance model. In this case, the ray interacts with a segmented or classified data volume. In a manner similar to surface rendering, the projected ray intersects the segmented object. If the object is opaque, then the color of the object is drawn into the 2D pixel location. In doing so, the local gradient (either from the binary surface or the grayscale volume) may be used to generate shading. If the object is defined with some translucence, then the color value is partially added to the 2D pixel location and the ray continues through the volume. Volume rendering, in this sense, has the benefit of working with the entire dataset (without need for surface parameterization or decimation) while still generating true object renderings. Figure 3.7c shows a gradient-shaded volume rendering. Other methods, such as shell rendering [Udupa and Odhner 1993], try to further improve upon the performance of volume rendering through data reduction while maintaining the integrity of the rendering as if from the full volumetric data.

There are several algorithmic techniques used to enhance performance of surface and volume rendering. This includes double frame buffering, depth buffering, surface culling, and multiple levels-of-detail. The use of these features is generally embedded within the visualization API and does not require additional development by the application programmer.

3.6.3 Fusion, Parametric Mapping, and Multi-Object Rendering

Because diverse imaging modalities provide different anatomical, pathological, and/or functional information, data fusion can play an important role in IGI. Upon registration, multiple volumes of data can be combined into a single volume using a variety of blending functions. In some cases, grayscale blending of the data is sufficient. For example, a CT scan of the head may be averaged with an MRI scan of the same head to visualize both the bony structures and the soft tissue. Grayscale blending, however, can reduce the contrast and sharpness of the image, resulting in poor image quality. Alternatively, color blending of data can preserve much of the data in each volume while generating a single fused volume for visualization. Using 24-bit RGB volumes, each color channel can be assigned a different image volume from the patient. A color-fused volume provides 8 bits of contrast for each dataset. Color-fused volumes require some understanding of color mixing in order to properly interpret the fused volume. Alternatively, as a hybrid of both grayscale and color blending, grayscale blending can be used in conjunction with a color map to provide enhanced contrast while maintaining the quantitative usefulness of each dataset. Figure 3.8a is an example fusion image for anatomical and functional neurologic data.

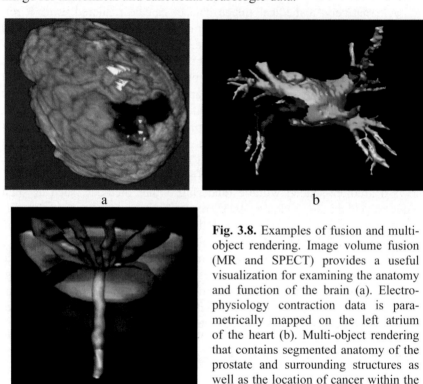

a

b

c

Fig. 3.8. Examples of fusion and multi-object rendering. Image volume fusion (MR and SPECT) provides a useful visualization for examining the anatomy and function of the brain (a). Electrophysiology contraction data is parametrically mapped on the left atrium of the heart (b). Multi-object rendering that contains segmented anatomy of the prostate and surrounding structures as well as the location of cancer within the prostate (c)

Parametric mapping is a form of data fusion; however, the term commonly refers to a specific mapping of color onto anatomical data. In particular, parametric mapping refers to fusing processed data (often 1D signals) into a 3D medical image volume. Processed data may be intrinsic image properties of the anatomical volume, such as regional thickness or displacement of the surface at different time points [Eusemann et al. 2001, 2003]. Another form of parametric mapping is the embedding of other biosensor data into a medical image dataset. For example, Fig. 3.8b shows cardiac electrical activity mapped onto the endocardial surface of the left atrium. These types of data are not directly acquired from a medical scanner. Instead, one or more datasets are acquired and processed to derive clinically important features.

Rendering multiple independent objects is important for several reasons. At a minimum, it is unlikely that the anatomy of interest is one object alone. Rather, multiple related anatomical objects are all relevant to an IGI procedure and should be visualized together. For example, in image-guided left atrium radio-frequency cardiac ablation, the esophagus is sometimes displayed together with the left atrium to ensure that the cardiologist avoids burning the esophagus. In some neurosurgeries, it is important to show different functional regions of a brain to ensure that critical structures are avoided. In addition, multi-object rendering for IGI includes visualization of surgical instruments and possibly the surgeon or patient, or both. Figure 3.8c is an example of rendering a prostate together with other associated anatomy such as the urethra and bladder. In addition, a suspected cancerous region is shown in red, as was confirmed by biopsy [Kay et al. 1998].

3.7   Systems for Visualization

3D visualization is now a mature technology utilizing the benefits of custom hardware and effective software application user interfaces (APIs). This section introduces some of the different programming libraries available; it is not intended to be a complete list. Each of the examples presented have, at a minimum, a C/C++ interface for programming; however, some also have interfaces to other programming languages including Visual Basic, C Sharp, Python, Tcl/tk, Java, and other proprietary languages.

3.7.1 Low-Level Interfacing to Hardware

OpenGL [Segal and Akeley 2006] and Direct3D [Microsoft 2006] are both low-level APIs for 2D and 3D visualization. OpenGL is derived from SGI's IRIS GL API, which was widely used in the 1980s for advanced visualization. The OpenGL standard is implemented in device drivers for all standard graphics cards, which allow a developer to take advantage of the hardware to draw both geometric and volume composite renderings in real time. Figure 3.9 is a rendering of DTI tractography data that was created with OpenGL.

Since the mid-1990s, Microsoft has been developing Direct3D to provide a low-level API for 3D visualization. Direct3D is also supported by the graphics card manufacturers and can be used to generate real-time 3D graphics. OpenGL is available on most major platforms, including various flavors of MS Windows, Mac OS, Linux, and other Unix systems. Direct3D was designed for MS Windows; however, there are some efforts to provide emulated support on other platforms.

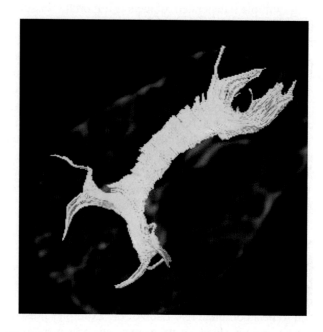

Fig. 3.9. DTI-identified fiber bundles rendering with OpenGL

3.7.2 Pipeline-Based APIs

The Visualization Toolkit [VTK] is a visualization API that uses a pipeline, or data-driven, model for generating renderings. VTK was developed at GE Corporate Research and Development, but it is now managed by Kitware, Inc. VTK supports many different platforms (MS Windows, Mac OS, Linux, and Unix) and can take advantage of graphics hardware, if available. In the pipeline approach, data objects are created and then inserted into the processing pipeline to be rendered. Data objects can be geometric primitives or volumetric data. In addition, VTK supports high-dimensional data, such as tensor fields. Several software packages have been developed using the VTK render engine including [Slicer] from the Surgical Planning Laboratory at Brigham and Women's Hospital. Other pipeline-based VTKs include Advanced Visualization Systems AVS package [AVS] and IBM's OpenDX library [OpenDX]. Figure 3.10 shows a rendering of a left atrium and intra-operative catheter measurements using the OpenDX library.

3.7.3 Scene-Graph APIs

Mercury Computer Systems OpenInventor is an example of a scene graph API for 2D and 3D visualization [OpenInventor]. Originally designed by

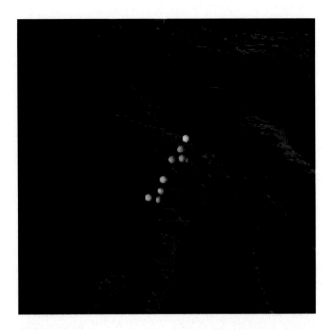

Fig. 3.10. OpenDX was used to generate this visualization of the left atrium together with points sampled with an intraoperative catheter. The red sphere is the location of a metal clip, as identified in CT data. The yellow and green spheres are catheter sample points taken with the Biosense CARTO system

SGI in the early 1990s, OpenInventor is a framework for combining multiple objects into a 3D scene. Each object can be either geometric or volumetric and may include object-specific properties such as transformations or color information. The scene can also contain lights and cameras. Upon rendering, all objects are transformed and rendered into the scene using a prespecified lighting and camera view. OpenInventor is built upon OpenGL which provides real-time rendering capabilities. An image of lung dynamics using OpenInventor is shown in Fig. 3.11 [Haider et al. 2005]. Other scene graph APIs include System In Motion's [Coin3D] and [OpenSceneGraph].

3.7.4 Software Rendering APIs

Mayo Clinic [ANALYZE] and University of Pennsylvania's [3DVIEWNIX] are two examples of software packages with embedded software-based rendering engines. For image-guided applications, the underlying programming interfaces can serve as the visualization engine during a procedure.

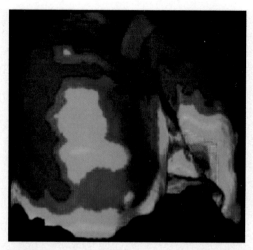

Fig. 3.11. OpenInventor was used to map lung surface deformation throughout the respiratory cycle onto an anatomical model

The programming interface for ANALYZE is AVW, a comprehensive cross-platform C library that contains several rendering algorithms for volumetric visualization of image processing functions. While neither a scene-graph nor a pipeline-based approach, AVW does allow multiple object rendering using different rendering algorithms and merging methods. AVW was used to generate Fig. 3.12, which shows a volume compositing image with cardiac functional data mapped onto the left atrium [Holmes et al. 2006].

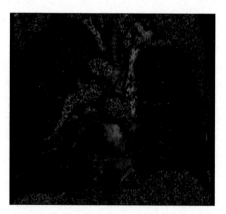

Fig. 3.12. Volume compositing was combined with functional mapping to create a rendering of cardiac anatomy and physiology using AVW

In contrast to many rendering engines, AVW and 3DVIEWNIX support other types of volume rendering beyond volume compositing, including gradient shaded rendering and t-shell rendering. Because neither package is tied to a particular hardware system or OS, cross-platform development is common and applications are ubiquitous.

3.7.5 Numerical Computing with Visualization

MATLAB, a product of The Mathworks (http://www.mathworks.com/), is a numerical computing package that is primarily designed for data processing [MATLAB]. It has, however, developed a quite extensive collection of visualization tools that can be used for medical image visualization. MATLAB also supports direct control of hardware via acquisition toolboxes that provide the necessary interface for data collection during IGIs. MATLAB provides a C programmable interface to allow embedding of MATLAB visualizations and processing in other software. IDL, by ITT Visual Information Solutions, is an example of another numerical processing package with visualization capabilities [Green 2002].

3.8   Real-Time Feedback and Hardware Interfacing

Visualization in IGI is intrinsically associated with a graphical user interface, and therefore, tied to the computer hardware necessary for receiving input and presenting output. The use of a keyboard, mouse, or touch screen are well-developed approaches for receiving input data from an operator. Intraoperative images and tracking data from spatial localizers are other examples of input data streams. Output data may be directly presented on a standard video monitor or an augmented reality display device. Data from the processing and visualization software also may be sent to robotic or haptic hardware. Figure 3.13 illustrates examples of input and display technologies as well as an augmented display example from a neurosurgical procedure.

3.8.1 Receiving Input

There are two basic approaches to receiving input – pulling data or pushing data. Pulling data suggests that the visualization software requests input to be provided by an external system. For example, a visualization system may call a function that queries a tracker and returns the current position and orientation of an instrument. Image data may be requested from a PACS server using a DICOM Query/Retrieve model. Alternatively, pushed data are initiated from an outside system and sent to the visualization system, either synchronously or asynchronously. For example, keyboard and mouse (or other pointer device) input can be considered pushed data because the input action is initiated outside of the application and placed in the event cue of the application. A data-acquisition board may push biosensor data to the visualization system during an intervention.

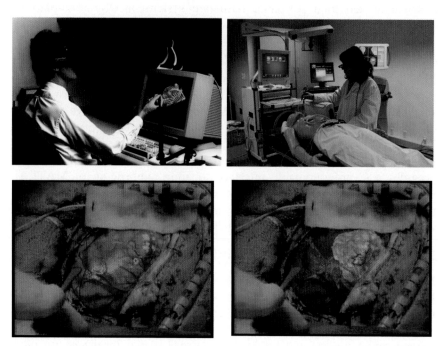

Fig. 3.13. Interfacing to a visualization system includes both input (signals) data and output (processed) data. In the *upper left* panel, a haptic device is used to input data, which is then visualized through an immersive display headset. In the *upper right* panel, the tracked instrument is used to input data while an augmented reality display is used to provide the visualization. The *bottom* two panels are an example of the use of augmented reality for visualizing a brain tumor. Preoperative images are processed to provide segmented renderings of tumor and blood vessels and then are fused (registered) in real time with video of the surgical opening during the intervention

Intraoperative image data may be pushed or pulled, and they may come from either digital or analog sources. For example, x-ray fluoroscopy data acquired with a digital detector can be pushed by the PACS management system to a visualization system, or can be requested by the guidance application. Analog image data, such as video from a camera or echo signals from an ultrasound system, can be recorded using a video capture card. Captured images can be stored and/or directly visualized during a procedure.

Localization and bio-signals can also be pushed or pulled, depending on the architecture of the acquisition system. Most visualization systems provide a means for receiving input through a pushing or pulling approach, or both. In the pushing model, events are generated in the application event cue that informs the application that data is available for processing. For example, in windows, an ActiveX component can be used to respond to an instrument position event from a localizer. In a pulling model, the application simply calls a query function through the localizer API.

3.8.2 Presenting Output

Output presentation is generally, but not always, visual. The most common display technology is a computer monitor; however, images can also be presented to less traditional displays such as fully immersive headsets and augmented-reality systems. A visualization system may support more than one display device based on the requirement of the intervention. Computer monitors, plus keyboards and pointers (e.g., mouse), are useful for presentation of many types of data, including patient 2D images and vital signs. Partially or fully immersive displays and touch screens are effective for presenting intraoperative 3D image data and rendering of merged images and bio-signals (data fusion). Nonvisual feedback can include audio signals to direct a procedure and tactile feedback via haptics devices to sense interfaces during a procedure.

3.9   Applications

3.9.1 Epilepsy Foci Removal

Epilepsy is a neurological disorder associated with seizure that affects up to 1% of the world population [Wiebe 2003]. Although drugs may help control epileptic seizures, one third of patients remain refractory to medications. For such patients, surgery is often a safe and effective treatment [Arango et al. 2004]. Surgical options include resection of a small section of the cortex, removal of a lobe, or in severe cases removal of an entire hemisphere. A critical component to surgical interventions is the pre-surgical planning for localization of seizure activity [Arango et al. 2004]. Traditional seizure localization is accomplished through EEG monitoring, which can be either noninvasive (i.e., electrodes placed on the scalp) or invasive (subdural electrode strips or grids). More recently, advances in imaging technologies provide noninvasive methodologies for mapping seizure activity utilizing radionuclide imaging. These include PET and SPECT imaging systems, used in combination with MRI.

PET or SPECT can be used to localize epileptic foci since blood flow increases in these areas during a seizure and the radioisotopes selectively sequester in tissue excited regions. It is difficult, however, to utilize the ictal (during seizure) scan alone to localize an epileptic focus, because these regions may be hypoperfused interictally (between seizures) thereby masking the ictal increase in blood flow. It is also challenging to anatomically localize the seizure focus due to the poor spatial resolution of PET or SPECT scans. A protocol called SISCOM (Subtraction Interictal SPECT COregistered to MRI), developed at the Mayo Clinic, utilizes both ictal and interictal function SPECT scans in conjunction with a structural MR scan to generate a fused visualization of the region of epileptic activity on high-resolution anatomical images [O'Brien et al. 1998].

SISCOM processing consists of several steps including interictal/ ictal volume registration, subtraction, and determination of locations with a significantly greater blood flow ictally versus interictally. The subtraction volume is registered to the structural MR volume providing a fusion of anatomic and functional data. This technique is especially important in nonlesional cases of epileptic seizure. The fused 3D images could potentially be used to guide the resection of brain tissue during a stereotaxic, image-guided neurosurgical procedure. Figure 3.14 demonstrates a fused visualization of the structure-function data, the seizure "hot spot" (shown as bright regions on the rendering), and the location of a tracked neurosurgical instrument.

3.9.2 Left Atrium Cardiac Ablation

Left atrial fibrillation is a condition in which the left atrium beats irregularly due to abnormal electrical pathways in the heart muscle. This condition becomes more prevalent with age, affecting approximately 6% of the population over 65 [Lin and Marchlinski 2003]. Pharmacological treatments are sometimes effective; however, they often do not work and/or have undesirable side effects. Open chest surgery, in which incisions are made in the heart tissue to interrupt aberrant electrical pathways, is highly effective but has high risk, morbidity, and cost associated with them. Over the past 20 years, minimally invasive cardiac catheter ablation has become the initial choice of therapy for many types of arrhythmias [Lin and Marchlinski 2003]. In this procedure, radiofrequency energy is delivered via a catheter to produce lesions in the left atrium that block the abnormal pathways and eliminate the arrhythmia. A major limitation of catheter-based procedures is the inability to precisely visualize and target the specific diseased anatomical structures giving rise to the arrhythmias.

Typical visualization tools available to the cardiologist for guidance include biplane fluoroscopy and real-time ultrasound. General 2D silhouettes of the cardiac structure can be visualized with fluoroscopy. Ultrasound provides 2D real-time visualization of the catheter tip and the local endocardial morphology. 3D ultrasound imaging devices have also been recently introduced. Catheter tip-tracking technologies have been incorporated into the

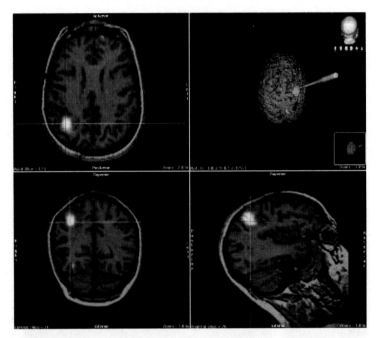

Fig. 3.14. Visualization system for localizing epilepsy seizure focus for resection. This software fuses preoperative 3D MR with processed (registered and subtracted) 3D SPECT data to generate a precise visualization of regional epileptic activity. The tracked probe is rendered into the 3D visualization and linked to the 2D views

procedure to provide 3D representations of the heart. Points on the endocardial surface are sampled by the cardiologist using a tracked catheter to build up a model of the left atrium and pulmonary veins [Gepstein et al. 1997].

Another approach [Peters et al. 1997] constructs a model using noncontact probes. Advances in the procedure include incorporation of detailed, patient-specific anatomical image data [Dickfeld et al. 2003; Reddy et al. 2004; Sra et al. 2005; Sun et al. 2005] where a model is built from preoperative CT or MR data. These models are then registered into the space of the patient during the procedure using landmark-matching and surface-based approaches.

A system is under development at Mayo Clinic to integrate in real time the various imaging modalities and electrophysiology mapping systems together with the position of the catheter tip into a single visual display [Rettmann et al. 2006]. The system utilizes a fast, distributed database model for communication between the system components for reading data streams, computing registrations, and visualizing fused images.

Figure 3.15 demonstrates a fused visualization of patient-specific data and real-time catheter positions during a procedure. The endocardial surface of the left atrium is embedded within a volume rendered from the patient CT data. This provides the cardiologist with information regarding relevant anatomic structures adjacent to the left atrium. The small red spheres represent positions of the catheter collected during the procedure and registered to the left atrial surface. These visualizations provide the cardiologist with detailed patient specific anatomic targets relative to the position of the catheter tip.

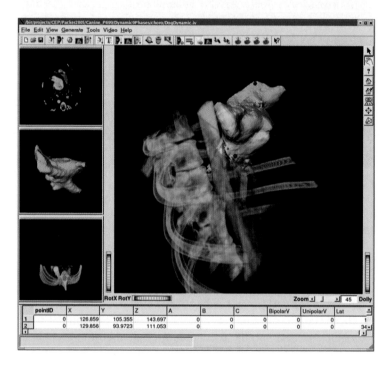

Fig. 3.15. Visualization system for cardiac ablation. In this software, multiple visualization methods are used to provide dynamic cues for guidance. Volume compositing of the thorax provides 3D context of the anatomy; a surface model of the left atrium shows the target anatomy of interest; and colored tags identify regions for ablation, all computed and fused in real time

3.9.3 Permanent Prostate Brachytherapy

According to the American Cancer Society (ACS), it is estimated that over 200,000 new cases of prostate cancer were diagnosed in 2006 [ACS 2006].

Fortunately, the ACS also notes that with proper detection and management of the disease, 5-year survival for men with prostate cancer is nearly 100%. Although there are several options for treating prostate cancer, prostate brachytherapy is an effective method for treating early-stage disease which can have minimal side-effects. In the procedure, up to 100 radioactive seeds are inserted with a needle into the prostate. In order to adequately cover the prostate with the recommended dose [Nath et al. 1995], the procedure requires significant 3D planning and precise execution of the plan. The planning procedure uses transrectal ultrasound images to determine the desired location of the sources that provide adequate dose to the prostate while avoiding collateral damage to adjacent tissues, such as the bladder, urethra, and rectum. The procedure is guided with fluoroscopy and/or transrectal ultrasound (TRUS). CT is used postoperatively to evaluate the outcome.

Permanent prostate brachytherapy must be guided with imaging because the prostate is not openly exposed. While both TRUS and fluoroscopy have been used effectively for several years, placement of the radioactive sources is challenging, since neither imaging modality can effectively provide a complete 3D description during the procedure. Fluoroscopy has low imaging contrast and provides only 2D images; TRUS can collect 3D data, however, due to image artifacts, the seeds cannot be easily resolved in the images. Several sites have developed new image guidance approaches to prostate brachytherapy implantation. One approach merges TRUS and fluoroscopy with transurethral ultrasound (TUUS) to provide a more effective description of the prostate and radioactive sources [Holmes et al. 2003]. The system under development at Mayo Clinic uses three-film x-ray images, as well as data collected from TRUS and TUUS to reconstruct the boundary of the prostate and the 3D position of the seeds [Su et al. 2006]. Using 3D visualization, the radiation oncologist can determine whether sources are placed accurately, and if there is a need for additional sources to fill voids, called "cold spots," in the prostate.

Figure 3.16 shows the images collected during a brachytherapy procedure together with a 3D rendering of the fused data. The system uses the Mayo AVW API for most of the data processing and an OpenInventor API for image display. The 3D rendering is based on surface models generated from a pre-procedural MRI and seed locations determined from ultrasound. Phantom, animal, and clinical data have been collected with the system and evaluated. The system is still under development for IGI and clinical validation.

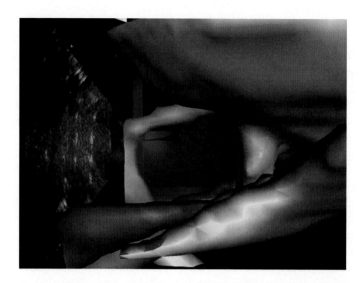

Fig. 3.16. Visualization system for Permanent Prostate Brachytherapy. In this image, 3D models segmented and rendered from preoperative MR have been fused with intraoperative trans-urethral ultrasound (TUUS). The MR images provide excellent soft tissue differentiation for accurate segmentation, while the TUUS images provide real-time feedback for localization of the seeds

3.9.4 Virtual and Enhanced Colonoscopy

Virtual endoscopy has been under development for well over a decade [Satava 2007]. The approach uses renderings of medical image data such that the resulting image is similar to one that might be seen with a real endoscope. One application in which virtual endoscopy may be helpful is the screening for colorectal cancer. According to the ACS, over 55,000 people in the USA will die from colon cancer in 2006 [ACS 2006]. Virtual colonoscopy can be used to visualize 3D CT data of the colon in order to detect polyps [Gallo et al. 2006]. In Fig. 3.17a, a virtual colonoscopy rendering is shown, which provides information on both the morphology and vascularity of the polyp obtained from mathematical processing of the 3D CT scan data.

As an enhancement to conventional colonoscopy for colon cancer screening, tracking technology can be used to determine the position of the colonoscope during the interventional procedure. The video data stream from the scope can be processed and analyzed to determine the quality of the images. Such information can be used to flag regions of the colon that may not have been adequately visualized during the first pass, and the gastro-enterologist is guided back for another look at these regions. This ensures that 100% of the colon is examined with acceptable images. Figure 3.17b shows the video and tracking data from a colonoscopy procedure. The location of the sphere delineates the position of the video data within the colon, while the color of the sphere can be used to convey the quality of the video data at that point. In addition to video analysis and tracking visualization, screening CT scans can be registered to the scope during the procedure to provide additional information to the gastroenterologist.

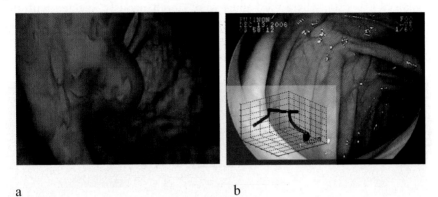

a   b

Fig. 3.17. Use of visualization in virtual and real colonoscopy procedures. (a) Volume compositing on a CT dataset is used to visualize vasculature within a polyp. (b) Visualization of the tracked colonoscope along with the video image stream provides feedback about the location and quality of the data collected during the procedure. This can be used to direct reexamination of regions of the colon inadequately visualized during the first pass

3.9.5 Surgical Separation of Conjoined Twins

Conjoined twins are identical twins with parts of their bodies physically joined at birth. This condition is quite rare, occurring in only 1 in 250,000 live births, with a higher frequency in females than males [Spitz 2005]. The first attempt to surgically separate conjoined twins occurred in A.D. 970 in Kappadokia, Armenai. The separation was attempted on male twins, age 30, after one of the men died. Unfortunately, this surgery was not successful and the second man died a few days after the separation. The first successful separation, dating back to 1689, was performed on twin girls in Basel, Switzerland. Current success rates of separation are promising, with an 80% success rate in planned surgeries and 10–30% success rate in emergency surgeries [Spitz and Kiely 2003]. Imaging data have become critically important in the surgical planning step for understanding the detailed anatomy of separate and shared organs and body structures.

A recent case of conjoined twins at the Mayo Clinic involved twin girls joined from the chest to the abdomen. Several organs were fused and/or tangled together, including the pancreases, livers, and intestines. The two hearts were overlapping and out of normal position. Of particular concern was the shared blood supply to the shared liver, as well as a shared common bile duct. Comprehensive imaging studies were conducted to provide details of anatomic structures as well as perfusion of the blood supply to the conjoint liver. Contrast-enhanced CT scans were performed on each baby separately to determine individual blood supplies to the liver. A joint contrast-enhanced CT scan, where the babies were simultaneously injected with the contrast agent, was utilized to delineate regions of the liver that were jointly perfused. CT colangiography was performed for in-depth visualization of the gall bladders, livers, and bile ducts.

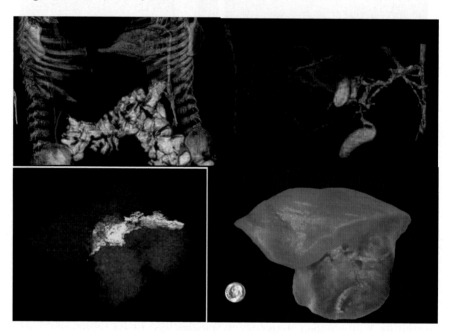

Fig. 3.18. *Top left*: Segmented 3D anatomic structures of conjoined twins. Shown are two hearts (red and blue), the liver (dark red), intestines (yellow), two gall bladders (green). *Top right*: Detailed view of blood vessel supply to liver from each baby. *Bottom left*: Perfusion map of liver, blood supply from one baby in red, other baby in blue, joint perfusion in yellow. *Bottom right*: Photo-graph of life-size physical model of liver produced from 3D CT segmentation

Anatomic structures were segmented from the various imaging studies, spatially registered and fused to create comprehensive 3D anatomic and functional visualizations for the surgeons. The top left panel in Fig. 3.18 illustrates the skeletal structure, the two hearts (red and blue), the joined liver (dark red), entangled intestines (yellow), and gall bladders (green). Each heart, together with the associated vessels, was segmented from the individual contrast-enhanced CT scans. The liver and gall bladders are produced from the colangiogram, and the intestines and bony structures came from the dual-injection CT scan. All segmented anatomy from the different imaging procedures was registered to a single volume to create this combined display.

The top right panel of Fig. 3.18 shows a more detailed view of the liver with the combined blood supply where the vessels from one baby are colored in red and the vessels from the other baby are in blue. The gall bladders and ducts of the biliary system (in green) can also be clearly seen.

The bottom left panel is a perfusion map of the liver where red indicates regions of the liver perfused by one baby, blue indicates regions perfused by the other baby, and yellow represents regions perfused by both babies. In order to provide additional visualization aids to the surgeons, life-size physical models were constructed of select anatomy from the 3D segmented data. A photograph of the physical model of the liver is shown in the bottom right panel. These visualizations and physical models were utilized primarily in the preplanning phases; however, it is entirely feasible to incorporate them into the surgical procedure for guidance.

3.10   Summary

This chapter has provided an introduction to some of the fundamental concepts and components used for visualization in IGI. Visualization in IGI involves an integration of software and hardware components interacting either synchronously or asynchronously during an interventional procedure. Because IGI visualization is inherently interactive, is often based on use of large image datasets, involves merging of relevant biosignals and device manipulations, and all these placed into a common framework for real-time display, meeting the computational demands of visualization systems in IGI is of paramount importance. Of secondary, but still critical, importance is the design and associated effectiveness of the interactive user interface. Successful integration requires unification of disparate coordinate systems and different types of multi-modality images, the fusion of real-time data and signal streams with both preoperative and intraoperative images, the necessary computational image processing that must be carried out (i.e., segmentation, registration, fusion), and the coherent presentation of all this information in a relevant, meaningful and interactive way. This is all to say that successful visualization in IGI is not a simple proposition, nor a readily achieved objective. One must take care that all of the interrelated components and concepts are integrated in an expedient, accurate, and facile way. When this is accomplished, however, visualization becomes the key component in the process of navigation, targeting, and monitoring during the interventional procedure. The potential results are improved outcomes, reduced risk and morbidity, reduced time in the procedure room, increased throughput, and reduced cost. However, at this point in the evolution of visualization in IGI, this panacea has yet to be fully achieved. Nonetheless, the rate of progress and improvement toward this goal over the past decade has been truly remarkable and portends significant potential for the future of visualization in IGI.

Acknowledgments

The authors would like to acknowledge the staff of the Mayo Biomedical Imaging Resource for their many technical contributions, their faculty colleagues in the Mayo Clinic College of Medicine, and many extramural collaborators whose interests and expertise have helped make possible many of the advances described in this chapter. The DTI data was obtained from the Johns Hopkins in vivo human data-base acquired under grants from the Human Brain Project and National Research Resource Center (ROI AG20012-01 / P41 RR15241-01A1).

References

3DVIEWNIX. "3DViewnix (http://www.mipg.upenn.edu/~Vnews/)."

ACS. (2006). "Cancer Facts and Figures 2006." American Cancer Society, Atlanta.

Aharon S, Cameron B, and Robb RA. (1997). "Computation of efficient patient specific model from 3-D medical images: use in virtual endoscopy and surgery rehearsal." *IPMI*, Springer, Pittsburgh, PA.

ANALYZE MC. "Mayo Clinic Analyze (http://www.mayo.edu/bir/Software/Analyze/Analyze1NEW.html)."

Arango MF, Steven DA, and Herrick IA. (2004). "Neurosurgery for the treatment of epilepsy." *Current Opinion in Anaesthesiology*, 17, 383–387.

AVS. "AVS: Advanced Visual Systems (http://www.avs.com)."

Baxendale S. (2002). "The role of functional MRI in the presurgical investigation of temporal lobe epilepsy patients: a clinical perspective and review." *Journal of Clinical & Experimental Neuropsychology: Official Journal of the International Neuropsychological Society*, 24(5), 664–676.

Blaimer M, Breuer F, Mueller M, Heidemann RM, Griswold MA, and Jakob PM. (2004). "SMASH, SENSE, PILS, GRAPPA: how to choose the optimal method." *Topics in Magnetic Resonance Imaging*, 15(4), 223–236.

Bronskill M, and Sprawls P. (1993). *The Physics of MRI: 1992 AAPM Summer School Proceedings*, American Institute of Physics, Woodbury.

Budoff MJ, Achenbach S, Blumenthal RS, Carr JJ, Goldin JG, Greenland P, Guerci AD, Lima JA, Rader DJ, Rubin GD, Shaw LJ, Wiegers SE, American Heart Association Committee on Cardiovascular I, Intervention, American Heart Association Council on Cardiovascular R, and American Heart Association Committee on Cardiac Imaging CoCC. (2006). "Assessment of coronary artery disease by cardiac computed tomography: a scientific statement from the American Heart Association Committee on Cardio-vascular Imaging and Intervention, Council on Cardiovascular Radiology and Intervention, and Committee on Cardiac Imaging, Council on Clinical Cardiology." *Circulation*, 114(16), 1761–1791.

Butler WE, Piaggio CM, Constantinou C, Niklason L, Gonzalez RG, Cosgrove GR, and Zervas NT. (1998). "A mobile computed tomographic scanner with intraoperative and intensive care unit applications." *Neurosurgery*, 42(6), 1304–1310; discussion 1310–1301.

Cameron BM, Manduca A, and Robb RA. (1996). "Patient-specific anatomic models. Geometric surface generation from three-dimensional medical images using a specified polygonal budget." *Studies in Health Technology & Informatics*, 29, 447–460.

Christian P, Bernier D, and Langan J. (2003). *Nuclear Medicine and PET: Technology and Techniques*, Mosby, St. Louis, MO.

Coin3D. "Coin3D (http://www.coin3d.org)."

Crouch D, and Robb RA. (1997). "A new algorithm for efficient polygon decimation for virtual reality applications in medicine." *Proceedings of SPIE*, 3031, 514–517.

Dickfeld T, Calkins H, Zviman M, Kato R, Meininger G, Lickfett L, Berger R, Halperin H, and Solomon SB. (2003). "Anatomic stereotactic catheter ablation on three-dimensional magnetic resonance images in real time." *Circulation*, 108(19), 2407–2413.

DICOM. (2006). *Digital Imaging and Communications in Medicine (DICOM)*, National Electrical Manufacturers Association, Virginia.

Eusemann CD, Ritman EL, Bellemann ME, and Robb RA. (2001). "Parametric display of myocardial function." *Computerized Medical Imaging & Graphics*, 25(6), 483–493.

Eusemann CD, Ritman EL, and Robb RA. (2003). "Parametric visualization methods for the quantitative assessment of myocardial motion." *Academic Radiology*, 10(1), 66–76.

Foley J, van Dam A, Feiner S, and Hughes J. (1990). *Computer Graphics: Principles and Practice*, Addision-Wesley, Reading, MA.

Gallo TM, Galatola G, Laudi C, and Regge D. (2006). "CT colonography: screening in individuals at high risk for colorectal cancer." *Abdominal Imaging*, 31(3), 297–301.

Gepstein L, Hayam G, and Ben-Haim SA. (1997). "A novel method for non-fluoroscopic catheter-based electroanatomical mapping of the heart. In vitro and in vivo accuracy results." *Circulation*, 95(6), 1611–1622.

Gray H. (1918). *Anatomy of the Human Body*, Lea & Febiger, Philadelphia, PA.

Green B. (2002). "The maze III surgical procedure." *AORN Journal*, 76(1), 134–146; quiz 147–150.

Guillonneau B. (2006). "Can TRUS guidance reduce the incidence of positive margins during laparoscopic radical prostatectomy?" *Nature Clinical Practice Urology*, 3(10), 518–519.

Gunneson TJ, Menon KV, Wiesner RH, Daniels JA, Hay JE, Charlton MR, Brandhagen DJ, Rosen CB, and Porayko MK. (2002). "Ultrasound-assisted percutaneous liver biopsy performed by a physician assistant [see comment]." *American Journal of Gastroenterology*, 97(6), 1472–1475.

Haider CR, Bartholmai BJ, Holmes DR, Camp JJ, and Robb RA. (2005). "Quantitative characterization of lung disease." *Computerized Medical Imaging & Graphics*, 29(7), 555–563.

Haydel MJ, Preston CA, Mills TJ, Luber S, Blaudeau E, and DeBlieux PM. (2000). "Indications for computed tomography in patients with minor head injury [see comment]." *New England Journal of Medicine*, 343(2), 100–105.

Hendee W, and Ritenour R. (1992). *Medical Imaging Physics*, Mosby, St. Louis, MO.

Holmes DR, 3rd, Davis BJ, Bruce CJ, and Robb RA. (2003). "3D visualization, analysis, and treatment of the prostate using trans-urethral ultrasound." *Computerized Medical Imaging & Graphics*, 27(5), 339–349.

Holmes DR, III, Rettmann ME, Cameron BM, Camp JJ, and Robb RA. (2006). "Cardioscopy: Interactive Endocardial Visualization to Guide RF Cardiac Ablation." *Proceedings of SPIE – Medical Imaging 2006*, San Diego, CA.

Hounsfield GN. (1973). "Computerized transverse axial scanning (tomography). 1. Description of system." *British Journal of Radiology*, 46(552), 1016–1022.

Hutton BF, Braun M, Thurfjell L, and Lau DY. (2002). "Image registration: an essential tool for nuclear medicine." *European Journal of Nuclear Medicine & Molecular Imaging*, 29(4), 559–577.

Kay PA, Robb RA, and Bostwick DG. (1998). "Prostate cancer microvessels: a novel method for three-dimensional reconstruction and analysis." *Prostate*, 37(4), 270–277.

Lattanzi R, Baruffaldi F, Zannoni C, and Viceconti M. (2004). "Specialised CT scan protocols for 3-D pre-operative planning of total hip replacement." *Medical Engineering & Physics*, 26(3), 237–245.

Le Bihan D. (2003). "Looking into the functional architecture of the brain with diffusion MRI." *Nature Reviews Neuroscience*, 4(6), 469–480.

Lin D, and Marchlinski FE. (2003). "Advances in ablation therapy for complex arrhythmias: atrial fibrillation and ventricular tachycardia." *Current Cardiology Reports*, 5(5), 407–414.

Lorensen W, and Cline H. (1987). "Marching cubes: a high resolution 3D surface construction algorithm." *Computer Graphics*, 21, 163–169.

Matlab. "Matlab (http://www.mathworks.com)."

Microsoft. (2006). "DirectX 9.0 (http://msdn.microsoft.com/directx/)."

Nath R, Anderson LL, Luxton G, Weaver KA, Williamson JF, and Meigooni AS. (1995). "Dosimetry of interstitial brachytherapy sources: recommendations of the AAPM Radiation Therapy Committee Task Group No. 43. American Association of Physicists in Medicine [see comment] [erratum appears in *Med Phys* 1996 Sep; 23(9), 1579]." *Medical Physics*, 22(2), 209–234.

Nicholls SJ, Tuzcu EM, Sipahi I, Schoenhagen P, and Nissen SE. (2006). "Intravascular ultrasound in cardiovascular medicine." *Circulation*, 114(4), e55–59.

NIFTI DFWG. "A (Sort of) New Image Data Format Standard: NIfTI-1(http://nifti.nimh.nih.gov/nifti-1/documentation/hbm_nifti_2004.pdf)."

O'Brien TJ, So EL, Mullan BP, Hauser MF, Brinkmann BH, Bohnen NI, Hanson D, Cascino GD, Jack CR, Jr., and Sharbrough FW. (1998). "Subtraction ictal SPECT co-registered to MRI improves clinical usefulness of SPECT in localizing the surgical seizure focus." *Neurology*, 50(2), 445–454.

OpenDX. "OpenDX: The Open Source Software Project Based on IBM's Visualizaiton Data Explorer (http://opendx.org/)."

OpenInventor. "Open Inventor by Mercury Computer Systems (http://www.tgs.com)."

OpenSceneGraph. "OpenSceneGraph (http://www.openscenegraph.org/)."

Pakin SK, Cavalcanti C, La Rocca R, Schweitzer ME, and Regatte RR. (2006). "Ultra-high-field MRI of knee joint at 7.0T: preliminary experience." *Academic Radiology*, 13(9), 1135–1142.

Peters NS, Jackman WM, Schilling RJ, Beatty G, and Davies DW. (1997). "Images in cardiovascular medicine. Human left ventricular endocardial activation mapping using a novel noncontact catheter." *Circulation*, 95(6), 1658–1660.

Pfister H, Lorensen B, Bajaj C, Kindlmann G, Schroeder W, Avila LS, Raghu KM, Machiraju R, and Lee J. (2001). "The transfer function bake-off." *IEEE Computer Graphics and Applications*, 21(3), 16–22.

Reddy VY, Malchano ZJ, Holmvang G, Schmidt EJ, d'Avila A, Houghtaling C, Chan RC, and Ruskin JN. (2004). "Integration of cardiac magnetic resonance imaging with three-dimensional electroanatomic mapping to guide left ventricular catheter manipulation: feasibility in a porcine model of healed myocardial infarction." *Journal of the American College of Cardiology*, 44(11), 2202–2213.

Rettmann ME, Holmes DR, 3rd, Su Y, Cameron BM, Camp JJ, Packer DL, and Robb RA. (2006). "An integrated system for real-time image guided cardiac catheter ablation." *Studies in Health Technology & Informatics*, 119, 455–460.

Ritman EL. (2003). "Cardiac computed tomography imaging: a history and some future possibilities." *Cardiology Clinics*, 21(4), 491–513.

Robb RA. (2008a). "Mayo Clinic Analyze 7.5 Format (http://www.mayo.edu/bir/PDF/ANALYZE75.pdf)." Biomedical Imaging Resource, Mayo Clinic.

Robb RA. (2008b). "Mayo Clinic Analyze Coordinate System (Analyze Help Documentation)." Biomedical Imaging Resource, Mayo Clinic.

Robb RA. (2000). "Virtual (Computed) Endoscopy: Development and Evaluation Using the Visible Human Datasets." *Visible Human Project Conference*, Bethesda, MD.

Robb RA. (2000). Biomedical Imaging, Visualization, and Analysis, Wiley-Liss, New York, NY.

Satava RM, Robb RA. (1997). "Virtual Endoscopy: Application of 3-D visualization to Medical Diagnosis." *Presence*, 6(2), 179–197.

Schenck JF, Jolesz FA, Roemer PB, Cline HE, Lorensen WE, Kikinis R, Silverman SG, Hardy CJ, Barber WD, and Laskaris ET. (1995). "Superconducting open-configuration MR imaging system for image-guided therapy." *Radiology*, 195(3), 805–814.

Segal M, and Akeley K. (2006). "The OpenGL Graphics System: A Specification (Version 2.0) (http://www.opengl.org/documentation/spec.html)."

Slicer. "3D Slicer (http://www.slicer.org/)."

Spencer JA. (2001). "Oncological radiology." *Clinical Radiology*, 56(7), 521–522.

Spitz L. (2005). "Conjoined twins." *Prenatal Diagnosis*, 25(9), 814–819.

Spitz L, and Kiely EM. (2003). "Conjoined twins." *JAMA*, 289(10), 1307–1310.

Sra J, Krum D, Hare J, Okerlund D, Thompson H, Vass M, Schweitzer J, Olson E, Foley WD, and Akhtar M. (2005). "Feasibility and validation of registration of three-dimensional left atrial models derived from computed tomography with a noncontact cardiac mapping system." *Heart Rhythm*, 2(1), 55–63.

Su Y, Davis BJ, Herman MG, and Robb RA. (2006). "TRUS-fluoroscopy fusion for intraoperative prostate brachytherapy dosimetry." *Studies in Health Technology & Informatics*, 119, 532–537.

Sun Y, Azar FS, Xu C, Hayam G, Preiss A, Rahn N, and Sauer F. (2005). "Registration of high-resolution 3D atrial images with elecroanatomical cardiac mapping: evaluation of registration methodology." *SPIE Medical Imaging*, 299–307.

Szabo T. (2004). *Diagnostic Ultrasound Imaging: Inside Out*, Academic Press, Burlington, MA.

Udupa J, and Odhner D. (1993). "Shell Rendering." *IEEE Computer Graphics and Applications*, 13(6), 58–67.

VTK. "The Visualization Toolkit (http://www.vtk.org)."

Wiebe S. (2003). "Brain surgery for epilepsy." *Lancet*, 362(Suppl), s48–s49.

Zimmerman R, Sirven J, Roarke M, Drazkowski J, Larson S, Dixit S, and Tollefson C. (2004). "SISCOM localization of a seizure focus within a heterotopia." *Neurology*, 62(12), 2328.

Chapter 4
Augmented Reality

Frank Sauer, Sebastian Vogt, and Ali Khamene

Abstract

Much of the visualization in image-guided interventions is achieved by creating a virtual image of the surgical or therapeutic environment, based upon preoperative images, and displaying it on a workstation that is remote from the patient. Linkages between the patient and the image are created through image registration and tracked tools. Such solutions are not always ideal, and result in a psychophysical decoupling of the actual and virtual therapeutic working spaces. Using augmented reality, these two spaces are fused into a single volume, which is typically viewed stereoscopically so that a preoperative or intraoperative patient image appears at the location of the actual patient anatomy. The surgeon has the perception that he is "seeing through" the patient or organ surface to observe the operative site. This chapter reviews the various approaches to augmented reality, and discusses the engineering and psychophysical challenges in developing user-friendly systems.

4.1 Introduction

4.1.1 What Is Augmented Reality?

Augmented reality (AR) is a visualization concept that enhances real images with virtual, computer-generated graphics. The term mixed reality is often used to describe the whole spectrum that ranges from AR, where the emphasis is on the real image, to augmented virtuality, where the virtual scene dominates and the real elements appear as add-ons [Milgram and Kishino 1994].

Interestingly, the general concept of enhancing real images with computer graphics is already ubiquitous in today's media. A photo with text annotation may be regarded as one, albeit very simple, example. Weather reports on TV go further and use blue screen technology to make a real

T. Peters and K. Cleary (eds.), *Image-Guided Interventions.*
© Springer Science + Business Media, LLC 2008

weather person appear in front of computer-generated weather maps. And, of course, all Hollywood action movies nowadays rely on a sophisticated combination of real shots with computer-generated imagery.

In contrast to these everyday examples, the concept of combining real and virtual images still needs to be established in medical practice. In this chapter, we want to put forward a specific understanding of medical AR as an advanced form of interventional image guidance. Based on that understanding, medical AR has very specific requirements.

For medical AR, it is useful to consider medical images as maps of a patient's anatomy. Instead of displaying these maps apart from the patient as in standard medical navigation systems, we overlay them directly onto the physician's view of the real patient. If, for example, there is a tumor in the map, we perceive this tumor now as a graphical object at the location of the actual tumor. Figure 4.1 illustrates this basic principle.

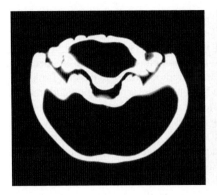 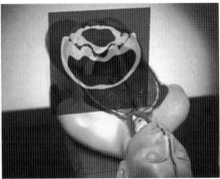

Fig. 4.1. *Left*: A cross-sectional CT image of a "patient." *Right*: Augmented view of the patient with the CT image appearing at the location of the actual anatomy (figures are from Sauer et al. 2000, © 2000 IEEE)

A central requirement for medical AR in the field of image guidance is precise registration between the map and the corresponding real patient. If the map does not align correctly with the patient, AR can become dangerous, as the physician would be guided to place instruments in incorrect locations. Furthermore, medical AR needs to be "on-line," which means it must be available in real time to the physician, who is acting on the information when performing a surgical or interventional procedure.

Figure 4.2 lists the components of a typical medical AR view. On the "real" side, we have an optical or video view of patient and instruments (and sometimes the physician's hands). On the "virtual" side, we have graphical models of the patient (the anatomical map), derived from a preoperative image (e.g., CT) or provided by a real-time modality (e.g., ultrasound), and models of surgical instruments and treatment plans.

To include virtual views of the surgical instruments, the locations of these instruments need to be tracked in the same way as for standard navigation systems. Treatment plans are optional and can be inserted as annotations in the patient map. A treatment plan shows, for example, entry point and path for a needle procedure, or shape and size of resection volume for a tumor operation. The AR view is then created as a fusion of the real view with a rendering of the virtual components.

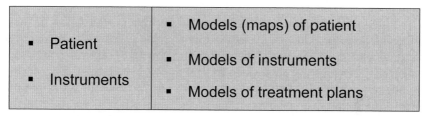

Fig. 4.2. Real and virtual components of medical AR visualization

4.1.2 Why AR for Interventional Guidance?

In general, image guidance systems help the physician to establish a correspondence between locations in a patient's medical images (the "patient map") and the patient's physical body.

In conventional image guidance systems, a pointer or an instrument is tracked and the location visualized in the medical images. The physician observes on a monitor where the pointer or the instrument is positioned with respect to the internal anatomical structures. Hence, the conventional image guidance system maps the instrument into the medical data set, and displays the relationship on a monitor separate from the patient.

In contrast, image guidance that incorporates AR places the patient map directly in the 3D context of the patient's body. AR visualization enables the physician to focus on the surgical site without dividing his attention between the patient and a separate monitor. AR visualization can facilitate hand-eye coordination as the physician observes real and virtual instruments from a consistent natural point-of-view. Furthermore, with stereoscopic AR visualization, the relationships between 3D anatomical structures and the patient are readily appreciated.

The conceptual advantages of AR have to be realized in a practical way. The next section describes a number of design options for building an AR system.

4.2   Technology Building Blocks and System Options

To generate an AR view, we can either combine the computer graphics with a direct view of the real scene in an optical manner, or with a video view electronically. This leads to a very fundamental distinction between AR systems. We call the former category of systems optical AR systems, the latter video AR systems. This nomenclature is most common when using head-mounted displays; here one distinguishes between optical see-through and video see-through systems. A special case of video AR systems is the endoscopic video system that overlays medical graphics onto the endoscopic video images.

Video systems always contain an optical system: the lenses in front of the video sensor. This results in a real image that is not well characterized and independent of the user. The same is true with an optical microscope system that contains a well-defined optical axis to which the user keeps his eye aligned. However, if one looks into the real world through a semitransparent screen that displays the virtual image, one experiences a viewpoint-dependent parallax shift between these two images. Both the screen and the user need to be tracked in this case to keep real and virtual images correctly aligned. Hence, a further important distinction is between AR systems that have an optical axis and those that do not.

Another distinction arises from the configuration and placement of the displays, affecting the ergonomics and usability of the system. An important basic difference is whether the user wears the displays in a head-mounted fashion, or whether the displays are attached to an external mount. A stereoscopic system, in contrast to a monoscopic system, provides the user with a 3D perception of the AR scene.

Figure 4.3 lists these basic design options for AR systems. In Section 4.4, we will use them to organize our overview of the systems that have been described in the literature.

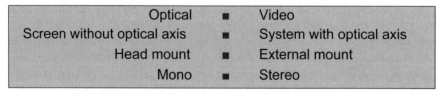

Optical	▪	Video
Screen without optical axis	▪	System with optical axis
Head mount	▪	External mount
Mono	▪	Stereo

Fig. 4.3. Important AR system design options

In the same way that tracking is an essential enabling technology for standard image guidance systems, we need tracking for AR image guidance. For AR, we not only must keep track of where the instruments may be positioned with respect to the patient, but more importantly we also must know the user's viewpoint, that is the viewpoint and viewing direction that determines how the patient is seen in the real view.

Based on this information of real viewpoint and viewing direction, we can place a virtual camera in the corresponding pose relative to the patient model (external camera parameters), and render the virtual image accordingly, making use of the internal camera parameters determined in a prior calibration step. If the patient model has been correctly registered to the real patient, the AR view will show the graphics view of the patient model in correct alignment with the real view of the patient.

Calibration and registration methods vary with different AR systems configuration. Sauer et al. [2000] and Vogt et al. [2006] describe the case of a video see-through system. Tuceryan and Navab [2000] present a calibration method for an optical see-through system.

4.3   System Examples and Applications

A relatively small number of groups have been active in developing AR systems for medical navigation. The credit for the first medical AR publication goes to Bajura et al. [1992], who describe the idea of overlaying live ultrasound images onto a live view of a patient using a head-mounted display.

In this section, we present an overview of the AR systems literature. This is not organized historically, but follows the design structure displayed in Fig. 4.3. The following survey describes examples of systems and applications that are based on optical microscopes (optical AR with optical axis), video-based technologies, large semitransparent screens (optical AR without optical axis), tomographic overlays as a special case of large-screen systems, and endoscopy (a special case of video based systems). We also briefly mention some methods that go beyond these AR approaches.

Applications targeted by AR systems include neurosurgery and otolaryngology, cranio- and maxillofacial surgery, breast and abdominal needle biopsies and tumor ablations, orthopedics, and cardiovascular and thoracic surgery.

After the examples in this section, we will list characteristic features of the different system types in Section 4.5 for an easier comparison.

4.3.1 Optical Microscope Systems

Operating microscopes are routinely used for many ENT and neuro-surgical procedures. AR image guidance can be achieved by overlaying precisely aligned 3D graphics derived from the patient's preoperative images onto the optical view of the microscope. Proof of principle and early phantom tests have been presented, for example, in Friets et al. [1989] and Edwards et al. [1995a,b].

4.3.1.1 Microscope (Optical System with Optical Axis);
External Mount

A prototype AR system, called *MAGI* (microscope-assisted guided interventions), has been developed at Guy's Hospital, London, England. It provides 3D AR visualization for microscope-assisted interventions in neurosurgery and otolaryngology [Edwards et al. 1999, 2000; King et al. 2000]. *MAGI* is based on a Leica binocular operating microscope. Medical image information derived from MRI or CT scans of the patient's head or neck is inserted into the optical paths of both eyepieces via two monochrome VGA (640 × 480) displays and beam-splitters. Figure 4.4 shows the system in use and the augmented view through one of the microscope's oculars.

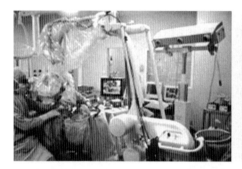 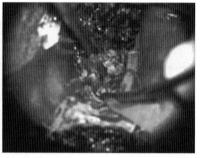

Fig. 4.4. *Left*: A device for microscope-assisted guided interventions (MAGI) developed at Guy's Hospital, London. *Right*: Augmented view through the microscope (pictures courtesy of Philip Edwards)

A set of infrared LEDs is attached to the microscope to mark its position, and then tracked by an optical tracking system (Optotrak, Northern Digital Inc., Waterloo, Ontario, Canada). For precise patient localization, the London group developed a locking, acrylic dental stent (LADS), which attaches to the patient's upper teeth, and contains LEDs for tracking with the Optotrak system. This LADS device replaces the standard surgical head clamp or bone implanted markers.

As has been shown in several clinical tests [Edwards et al. 1999], an operating microscope with AR image guidance can be used to perform difficult surgical interventions on both head and neck. For instance, the removal of a petrous apex cyst, where a more anterior approach was necessary to preserve hearing, was guided successfully using the MAGI device. The precision of the graphics overlay was reported to be better than 1 mm throughout the procedure.

4.3.1.2 Microscope (Optical System with Optical Axis); Head Mount

An approach similar to MAGI has been taken at the Allgemeines Krankenhaus Wien (AKH) Hospital in Vienna, Austria (intermittently the CARCAS Group at the University Hospital Basel, Switzerland), now using a head-mounted microscope instead of a free-standing, externally mounted micro-scope. The commercially available *Varioscope* is a head-mounted, lightweight operating binocular (Life Optics, Vienna) with autofocus, automatic parallax correction, and zoom. The group in Vienna has modified the *Varioscope* for stereoscopic AR visualization [Birkfellner et al. 2000a,b, 2002]. Clinical appli-cations of operating binoculars, which typically have a 3x–7x magnification, include oral and cranio-maxillofacial surgery, plastic and reconstructive surgery, and also orthopedics.

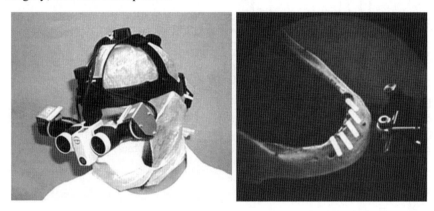

Fig. 4.5. *Left*: The Varioscope AR, a head-mounted operating microscope with AR visualization, developed at the AKH, Vienna, Austria. *Right*: Augmented view through one of the oculars, for the scenario of endosteal implant insertion (left picture Birkfellner et al. 2002, © 2002 IEEE; Pictures courtesy of Wolfgang Birkfellner)

Figure 4.5 shows pictures of the prototype device, also referred to as the *Varioscope AR*, and the augmented view through one of the oculars. The original *Varioscope* contains prisms for image rectification to correct for image inversion in both optical paths. In the *Varioscope AR*, these prisms are modified on one side with a thin semitransparent coating and act as beam combiners. Two miniature LCD displays with VGA (640 × 480) resolution provide the computer-generated virtual images, and these images and the optical images of the real scene are focused into a common focal plane, avoiding focal disparity in the AR view (Fig. 4.6).

Calibration of the *Varioscope AR* has to take into account the variable zoom, and the variable convergence of the two individual optical paths [Birkfellner et al. 2001; Figl et al. 2005]. The *Varioscope AR* was designed to work with existing CAS systems. To study this AR device, it was integrated into a surgical navigation system for cranio- and maxillofacial surgery, also developed at AKH Vienna. The navigation system was based on optical tracking, and the same optical tracking was used to also keep track of the head-mounted *Varioscope AR's* pose.

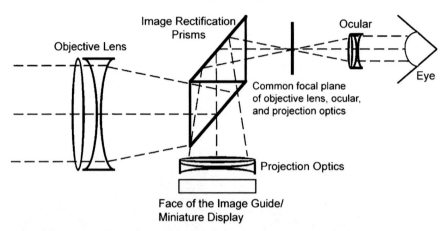

Fig. 4.6. The image rectification prisms of the Varioscope are used as beam combiners. Both the image from the real scene and the computer-generated image from the miniature display are focused into the same plane (picture Birkfellner et al. 2002, © 2002 IEEE; picture courtesy of Wolfgang Birkfellner)

4.3.2 Video AR Systems

Video-based AR systems capture the real view of a scene with video cameras and use a computer to augment it with virtual graphics. Head-mounted systems of this type are commonly called video see-through systems.

4.3.2.1 Video AR (Optical System with Optical Axis); Head Mount

AR for medicine was first proposed at the University of North Carolina (UNC), Chapel Hill, NC, USA, and its first implementation was in the form of a video see-through HMD system for ultrasound image guidance [Bajura et al. 1992; State et al. 1994]. The centerpiece of this system is a stereoscopic HMD, equipped with two miniature video cameras. The AR view is presented stereoscopically so the user has 3D perception based on stereo depth cues. Being able to change viewpoints, the user also experiences parallax depth cues, seeing objects in the foreground move faster than objects in the background. In this system, the HMD (and thereby the user's viewpoint) is tracked.

Early developments of the UNC system were targeted toward visualization of ultrasound images within a pregnant woman's womb (left image in Fig. 4.7). A 3D representation of the fetus could be seen in its actual location. Further research adapted this head-mounted video see-through approach for ultrasound-guided needle biopsies [Fuchs et al. 1996; Rosenthal et al. 2001, 2002; State et al. 2003, 1996].

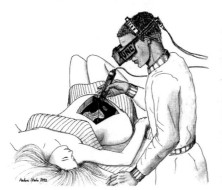 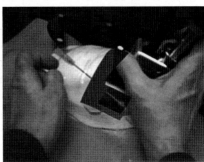

Fig. 4.7. UNC's approach for head-mounted video see-through augmented reality, which provides stereoscopic and parallax (kinesthetic) depth cues of the AR scene. *Left*: Schematic representation of AR fetus visualization. *Right*: AR view through the HMD during ultrasound-guided needle biopsies on breast phantom (right picture State et al. 1996, ©1996 ACM Inc., reprinted with permission; left artwork and right picture courtesy of Andrei State)

A version of UNC's AR system adapted for laparoscopic surgery is described in Fuchs et al. [1998]. As presented in Rosenthal et al. [2001], the UNC system uses optical tracking (FlashPoint 5000, Image Guided Technologies) of the HMD, ultrasound probe, and biopsy needle. The ultrasound image is visualized in its actual location within the patient. The AR view combines these ultrasound images with the video view of the patient, plus additional computer graphics, for example, a virtual object that identifies the location of a breast tumor (right image in Fig. 4.7). A randomized, controlled trial to compare standard ultrasound-guided needle biopsies to biopsies performed with UNC's AR prototype guidance system was used for evaluation of the system. Fifty biopsies of breast phantoms were performed by an interventional radiologist, and the method using AR visualization resulted in a significantly smaller mean deviation from the desired target compared with the standard ultrasound-guided method (1.62 mm for AR versus 2.48 mm for standard).

4.3.2.2 Video AR (Optical System with Optical Axis); Head Mount – Example 2

A stereoscopic video see-through AR system similar to the UNC system has been developed at Siemens Corporate Research in Princeton, NJ [Sauer et al. 2002c, 2000]. This system has been presented as the RAMP system, where RAMP stands for "Reality Augmentation for Medical Procedures."

An ergonomic difference between RAMP and the UNC system consists in the downward tilt of the camera pair mounted on the RAMP HMD. This camera tilt allows the user to assume a more upright, relaxed position when looking down at the workspace. Another difference lies in the tracking systems. Whereas the UNC system initially used the color cameras for tracking, which provided the real view of the scene, it was later equipped with a commercial tracking system for "outside-in" tracking. In contrast, the RAMP system was developed with a third camera on the HMD dedicated to inside-out tracking. This tracking camera is a black-and-white camera with a wide angle lens and is equipped with an infrared LED flash, placed as a ring around the lens. The tracking camera works in conjunction with retro-reflective optical markers that are framing a surgical workspace. Using this head-mounted tracker camera, the user cannot accidentally step in the way of the tracking system, making the typical line-of-sight restriction of optical tracking systems less limiting. Having the camera on the head also optimizes the perceived accuracy of the augmentation. Movements along the optical axis are tracked with a lower accuracy than transverse movements, but at the same time, a depth error of a virtual object's position is also less perceptible than a lateral error. In other words, when scene and tracker camera look in the same direction, the camera detects just what the user can see. What the camera cannot detect, the user cannot see either. The head-mounted tracking system was extended later beyond head-tracking to include also instrument tracking [Vogt et al. 2002]. As in the UNC system, the user's spatial perception is based on stereoscopic depth cues, and on parallax depth cues from viewpoint variations.

The three cameras are genlocked to each other, with the benefit that tracking information is available exactly for each frame that needs to be combined with computer graphics. This synchronization eliminates any time lag between the real and virtual components of the AR view. The Registration accuracy of the augmentation measured in object space is around 1 mm. The augmented images also appear stable, with no apparent jitter. Overall, there is a time latency of about 0.1 s between an actual event and its display. The RAMP system runs in real time at 30 frames per second and displays an augmented stereoscopic video view with XGA resolution for each eye. A new system design replaced the three networked SGI workstations of of the initial RAMP system with a single PC and improved the overall performance [Vogt et al. 2006, 2003].

Figure 4.8 shows the RAMP HMD and an augmented view in preparation of a neurosurgical procedure. The system has been put into a neurosurgical context [Maurer et al. 2001; Wendt et al. 2003], adapted to an interventional MRI operating room [Sauer et al. 2001a, 2002b], tested for CT- and MRI-guided needle placements on phantoms [Das et al. 2006; Khamene et al. 2003b; Sauer et al. 2002c, 2003] and pigs [Vogt et al. 2004b; Wacker et al. 2006], integrated with an ultrasound scanner [Khamene et al. 2003a; Sauer et al. 2001b, 2002a], and transformed into a 3D medical data exploration tool [Vogt et al. 2004a].

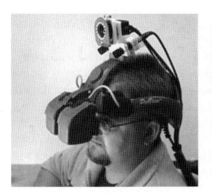 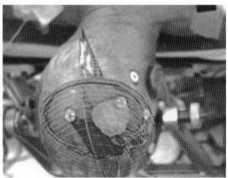

Fig. 4.8. RAMP system developed by Siemens Corporate Research Inc. *Left*: Stereoscopic video see-through HMD for interventional AR visualization with a dedicated third camera for tracking. *Right*: Augmented view of patient's head before neurosurgery (left figure is from Khamene et al. 2003b, with kind permission from Springer Science and Business Media)

At the Technische Universität of Munich, the RAMP system has been adapted to new applications [Heining et al. 2006; Sielhorst et al. 2004a,b], such as a birth simulator, where AR visualization may increase the efficiency of the training and provide support during a difficult procedure such as a forceps delivery.

4.3.3 Large Screens

A category of AR system uses large, stationary screens for display of the AR view. Opaque displays are used for video AR systems and semitransparent screens are required for optical AR systems.

4.3.3.1   Large-Screen Video AR (Optical System with Optical Axis); External Mount, Monoscopic

A large-screen video AR system was developed at the MIT AI Lab for the purpose of image-guided neurosurgery, and studied in close collaboration with the Surgical Planning Laboratory at Brigham & Women's Hospital, Boston, MA [Grimson et al. 1995, 1998, 1999].

In this system, a video camera placed close to the surgical scene provides the live video images of the patient. The patient's head, as well as the surgical instruments, are tracked by an optical tracking system (Flashpoint, Image Guided Technologies Inc.), for which LEDs are attached to the neurosurgical head clamp and the surgical instruments. To register the medical information from the MRI scan to the actual patient position in the head clamp, 3D surface points of the patient's scalp are collected with a laser scanner or a tracked pointer. The collected points are registered with the skin surface, which is extracted from the patient's MRI scan [Grimson et al. 1994, 1996]. During the interventional procedure, these registration parameters are used to align medical images from the MRI scan with the video image of the patient's head. The augmented video image on the monitor screen displays the patient in a transparent fashion, with internal anatomical structures from the MRI dataset overlaid on the video of the head. A tracked pointer is also visualized in this augmented view. Besides the augmented view, the system can display three orthogonal MRI slices in separate windows, selected with the tracked pointer as in traditional navigation systems. Figure 4.9 shows a neurosurgical intervention with the AR monitor screen above the surgical site and an example image of an argumented view of the patient. The AR system is set up in an interventional GE SP/i MR scanner (General Electric Medical Systems, WI).

Grimson and his colleagues [1998] at Brigham and Women's Hospital report that this AR image guidance system for neurosurgery has been used on 70 patients. It effectively supported the surgery in planning the craniotomy, identifying margins of tumor, and localizing key blood vessels. A wide range of neurosurgical cases were selected to evaluate the efficiency of the system, including tumor resection, pediatric epilepsy, meningioma, and biopsy cases. Limitations of the system are its fixed viewpoint, which does not coincide with the surgeon's direct viewpoint, and its monoscopic function, which does not provide 3D perception.

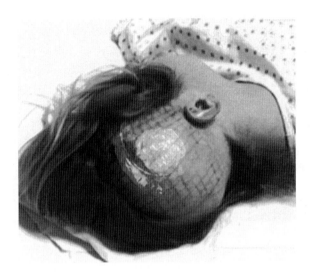

Fig. 4.9. Monitor-based video AR system for image-guided neurosurgery. Patient's head augmented with internal structures, which were extracted from an MRI scan (picture Grimson et al. 1996, © 1996 IEEE; Picture courtesy of W. Eric L. Grimson)

4.3.3.2 Large-Screen Optical AR (No Optical Axis); External Mount, Monoscopic/Stereoscopic

At the Carnegie Mellon University (CMU) Robotics Institute, Pittsburgh, PA, the MRCAS group (Medical Robotics and Computer Assisted Surgery) developed an image overlay system based on a semitransparent mirror placed above the surgical workplace [Blackwell et al. 1998a,b, 2000]. A high-resolution flat LCD panel is mounted above the half-silvered mirror, which acts as a beam combiner. The physician looks through this screen at the patient and simultaneously sees the reflection of the LCD display. This configuration creates the illusion of perceiving the virtual image below the screen inside the surgical workplace. Display and mirror are jointly attached to an articulated arm. An optical tracking system (OptoTrak, Northern Digital, Waterloo, Ontario, Canada) tracks patient, display/monitor setup, and the user by means of attached LEDs. Figure 4.10 illustrates the concept and its realization as a prototype system.

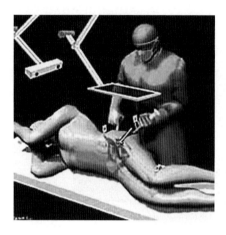 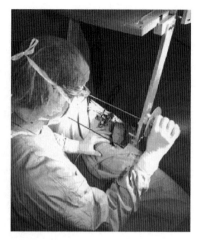

Fig. 4.10. Large-screen image overlay system for interventional image guidance or surgical education, developed at CMU's Robotics Institute. *Left*: Illustration of the concept. *Right*: Prototype system in use (pictures courtesy of the Carnegie Mellon Robotics Institute)

Potential applications include orthopedic surgery, neurosurgical procedures, and surgical education [Blackwell et al. 1998b]. Blackwell et al. [1995] describe an earlier prototype system from CMU based on a CRT monitor, which provided proof of concept of the monitor/mirror approach. It was the CRT monitor that made stereoscopic visualization possible. To create 3D perception, shutter glasses were used, with the monitor rendering a different view for each eye synchronized to the shutter glasses. In this way, the system provided stereoscopic depth cues for the virtual scene. As the real scene was observed directly through the semitransparent mirror, it appeared naturally in three dimension anyway.

4.3.3.3 Large-Screen Optical AR (No Optical Axis); External Mount, Stereoscopic – Example 2

Figure 4.11 shows another AR system that follows the transparent screen approach [Goebbels et al. 2003].

The *ARSyS-Tricorder* has been developed in Germany by multiple institutions in collaboration with the Fraunhofer-Gesellschaft, and utilizes a setup with a stereoscopic projector instead of a monitor to display the virtual graphics. The graphics appear on a polarization preserving projection screen, and are reflected to the eyes of the user by a half-transparent mirror.

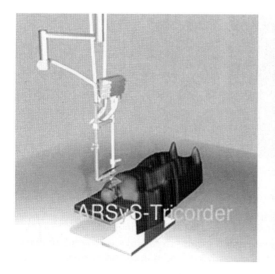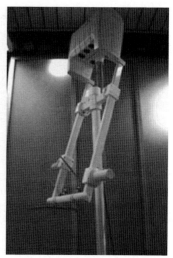

Fig. 4.11. ARSyS-Tricorder – AR system with projection system and semi-transparent mirror. *Left*: Illustration of the concept. *Right*: ARSyS-Tricorder prototype system (pictures © Fraunhofer Institut Intelligente Analyse- und Informations-syteme (IAIS), Sankt Augustin, Germany)

The user wears polarized glasses, which allow him to perceive the virtual images in stereo through the mirror. User, patient, and the combination of projector, projection screen, and mirror must be tracked for proper registration between the real view of the patient and the overlaid virtual medical graphics.

4.3.3.4 Large-Screen Video AR (Optical System with Optical Axis); External Mount, Monoscopic – More Examples

Lorensen et al. [1993, 1994] described an early prototype of a monitor-based video AR system for neurosurgical procedures. There still is current interest in the concept of a single stationary monitor displaying an augmented video view of the patient.

Hayashibe et al. [2005] describe a prototype system, which has been developed at Jikei University School of Medicine in Tokyo, Japan. Intra-operatively acquired volumetric images from a mobile C-arm x-ray system are used to overlay the patient's internal anatomy onto the camera view of the patient in the operating room (left image of Fig. 4.12).

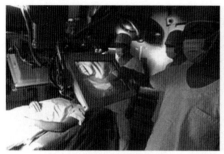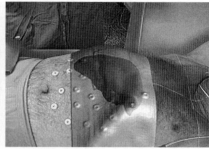

Fig. 4.12. *Left*: An AR system that combines a video view of the patient with intraoperatively acquired scans of a mobile X-ray C-arm, developed at Jikei University School of Medicine, Tokyo, Japan. *Right*: Augmented reality guidance for liver punctures with a prototype of a screen-based video AR system developed at IRCAD University Hospital, Strasbourg, France (left picture from Hayashibe et al. 2005 and right picture from Nicolau et al. 2005a, with kind permission of Springer Science and Business Media)

A screen-based video AR system to guide liver punctures for radio-frequency tumor treatment is being developed at IRCAD University Hospital, Strasbourg, France, in collaboration with INRIA Sophia-Antipolis, France [Nicolau et al. 2005a]. As the right side of Figure 4.12 shows, a larger number of skin markers are used for patient to image registration. In a stationary abdominal phantom, the system achieves a target precision of 3 mm. The first *in vivo* experiments have been presented in Nicolau et al. [2005b]. The common problem of respiratory motion for interventional guidance of abdominal procedures remains, and currently restricts the application of this system to larger targets with a diameter above 3 cm.

A unique AR video system has been reported in Mitschke et al. [2000] and Navab et al. [1999]. The CAMC system, short for Computer Augmented Mobile C-arm, attaches a video camera next to the x-ray source in a mobile C-arm, and by means of two mirrors aligns viewpoint and optical axis of the video camera to those of the x-ray system (Fig. 4.13). The result is a "dual energy imaging system"; both x-ray and video camera images of the patient are taken from the same viewpoint, but with different energy spectra. The video image shows the surface of the patient's body and objects located in front of it, while the x-ray image shows the inside of the body. The whole system is calibrated so that x-ray and video images can be overlaid in a registered way.

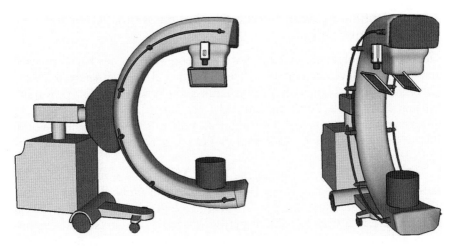

Fig. 4.13. Schematic drawing of CAMC. A mobile C-arm is equipped with a video camera and a double mirror system, aligning the video view with the X-ray view (pictures courtesy of Joerg Traub)

One application for CAMC is to guide needle placement during biopsies, as the x-ray image helps to identify an internal target. The initial alignment of the needle (outside of the patient) can then be performed under AR guidance without the need for additional x-ray radiation. The video image shows the external needle, which needs to be aimed at the target, and the overlaid x-ray image shows the location of the internal target.

4.3.4 Tomographic Overlays

Tomographic overlays are a special case of screen-based optical AR systems. Again, the user looks through a semitransparent mirror and sees the reflection of a monitor overlaid onto the view of the real scene. The feature of tomographic overlays is that, independent of the user's viewpoint, the mirror image of the monitor appears in a fixed position within the real scene. The physical monitor is just an object in the real environment, and the location of its mirror image depends only on the position of the mirror, not on the viewer. While the planar image on the monitor limits the AR view to the overlay of flat 2D virtual images, proper positioning of monitor and mirror and appropriate system calibration ensure that the 2D virtual image appears in the correct position with the appropriate scale within the 3D AR scene. This simple concept enables the augmented scene to be properly appreciated by multiple untracked observers, without the requirement of special eyewear.

4.3.4.1 Optical AR with Screen (No Optical Axis), 2D Virtual Images Only

The use of tomographic overlays for ultrasound imaging has been proposed and is being developed at the Visualization and Image Analysis (VIA) Laboratory at the University of Pittsburgh and Carnegie Mellon University [Stetten et al. 2000, 2001; Stetten and Chib 2001b]. Real-time ultrasound images appear in the actual position of the patient's anatomy, and the term *Real Time Tomographic Reflection (RTTR)* has been introduced for this approach.

Figure 4.14 shows a prototype of the VIA Lab's *sonic flashlight*. A flat-panel display attached to a B-mode ultrasound probe displays the live ultrasound image. This image is reflected in a half-silvered mirror, attached to the probe in a way that the displayed image of the ultrasound scan appears at the actual scan location. It provides the AR view with the correctly positioned 2D ultrasound image without the need of a tracking device. Figure 4.15 illustrates this principle.

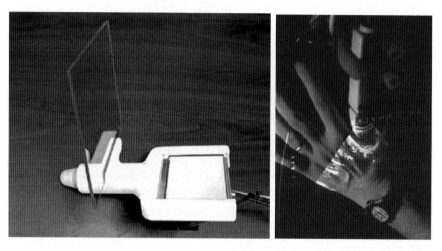

Fig. 4.14. A prototype of the *sonic flashlight*, developed at VIA Lab, Pittsburgh, PA. *Left*: A small flat-panel monitor is attached to the handle of an ultrasound probe. A half-silvered mirror bisects the angle between ultrasound plane and display. *Right*: Example of a tomographic overlay with the sonic flashlight (pictures courtesy of George Stetten)

Subsequent research has adapted this concept to develop magnified real-time reflection of ultrasound for remote procedures [Stetten and Chib 2001a], a C-mode sonic flashlight for a matrix array ultrasound probe [Stetten

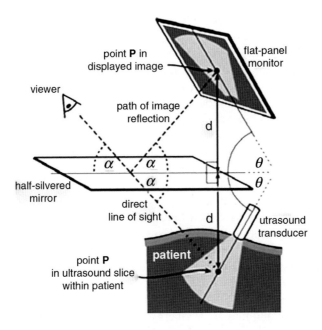

Fig. 4.15. The principle of real-time tomographic overlay as implemented in the sonic flashlight. Due to the geometric relation among half-silvered mirror, flat-panel display, and ultrasound transducer, each point in the virtual ultrasound image is precisely located at its corresponding physical 3D location (picture courtesy of George Stetten)

et al. 2003, 2005], and integrated the sonic flashlight with a laser guide for needle procedures [Wang et al. 2005]. Chang et al. [2005a] describe how the sonic flashlight was used for a cadaver study in a neurosurgical context, where the users localized a brain lesion with a needle, supported by ultrasound guidance. Compared to conventional ultrasound guidance, where the ultrasound image appears on a separate screen apart from the ultrasound probe and the patient, they reported that the sonic flashlight improved hand–eye coordination and helped to place the needle easily and intuitively into the lesion. Chang et al. [2005b, 2006] report on the successful use of the sonic flashlight for catheter placement.

4.3.4.2 Optical AR with Screen (No Optical Axis), 2D Virtual Images Only; External Mount – Example 2

The tomographic overlay concept, where no tracking is needed and which has been realized for ultrasound in the form of the sonic flashlight, can be adapted to other imaging modalities. At the CISST Lab at Johns Hopkins University, in collaboration with Tokyo Denki University, a prototype system has been developed to support percutaneous therapy performed inside a CT scanner [Fichtinger et al. 2005a,b, 2004; Masamune et al. 2002].

The overlay system comprises a flat-panel LCD display and a half-silvered mirror, attached to the gantry of a CT scanner.

Figure 4.16 shows the system on the left side. This prototype system has been evaluated for needle placements in phantoms and cadavers, guided by the tomographic overlay of CT slices in the scanner. Skeletal targets could be reached with one insertion attempt, and liver targets could be assessed successfully, although tissue deformations posed some challenges. By providing accurate and intuitive image guidance, the system can improve the learning curve for physicians in training, and help reduce the procedure time and x-ray dose for CT-guided needle procedures.

The right side of Fig. 4.16 shows a similar approach to AR from the same group at the CISST Lab at Johns Hopkins University, to guide needle placement procedures on a closed bore MRI scanner [Fischer et al. 2006, 2007]. A target application is MR arthrography (MRAr), where a needle is driven under fluoroscopy or CT guidance into a joint, and a diagnostic assessment is made based on MRI images of the contrast-injected joint. Preclinical trials of the proposed AR-guided procedure on the MRI scanner bed resulted in repeatedly successful first-attempt needle placements into the joint of porcine and human cadavers and show the system's potential to effectively support and simplify the overall arthrography procedure by eliminating radiographic guidance during contrast injection.

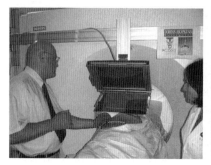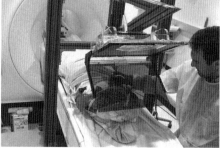

Fig. 4.16. Tomographic overlay systems for percutaneous therapy inside a CT or MRI scanner developed at CISST Lab at Johns Hopkins University. *Left*: The prototype system with monitor and half-silvered mirror attached to the CT gantry during a cadaver needle placement experiment. All observers see the 2D cross-sectional CT image in the same correct position. A marker is attached to the needle, indicating the length of the needle that has to be inserted to reach the target at the correct depth. Otherwise, the needle is not being tracked, and its actual position inside the patient can only be assessed with a CT control scan. *Right*: The overlay system constructed around an MRI scanner bed guiding a needle placement procedure (pictures courtesy of Gabor Fichtinger and Gregory Fischer)

4.3.4.3 Optical AR with Screen (No Optical Axis), Tomographic Overlay for 3D

The concept of the tomographic overlay is limited to the overlay of 2D images because of practical reasons. We display a 2D image as a light distribution on a 2D monitor, and perceive it consistently at the monitor's position in space. If we had true 3D monitors giving a consistent image of a 3D object independent of our viewpoint, we could as well employ a semi-transparent mirror and perceive the reflection of this 3D virtual object as part of the 3D real scene. Unfortunately, a stereo display does not produce a true 3D image. When the user moves the head to the side, the 3D image moves along and does not stay in a fixed position in space as would a real object.

Masamune et al. [2000] present a mirror-based AR system where the 3D display is implemented as a flat 2D display screen scanning through a volume, building up the 3D image slice by slice. Accordingly, the display system is called the "slice-display." A similar 3D display with a rotating screen is commercially available from the company Actuality Systems (Bedford, MA). Currently, such a 3D display system is still expensive and has limited resolution and contrast.

An earlier approach to augment a neurosurgical site with 3D images was based on integral photography [Iseki et al. 1997; Masutani et al. 1995, 1996]. Integral photography is a 3D imaging method that uses a lenslet array to record and display an object from a range of viewpoints within a given viewing angle. Integral photography images of three-dimensional medical data were recorded on film, which took several hours. During surgery, those integral photographs were superimposed on the patient with a half-silvered mirror. Since this *Volumegraph* does not involve computer screens, but uses conventional film, the image could not be altered during the surgery.

At the University of Tokyo, researchers introduced integral videography (IV) for medical AR, replacing the film in the Volumegraph with one or more high-resolution LCD displays [Liao et al. 2001, 2004, 2006; Nakajima et al. 2000]. Figure 4.17 illustrates the principle and shows a prototype system.

An optical tracking system (Polaris, Northern Digital Inc.) keeps track of the positions of surgical instruments and patient. Both models of the surgical instruments and the 3D patient data are overlaid as IV images during the surgery. The first phantom experiments showed that needle placement procedures could be guided with this system, with a mean error below 3 mm [Liao et al. 2004]. The pixel density of the display and the lens pitch are the main factors for the quality of the IV image. The virtual scene has to be rendered and displayed simultaneously for all the different viewpoints within the viewing range. This not only requires a very high display resolution to spatially multiplex all the different views, but also a correspondingly high processing power to render all the images. Approaches to build higher-resolution IV displays are being investigated and described in Liao et al. [2002].

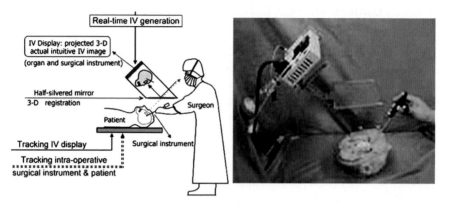

Fig. 4.17. Surgical navigation by integral videography image overlay, developed at the University of Tokyo. *Left*: Illustration of the concept, where the surgeon perceives 3D image overlay without the need for stereo glasses. *Right*: Prototype system (picture Liao et al. 2004, © 2002 IEEE)

4.3.5 Video Endoscope Systems

Endoscopes and laparoscopes are viewing instruments for minimally invasive surgery. They are equipped with video cameras and acquire "real" images from within cavities in the patient. These video views can also be augmented with corresponding medical images. Although the video view can only show outer surfaces, the medical images add information on anatomical structures that lie behind the surfaces.

The system described in Shahidi et al. [1998], developed at the Image Guidance Laboratory at Stanford University (Palo Alto, CA), tracks an endoscope with an optical tracking system and presents a side-by-side display of the endoscopic video view and a corresponding virtual endoscopic view, generated by volume rendering of preoperatively acquired CT or MR data. The virtual endoscope can make opaque tissue transparent and give the surgeon a look beyond the visible surface captured by the real endoscope. Both images, from surgical and virtual endoscopes, can be blended together to show an AR view on the monitor.

A similar approach has been described in De Buck et al. [2001] for laparoscopic procedures. A laparoscope is a rigid endoscope for procedures in the abdomen. The prototype system overlays the video images from the laparoscope with virtual graphics extracted from preoperative CT scans. An optical tracking system keeps track of the laparoscope's position with respect to the patient. One potential application is the visualization of the ureter as a virtual object in the laparoscopic view of the pelvis. Locating the ureter is a common challenge in laparoscopic surgery.

The augmented visualization of endoscopic images during robot-assisted coronary artery bypass graft (CABG) surgery is described in Coste-Maniere et al. [2004] and Mourgues et al. [2001, 2003]. The ChIR Medical Robotics Group at INRIA developed the system on the *da Vinci* platform (Intuitive Surgical Inc., Sunnyvale, CA) and tested it in animal trials. Figure 4.18 shows the setup and an AR visualization of the coronary tree. A model of the coronary tree, extracted from preoperative angiograms and CT data, is overlaid on the endoscopic images for extra guidance during the minimally invasive procedure. Registration of the real images and computer models poses a particular challenge for the beating heart. An initial registration is based on skin markers, and an interactive method during the procedure allows the surgeon to correct the overlay in real time. The system's evaluation on a dog and a sheep model showed its effectiveness in helping the surgeon localize target structures during the robot-assisted CABG procedure. In addition, Traub et al. [2004] report on the use of AR visualization in robot-assisted minimally invasive cardiovascular surgery.

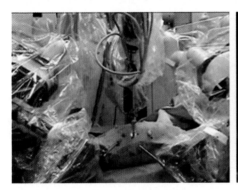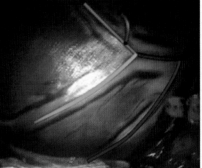

Fig. 4.18. Method for augmentation of endoscopic images during robot-assisted coronary artery bypass graft surgery with the *da Vinci* system, developed at INRIA. *Left*: Setup of the da Vinci system for an animal study of the proposed method. *Right*: Overlay of the coronary tree model on an endoscopic image of the da Vinci system (pictures reproduced with permission from Coste-Maniere et al. 2004, © 2004, by permission of SAGE Publications Ltd)

Endoscopy plays an important role in the further development of minimally invasive techniques. The combination with 3D medical imaging can not only extend the endoscopic view beyond the surface, but can also provide a global context for the local endoscopic views. AR visualization is just one possibility for displaying the combined information. Dey et al. [2000] describe a method of extracting surface shapes from preoperative images and mapping endoscopic images onto these 3D shapes.

4.3.6 Other Methods: Direct Projection

Graphical information can be directly projected onto the patient, also augmenting the physician's view. For practical reasons, the direct projection approach is limited to simple 2D graphics that appear on the skin surface: points, lines, and outlines. The patient is usually draped around the surgical site and does not provide a good projection screen. As a projected image moves and gets distorted when location and shape of the screen change, precise measurement of location and shape of the skin surface is necessary to make the guiding graphics appear correctly registered to the patient.

Glossop et al. [2003] describe a system with infrared and visible lasers. The infrared lasers assist with the registration, and the visible lasers project graphics guides onto the patient's skin, such as an entry point or a surgical plan [Marmurek et al. 2006].

A similar approach has been described by Hoppe et al. [2002, 2003] and Worn and Hoppe [2001]. Here a video projector projects the surgical plan onto the patient. For registration, the surface shape is measured using structured light and two video cameras that evaluate the projected patterns on the patient.

4.4   System Features Overview

The different types of systems have unique characteristics. In this section, we are listing the important features of the standard systems in bullet point format for a comparative overview.

4.4.1 Microscope Systems

1. They exhibit excellent quality of the optical images. To preserve the brightness of the optical image, one usually uses an interferometric beam combiner to inject the virtual image into the optical path. This limits the electronic display to be monochromatic.
2. By injecting the graphics into an intermediate focal plane of the optical system, focal disparity can be avoided – the user can see real image and virtual graphics in the same focal plane.
3. The system can be equipped with a beamsplitter to acquire video images of the AR view so that the camera sees the same image as the user. The resulting hybrid system shares important characteristics of a video AR system. The AR view can be displayed live for additional observers, or can be recorded for documentation. Furthermore, system calibration (see Section 4.4.5) can be performed in a user-independent way by processing the video images in the computer.

4. If a microscope is already a standard tool for a procedure, AR can be introduced in a very evolutionary and unobtrusive way. Physicians can continue to work as usual, and can consult AR visualization optionally without the need for extra equipment.

4.4.2 Video AR HMD Systems

1. Video AR systems can be readily equipped with good displays. This leads to very good quality virtual images (whereas the quality of the real images may be compromised by the intermediate video process).
2. Real and virtual images are blended electronically, which allows an optimal control of the resulting AR view. For example, one can reduce disturbing highlights in the real image, or adapt the brightness and contrast of the virtual image to the brightness of the real image for improved visibility.
3. The AR view is available in electronic form and can be stored for documentation. It can also be shared in real time with a larger audience.
4. As the AR view is available in electronic format, registration between real and virtual images can be calibrated in an "objective" (user-independent) manner. In addition, the registration accuracy can be monitored online.

4.4.3 Semitransparent Screens

1. Calibration is subjective as only the user can see the AR view, resulting in a user-dependent calibration procedure of limited accuracy.
2. For correct perception of the virtual scene, the user must assume a well-defined eye position with respect to both the display screen and the patient anatomy. This makes tracking more challenging compared to the systems discussed above and below, since the introduction of three independent coordinate systems, namely the user (viewpoint), the patient, and the screen, introduces more errors.

   In contrast, for microscope-based systems, the user does not have the freedom to assume an arbitrary viewpoint, as a well-defined eye-position is given by the exit pupil of the microscope – so the user does not have to be tracked. For video-based AR systems, the location of the electronic display does not influence the registration and need not be tracked. The position of the user's eyes relative to the display does not matter either; only the cameras need to be tracked, as they provide the real images in relation to the patient.
3. Stereo visualization is required not only to perceive the virtual graphics at the appropriate depth, but also to provide correct alignment of the

virtual features to the real scene. A practical implementation of stereo imaging requires that the user to wear glasses that separate the left and right eye images, for example, shutter glasses to separate temporally multiplexed stereo images.

4. Screen and patient are not in the same plane. The user needs to focus on virtual and real images separately, which diminishes the AR experience.

5. Sterility of the semitransparent screen is an issue that needs to be considered for practical surgical applications.

4.4.4 Tomographic Displays

1. Tomographic displays provide AR visualization without the need to track the user, who can still move and change viewpoints. This makes this concept simple and robust.

2. In practice, virtual images are limited to two dimensions. With a true 3D display – not just stereo – 3D imaging would be possible. But there are, at least currently, no practical solutions for a suitable 3D display.

4.4.5 Optical See-Through HMD Systems

1. Optical see-through HMD systems without an optical axis have not been discussed in this chapter, as they are basically unsuitable for medical AR applications (which require precise registration between real and virtual images according to our understanding of medical AR). However, the comparison of optical versus video see-through systems has been a topic of discussion, so we list some of the arguments here.

2. Calibration of the registration can only be performed by the user, subjectively aligning virtual and real structures. The accuracy of such a subjective calibration method is limited.

3. The registration between the real and the virtual images depends critically on the position of the user's eyes behind the small screen. Movement of the head-mounted display on the user's head can result in large registration errors, which can go unnoticed by the user and are not detectable by external means. This is a big safety concern in the context of medical image guidance.

4. Furthermore, as a head-mounted display cannot be put onto the user's head in a precisely reproducible position, the calibration process has to be repeated each time it is put on.

4.5   Technical Challenges and Fundamental Comparisons

For practical applications, there should be three basic requirements to perform meaningful comparisons: right place, right time, and right way.

4.5.1 Right Place: Calibration

Medical AR requires that the real images and the virtual images are spatially well registered. For this, the AR system needs to be calibrated before use, and objective calibration is necessary to achieve precise, user-independent results. For objective calibration, video images of a real scene are acquired and brought into correspondence with a corresponding virtual model. This is straightforward with video AR systems, as video images are readily available. Sauer et al. [2000] and Vogt et al. [2006] describe this calibration process in more detail. For optical AR systems that have an optical system with optical axis, a camera can be inserted instead of the user's eye, and objective calibration can be performed. A major drawback of the screen-based systems, where the user's eye position is variable, is that only the users can calibrate the system for their own use. This subjective calibration [Tuceryan and Navab 2000] provides results that are less precise than that in the case of objective, completely computer-based user independent calibration.

4.5.2 Right Time: Synchronization

We also need the correct registration to persist when movement is present. When the user moves and changes his viewpoint or moves an instrument, the image update in the real view and the virtual view should be synchronized. At any given time, the objects in the real view and in the virtual view should be correctly aligned.

It is in the nature of optical AR systems that the real view appears instantaneously. The information in the virtual view, however, is necessarily delayed because of the finite speed of tracking and rendering. This results in an unavoidable time lag between real and virtual images.

Video AR systems exhibit a delay for both real and virtual images. The real images are recorded by a video camera, transferred to the computer, and rendered in combination with the virtual images. This process takes the time of about 2–3 video frames or 60–90 ms. With proper synchronization of video acquisition and tracking, one can eliminate any time lag between real and virtual images and create a consistently correct AR view, but of course, at the price of an unavoidable overall delay [Sauer et al. 2000].

4.5.3 Right Way: Visualization and Perception

We need to show accurate information in the AR view, and we need to visualize it in the right way to achieve optimal perception. Even if real and virtual images are combined in correct alignment, the user does not necessarily *perceive* their correct spatial relationship.

The virtual view cannot provide all the depth cues that we experience in the real world. If a direct optical view is substituted with a video view, in place of the real view, we lose further depth cues. With the video view, we are limited to stereoscopic depth cues (if we have a stereoscopic AR system), parallax cues (if we wear a head-mounted display or can vary our viewpoint behind a large screen), and sharpness cues. The sharpness depth cue leads already to a perception mismatch between the real and virtual views. The real view has always a limited depth of focus; real objects too close to the user, or too far away are out of focus and appear blurred. In contrast, a practical rendering of the virtual view is sharp throughout and does not include a depth-dependent defocusing. This mismatch contributes to the difficulty of perceiving the correct spatial relationship between real and virtual views.

More important in this respect, however, is the issue of occlusion. When real and virtual objects are overlapping in a way that does not reflect their correct spatial relationship, depth perception becomes more difficult. We know the viewer's viewpoint and can make the graphics objects appear at the desired 3D locations. However, correct interaction between real and graphics objects would require 3D information about the real objects as well. Is a real object in the scene in front of or behind the location of an overlapping virtual object? This 3D information is usually not available; the graphics objects are simply superimposed onto the 2D images of the real scene. In this way, real objects can be hidden by virtual objects, but not vice versa. However, closer objects are not supposed to occlude objects that are farther away, which is the well-known occlusion problem in AR. Wrong occlusion triggers conflicting depth cues: if stereo depth cues suggest that a virtual object is farther away than a real object, but at the same time the virtual object occludes the real object, the brain's depth perception is confused. The brain may still accept a transparent patient (Fig. 4.19), but will not process the transparent physician scenario properly.

For correct occlusion, one needs to obtain 3D information of the real scene. Sauer et al. [2001a] report, however, that one can reduce the disturbing effect of wrong occlusion cues significantly with appropriate rendering of the graphics; showing segmented structures not as solids

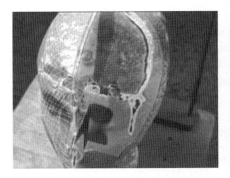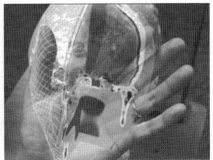

Fig. 4.19. AR view of head phantom. *Left*: Transparent patient. *Right*: Transparent physician (left figure is from Vogt et al. 2002, © 2001 IEEE)

but as wire frames; not with thick lines but with thin lines; not opaque but semi-transparent. The overall guideline is to show only the relevant structures in a sparse representation, avoiding occlusion as much as possible. This approach is very much in line with regarding the virtual images as maps, as relevant information abstracted from the original medical images that contain irrelevant details.

Another approach is to avoid the occlusion problem altogether by making all the relevant information available in the virtual images. This requires tracking of the surgical instruments in the same way as for standard navigation systems. Sauer et al. [2002b] describe an experiment in which a neurosurgeon used an elongated surgical tool called a rongeur, the position of which was not tracked, to extract hidden targets from a phantom. As long as the targets were only 2–3 cm below the surface, the neurosurgeon was successful in locating them with his rongeur, based on an AR view with a real view of the instrument only. For very deep-lying targets, however, the AR view did not sufficiently support the minimally invasive approach. The main reason, of course, was that the surgeon lost sight of the instrument tip once it was inserted into the phantom, and could not accurately extrapolate its location from the external part of the instrument. He could see the location of the target, but not the location of the instrument. The same paper describes another experiment, where a tracked needle was used to locate deep-lying targets in a similar phantom. The AR view now included a virtual model of the instrument, and the task became very easy as the surgeon could consistently and accurately see the spatial relationship of instrument and target throughout the procedure.

Not only is instrument tracking necessary to visualize a hidden instrument, it also helps to get around the AR occlusion problem. As both target and instrument locations are known in three dimension, they can be visualized and perceived with correct occlusion in the virtual scene. The real part of the AR view becomes less important and mainly serves to keep the surgeon connected to the patient and observe complications. This visualization moves more toward an augmented virtuality scenario, where the virtual scene essentially contains all the important information. Video-based AR systems are a good option here, as one can easily introduce excellent color graphics with them, and a potentially lower-quality video image is of lesser importance.

4.6   Concluding Remarks and Outlook

We have described medical AR as a form of advanced surgical image guidance. It enables physicians to look beyond the surface of the patient, and see anatomy and instruments that would otherwise be hidden from direct view. Standard image guidance systems provide essentially the same information, but removed from the patient. AR visualization includes this patient context and allows the physician to focus on the surgical site where all supporting information now become available. Hand–eye coordination becomes more straightforward, and understanding of the 3D topology becomes easier. However, AR comes at the price of added calibration and tracking complexity.

An important question is whether AR also provides a corresponding increase in clinical value. There is, of course, no general answer. It depends on the particular surgical or interventional procedure. At the current time, even though there are a variety of commercial surgical navigation systems on the market, none of them has an AR visualization option. The question about the actual clinical value of medical AR is still an open and important question.

To advance AR in general, two areas in particular will require more attention. AR perception studies [Johnson et al. 2002; Lerotic et al. 2007] will help to better understand how to fuse real and virtual images in an optimal way so that they register correctly in the user's brain. AR usability studies will help to better understand the potential user benefits of AR visualization in comparison to other visualization approaches. For medical AR, however, one needs to build medical AR prototypes and evaluate them in collaboration with clinicians to ultimately answer the question about its value as a clinical tool.

Building a basic AR system has become relatively easy. Hardware components, and in particular tracking systems, are available off the shelf. Computers have reached a performance level that makes real-time AR visualization possible in a straightforward way. Software modules for a variety of AR-related functions can be downloaded for reuse from the Internet, notably from the AR-toolkit [Billinghurst and Kato 1999; HITLab 2007] and ARTag [Fiala 2004]. In addition, the literature listed in this chapter's bibliography contains many of the technical details on how to design and test AR systems.

On the other hand, simply building a basic AR system is unlikely to make an impact on the field of medical AR. For clinical evaluation, a well-engineered system, not only with accurate and robust tracking, good display, and convincing visualization is required, but, importantly, one that also fits into the clinical environment, supports a smooth data transfer, and provides an efficient workflow. Anybody interested in medical AR research should be aware of this hurdle: it may be easy to get started, but it is a substantial effort to develop a clinically meaningful AR system. Evaluation of a prototype system will be an evaluation of the AR concept as much as an evaluation of the particular implementation. Without a convincing implementation, the clinician may develop a negative bias toward the whole AR concept, or at least quickly lose interest in further tests.

To make medical AR successful, one needs to pick the right applications (and let clinical requirements determine the design choices). If the clinical task is too simple, AR guidance may just be unnecessary. If the clinical task is truly challenging, the physician can appreciate the support of the AR system. Then the AR system needs also to provide value beyond that of a standard image guidance system. Our main expectation is that AR can be shown to be the more ergonomic tool and permit an easier, more efficient workflow.

AR is in fact entering clinical practice unobtrusively. The company, Carl Zeiss Inc. (Thornwood, NY) offers a surgical microscope MultiVision™, with image overlay [http://www.meditec.zeiss.com]. Here the physicians do not need to be introduced to new equipment, but they receive increased functionality and value from existing tools. Other types of medical AR will follow, driven by prior demonstration of their clinical value. Endoscopy-based AR systems also may not require a change in instrumentation for the user, and conventional navigation systems could easily be equipped with AR as a high-end visualization option. There are no real technical barriers to build practical medical AR systems. The bottleneck is primarily the current lack of a market driver, and the amount of effort and resources required to develop and prove a practical medical AR system. Ultimately, medical AR promises practical, easy-to-use tools, with applications not only in interventional image guidance, but also in training and education [Sielhorst et al. 2004a]. The field is sufficiently exciting that it should continue, turning the promises into real systems.

References

Bajura M, Fuchs H, and Ohbuchi R. (1992). "Merging virtual objects with the real world: Seeing ultrasound imagery within the patient." *Comput Graph*, 26(2), 203–210.

Billinghurst M, and Kato H. (1999). "Collaborative Mixed Reality." *Proceedings of International Symposium on Mixed Reality (ISMR '99). Mixed Reality – Merging Real and Virtual Worlds*, 261–284.

Birkfellner W, Figl M, Huber K, Hummel J, Hanel RA, Homolka P, Watzinger F, Wanschitz F, Ewars R, and Bergmann H. (2001). "Calibration of projection parameters in the varioscope AR, a headmounted display for augmented-reality visualization in image-guided therapy." *Proceedings of SPIE's Conference of Medical Imaging 2001: Visualization, Display, and Image-Guided Procedures*, 471–480.

Birkfellner W, Figl M, Huber K, Watzinger F, Wanschitz F, Hanel R, Wagner A, Rafolt D, Ewars R, and Bergmann H. (2000a). "The varioscope AR – a head-mounted operating microscope for augmented reality." *Proceedings of the Third International Conference on Medical Image Computing and Computer-Assisted Intervention (MICCAI)*, Pittsburg, PA, 869–877.

Birkfellner W, Figl M, Huber K, Watzinger F, Wanschitz F, Hummel J, Hanel RA, Greimel W, Homolka P, Ewars R, and Bergmann H. (2002). "A head-mounted operating binocular for augmented reality visualization in medicine–design and initial evaluation." *IEEE Trans Med Imaging*, 21(8), 991–997.

Birkfellner W, Huber K, Watzinger F, Figl M, Wanschitz F, Hanel R, Rafolt D, Ewars R, and Bergmann H. (2000b). "Development of the Varioscope AR, a see-through HMD for computer-aided surgery." *Proceedings of the IEEE and ACM International Symposium on Augmented Reality (ISAR)*, 54–59.

Blackwell M, Morgan F, and DiGioia AM, 3rd. (1998a). "Augmented reality and its future in orthopaedics." *Clin Orthop Relat Res* 354, 111–122.

Blackwell M, Nikou C, DiGioia AM, and Kanade T. (1998b). "An image overlay system for medical data visualization." *Proceedings of the First International Conference on Medical Image Computing and Computer-Assisted Intervention (MICCAI)*, 232–240.

Blackwell M, Nikou C, DiGioia AM, and Kanade T. (2000). "An image overlay system for medical data visualization." *Med Image Anal*, 4(1), 67–72.

Blackwell M, O'Toole RV, Morgan F, and Gregor L. (1995). "Performance and accuracy experiments with 3D and 2D image overlay systems." *Proceedings of the Medical Robotics and Computer Assisted Surgery (MRCAS)*, 312–317.

Chang WM, Horowitz MB, and Stetten GD. (2005a). "Intuitive intraoperative ultrasound guidance using the Sonic Flashlight: a novel ultrasound display system." *Neurosurgery*, 56(2 Suppl), 434–437.

Chang W, Amesur N, Wang D, Zajko A, and Stetten G. (2005b). First Clinical Trial of the Sonic Flashlight – Guiding Placement of Peripherally Inserted Central Catheters, *2005 meeting of the Radiological Society of North America*, November 2005, Chicago, Illinois. Paper Number SSJ03-02.

Chang W, Amesur N, Klatzky R, Zajko A, and Stetten G. (2006). Vascular Access: Comparison of US Guidance with the Sonic Flashlight and Conventional US in Phantoms, *Radiology*, 241, 771–779.

Coste-Maniere E, Adhami L, Mourgues F, and Bantiche O. (2004). "Optimal planning of robotically assisted heart surgery: Transfer precision in the operating room." *Int J Robot Res*, 23(4), 539–548.

Das M, Sauer F, Schoepf UJ, Khamene A, Vogt SK, Schaller S, Kikinis R, vanSonnenberg E, and Silverman SG. (2006). "Augmented reality visualization for CT-guided interventions: system description, feasibility, and initial evaluation in an abdominal phantom." *Radiology*, 240(1), 230–235.

De Buck S, Van Cleynenbreugel J, Geys I, Koninck T, Koninck PR, and Suetens P. (2001). "A system to support laparoscopic surgery by augmented reality visualization." *Proceedings of the Fourth International Conference on Medical Image Computing and Computer-Assisted Intervention (MICCAI)*, Springer-Verlag, 691–698.

Dey D, Slomka P, Gobbi D, and Peters T. (2000). "Mixed reality merging of endoscopic images and 3-D surfaces." *Proceedings of the Third International Conference on Medical Image Computing and Computer-Assisted Intervention (MICCAI)*, Springer-Verlag, 797–803.

Edwards PJ, Hawkes DJ, Hill DL, Jewell D, Spink R, Strong A, and Gleeson M. (1995a). "Augmentation of reality using an operating microscope for otolaryngology and neurosurgical guidance." *J Image Guid Surg*, 1(3), 172–178.

Edwards PJ, Hill DL, Hawkes DJ, Spink R, Colchester A, Strong A, and Gleeson M. (1995b). "Neurosurgical guidance using the stereo microscope." *Proceedings of Computer Vision, Virtual Reality, and Robotics in Medicine '95 (CVRMed)*, 555–564.

Edwards PJ, King A, Maurer C, De Cunha D, Hawkes DJ, Hill DL, Gaston R, Fenlon M, Chandra S, Strong A, Chandler C, Richards A, and Gleeson M. (1999). "Design and evaluation of a system for microscope-assisted guided interventions (MAGI)." *Proceedings of the Second International Conference on Medical Image Computing and Computer-Assisted Intervention (MICCAI)*, Springer-Verlag, 843–851.

Edwards PJ, King A, Maurer C, De Cunha D, Hawkes DJ, Hill DL, Gaston R, Fenlon M, Jusczyzck A, Strong A, Chandler C, and Gleeson M. (2000). "Design and evaluation of a system for microscope-assisted guided inter-ventions (MAGI)." *IEEE Trans Med Imag*, 19(11), 1082–1093.

Fiala M. (2004). ARTag Revision 1, A Fiducial Marker System Using Digital Techniques NRC/ERB-1117, November 24, 2004. NRC Publication Number: NRC 47419.

Fichtinger G, Deguet A, Fischer G, Iordachita I, Balogh E, Masamune K, Taylor RH, Fayad LM, de Oliveira M, and Zinreich SJ. (2005a). "Image overlay for CT-guided needle insertions." *Comput Aided Surg*, 10(4), 241–255.

Fichtinger G, Deguet A, Masamune K, Balogh E, Fischer G, Mathieu H, Taylor RH, Fayad LM, and Zinreich SJ. (2004). "Needle insertion in CT scanner with image overlay – cadaver studies." *Proceedings of the Seventh International Conference on Medical Image Computing and Computer-Assisted Intervention (MICCAI)*, Springer-Verlag, 795–803.

Fichtinger G, Deguet A, Masamune K, Balogh E, Fischer G, Mathieu H, Taylor RH, Zinreich SJ, and Fayad LM. (2005b). "Image overlay guidance for needle insertion in CT scanner." *IEEE Trans Biomed Eng*, 52(8), 1415–1424.

Figl M, Ede C, Hummel J, Wanschitz F, Ewers R, Bergmann H, and Birkfellner W. (2005). " A fully automated calibration method for an optical see-through head-mounted operating microscope with variable zoom and focus". *IEEE Trans Med Imaging*, 24, 1492–1499.

Fischer GS, Deguet A, Csoma C, Taylor RH, Fayad L, Carrino JA, Zinreich SJ, and Fichtinger G. (2007). "MRI image overlay: Application to arthrography needle insertion." *Comput Assist Surg*, 12(1), 2–14.

Fischer GS, Deguet A, Schlattman D, Taylor RH, Fayad L, Zinreich SJ, and Fichtinger G. (2006). "MRI image overlay: Applications to arthrography needle insertion." *Proceedings of the 14th Annual Medicine Meets Virtual Reality Conference (MMVR)*, 150–155.

Friets E, Strohbehn J, Hatch J, and Roberts D. (1989). "A frameless stereotaxic operating microscope for neurosurgery." *IEEE Trans Biomed Eng*, 36, 608–617.

Fuchs H, Livingston M, Raskar R, Colluci D, Keller K, State A, Crawford J, Rademacher P, Drake S, and Meyer A. (1998). "Augmented reality visualization for laparoscopic surgery." *First International Conference on Medical Image Computing and Computer-Assisted Intervention (MICCAI)*, 934–943.

Fuchs H, State A, Pisano E, Garrett W, Hirota G, Livingston M, Whitton M, and Pizer S. (1996). "Towards performing ultrasound guided needle biopsies from within a head-mounted display." *Proceedings of the Fourth International Conference on Vizualization in Biomedical Computing (VBC)*, 591–600.

Glossop N, Wedlake C, Moore J, Peters T, and Wang Z. (2003). "Laser projection augmented reality system for computer assisted surgery." *Proceedings of the Sixth International Conference on Medical Image Computing and Computer-Assisted Intervention (MICCAI)*, Springer-Verlag, 239–246.

Goebbels G, Troche K, Braun M, Ivanovic A, Grab A, von Lubtow K, Sader R, Zeilhofer F, Albrecht K, and Praxmarer K. (2003). "ARSyS-Tricorder – Entwicklung eines Augmented Reality System für die intraoperative Navi-gation in der MKG Chirurgie." *Proceedings of the 2. Jahrestagung der Deuts-chen Gesellschaft für Computer- und Roboterassistierte Chirurgie e.V.*, 1619–1627.

Grimson E, Leventon M, Ettinger G, Chabrerie A, Ozlen F, Nakajima S, Atsumi H, Kikinis R, and Black P. (1998). "Clinical experience with a high precision image guided neurosurgery system." *Proceedings of the First International Conference on Medical Image Computing and Computer-Assisted Intervention (MICCAI)*, 63–73.

Grimson W, Ettinger G, White S, Gleason P, Lozano-Perez T, Wells W, and Kikinis R. (1995). "Evaluating and validating an automated registration system for enhanced reality visualization in surgery." *Proceedings of Computer Vision, Virtual Reality, and Robotics in Medicine '95 (CVRMed)*, 3–12.

Grimson W, Ettinger G, White S, Lozano-Perez T, Wells W, and Kikinis R. (1996). "An automatic registration method for fram eless stereotaxy, image guided surgery, and enhanced reality visualization." *IEEE Trans Med Imag*, 15, 129–140.

Grimson W, Kikinis R, Jolesz F, and Black P. (1999). "Image guided surgery." *Sci Am*, 280(6), 62–69.

Grimson W, Lozano-Perez T, Wells W, Ettinger G, White S, and Kikinis R. (1994). "An automatic registration method for frameless stereotaxy, image guided surgery, and enhanced reality visualization." *Proceedings of the IEEE Computer Vision and Pattern Recognition Conference (CVPR)*, 430–436.

Hayashibe M, Suzuki N, Hattori A, Otake Y, Suzuki S, and Nakata N. (2005). "Data-fusion display system with volume rendering of intraoperatively scanned CT images." *Proceedings of the Eigth International Conference on Medical Image Computing and Computer-Assisted Intervention (MICCAI)*, Springer-Verlag, 559–566.

Heining S-M, Stefan P, Omary L, Wiesner S, Sielhorst T, Navab N, Sauer F, Euler E, Mutzler W, and Traub J. (2006). "Evaluation of an in-situ visualization system for navigated trauma surgery." *J Biomech*, 39(Supplement), 209.

HITLab. (2007). http://www.hitl.washington.edu/home/

Hoppe H, Eggers G, Heurich T, Raczkowsky J, Marmuller R, Wörn H, Hassfeld S, and Moctezuma L. (2003). "Projector-based visualization for intraoperative navigation: first clinical results." *Proceedings of the 17th International Congress and Exhibition on Computer Assisted Radiology and Surgery (CARS)*, 771.

Hoppe H, Kuebler C, Raczkowsky J, Wörn H, and Hassfeld S. (2002). "A clinical prototype system for projector-based augmented reality: Calibration and projection methods." *Proceedings of the 16th International Congress and Exhibition on Computer Assisted Radiology and Surgery (CARS)*, 1079.

Iseki H, Masutani Y, Iwahara M, Tanikawa T, Muragaki Y, Taira T, Dohi T, and Takakura K. (1997). "Volumegraph (overlaid three-dimensional image-guided navigation). Clinical application of augmented reality in neurosurgery." *Stereotact Funct Neurosurg*, 68(1–4 Pt 1), 18–24.

Johnson L, Edwards PJ, and Hawkes DJ. (2002). "Surface transparency makes stereo overlays unpredictable: the implication for augmented reality." *Stud Health Technol Inform*, 94, 131–136.

Khamene A, Vogt S, Azar F, Sielhorst T, Sauer F, and Niemann H. (2003a). "Local 3D reconstruction and augmented reality visualization of free-hand ultrasound for needle biopsy procedures." *Proceedings of the Sixth International Conference on Medical Image Computing and Computer-Assisted Intervention (MICCAI)*, 344–355.

Khamene A, Wacker F, Vogt S, Azar F, Wendt M, Sauer F, and Lewin J. (2003b). "An Augmented Reality system for MRI-guided needle biopsies." *Proceedings of the 11th Annual Medicine Meets Virtual Reality Conference (MMVR)*, 151–157.

King A, Edwards PJ, Maurer C, De Cunha D, Gaston R, Clarkson M, Hill DL, Hawkes DJ, Fenlon M, Strong A, TCS C, and Gleeson M. (2000). "Stereo augmented reality in the surgical microscope." *Presence*, 9(4), 360–368.

Lerotic M, Chung A., Mylonas G, Yang G-Z. (2007). "pq-space Based Non-Photorealistic Rendering for Augmented Reality". *Proc MICCAI 10 part II*, Lecture Notes in Computer Science 4792, 102–109.

Liao H, Hata N, Iwahara M, Nakajima S, Sakuma I, and Dohi T. (2002). "High-resolution stereoscopic surgical display using parallel integral videography and multi-projector." *Proceedings of the Fifth International Conference on Medical Image Computing and Computer-Assisted Intervention (MICCAI)*, Springer-Verlag, 85–92.

Liao H, Hata N, Nakajima S, Iwahara M, Sakuma I, and Dohi T. (2004). "Surgical navigation by autostereoscopic image overlay of integral videography." *IEEE Transactions on Information Technology in Biomedicine*, 114–121.

Liao H, Iwahara M, Koike T, Momoi Y, Hata N, Sakuma I, and Dohi T. (2006). "Integral videography autostereoscopic display using multiprojection". *Systems and Computers in Japan*, 37, 34–45.

Liao H, Nakajima S, Iwahara M, Kobayashi E, Sakuma I, Yahagi N, and Dohi T. (2001). "Intra-operative real-time 3-D information display system based on integral videography." *Proceedings of the Fourth International Conference on*

116   F. Sauer et al.

Medical Image Computing and Computer-Assisted Intervention (MICCAI), Springer-Verlag, 392–400.

Lorensen W, Cline H, Kikinis R, Altobelli D, Gleason L, and Jolesz F. (1994). "Enhanced reality in the operating room." *Proceedings of the Second Annual Medicine Meets Virtual Reality Conference (MMVR)*, 124–127.

Lorensen W, Cline H, Nafis C, Kikinis R, Altobelli D, and Gleason L. (1993). "Enhancing reality in the operating room." *Proceedings of IEEE Visualization '93*, 410–415.

Marmurek J, Wedlake C, Pardasani U, Eagleson R, and Peters TM. (2006). "Image-guided laser projection for port placement in minimally invasive surgery" *Stud Health Technol Inform*, 119, 367–372.

Masamune K, Fichtinger G, Deguet A, Matsuka D, and Taylor RH. (2002). "An image overlay system with enhanced reality for percutaneous therapy performed inside ct scanner." *Proceedings of the Fifth International Conference on Medical Image Computing and Computer-Assisted Intervention (MICCAI)*, Springer-Verlag, 77–84.

Masamune K, Masutani Y, Nakajima S, Sakuma I, Dohi T, Iseki H, and Takakura K. (2000). "Three-dimensional slice image overlay system with accurate depth perception for surgery." *Proceedings of the Third International Conference on Medical Image Computing and Computer-Assisted Intervention (MICCAI)*, 395–402.

Masutani Y, Dohi T, Nishi Y, Iwahara M, Iseki H, and Takakura K. (1996). "Volumegraph – an integral photography based enhanced reality visualization system." *Proceedings of the Tenth International Symposium on Computer Assisted Radiology (CAR)*, 1051.

Masutani Y, Iwahara M, Samuta O, Nishi Y, Suzuki M, Suzuki N, Dohi T, Iseki H, and Takakura K. (1995). "Development of integral photography-based en-hanced reality visualization system for surgical support." *Proceedings of the Second International Symposium on Computer Aided Surgery (ISCAS)*, 16–17.

Maurer C, Sauer F, Brown C, Hu B, Bascle B, Geiger B, Wenzel F, Maciunas R, Bakos R, and Bani-Hashemi A. (2001). "Augmented reality visualization of brain structures with stereo and kinetic depth cues: System description and initial evaluation with head phantom." *Proceedings of SPIE's Conference of Medical Imaging 2001*, 445–456.

Milgram P, and Kishino FA. (1994). "Taxonomy of Mixed Reality Visual Displays," Institute of Electronics, Information, and Communication Engineers Trans. Information and Systems (IECE special issue on networked reality), vol. E77-D, 12, 1321–1329.

Mitschke M, Bani-Hashemi A, and Navab N. (2000). "Interventions under video-augmented X-ray guidance: Application to needle placement." *Proceedings of the Third International Conference on Medical Image Computing and Computer-Assisted Intervention (MICCAI)*, 858–868.

Mourgues F, Devernay F, and Coste-Maniere E. (2001). "3D reconstruction of the operating field for image overlay in 3D-endoscopic surgery." *Proceedings of the IEEE and ACM International Symposium on Augmented Reality (ISAR)*, 191–192.

Mourgues F, Vieville T, Falk V, and Coste-Maniere E. (2003). "Interactive guidance by image overlay in robot assisted coronary artery bypass." *Proceedings of the Sixth International Conference on Medical Image Computing and Computer-Assisted Intervention (MICCAI)*, Springer-Verlag, 173–181.

Nakajima S, Orita S, Masamune K, Sakuma I, Dohi T, and Nakamura K. (2000). "Surgical navigation system with intuitive three-dimensional display." *Proceedings of the Third International Conference on Medical Image Computing and Computer-Assisted Intervention (MICCAI)*, 403–411.

Navab N, Bani-Hashemi A, and Mitschke M. (1999). "Merging visible and invisible: Two camera-augmented mobile C-arm (CAMC) applications." *Proceedings of the Second International Workshop on Augmented Reality (IWAR)*, 134–141.

Nicolau S, Garcia A, Pennec X, Soler L, and Ayache N. (2005a). "An augmented reality system to guide radio-frequency tumor ablation." *J Comput Animation Virtual World*, 16(1), 1–10.

Nicolau S, Pennec X, Soler L, and Ayache N. (2005b). "A complete augmented reality guidance system for liver punctures: First clinical evaluation." *Proceedings of the Eighth International Conference on Medical Image Computing and Computer-Assisted Intervention (MICCAI)*, pp 539–547. Springer-Verlag.

Rosenthal M, State A, Lee J, Hirota G, Ackerman J, Keller K, Pisano E, Jiroutek M, Muller K, and Fuchs H. (2001). "Augmented reality guidance for needle biopsies: An initial randomized, controlled trial in phantoms." *Proceedings of the Fourth International Conference on Medical Image Computing and Computer-Assisted Intervention (MICCAI)*, Springer-Verlag, 240–248.

Rosenthal M, State A, Lee J, Hirota G, Ackerman J, Keller K, Pisano E, Jiroutek M, Muller K, and Fuchs H. (2002). "Augmented reality guidance for needle biopsies: An initial randomized, controlled trial in phantoms." *Med Image Anal*, 6(2), 313–320.

Sauer F, Khamene A, Bascle B, and Rubino G. (2001a). "A headmounted display system for augmented reality image guidance: Towards clinical evaluation for iMRI-guided neurosurgery." *Proceedings of the fourth International Conference on Medical Image Computing and Computer-Assisted Intervention (MICCAI)*, Springer-Verlag, 707–716.

Sauer F, Khamene A, Bascle B, Schimmang L, Wenzel F, and Vogt S. (2001b). "Augmented reality visualization of ultrasound images: System description, calibration, and features." *Proceedings of IEEE and ACM International Symposium on Augmented Reality (ISAR '01)*, 30–39.

Sauer F, Khamene A, Bascle B, and Vogt S. (2002a). "An augmented reality system for ultrasound guided needle biopsies." *Proceedings of the Tenth Annual Medicine Meets Virtual Reality Conference (MMVR)*, 455–460.

Sauer F, Khamene A, Bascle B, Vogt S, and Rubino G. (2002b). "Augmented reality visualization in iMRI operating room: System description and pre-clinical testing." *Proceedings of SPIE's Conference of Medical Imaging 2002: Visualization, Image-Guided Procedures, and Display*, 446–454.

Sauer F, Khamene A, and Vogt S. (2002c). "An augmented reality navigation system with a single-camera tracker: System design and needle biopsy phantom trial." *Proceedings of the Fifth International Conference on Medical Image Computing and Computer-Assisted Intervention (MICCAI)*, 116–124.

Sauer F, Schoepf J, Khamene A, Vogt S, Das M, and Silverman SG. (2003). "Augmented reality system for CT-guided interventions: System description and initial phantom trials." *Proceedings of SPIE's Conference of Medical Imaging 2003: Visualization, Image-Guided Procedures, and Display*, 384–394.

Sauer F, Wenzel F, Vogt S, Tao Y, Genc Y, and Bani-Hashemi A. (2000). "Augmented workspace: Designing an AR testbed." *Proceedings of the IEEE and ACM International Symposium on Augmented Reality (ISAR)*, 47–53.

Shahidi R, Wang B, Epitaux M, Grzeszczuk R, and Adler J. (1998). "Volumetric image guidance via a stereotactic endoscope." *Proceedings of the First International Conference on Medical Image Computing and Computer-Assisted Intervention (MICCAI)*, 241–252.

Sielhorst T, Obst T, Burgkart R, Riener R, and Navab N. (2004a). "An augmented reality delivery simulator for medical training." *Proceedings of the International Workshop on Augmented Environments for Medical Imaging (AMIARCS 2004) – MICCAI Satellite Workshop*, 11–20.

Sielhorst T, Traub J, and Navab N. (2004b). "The AR apprenticeship: Replication and omnidirectional viewing of subtle movements." *Proceedings of the Third IEEE and ACM International Symposium on Mixed and Augmented Reality (ISMAR)*, 290–291.

State A, Chen D, Tector C, Brandt A, Chen H, Ohbuchi R, Bajura M, and Fuchs H. (1994). "Case study: Observing a volume rendered fetus within a pregnant patient." *Proceedings of IEEE Visualization '94*, 364–368.

State A, Keller K, Rosenthal M, Yang H, Ackerman J, and Fuchs H. (2003). "Stereo imagery from the UNC augmented reality system for breast biopsy guidance." *Proceedings of the 11th Annual Medicine Meets Virtual Reality Conference (MMVR)*, 325–328.

State A, Livingston M, Hirota G, Garrett W, Whitton M, Fuchs H, and Pisano E. (1996). "Technologies for augmented-reality systems: realizing ultrasound-guided needle biopsies." *SIGGRAPH, 96 Computer Graphics Proceedings, Annual Conference Series*, 439–446.

Stetten G, and Chib V. (2001a). "Magnified real-time tomographic reflection." *Proceedings of the Fourth International Conference on Medical Image Computing and Computer-Assisted Intervention (MICCAI)*, Springer-Verlag, 683–690.

Stetten G, Chib V, and Tamburo R. (2000). "Tomographic reflection to merge ultrasound images with direct vision." *Proceedings of the Applied Imagery Pattern Recognition Annual Workshop (AIPR)*, 200–205.

Stetten G, Chib VS, Hildebrand D, and Bursee J. (2001). "Real time tomographic reflection: Phantoms for calibration and biopsy." *Proceedings of the IEEE and ACM International Symposium on Augmented Reality (ISAR)*, 11–19.

Stetten G, Cois A, Chang W, Shelton D, Tamburo R, Castellucci J, and Von Ramm O. (2003). "C-mode real time tomographic reflection for a matrix array ultrasound sonic flashlight." *Proceedings of the Sixth International Conference on Medical Image Computing and Computer-Assisted Intervention (MICCAI)*, Springer-Verlag, 336–343.

Stetten G, Cois A, Chang W, Shelton D, Tamburo R, Castellucci J, and von Ramm O. (2005). "C-mode real-time tomographic reflection for a matrix array ultrasound sonic flashlight." *Acad Radiol*, 12(5), 535–543.

Stetten GD, and Chib VS. (2001b). "Overlaying ultrasonographic images on direct vision." *J Ultrasound Med*, 20(3), 235–240.

Traub J, Feuerstein M, Bauer M, Schirmbrck E, Najafi H, Bauernschmitt R, and Klinker G. (2004). "Augmented reality for port placement and navigation in robotically assisted minimally invasive cardiovascular surgery." *Proceedings of the 18th International Congress and Exhibition on Computer Assisted Radiology and Surgery (CARS)*, 735–740.

Tuceryan M, and Navab N. (2000). "Single point active alignment method (SPAAM) for optical see-through HMD calibration for AR." *Proceedings of IEEE and ACM International Symposium on Augmented Reality (ISAR'00)*, Munich, Germany, 149–158.

Vogt S, Khamene A, Niemann H, and Sauer F. (2004a). "An AR system with intuitive user interface for manipulation and visualization of 3D medical data." *Proceedings of the 12th Annual Medicine Meets Virtual Reality Conference (MMVR)*, 397–403.

Vogt S, Khamene A, and Sauer F. (2006). "Reality augmentation for medical procedures: System architecture, single camera marker tracking, and system evaluation." *Int J Comput Vis*, 70(2), 179–190.

Vogt S, Khamene A, Sauer F, Keil A, and Niemann H. (2003). "A high performance AR system for medical applications." *Proceedings of the Second IEEE and ACM International Symposium on Mixed and Augmented Reality (ISMAR)*, 270–271.

Vogt S, Khamene A, Sauer F, and Niemann H. (2002). "Single camera tracking of marker clusters: Multiparameter cluster optimization and experimental verification." *Proceedings of the IEEE and ACM International Symposium on Mixed and Augmented Reality (ISMAR)*, 127–136.

Vogt S, Wacker F, Khamene A, Elgort D, Sielhorst T, Niemann H, Duerk J, Lewin J, and Sauer F. (2004b). "Augmented reality system for MR-guided interventions: Phantom studies and first animal test." *Proceedings of SPIE's Conference of Medical Imaging 2004: Visualization, Image-Guided Procedures, and Display*, 100–109.

Wacker FK, Vogt S, Khamene A, Jesberger JA, Nour SG, Elgort DR, Sauer F, Duerk JL, and Lewin JS. (2006). "An augmented reality system for MR image-guided needle biopsy: initial results in a swine model." *Radiology*, 238(2), 497–504.

Wang D, Wu B, and Stetten G. (2005). "Laser needle guide for the sonic flashlight." *Proceedings of the Eighth International Conference on Medical Image Com-puting and Computer-Assisted Intervention (MICCAI)*, Springer-Verlag, 647–653.

Wendt M, Sauer F, Khamene A, Bascle B, Vogt S, and Wacker F. (2003). "A head-mounted display system for augmented reality: Initial evaluation for interventional MRI." *RöFo – Fortschritte auf dem Gebiet der Röntgenstrahlen und der bildgebenden Verfahren*, 175(3), 418–421.

Worn H, and Hoppe H. (2001). "Augmented reality in the operating theatre of the future."*Proceedings of the Fourth International Conference on Medical Image Computing and Computer-Assisted Intervention (MICCAI)*, Springer-Verlag, 1195–1196.

Chapter 5
Software

Luis Ibanez

Abstract

Software is a core component of any system intended to support image-guided surgery interventions. This chapter describes some of the important considerations that should be kept in mind when designing, implementing, and using software as a component of an image-guided surgery system. Particular emphasis is given to quality control and the principles of software design for safety-critical applications.

5.1 Introduction

Providing support for the difficult tasks that surgeons face during medical interventions is a delicate balancing act in ensuring that valuable help is actually provided to the clinician, without compromising the safety of the patient subjected to the intervention. The combination of hardware, software, and well-defined practices has the potential to provide such help. For this potential to become a reality, it is essential to create the proper balance between the capabilities of the hardware, the functionalities of the associated software, and the procedures established in the clinical practices that have proved to provide benefits to the patient. When any of the three components fails to integrate properly with others, the capabilities of the entire IGI system for providing benefits to the patient decrease rapidly.

5.1.1 The Need for Software

The fundamental role of an IGI system is to provide information processing capabilities. It involves information acquisition via image scanners, tracking systems, respiratory and cardiac gating, as well as video and voice recording. The information gathered from all these different sources must be integrated in a consistent manner and then must be used for generating informative displays to be presented to clinicians, with the goal of facilitating the execution of the surgical intervention. The types of information to be gathered and

T. Peters and K. Cleary (eds.), *Image-Guided Interventions.*
© Springer Science + Business Media, LLC 2008

the kind of displays to be generated at every given moment depend on the current specific stage of the surgical intervention. In an IGI system, software plays the role of integrator of the information provided by multiple hardware devices. It analyzes incoming information and also generates the output to be presented to the surgeons. Software must do all this by following the workflow of the surgical procedure. Without software to perform these tasks, the clinician would have to mentally integrate all the different sources of information; a daunting task that in many cases involves demanding mathematical computations, as well as the management of high rates of information flow. The surgeon's attention and focus need to be fully engaged in the medical aspects of the intervention, and not overwhelmed with tasks of information manipulation for which software can perform efficiently.

5.1.2 Software as a Risk Factor

The very same characteristics that make software such a good fit for processing IGI information, also make it a significant risk factor when it has been integrated into the information processing flow guiding a surgical procedure. In particular, the enormous flexibility of software may make it an unpredictable element in the ensemble of IGI components. In practical terms, we must continuously ask the question: "what can go wrong?" The answers to this question will suggest measures to reduce the occurrence of bad outcomes, as well as mitigating the detrimental effects that may result to the patient.

The following list specifies some of the worst situations, where the software of an IGI system may compromise patient safety:

1. Design flaws that may result in the software not fitting the workflow of the surgical intervention. For example, failing to provide the necessary information, or expecting information that is not going to be available until much later in the intervention.
2. Failure to verify the validity of information presented to the surgeon. For example, displaying images that correspond to a different patient or failing to use the correct left–right orientation labeling in a display.
3. Inability to deal with unanticipated situations during an intervention, such as the accidental disconnection of a tracker cable.
4. Coding errors that escaped notice during the software implementation phase, which result in quality defects. For example, memory leaks, noninitialized variables, dangling pointers, and past-the-end access in arrays.
5. Unfounded assumptions that were presumed during the design and implementation phases of the software, which prove to be wrong in the specific circumstances of the intervention. For example, assuming that an intervention will never last more than 8 h, or assuming that a certain calibration procedure needs to be performed only once.

Some of these detrimental characteristics can be reduced by closely involving clinical partners in the design of IGI systems; others can be reduced by applying engineering techniques for quality control, while eliminating others requires the use of design techniques suitable for safety-critical applications.

5.1.3 Quality Control

One of the characteristics that makes software a significant risk factor in an IGI system is the extreme ease with which the lines of code of a program can be modified, and the large number of unintended effects that such changes may have. Software systems are by nature extremely complex. Therefore, it is easy for developers to focus on the logic of a local task and to overlook the global effects that local changes in the software may have in the long-term behavior of the system, or in the behavior of other software components. In many cases, these unintended effects may pass unnoticed for long periods of time, and by the time they are discovered it is very laborious to track them down to the original change.

Having a quality control system in place that continuously verifies the correct behavior of the software helps to prevent such unintended effect from passing unnoticed, and helps to warn developers about the need to correct them immediately.

There are three main levels at which quality control system should act to be effective in protecting developers from introducing defects in software packages: code reviews, unit testing, and application testing. They are discussed further in Section 5.2.4.

5.1.4 The Cost of Software Maintenance

The cost of software development, that is, writing the initial working version of an application, is just the tip of the iceberg when it comes to evaluating the cost of software development. The largest portion of the iceberg is the cost associated with the maintenance and evolution of the code over the years.

The longevity of software tends to be largely underestimated. Most software packages have useful lives in the range of decades, and it is not uncommon to find routines that keep being reused after half a century, for example, www.netlib.org, sometimes by being rewritten in the form of multiple reincarnations. In acknowledging the expected longevity of software, it becomes easier to prepare for the long-term challenge of the continuous addition of new functionality, and for the continuous repair of software defects resulting not only from these additions, but also from unintended effects from fixing previous defects. All in all, software maintenance easily accounts for 80% of the total cost of a software development endeavor.

Keeping software longevity in mind provides guidelines that may help when making decision on topics such as coding style, performance improvements versus code readability, and will help to allocate the appropriate amount of resources to testing and validation versus initial development of software.

5.1.5 Open Source Versus Closed Source

The arguments for and against the use of Open Source or Closed Source software are extensive and passionate.

Closed Source software is promoted by commercial and academic institutions that highly value the intellectual property associated with the source code. There are two intellectual property aspects that can be associated with the software: patents and copyrights. In the case of patents, the subject of a patent is actually a matter of public knowledge, given that the patent offices make the content of an assigned patent public. In that regard, hiding the source code that implements a patented method does not directly provide a protection from infringement of intellectual property. In the case of copyrights, keeping the source code closed prevents the material from being copied and reused in the form of derivative work. Supporters of closed source tend to argue that by creating a commercial enterprise around the software development and maintenance, and by gathering revenue from the licensing of the software, they are able to maintain high standards of quality in a well-controlled environment of software development.

Open Source is an engineering approach in which anybody is allowed to read the source code. In this context, the user community is informally recruited as a large quality control team that continuously performs code reviews. The community also provides feedback for driving the future evolution of the software. When the proper infrastructure is put in place for supporting the user community, it is possible to benefit from the high-quality feedback from domain experts. There are many misconceptions of what open source actually means, and probably the most significant of these in the domain of IGI are that (1) anyone can change the software and (2) users can do anything with the software.

The first misconception, namely that anybody can modify the software, is mostly the result of a limited public knowledge on how the communities of open source software developers actually operate. In practice, these communities tend to be quite small, rarely reaching more than 50 individuals at any given time. These groups usually maintain control of a source code repository, where read access is granted to anybody, and write access is reserved to very few individuals who have proved their qualities as software developers and as positive team players. For a newcomer to gain write access in an open source project, they must first demonstrate to the core developers an understanding of the code, display expertise in software development, and maintain a good attitude in dealing with other members of the team in a positive fashion. All these characteristics usually can only be displayed in the online forums, blogs, and mailing lists associated with the communities of users and developers of the software in question. In part, this misconception has been fueled by the fact that in many cases anyone is allowed to modify their *local* copy of the software. This aspect will be discussed in more length in the following section on licensing. The second misconception, that anybody can use the software for any purpose, is the unfortunate consequence of failing to read in detail the terms of the licenses under which open source software packages are distributed. This is also discussed in the following section.

It has been said that benefits to society can be maximized by promoting the proper balance between closed source and open source software. In particular, open source should be used for common infrastructure where maximizing the reuse of code will result in distributing the effort of software development and maintenance over a large community. Open source is also appropriate for applications such as government, voting, and security where the source code must be made available for audit purposes. Closed source, on the other hand, is more appropriate for promoting commercial activity in specific niches where software applications should be highly customized in order to suit a specialized community. This balance is usually compared with the road network in a city, where highways and large roads are part of the public space and are developed as shared community resources, while private business are located along the highways and benefit from the access through the public roads.

5.1.5.1 Licensing

Licensing conditions are one of the first aspects that should be considered when adopting software. In general, software is considered to be the property of the company that develops it. Mostly, software development companies maintain ownership of the software and only sell licenses to users. The license specifies what the user may and may not do with the software. This includes whether the software may be used in one or multiple computers, if the user may make copies of the software, sell or transfer his or her license to third persons, redistribute software, etc. Licenses fall under the domain of intellectual property lawyers and as such they are usually not read carefully by users during the installation process of software packages. The failure to read software licenses is the largest contributing factor in the abundant misconceptions regarding closed source and open source.

In the domain of commercial software, licenses usually preclude the creation of derivative work, the redistribution of the software, and the creation of copies for any purpose other than backups. It is common for them to forbid reverse engineering, de-compilation, and disassembly. For an example, please see the license of Windows XP home edition [Microsoft 2004].

In the domain of Open Source there are also a variety of licenses [Open Source Initiative]. The open source initiative web site maintains a list of about 60 approved licenses. The most popular open source licenses are the GPL and LGPL licenses, followed by the BSD, MIT, and Apache licenses. One of the controversial aspects of the GPL license is that it requires derivative work to be distributed under the same license. This requirement is softened in the LGPL license when the derivative work is linking shared libraries of the LGPL licensed software. The GPL license does not preclude the use of the software for commercial applications. In fact, they encourage commercial vendors to use open source software in products, as long as the final code is redistributed under the conditions of the GPL license.

Regardless of whether your IGI application uses closed or open source software, it is important to become familiar with the specific terms and conditions stated in the licenses of each package on which your application is based.

5.1.5.2 Liability

Liability has often been mentioned as a reason for not using open source software. This is also a misconception resulting from not reading the license agreement of software products. In general, no software package provides any liability in case the software does not perform as expected. In most cases, the liability terms of the license are only related to the media in which the software is distributed. In other words, if you received a DVD with a scratch that prevents you from installing the software, then you are entitled to receive a replacement DVD, but if you install the software and it does not perform the functionalities that are described in the documentation, then you are not entitled to any compensation.

An attentive reading of the Microsoft End User License Agreement (EULA) [Microsoft 2004] will reveal that

> LIMITATION ON REMEDIES; NO CONSEQUENTIAL OR OTHER DAMAGES. Your exclusive remedy for any breach of this Limited Warranty is as set forth below. Except for any refund elected by Microsoft, YOU ARE NOT ENTITLED TO ANY DAMAGES, INCLUDING BUT NOT LIMITED TO CONSEQUENTIAL DAMAGES, if the Software does not meet Microsoft's Limited Warranty, and, to the maximum extent allowed by applicable law, even if any remedy fails of its essential purpose.

The software warranty is quite limited, as can be seen from the following excerpt:

> LIMITED WARRANTY FOR SOFTWARE ACQUIRED IN THE US AND CANADA. Microsoft warrants that the Software will perform

substantially in accordance with the accompanying materials for a period of ninety (90) days from the date of receipt.

Microsoft declines any responsibility for the suitability of its products for a particular purpose:

DISCLAIMER OF WARRANTIES. The Limited Warranty that appears above is the only express warranty made to you and is provided in lieu of any other express warranties or similar obligations (if any) created by any advertising, documentation, packaging, or other communications. Except for the Limited Warranty and to the maximum extent permitted by applicable law, Microsoft and its suppliers provide the Software and support services (if any) AS IS AND WITH ALL FAULTS, and hereby disclaim all other warranties and conditions, whether express, implied or statutory, including, but not limited to, any (if any) implied warranties, duties or conditions of merchantability, of fitness for a particular purpose, of reliability or availability, of accuracy or completeness of responses, of results, of workmanlike effort, of lack of viruses, and of lack of negligence, all with regard to the Software, and the provision of or failure to provide support or other services, information, software, and related content through the Software or otherwise arising out of the use of the Software. ALSO, THERE IS NO WARRANTY OR CONDITION OF TITLE, QUIET ENJOYMENT, QUIET POSSESSION, CORRESPONDENCE TO DESCRIPTION OR NON-INFRINGEMENT WITH REGARD TO THE SOFTWARE.

The complexity of software simply makes it too risky for software development companies to dare to offer any warranties regarding the performance of their products.

In the context of IGI applications, this absence of warranties from software providers emphasizes the need to perform extensive testing and validation of the applications that are brought to the operating room.

5.2   Software Development Process

The fragile nature of software and its inherent complexity makes it necessary to put rigorous practices of software development in place to ensure high quality and robustness of the resulting software. The following sections describe some of the software development practices that are recommended by regulatory agencies, as well as practices that have been adopted as industry standards.

5.2.1 FDA Guidelines

The U.S. Food and Drug Administration (FDA) is an agency of the United States Department of Health and Human Services that is responsible for regulating food (humans and animal), dietary supplements, drugs (human and animal), cosmetics, medical devices (human and animal), radiation emitting devices (including nonmedical devices), biologics, and blood products in the USA. As part of this role in regulating the manufacturing of medical devices, the FDA provides guidelines regarding the development practices of software used in medical devices.

Three main documents published by the FDA in this regard are

1. General Principles of Software Validation; Final Guidance for Industry and FDA Staff (FOD# 938, 01-11-2002) [FDA 2002]
2. Guidance for Off-the-Shelf Software Use in Medical Devices (FOD# 585, 09-09-1999) [FDA 1999]
3. Guidance for the Content of Premarket Submissions for Software Contained in Medical Devices—Guidance for Industry and FDA Staff (FOD# 337, 05-11-2005) [FDA 2005].

The first document provides guidance on the validation of software contained in medical devices or software used for designing and manufacturing medical devices. The second document provides guidelines for validating software provided by third parties, but is not inherently intended for use in medical devices. The third document describes how to prepare a submission for the approval of a medical device that incorporates software.

The main aspects of these documents are summarized in the following sections. Note however that these summaries are only intended to motivate you to read the original documents, and in no way should be assumed to be a comprehensive reduction of the original material. The main point here is that the FDA guidelines, despite being somewhat cumbersome, make a lot of sense when we keep in mind that the patient safety is the primary concern. In many cases, the guidelines are also applicable to any software product of professional quality.

5.2.1.1 Software Validation Guidelines

The central aspect of the guidelines is to encourage the integration of the software development process and the risk management activities typical of medical devices manufacturing. The purpose of these guidelines is to validate the functionalities of the software to make sure that once the medical devices are deployed they will perform as intended. The following excerpt from the report shows the need for rigorous software development:

The FDA's analysis of 3140 medical device recalls conducted between 1992 and 1998 reveals that 242 of them (7.7%) are attributable to software failures. Of those software related recalls, 192 (or 79%) were caused by software defects that were introduced when changes were made to the software after its initial production and distribution. Software validation and other related good software engineering practices discussed in this guidance are a principal means of avoiding such defects and resultant recalls. [FDA 2002]

As stated earlier in this chapter, when it comes to quality control, it is not the initial software development that is of most concern. Instead, it is the subsequent continuous stream of modifications, fixes, and "*improvements*" that tend to degrade the quality of the software. These modifications can introduce defects that pass unnoticed by the developers because of the lack of systematic validation procedures. The guidelines provided in the FDA document are intended to (a) prevent unnecessary changes from being introduced in the software, (b) properly define the specific changes that are considered necessary, and (c) specify exactly how to verify that the modifications have been integrated successfully with the software.

The software used in a medical device may be produced by different providers. It may have been developed in house by the medical device manufacturer itself, it may have been developed under specifications by a subcontractor, or it may have been taken from an off-the-shelf product. Regardless of the source of the software, the final responsibility of validating and verifying that the software performs as expected lies with the medical device manufacturer.

Given that the validation of the software is necessarily performed under a specific version of the code, it is of utmost importance to keep track of the versions that are approved, as well as to fully specify the dependencies that a software application may have on other, presumably third-party, pieces of software, such as libraries, drivers, and compilers. The precise procedure for building an application must also be documented to ensure that future builds are performed in a consistent way. This documentation is intended to prevent developers from using a different, nonvalidated, version of dependent libraries; or from using nonvalidated compiler flags that may result in the final medical device behaving in a way that does not satisfy its requirements.

Risk analysis is an activity to be integrated as part of the software development process. It should be an integral part of the code reviews and design reviews, and it should be reflected in the testing infrastructure by generating specific tests that verify that the system behaves correctly. Programming techniques described in Section 5.3 can also be used as a daily mechanism of low-level risk analysis and mitigation that overall will raise the entire application level of quality.

Regulatory agencies will rarely look at the source code developed by a medical device manufacturer. Instead, they require the manufacturer to have a documented procedure of how the software has been developed and a documentation trail demonstrating that those procedures are followed as defined in the documentation.

Traceability plays a central role in the enforcement that the FDA exerts when reviewing a medical device for approval. In the particular case of software, the FDA expects the manufacturer to maintain documentation demonstrating that

1. each element of the software design specification has been implemented in code;
2. modules and functions implemented in code can be traced back to an element in the software design specification and to the risk analysis;
3. tests for modules and functions can be traced back to an element in the software design specification and to the risk analysis; and
4. tests for modules and functions can be traced to source code for the same modules and functions [FDA 2002].

5.2.2 Requirements

As emphasized in the FDA guidelines, one of the main mechanisms to ensure that no unnecessary functionalities are introduced in the software is to gather and maintain a collection of requirements. These requirements describe the set of needs and expectations of the users of the final medical device. Requirements are the initial input for the design of the device and its software. Only functionalities that are intended to satisfy a specific requirement should be added to the system. The requirements collection helps to keep the focus on the application, by making sure that all the expected functionalities are provided, and that no unnecessary functionalities are introduced. Software requirements are a subset of the entire requirements collection of the medical device. In some cases, a software requirement is elaborated with the purpose of addressing two or more requirements of the medical device. In either case, a system must be put in place so that requirements are managed through a careful review process that ensures they are meaningful and justified, and that no requirements are added or removed from the collection without a judicious consideration of the consequences.

Requirements also provide the basis of the quality validation for the medical device. To that end, requirements should be written in such a way that they can be tested and verified. In this way, the validation process should include a walkthrough of the set of tests that verify the successful implementation of functionalities described in the requirements. Writing requirements as testable statements also prevents them from being too nebulous or too generic, and in this way, reduce their potential ambiguity. The requirements collection is also referred to as the "specification" of the system.

5.2.3 *Validation and Verification*

Quality system regulations differentiate the two concepts of validation and verification. Validation is the confirmation that the requirements collection actually conforms to user needs and the intended uses of the medical device and its software. The process of software validation includes evidence that all software requirements have been implemented correctly, and that they can be traced back to specific system requirements. Testing the software in an environment that simulates the conditions under which the device is expected to be used, as well as testing the device on the deployment site, is a typical validation activity. Verification is the process of gathering evidence that the final device satisfies the requirements collection. This involves a number of tests that will attempt to exercise the expected functionalities in the device, and that will verify the correctness of the resulting outcome. Other verification activities include dynamic analysis, code reviews, and code coverage analysis.

5.2.4 *Testing*

From the practical point of view, testing is probably the aspect of the validation activity that can be better specified and quantified. The following sections describe the main activities that are considered industry standards for software testing.

5.2.4.1 Code Reviews

Code reviews are a standard practice by which the code written or modified by one developer is to be reviewed by other developers. The review process is usually based on a predefined checklist of commonly introduced defects as well as on the verification of an appropriate coding style. The reviewers are part of the same development team and must be familiar with the inner workings of the software, as well as with the particular programming techniques and design style used in the project. During the review process, reviewers list all the defects encountered and bring them to the attention of the original developers. This feedback is intended to prevent similar defects from being introduced in future developments. Important defects are also registered in a bug-tracking or defect-tracking database to make sure that they are addressed appropriately. Code reviews also serve the purpose of ensuring that the software has a uniform style, to the point where it appears to be written by a single person. Uniformity of style reduces the risk that future modifications of the software will introduce defects because of ambiguities in the programming techniques used.

One of the cruel paradoxes of software quality control is that a large proportion of bugs in a system are introduced as a side effect of fixing a known bug. Code reviews are one of the tools that help to break this pernicious cycle. By having the eyes of a second developer review the code changes, the opportunities for detecting pernicious side effects are multiplied. A similar effect is achieved in some programming methodologies, such as Agile programming, by having developers work in pairs. In this context, one developer can focus on the syntactic aspects of writing the code, while the observing developer considers a more global view of how the modifications fit in the larger scheme of the software. The practice of pair development is not intended to be a replacement for code reviews. It is rather an earlier code review that facilitates catching many of the potential defects before they are even typed into the system, while the logic of the problem is still fresh in the mind of both developers.

Another important product of the code review process is the documented trace of the software development process. When maintained in an appropriate format, the code review reports provide a background that will help future developers to understand why some changes were made in the system in a particular way.

5.2.4.2 Unit Testing

As much as reading and reviewing a piece of software may build confidence in its quality, there is nothing to substitute for executing the software using realistic input and then verifying the output against well-established results. For this approach to be effective, it must be implemented using a large number of tests, each one addressing a small portion of the functionalities of a total system. This approach, also known as "unit testing," is fundamental for any software development enterprise.

Unit testing is a natural fit for software that has been implemented as a collection of small units; whether they are functions, as in procedural programming, or classes, as in object-oriented programming, the fundamental idea of "divide and conquer" applies equally. A unit testing framework requires multiple components, including a test suite, a collection of validated input data, a collection of validated output data, an infrastructure for running tests, and an infrastructure for summarizing test results and tracking failures.

A test suite is a collection of small, minimalist programs that exercise the functionalities of each one of the software units, regardless of whether they are classes or functions. A typical element of a test suite will be a small program that sets up appropriate input data for the software unit, then invokes the unit's execution, and finally reports the resulting output. Ideally, the test program must be written before writing the software unit, or at least simultaneously with it. The test program must also be maintained along with the software, in the sense that, as the software is modified over the years, the testing code must also be adapted accordingly. Moreover, when defects are found in a unit, the circumstances that made detection of the defect possible must be repeated in the form of a new test, with the purpose of preventing the same defect from reappearing and passing unnoticed in a future instance of the software.

In a typical test suite, it is reasonable to expect to have as many lines of testing code as lines of unit code. A well-constructed test suite will greatly simplify the task of fixing defects, because it naturally partitions the complexity of the software into smaller pieces that can be verified easily. By continuously running the test suite, it also becomes possible to detect problems as soon as they are introduced in the system, and therefore the greatly reduce the time that it takes to fix them.

A collection of validated input data provides a realistic context for executing the unit tests. It would be pointless to use trivial data as the input of the tests, or to use data that does not reflect the variability of the input data that is likely to be found when deploying the software in the field. The best collection of data is, of course, the one that can be constructed over the years by storing real data into an annotated database. Such data collection must follow practices that respect patient confidentiality and follow the guidelines for research on human subjects. The data should be validated by domain experts with the purpose of ensuring that the annotations are appropriate, and that the data represent the actual information likely to be encountered in the field. For example, it is not appropriate to use a radiograph as a testing input for a software unit that is designed to work on fluoroscopy images. The characteristics of noise, geometry, intensity range, and field of view of these two image modalities are not sufficiently similar to state that the software unit will perform as well with a fluoroscopy image as with a radiograph. Just as with the software and the testing suite, image collections must be maintained over the years to ensure they are still relevant and sufficient for the applications for which the software is intended.

A collection of validated output data is constructed by initially running the elements of the test suite and then domain experts judge whether the resulting output is correct or not. Once the data have been approved by domain experts, they are annotated and stored in a database. Future runs of the test suite will generate new output data that should be compared with the approved data stored in the database. Discrepancies between the new and the approved data will be flagged as failures of the associated unit tests. This practice is also known as "*regression testing*," and it is particularly important because it closely verifies the correctness of the results produced by the system. Given the nature of some of the data, the resulting outputs may still have acceptable differences with the approved output. It is therefore necessary to set up comparison tools that involve a certain level of tolerance when comparing two instances of output data. A collection of annotated output data also must be maintained over the years, and must be updated when new data are added to the input collection. Occasionally, it will be found that modifications of the software require replacing an existing valid output with a new one to get a test to pass. This replacement should only be done after a careful verification that it is indeed the correct way of addressing the problem. Otherwise, it would be trivial to continuously fake all tests to pass by simply modifying the collection of validated output data, and thereby making the entire testing system pointless. Regression testing provides the most benefit to the development team when it is executed on a regular basis. Preferably, it should be run on an hourly basis and in the worst case on a daily basis. To reach such frequency of execution, an appropriate infrastructure must be put in place for running the tests automatically or at least with minimal human intervention.

An infrastructure for running tests may appear as a simple convenience but, in practice, it is an absolute necessity, given that the number of tests for a software system can easily reach the hundreds, and it is not uncommon for it to reach the thousands. Expecting developers to run the tests manually is unrealistic, and will simply result in the testing process being ignored. The infrastructure does not have to be too sophisticated. In its simplest form, it may be a shell script that contains the names of the tests and their list of parameters, including sources of input data and destinations for output data. It also may take more complete forms, such as the CTest module of CMake [CMake] or the Junit [JUnit]. These testing frameworks simplify the task of dealing with hundreds of tests and the intricacies of their multiple input and output parameters.

An infrastructure for summarizing results is needed for presenting the output of hundreds or even thousands of tests in a concise manner. As a test suite reaches its appropriate size, it is important to be able to count on a scalable system that can keep up with a larger number of tests, yet still be usable enough to encourage developers to run the test suite as a friendly development companion. Examples of such infrastructures are the Dart quality dashboard [Dart] and JUnit [JUnit].

One important feature in these infrastructures is the capability to track the state of a test over time and associate it to changes in the code. The purpose of such a linkage is that once a developers notice that a test is failing, it is important to identify when it started to fail. By answering the "when" question, the developer will arrive at the date when changes happened in the source code repository, and in this way it will be possible to answer the question of "who" made the changes. With the "when" and the "who," it becomes possible to answer the question of "why" the changes in the source code resulted in a failure of the associated test, and the developer will be a step closer to solving the problem.

This hypothetical scenario also reveals some weaknesses in software development management. In particular, it raises the question as to why the developer who introduced the change and produced the test failure in the first place did not notice that the test was failing. Three possible answers come to mind: (a) the developer did not run the test suite; (b) the developers did not monitor the summarizing infrastructure; or (c) the failure was the result of a combination of two apparently unrelated changes.

Good unit tests must be written with the intention of making the software fail, by exercising it under a variety of conditions likely to cause failure. If, despite the efforts made in the test, the software unit still passes the test, then the test is significant. In other words, a test is as significant (strong) as its effort in making the software fail. One aspect of this test strength is the code coverage.

5.2.4.3 Code Coverage

The code coverage is the percentage of lines of code from the software unit that are exercised in a test. A test that exercises only 27% of the lines of code from a software unit is not as significant as one that exercises 85% of the lines of code. One of the common difficulties in reaching a 100% code coverage is the fact that a certain portion of lines of code are intended for managing error conditions, but it is difficult to create some of the error conditions artificially. This difficulty can be addressed by a combination of two techniques. One technique is to use an architectural design for error management that allows building error conditions into the logic of the software units, instead of having them scattered as occasional *if* conditions and *assertions* all over the code. The other is to use input simulators, which will produce the appropriate offending input that will exercise the error management code.

Code coverage percentage has the unusual property of being exponentially hard to increase. That is, increasing the code coverage by 5% from 90% to 95% can be twice as hard as increasing it from 85% to 90%. Many systems can easily reach 70% of code coverage, and with adequate discipline can raise it to 80%. Levels of code coverage in the range of 90–100% are still only reached by the strict application of specific programming techniques that avoid the creation of *"hard to test"* pockets of code. Some of these techniques are discussed in Section 5.3. Higher levels of code coverage can be reached with more ease when developers consciously integrate the notion of testing into the hourly activity of software development, in particular, by incrementally developing the tests as the software is being written.

5.2.4.4 Application Testing

If unit testing appears to be a monumental task, application testing presents even larger difficulties. In unit testing, developers have the advantage of having most of the testing conditions under control, particularly in eliminating the need for external inputs from users or from hardware devices. In the case of application testing, developers are faced with the challenge of having a complex system exposed to a large variety of inputs from different sources. Automating this task is of utmost importance, or the test suite will not be run sufficiently often to provide an effective defect detection system.

One of the common challenges of application testing is how to simulate the interactions of a user with a graphical user interface (GUI), that is, being able to simulate a user actually clicking on the buttons and moving the sliders in the application. Several methods are commonly used to address this problem. Some applications provide tracking for the events of their own GUI and allow replaying of these events as a simulated session. This approach requires intercepting and customizing the event loop of the application. Other applications intercept the GUI events at the level of the operating system and also replay them as a simulated session. The first approach has the disadvantage that the replay sessions are always tested at a layer that is one level below the actual GUI code. The second approach has the disadvantage of being platform specific.

5.2.4.5 Level of Testing

The level of testing that must be exercised in an application should commensurate with the complexity of the application and the level of risk it presents to the patient. More thorough test suites and reviews are expected to be applied to aspects of the medical device that present the higher risk to the patient. More complete tests should also be used for validating the more complex aspects of the applications.

5.2.4.6 Independent Reviews

Software developers are well qualified to perform unit testing, but not application-wide testing. This is because developers form a mental framework of the application, which influences them to use software applications in ways that they know are the most stable. It is a common mistake for software developers to "*test*" their applications by running them through well-known sequences of interactions. Those sequences, of course, end up being the ones that work the best and are more reliable. When the applications are tested by users who are unaware of the implementation details, they will interact with the applications using paths that were never anticipated by the developers.

This fundamental difference in how users interact with the application makes the test more valuable when it is performed by a team that is independent of the development team. It is important to establish communication mechanisms between the testing team and the development team that will not interfere with their independence over time. For example, developers should avoid explaining to the testing team that the behavior of the application is actually the result of a particular software implementation technique. Their conversation should be limited to the visible behavioral aspects of the software, so that the testing team performs as closely as possible to the end users of the final system.

5.2.4.7 Performance

There are several measures of performance that are applicable to software. These measures are sometimes contradictory and may require the development team to evaluate trade-offs and establish some compromises. The typical measures are run time speed, memory requirements, mathematical precision, robustness, and repeatability. Speed and memory form a typical pair of performance measures that are difficult to improve simultaneously. Many of the techniques used for reducing memory consumption result in an increase of computation time, and vice versa.

Mathematical precision and computation time form another pair that is difficult to optimize simultaneously. In many cases, it is necessary to refer to the system requirement to find guidelines that will allow finding the appropriate compromise between two performance measures.

Computation time and mathematical precision are easily measured by the testing infrastructure without requiring sophisticated tools. There are, however, cases where profiling tools are needed. Commonly used tools are GNU **gprof** in Unix systems [GNU 1998] and **VTune** in systems based on Intel processors [VTune].

Measurements of memory usage are harder to collect and usually require the software to have a built-in mechanism for quantifying its memory usage. This is typically done by implementing memory allocation as a service provided by a customized software routine or class. This customized service integrates book-keeping capabilities that report on the memory usage at different stages of the program execution. Such built-in mech-anisms are also helpful for detecting and preventing memory leaks.

An important rule of performance analysis is to make sure that metrics are generated from well-defined tests, which can be repeated consistently. In general, it is desirable to integrate such tests with the daily test suite of the system. Unfortunately, performance tests usually require longer computation times, and may force developers to run these specific tests on a lower frequency basis, for example, weekly or biweekly. Postponing tests is a decision that must be taken with careful consideration, because the time interval between two tests also becomes the response time for detecting serious defects. This is important because the longer a defect is allowed to exist in the system, the harder it becomes to fix. Developers will have to put a lot more effort in just tracking the problem back to the original source, and then finding a fix that does not conflict with the myriad of other changes that have been inserted for other reasons during the same period of time.

5.2.5 Bug Tracking

Given the inherent complexity of software, it is expected that a large number of defects are always latent in the code. They may be the result of misunderstood specifications, flawed programming techniques, lack of synchronization in API changes, and unintended lateral effects from other changes, among many other situations. It is extremely hard to find all defects in a piece of software, which makes it very important to ensure that whenever a suspicious behavior is observed, its appearance is recorded so that it can be thoroughly investigated.

A suspicious behavior can be a manifestation of a software defect. Registering the circumstances that led to the observation of the suspicious behavior in a database is a good mechanism for making sure that the testing team and the developing team will investigate further, and to make sure that if a defect is present, it is characterized and fixed.

Database systems for tracking software defects are usually called "*bug trackers.*" There are many of them to choose from, both as commercial products and as open source software. It is important, however, when developing software that is to be submitted for approval to a regulatory agency such as the FDA, to use bug tracking software that satisfies the same requirements of all software used for supporting the manufacturing of medical devices. In particular, a bug tracker must satisfy the guidelines of the Code of Federal Regulations 21 CFR Part 11, which relates to the management of electronic records and electronic signatures. The rules are intended to formalize the procedures for keeping electronic records in such a way that their authenticity, integrity, and security are guaranteed. One fundamental aspect of these guidelines is to make sure there is accountability in the system. That is, that any modification made to an entry in the bug database can be traced back to a specific user, at a specific date, and can have an annotation describing a justification for the change. More details on the regulations regarding electronic records can be found at FDA [2000].

In the context of developing software for a medical device, a bug tracking database is expected to guarantee that when defects are found in the software, they are reported and fully tracked through the process discussed among the developers and then fixed. Those fixes should then be tested to make sure that they do not introduce further defects in other sections of the code. Bug tracking databases that satisfy 21 CFR Part 11 should provide industry standard mechanisms for secure login of users, and must define roles for those users. For example, developers are allowed to enter additional information in a bug report, but they are not allowed to delete a bug. Developers should not be allowed to mark a bug as resolved, and only a verification provided by the testing team should lead to labeling a bug entry as a solved problem.

As with other procedures, the FDA does not enforce a particular mechanism for managing bug tracking. Instead, it expects manufacturers to define documented procedures and to demonstrate that these procedures are followed. Precise rules must be defined on how to enter a new bug, review it, apply fixes to the code based on the discussion of a bug report, and finally to mark the bug as a solved problem.

The procedures for managing bug reports must also include how to receive reports from users of systems that are already deployed in the field. These user reports are particularly important, because the defects in question may already be affecting a large number of patients, and because they signal defects that escaped the quality controls of the manufacturing process, which indicates a breach in the quality control system itself.

During the life cycle of the software, the number of defects found during a given unit of time is expected to decrease, without ever reaching a null value. The decrease in the number and severity of identified bugs is sometimes used as a measure of how ready the product is to be released in the field.

5.2.6 Coding Style

When writing source code, developers have a lot of latitude regarding the ways they can arrange the variable names, function names, and names of classes, as well as the way they arrange specific elements of the language statements. The set of rules that defines those arrangements is the coding style. Since following their coding style increases their productivity, developers have strong feelings about sticking to their coding style and are very reluctant to adopt any other.

Encountering a familiar coding style greatly facilitates the developer's task of understanding what the source code is doing, and therefore is a key element in the long-term maintenance and evolution of the code. Using a consistent coding style across the software generates familiarity and makes it possible for future developers and maintainers to navigate effortlessly through different sections of the code.

The FDA guidelines document FOD# 938 states

> Firms frequently adopt specific coding guidelines that establish quality policies and procedures related to the software coding process. Source code should be evaluated to verify its compliance with specified coding guidelines. Such guidelines should include coding conventions regarding clarity, style, complexity management, and commenting. Code comments should provide useful and descriptive information for a module, including expected inputs and outputs, variables referenced, expected data types, and operations to be performed. Source code should also be evaluated to verify its compliance with the

corresponding detailed design specification. Modules ready for integration and testing should have documentation of compliance with coding guidelines and any other applicable quality policies and procedures.[FDA 2002]

The process of adopting a specific coding style has two main challenges: first, to get a group of developers and managers to agree on a specific set of rules, and second, to enforce these rules without impinging on the efficacy of the software development process. The first challenge can be better addressed when technical justifications are provided for specific coding style rules. Unfortunately, in many cases, developers are strongly accus-tomed to the coding style of previous projects where they may have worked, and tend to defend those styles with some passion.

The second challenge, that of enforcing the coding style once the rules have been defined, requires the introduction of automatic parsing and style verification tools. One of such tools is the open source application KWStyle [Kitware]. These tools can be configured to verify whether the source code complies or not with the coding style rules, and produces summaries of style violations in a format that make it easier for developers to fix the source code. The tools are very effective when used as check points of the process for committing code in the source code repositories. In this way, only the code that satisfies the coding style will enter the official version of the code. This mechanism, by being annoying to developers who do not abide by the coding rules, forces them to straighten their ways, because until they fix their code, they cannot put it in the repository. The alternative approach of performing a posteriori code reviews, and then requesting developers to fix functional code that has existed in the system for a long time, has a very mild chance of success.

Most text editors designed to facilitate code writing have options for helping developers follow a particular coding style. It is a good investment of time to customize the editors of all developers in the team. In this way, the coding style is applied in the most natural way, and simply becomes part of the daily activity of writing code. The less effort developers need to expend to bring the code to accepted coding style standards, the more likely they are to actually follow the rules.

5.2.7 Documentation

Software documentation should address two aspects. On one hand, it should provide information for future developers and maintainers regarding the technical details of the software, including the overall design and architectural choices, as well as the details of the particular programming techniques adopted for the implementation. On the other hand, there should be documentation addressed to the users of the system, explaining how the software is intended to be used. In the case of a medical device, this documentation ends up being merged with the general documentation of the device, and the software is not exposed as an individual component, but rather as an integral aspect of the interface that the medical device presents to the user.

As with the software itself, there are two stages to the process of producing documentation, beginning with the generation of the initial documentation that matches the first version of the software. This is followed by the stage of maintaining the documentation to update it with any changes or additions, including correcting any documentation mistakes that may have slipped through the quality control revisions of the first version.

The documentation intended for developers is more effective when it is scattered through the code in the form of meaningful and well-located comments. There are documentation tools such as Doxygen [Doxygen], Doc++ [Doc++], and JavaDoc [Sun Microsystems] that will parse the source code and collect these documentation comments in order to organize them and reformat them in the form of an HTML page, a Windows Help file, an RTF file, or a LaTeX file that can be converted to PostScript and PDF formats.

The task of maintaining documentation is complicated by the fact that there is no automatic way of ensuring that it matches the source code. After all, compilers will simply ignore the content of any comment added to the code. It is therefore quite easy to end up with source code that has evolved over the years and still carries comments introduced for the initial development, which no longer apply to the new state of the software. Such a situation makes the code very fragile to new modifications, because new developers will read the comments and judge how to further modify the code. Outdated comments will mislead the developers and will make them prone to introduce new bugs in the code.

The documentation to be presented to users passes through a more rigorous quality control, but it is still necessarily based on visual review by members of the team, making the documentation vulnerable to human error. Problems that users report regarding the documentation of the medical device are also to be managed as bugs and should be entered in the database, to make sure that they are solved in future releases of the product.

5.2.8 Refactoring

It is an accepted fact that the source code will never perfectly match the goals described in the requirements collection. The development team must continually introduce changes in the system to bring it closer to the requirements contained in the specification. Many of these changes may be small and well-localized modifications. On other occasions, however, it may be found that a major overhaul of the software is needed to fix a mismatch between the expected behavior of the software and the actual set of functionalities that it currently provides. In those cases, the developers must return to the design board and plan a new structure that will be more appropriate for addressing the requirements. They must also plan a strategy for replacing the old code with the new code. This pair of actions is also known as "*refactoring*" and is an integral part of the software life cycle. Neglecting the need for occasional refactoring is a denial of the ever-changing nature of software and of the complexity of satisfying a large set of requirements, with software implementation in just the initial pass.

The process of refactoring must be followed by a validation of the system, to make sure that all tests work as earlier. The refactoring may indeed require the addition of new tests to cover pieces of source code that have been added as part of the refactoring effort. FDA guidelines require that a design review should be performed before the team engages in implementing a refactoring process. The purpose of the design review is to make sure that the modifications are consistent with the operation of other parts of the software and that there will be a documented trail of why these changes were necessary.

5.2.9 Backward Compatibility Versus Evolution

The need for continuously modifying pieces of the software brings the challenge of how to isolate these changes from other pieces of the code, that is, preventing the changes from propagating through the entire code base. This is particularly important when the software has been organized into multiple libraries or modules that are then used by the final application. When the source code of one of the libraries changes, it may require changes to be propagated to the application. In most cases, when a new version of the application is being developed, the team will usually try to take advantage of the occasion for also updating the many libraries that the application depends upon. This desire is motivated by the expectation that the version of those libraries may have bug fixes for defects existing in previous versions. When the team updates the version of the libraries, they may find that the application programming interface (API) of the library has changed. Functions may have been deprecated, or renamed classes may have been replaced with new ones. This rupture of the API prevents the library from being "*backwards compatible*," meaning that the new library cannot be used directly with software that was using the previous version of the library.

It is usually an expensive task to modify an application to fix the backward compatibility deficiencies of a library. In most cases, this is expensive because the libraries fail to provide easy mechanisms for letting developers know about the API changes, and, in particular, teach them about the "*new ways*" of doing things. Developers discover the API changes by simply encountering compiler and linker errors while they are building the software.

The most dangerous scenario of API changes is when the modifications are not reflected in the syntax of the software, but in the semantics. That is, when the application will still compile and link with the new version of the library, but at run time, the new version behaves differently from the previous version. In these cases, the developers rely entirely on the capacity of their testing and validation system to catch the misbehaviors of the software, so that it can be fixed before it is deployed in the field.

Developers of libraries try, in general, to maintain backwards compatibility, but this is not always possible. Sometimes the old API is inappropriate, or it is so misleading that it can easily induce developers to misuse the software. In such cases, breaking the API has actually a healthy benefit. What is important to avoid is the introduction of capricious changes, or minor modifications that are not justified by major technical benefits. Developer teams that follow FDA guidelines will usually avoid such a situation by having to justify the source code changes in terms of how they address new or established requirements, which have been discussed during design reviews. Maintaining backwards compatibility at "*any price*" is not a healthy behavior either, because it can lead developers to provide functionalities in awkward ways that lead to confusion and misuse of the software.

Finding the appropriate balance between stability and evolution of the software is not a trivial task. In the context of IGI applications, it is usually better to err on the conservative side, and to always provide solid justifycations for introducing changes in the code.

5.3   Design

Design is a fundamental aspect of software development. It defines the essential characteristics of the software, and it provides guidelines for the duration of the software development effort. The design process is initiated by the collection of requirements based on the final application scenarios of the software and the constraints of its expected use.

5.3.1 Safety by Design

Safety is the most fundamental characteristic to be cultivated in software intended to be used in the domain of image-guided interventions. Design methodologies suitable for fostering the safety levels of the final application must be adopted early on in any IGI project. One of such methodologies is known as "*safety by design*," which encompasses the use of design decisions that remove risk opportunities from the features of the software.

Safety by design blends methodologies at multiple different levels; some of which are related to the high-level architecture of the software, while others are related to specific programming techniques, and even to the basic coding style. The fundamental ideas of safety by design are applied to everyday products such as child-proof caps for prescription medication, asymmetrical shape design for electronic connections to prevent users from connecting cables in wrong polarities, and electrical devices that auto-matically turn off when they are open.

Examples of safety-by-design techniques that are commonly used in C++ programming are the following:

1. Replacing pointer with references in arguments of functions
2. Using const-correctness in the API of functions
3. Using unsigned types whenever no negative values are expected
4. Enforcing the initialization of variables before they can be used
5. Enforcing encapsulation by using private members
6. Avoiding duplication of data, because it usually leads to inconsistent copies
7. Constructing hierarchical modules that expose only the minimal elements to their API
8. Whenever two or more concepts must be consistent, then they are grouped in a single class where their consistency can be enforced
9. Verifying versions of dependent libraries before using them

Safety by design is an extremely useful and effective tool in IGI software, because it removes the risk before it can be introduced in the software. Any amount of effort that can be invested in safer design will pay off by removing the burden of the need to perform testing and validation. By simply making it impossible to take wrong actions, it becomes unnecessary to test for wrong results.

In most cases, safety by design comes down to removing unnecessary "*flexibility*" from the system. The more restrictive is the software interface, the lower the risk it offers to users. There is, of course, a balance to be found between minimizing the flexibility of the system while still providing the functionalities that are specified in the requirements.

5.3.2 Architecture

Given the ease with which software code can be modified, it is very important to have an architectural structure that will give shape to the overall software development effort. This overall architecture should be suitable to accommodate the evolution of the software as it progresses through its life cycle. That is, it must acknowledge the elemental fact that software is never completed and is subject to continuous change. The architecture must address the long-time expectancy of the software by creating a structure that is easy to maintain, refactor, and extend. Nearsighted architectures that do not take the evolvement of the software into account force future developers and maintainers of the software to add inconsistent patches, and to graft additional functionalities that do not harmonize with the rest of the system.

The more these patches are added, the more the system will degrade over time, and the easier it will become for maintainers to introduce defects in the system as the result of unintended lateral effects of requested modifications.

Identifying the elements of the system that are, and are not, expected to evolve requires extensions and is one of the most important tasks of the architectural design. The elements that are not to be changed are locked down using safety-by-design techniques, and the elements that are expected to be added are designed in a modular fashion, which will facilitate the addition of many different modules in the future.

In the context of IGI, the architecture should account for the many different image modalities that are used for carrying image data, the many different types of tracking devices in the market, and the new devices to come. The architecture also should account for the management of patient information to ensure that data from one patient are not accidentally used for another patient.

The architecture of an IGI system should also define a safe mechanism for moving information between the different components of the system in such a way that the components are as decoupled as possible from one another. Using *events* as information carriers is one such technique, but certainly not the only one.

A safe architecture for IGI should also incorporate somehow the notion of the workflow of the intervention. This may be done by introducing state machines, or workflow support classes such as Petri nets. It also can be done by simply using state diagrams as part of the architectural design tools of each one of the components of the system, and later as part of the user–system interaction design. By formalizing and enforcing the order in which actions are to be performed in the system, much of the risk is removed and a variety of potential software defects are avoided.

5.3.3 *User Interaction*

The FDA guidelines document (FOD# 938) states

> The software design needs to address human factors. Use error caused by designs that are either overly complex or contrary to users' intuitive expectations for operation is one of the most persistent and critical problems encountered by FDA. Frequently, the design of the software is a factor in such use errors. Human factors engineering should be woven into the entire design and development process, including the device design requirements, analyses, and tests. [FDA 2002]

One of the most remarkable success stories of safety record improvements in the area of surgery is that of anesthesiology. Starting in the 1980s, the FDA and the American Association of Anesthesiologists (ASA) and equipment manufacturers analyzed videos of the interaction between the anesthesiologist and the equipment used in surgery. A surprising number of fundamental issues were found in that study. For example, some manufacturers provide dials that increase dosages by turning clockwise, while others increase dose by turning the dials counterclockwise. When an anesthesiologist went from one intervention, using one type of equipment, to another surgical suite, where a different type of equipment was present, it was very easy to move the dial in the wrong direction, simply due to the inconsistency of the user interaction.

Another area where the standardization of user interface improves the safety of users is the design of automobile dashboards. There are very small variations in the distribution and form of interaction of the pedals and levers found in most modern automobiles. It is easier to imagine the catastrophic consequences resulting from a car manufacturer exchanging the position of the accelerator pedal and the brake pedal in a car.

These simple aspects of user interaction are an essential element of the design of an image-guided surgery software application.

5.3.4 Keeping It Simple

Minimizing the number of features helps to reduce risk in the software. The practice of focusing on satisfying the specification requirements is one mechanism for making sure that only necessary features are included in the software. When implementing those features and designing the interactions that the user will have with the system, simplicity is of paramount importance. Offering a simple and natural interaction to the user will reduce the opportunities for the user to become confused and unintentionally taking incorrect actions.

Users of an image-guided intervention system will interact with the system under preexisting conditions of pressure and stress. They may do so also in conditions of fatigue and haste, since it is not unusual for surgical interventions to take many hours. Given such conditions, the simplicity of the system and its user interface become an important asset for preventing users from misusing the system.

Designing a user interface is not a trivial task, and in general it should not be left to engineers. This is as unwise as hiring a civil engineer to design a house, instead of hiring an architect. The user interface must be designed by team members with experience in the management of human factors, and in collaboration with the final users of the system. The interactions must ultimately be very intuitive to the final users.

One of the mechanisms that can be used to simplify the user interface is to map the workflow of the surgical intervention into the IGI software application itself. In this way, at every given stage of the intervention, the application will only expose the aspects that are relevant to that particular stage. For example, if the intervention requires an initial stage where optical trackers are calibrated and a subsequent stage where a tracked instrument is presented in a 3D display, then in the first stage the system will present in its user interface only the widgets associated with options relevant to the calibration procedure. Once the user determines that the calibration has been completed, then the system will move to the tracking stage and replace all those widgets in the user interface with new widgets that are now relevant to the instrument tracking stage. By selectively presenting only the GUI items relevant to a specific stage of the surgery, it is possible to avoid cluttering the user interface with too many widgets, and it becomes easier to present a simplified set of interactions containing options that are intuitive to users.

It is unlikely that a natural interface could be designed in a single pass, without observing the users interacting with the system, studying their behavior, and listening to their feedback. Developers of IGI software should take any opportunity to observe how a surgical intervention progresses. Witnessing the environment and the behavior of the clinical team in the surgery room provides much valuable insight into how the software application may make things easier for users.

5.3.5 Risk Analysis

The safety-critical nature of IGI applications requires the software team to develop a risk-based mentality. This involves continuously considering what can go wrong in the use of the application, and continuously introducing software elements that will prevent an adverse event from happening. These elements can be taken from safety-by-design principles or from safe programming techniques such as defensive programming. The FDA guidelines emphasize the recommendation that risk analysis should not be left as a final step of the revision of a software application. Instead, risk analysis is a continuous task that must be integrated in the day-to-day activities of the design, development, and testing teams.

Risk analysis, unfortunately, is not part of the standard education of software engineers or researchers, who usually make up most of the IGI team. It is therefore important to introduce them to the notion that even seemingly innocuous pieces of source code may result in catastrophic events when they are left unchecked. A very effective way of training developers in the concepts of risk analysis is to show them case studies of previous adverse events for which software has been identified to be responsible. Many of these events show that the problems are caused by rather small design flaws or small implementation oversights. In many of these cases, the decisions made during the design and implementation seem to make sense, but simply failed to have a more continuous and ubiquitous application of the question: *"what can go wrong with this section of source code."* Developers are very result oriented and therefore tend to think in terms of how to produce the source code that will achieve a result. In the context of IGI, however, the task is focused on producing source code that will not result in any adverse event.

There are formal methods for risk analysis that have been used over the years in fields such as aeronautics and nuclear power generation. One of these methods is Probabilistic Risk Analysis (PRA). In this methodology, risk is characterized by two metrics: the magnitude and the likelihood. The magnitude is the severity of the possible adverse consequences, and the likelihood is the probability of occurrence of each consequence. Two specific methodologies that are commonly used are Failure Mode and Effect Analysis (FMEA), and Fault Tree Analysis (FTA). In FMEA, the system is first described in a block diagram and then the team analyzes what happens if each block of the diagram fails. Then a table is created pairing the failures and their effects. Based on this table, corrective or mitigating actions are taken in the design and implementation of the system, and the risk analysis table is updated. The process is repeated until the remaining risk is considered to be acceptable. In FTA, an undesired event is placed at the top of an analysis tree. An example would be confusing the left and right sides of the patient, an event that, unfortunately, still accounts for 2% of the adverse events reported in US hospitals. Using FTA, a tree is drawn by capturing the logic of all the elements that may lead to the occurrence of the wrong event. Branches of the tree contain Boolean operators (AND, OR), and the leaves of the tree are potential faults in the system.

These analysis techniques are important at the high level of the implementation of an IGI system, but they are ineffective if they are not accompanied by a risk-awareness indoctrination of the design and development team. Given the complexity of software, and the ease with which a single weak statement of source code can propagate and produce catastrophic results, it is unlikely that a top-level analysis alone can reveal all potential risk situations. A team of conscientious developers, on the other hand, have a much better chance of hardening the system at every line of code.

Note that this is not to discredit formal risk analysis techniques. On the contrary, the point to be made here is that risk analysis must permeate the entire design, implementation, and maintenance process for it to be effective. That involves a combination of high-level risk analysis, and day-to-day risk awareness in the actions of the team developing an IGI system.

5.3.6 State Machines

Computers *are* state machines. Unfortunately, their state is defined by a large number of variables that include among others: the content of their main RAM memory, the values of the registers in the microprocessor(s), and the state of registers in their IO devices. This large number of variables makes it impractical to model the computer as a state machine. Any software program running in a computer is also a state machine, but with a much smaller set of state variables. When conventional programming techniques are used, the state of the program is largely distributed across many different sections of the code in many different variables. In this condition again, despite the fact that the program is a state machine, it becomes intractable in practice. A large number of behavioral disorders exhibited by software applications are the consequence of disregarding their state machine nature.

In procedural programming, for example, the state-base nature of the program is almost completely ignored, mostly because of the assumption that the program is executed only once in a mostly linear pattern. In object-oriented programming on the other hand, the state-based nature of software is much better represented, thanks to the use of member variables that represent the state of a class. Object-oriented programming, combined with event-based architectures, is one of the best fits for designing and implementing applications that offer a GUI, and that continuously interact with a user. Applications of this type typically have an idle cycle in which they are waiting for the user to make choices. Once the user selects options in the user interface, the application executes the corresponding actions, produces result for the user, and returns to the state of waiting for further user requests. Software applications intended for image-guided interventions largely fall in this category of GUI applications. The application itself, at the highest level, can be modeled as a state machine where the inputs are provided by user interactions. Depending on the current state of the application, different actions may be taken in response to the user request, and the application will move into a different final state. Modeling the entire application as a state machine facilitates the achievement of two goals; first to fully specify what the program should do in response to every possible request, and second to prevent certain logical paths from becoming available to the user. In the first aspect, the state machine model of the application ensures that all the functional requirements are addressed. In the second aspect, the state machine model facilitates implementation of the preventive actions resulting from the risk analysis of the application. Both of these qualities are so important in an IGI application that the use of state machines modeling should be considered a fundamental feature in this domain.

State machine modeling is a standard methodology in almost all safety-critical applications, and in most embedded system applications. There are multiple levels at which the state machine paradigm can be applied to the design and implementation of the software. At a very high level, the design team can simply use state diagrams, such as those specified in UML, for supporting and facilitating the design tasks. This is a great help for ensuring that all required behaviors of the system are addressed, and that the system does not skip any stages before engaging in a particular process. The design can then be implemented using traditional object-oriented methodologies without explicitly representing the state machine concept at the software level. This approach has the disadvantage that it is very easy to fail to map the state diagram design into the implementation, and discovering where the mapping is faulty becomes an arduous debugging task.

A more complete approach is to use state diagrams in the design phase, and also to use explicit state machine modeling in the implementation phase of the code. In particular, this can be done by creating specific classes that represent the state machine abstraction, which explicitly map the actions of the state machine into class methods, and the states of the state machine into class variables. This approach greatly simplifies the mapping between the top-level design of the application and the actual implementation of the source code.

The mapping between design and implementation can be verified further by incorporating in the state machine class the ability to export its own state diagram. In this way, the design and development teams can compare the state machine programming that was actually implemented against the intended state diagram produced during the design phase.

The concept of state machine programming can be brought further to the level of every individual class of the application. The purpose of propagating the state machine modeling to the smaller granularity of the source code is that the top-level components are as safe and as predictable as the combination of its elemental components. If a top-level action of the IGI application is executed in practice by a conglomerate of 10 or 20 class instances, then the possibilities for failure of that top-level action are the nonlinear combinations of the possible failures of every single elemental component.

By explicitly defining state diagrams for the behavior of every component of an IGI application, and mapping that design in the form of a state machine at the coding level, it becomes possible to restrict and control the behavior of the specific component, and therefore the global behavior of the IGI application.

Applying a state machine paradigm facilitates the unit testing of the basic classes, because specific paths of the state diagram can be evaluated as usual test cases. The order in which operations of a class must be executed can also be enforced when a state machine programming approach is used. This prevents one of the common causes of software failure, which is the assumption made by developers that the methods of a class will be invoked in a particular order. In practice, however, interactive applications can easily invoke class methods in orders that were not anticipated by developers, which can easily result in incorrect behaviors due to variables being set incorrectly.

From the point of view of testing, one of the major advantages of using the state machine approach is that the logic of the classes is concentrated in a single location: the transition matrix of the state machine. This concentration of the logic makes it easier to test the software up to 100% code coverage, because there is a minimal amount of branching logic scattered across the code. When state machines are implemented correctly, the typical conditional statements are removed from the code and brought in the form of transitions logical to the state machine. This process of concentrating the logic also involves incorporating the management of error conditions in the state diagram just as normal transitions, instead of managing them as exceptional events. By explicitly spelling out the expected error conditions and explicitly addressing the appropriate actions that must be executed in response, the code becomes robust in a very natural way. The reactions to error events, in this case, can be fully tested and verified. This is very different from what happens in traditional object-oriented programming where errors are managed as exceptions, or have to be carried along as conditional statements and are rarely tested.

State machines, however, do not come without a price. In practice, the hardest aspect of using this programming methodology is in the training of developers. When developers who are accustomed to traditional procedural programming and traditional object-oriented programming start developing a state machine paradigm, they find it frustrating to be unable to write the free-style code with which they are familiar. When engaging in an IGI project, it is important to properly train developers in programming techniques adapted for the application. Given a properly trained team, mapping state machine diagrams from design to the implementation should be a straightforward task. Whenever the state machine implementation seems difficult, this is an indication of a design or an implementation flaw, most likely due to misrepresenting the circumstances of the problem into a state diagram paradigm.

State machines are not the only programming methodology that can bring to the code the benefits of explicitly stating the logic, and explicitly incorporating the management of error conditions. Other technique models such as Petri Nets can also be used to achieve similar purposes.

5.3.6.1 Guidance for Critical Applications

State machines are a natural fit for critical applications, because they avoid implicit assumptions on the state and behaviors of the code. The sequence of design, implementation, and validation can be expressed in the common language of state diagrams, where every possible input to the system and every system response are defined explicitly.

Following the behavior of the system at run time also becomes easier, as it results in having the state machine report their transitions into a logging system, which can be analyzed retrospectively to compare the actual unfolding of the surgical intervention against the sequences that were anticipated during the design stages.

An additional advantage of state machine programming is that it simplifies the serialization of the elemental classes and the serialization of the application as a whole, reducing the process into serializing the state variables of each one of the state machines in the system. Restoring the state of the system from the serialized version means recreating all class instances and recovering the values of all their state variables. This, although not a trivial task, is certainly a lot easier than when state machine programing is not used.

The capability of restoring a system after a failure is extremely important in critical applications, and certainly in IGI. A typical scenario is an accidental power-down of the computer that is running an IGI application. The system should be able to resume the task it was performing before the power failure, or come very close to it. The property of failure recovery is simply an acknowledgment that, regardless of how much care is exerted to make the system failure free, circumstances will occur that are outside the control of the system, and therefore it is desirable to be able to gracefully recover from such events. As with any other property of a software system, the behavior of failure recovery must be tested and validated often to ensure it is performing as expected.

5.3.6.2 Multi-Threading

The user interactive nature of most IGI applications requires that the application should always be responsive to user input. This conflicts with the need of the application to be simultaneously performing the actions that the user may have requested. A common mechanism for addressing this conflict is the use of multiple threads. Another common mechanism is to design the application to be executed as multiple collaborating processes. In either case, the basic concept is that two or more tasks are being executed simultaneously and that data is being passed between them.

One of the challenges in using multiple threads is to ensure that they do not attempt to write simultaneously in the same variables. This is usually prevented by using mutual exclusion mechanisms. Open source toolkits such as ITK [ITK], VTK [VTK], and IGSTK [IGSTK] offer basic classes for managing multiple threads and mutual exclusion guards. These mechanisms have been perfected to work in multiple different platforms. The drawback of mutual exclusion is that it takes a toll in computing time, and therefore, it should not be used in operations that are performed at high frequencies.

In the context of state machines, it is a natural fit to have different state machines running in different threads or in different processes. The communication between multiple state machines must cross the different threads or process boundaries. This can be done in multiple ways, but usually involves defining shared sections where events are sent from one state machine and translated into inputs to another state machine. When using multiple threads, this can be done by implementing "request" methods in the classes based on state machines, and having these request methods translate the request into an input to the state machine. The input is pushed out to a queue of inputs under the control of mutual exclusion guards. In this way, the input queue becomes the communication mechanism in the frontier between two different threads.

Another implementation option is to use pipes to implement the queue of state machine inputs. In this option, there is no need to use mutual exclusion guards, because the operating system level functions will manage the alternative access to the pipes. This implementation mechanism is also an option when the state machines are set into different processes instead of different threads.

Regardless of the implementation mechanism, the introduction of multiple threads or multiple processes may result in deadlock situations. Since these situations are the result of systemwide interactions, they cannot be prevented at the level of individual software components. Instead, this is usually addressed by analysis tools that can explore the interaction between multiple components. This type of analysis, also known as concurrency analysis, is a standard practice in the domain of embedded systems, and several software tools are available for addressing it.

Concurrency problems are rarely caught by testing frameworks because they appear only under very specific and unusual timing conditions. A design level analysis of the interactions between multiple state machine classes is the only way to clear out the possibility of deadlock situations appearing at run time.

5.3.6.3 Real Time

The term "*real time*" is commonly misused to express the notion that a system responds at interactive rates with its input. The formal meaning of real time actually corresponds to the property of a system offering guaranteed response times. These times are not necessarily short, but the value is the fact they are guaranteed. A real-time system incorporates two types of processes: first it has processes that are guaranteed to finish in a given time; second, it has processes that are interruptible. By combining these two types of processes, a real-time system can schedule the execution of these processes to ensure that certain actions will be executed with a given periodicity subject to a limited tolerance.

In the context of an IGI system, the notions of real time are relevant when it comes to ensuring that clinicians will receive data from the system at a given rate. For example, during a particular stage of the intervention, the system should be refreshing the display of the surgical scene at a frequency of 30 Hz, while simultaneously gathering input from an optical tracker at a frequency of 10 Hz. To guarantee that both actions, along with all the necessary intermediate computations, are kept at the claimed rates, the operating system may need to ensure that the program is not going to be delayed because of some input/output operation, or because of the execution of other background tasks. Real-time IGI systems must be implemented on a real-time operating system, with the operating system scheduler ensuring that the different processes receive processor time at the rate they require.

Systems that have been implemented using state machine programming are well suited to be ported to a real-time implementation. The most direct way of doing so is by running every instance of a state machine as an operating system process, and to use operating system queues as the communication mechanism between different state machine classes. In this context, for example, a class instance that manages an optical tracker device will run as process A, while the class instance that manages the display will run as process B. Information about the position of a tracked surgical instrument will be produced by process A and push into a queue that process B can read.

Most IGI systems, in practice, are not run on top of real-time operating systems. This is an unfortunate choice in the IGI field, where confidence is placed on the high speed of modern computers. The availability of open source versions of real-time operating systems makes it difficult to justify this choice of IGI developers. Hopefully this trend will change in the near future, as common platforms for performing IGI are adopted by the larger research and clinical communities.

5.3.7 Devices

IGI systems usually integrate a number of different hardware devices such as trackers, pedals, touch screens, video, and audio. The challenge in integrating many different devices must be addressed with modular architectures that facilitate replacing one device with another.

5.3.7.1 Trackers (Software Aspects)

Despite the fact that IGI stands for "*image-guided interventions*," the reality of the field is that much of it depends on tracking surgical instruments and fiducials placed on the patient. Tracking is performed by different types of physical devices connected to the system. Interfacing with the many different tracking devices available in the market is a challenge that IGI systems should address. In particular, it should be considered that the life expectancy of software is 5–10 times longer than the life expectancy of hardware. In such conditions, most of the tracking devices commonly used today probably will be replaced in the next 5 years. This means that the architecture of IGI systems should account for easy ways of replacing the modules that interface with tracking devices. This will make it relatively easy to extend an existing IGI system to use any new tracking device that appears in the market.

Manufacturers of tracking devices have had the good judgment to offer open interfaces to their products, and most of them are based on interface connections through serial RS-232, USB, and Ethernet links. This makes it very easy for developers of IGI systems to interface with many different tracking devices.

5.3.7.2 Screens

The most common output of an IGI system is a graphical display on a screen. This is not necessarily the only output that a system should produce, but in practice it is what is most commonly presented to the clinician. This in part is due to the fact that the IGI system is intended to provide additional helpful information to the surgeon, without intending to remove control from the physician. In addition to graphic displays, one can easily imagine that audio alarms might be helpful for indicating exceptional conditions, such as the loss of signal from a tracker or the failure to register a set of fiducials to a preoperative image.

Since the graphic display is the most common output presented to the clinician, and sometimes it is the *only* output of the IGI system, a great deal of attention must be dedicated to its design and its validation. First of all, the graphic display must be designed in close collaboration with the clinician and by continuously considering the workflow of the intervention. The surgeon, being the ultimate user of the graphic display, should find it intuitive, clear, and informative. Developers, on the other hand, may tend to overload displays with graphic features, especially if they have a back-ground in computer graphics or image processing. The graphic display must be a complement to the mental picture that the surgeon maintains of the clinical scene. The closest the display matches that mental picture, the more direct will be the benefit to the surgeon, and therefore to the patient. In particular, a graphic display should avoid forcing the surgeon to go through the continuous mental exercise of converting or translating information. For example, if the surgeon is used to thinking about the position of the surgical instrument from his visual perspective, and not from the perspective of an anatomical coordinate system, then the display should match the surgeon's perspective. Design decisions are hard to generalize and they will strongly depend on the type of surgical intervention, and even the particular stage of the workflow in the intervention. Gathering feedback from clinicians and encouraging developers to attend surgical interventions is the best way to bridge the communication gap between the surgical world of the clinician and the computer graphics world of the software developers.

5.3.8 Realism Versus Informative Display

It is a common mistake on the part of developers to introduce advanced graphics into IGI systems. Good-looking displays are not necessarily informative and can distract the attention of the development team from the essential features of the system. Many times, the surgeon will greatly benefit from summarized information that the IGI system can easily compute and display in simple line diagrams. The same information when presented in an impressive volume rendering display may be ambiguous and distractive. For example, in a needle biopsy application, one of the most important pieces of information that the surgeon needs is the distance between the tip of the needle and the target inside the patient. Although it can be claimed that this information could be derived from a 3D graphic display of the surgical instrument and the anatomical target, in practice such a display will have the ambiguity of the scale, perspective projection, and the orientation of the screen plane with respect to the axis of the needle. In this case, an IGI system can be more informative by explicitly displaying a graduated bar on the screen that indicates the distance between the tip of the needle and the target.

A view of the typical instruments found in the dashboard of an airplane provides insight into how the aeronautical industry has provided easy-to-use information for pilots. For example, the altitude position of an aircraft is displayed by a minimalist drawing of a plane with a set of reference lines that indicate the horizon.

The IGI field can learn from the experience of the aeronautical and automotive industries, which have succeeded in creating a communication link between the user and the system, where the system becomes abstracted in the mind of the user. In that ideal situation, navigation becomes intuitive, and this is the goal that software developers should strive to attain.

References

CMake. "CMake Cross Platform Make." <http://www.cmake.org/HTML/Index.html> (October 15, 2007).

Dart. "Dart: Tests, Reports, and Dashboards." <http://public.kitware.com/Dart/HTML/Index.shtml> (October 15, 2007).

DOC++. "DOC++." <http://docpp.sourceforge.net/> (October 15, 2007).

Doxygen. "Doxygen: Source Code Documentation Generator Tool." <http://www.stack.nl/~dimitri/doxygen/> (October 15, 2007).

FDA. (1999). "Guidance for Industry, FDA Reviewers and Compliance on Off-the-Shelf Software Use in Medical Devices." Services USDoHaH, ed., FDA Office of Device Evaluation, 1–29.

FDA. (2000). "Title 21 Code of Federal Regulations (21 CFR Part 11) Electronic Records; Electronic Signatures." Affairs OoR, ed.

FDA. (2002). "General Principles of Software Validation; Final Guidance for Industry and FDA Staff." U.S. Department of Health and Human Services, Center for Devices and Radiological Health.

FDA. (2005). "Guidance for the Content of Premarket Submissions for Software Contained in Medical Devices – Guidance for Industry and FDA Staff." Administration USDoHaHSFaD, ed., 23.

GNU. (1998). "GNU gprof Free Software Foundation." <http://www.gnu.org/software/binutils/manual/gprof-2.9.1/gprof.html>.

IGSTK. "IGSTK: The Image-Guided Surgery Toolkit." <http://www.igstk.org/index.htm> (October 15, 2007).

ITK. "ITK: The National Library of Medicine Insight Segmentation and Registration Toolkit." <http://www.itk.org/> (October 15, 2007).

JUnit. "JUnit.org." <http://www.junit.org/> (October 15, 2007).

Kitware. "KWStyle the Source Checker." <http://public.kitware.com/KWStyle> (October 15, 2007).

Microsoft. (2004). "Microsoft Windows XP Home Edition (Retail) End-User License Agreement for Microsoft Software." <http://www.microsoft.com/windowsxp/home/eula.mspx> (October 15, 2007).

Open Source Initiative. <www.opensource.org> (October 15, 2007).

Sun Microsystems. "Javadoc Tool Version 1.5." <http://docpp.sourceforge.net/> (October 15, 2007).

VTK. "The Visualization Toolkit." <http://www.vtk.org/> (October 15, 2007).

VTune. "Intel VTune Performance Analyzer." <http://www.intel.com/cd/software/products/asmo-na/eng/vtune/239144.htm> (October 15, 2007).

Chapter 6
Rigid Registration

Ziv Yaniv

Abstract

Rigid registration is a key component of all image-guided surgical applications, either as an end in itself or as a precursor to nonrigid registration. This chapter reviews common methods used for rigidly registering pairs of three-dimensional data sets (3D/3D registration), and three-dimensional data to two-dimensional data (2D/3D registration). The chapter defines five criteria that should be addressed when evaluating a registration algorithm. These include execution time, accuracy in the region of interest, breakdown point, automation, and reliability. On the basis of these criteria, one can assess whether an algorithm is applicable for a specific medical procedure, where acceptable bounds on algorithm performance are defined subjectively by physicians. Currently, the only registration algorithms that address these criteria analytically are the paired-point registration methods. All other algorithms have been evaluated empirically, usually using proprietary data sets whose transformations were estimated using paired-point registration. Future efforts should thus focus on addressing the evaluation criteria analytically, and on the establishment of publicly available data sets with known gold standard transformations, enabling objective empirical evaluations.

6.1   Introduction

Rigid registration has been studied extensively over the past several decades, both for medical and nonmedical applications [Goshtasby 2005; Hajnal et al. 2001], and somewhat surprisingly, this is still an active area of research [Gong et al. 2006; Ma and Ellis 2006; Moghari and Abolmaesumi 2006].

In the medical context, the use of a rigid transformation to align data is particularly important. The transformation itself is the simplest useful transformation with only six degrees of freedom. It is invertible, has a simple composition rule, and, most importantly, there are rigid registration tasks that have analytic solutions with well-understood error predictors.

T. Peters and K. Cleary (eds.), *Image-Guided Interventions.*
© Springer Science + Business Media, LLC 2008

This is why the majority of image-guided navigation systems currently model *whole* anatomical structures as rigid bodies and employ rigid registration. Although this model is only correct for registration of intrapatient osseous structures, there are cases where it is *sufficiently accurate*[1] for procedures concerned with soft tissue, most notably neurosurgical procedures.

Registration methods are categorized according to many criteria that broadly fall into two general classes, related to both input and the employed algorithm [Maintz and Viergever 1998]. We describe rigid registration algorithms by first classifying them according to the data dimensionality, an input-related criterion, and then classifying them according to the data type used by the registration process, an algorithm-related criterion.

Currently, the available input sources for registration include three-dimensional (3D) images (e.g., CT), two-dimensional (2D) projective images (e.g., X-ray fluoroscopy), 2D tomographic images (e.g., ultrasound), and 3D digitized points obtained in several ways including, contact-based digitization with a tracked probe, laser range scanning, and stereo imaging using standard video images.

Data types used for registration can be classified as either geometric objects or image intensity data. The rationale for using geometric objects is that using sparse, accurately segmented, geometric data results in fast running times, and that intramodal and intermodal registration are not distinct cases. The rationale for using image intensities is that they do not require accurate segmentation and that the use of more information potentially results in robustness to outlying intensity values.

Using the criteria described earlier, we first classify algorithms as either three-dimensional to three-dimensional (3D/3D), or two-dimensional to three-dimensional (2D/3D) and then classify them into geometry or intensity-based algorithms. Algorithms that do not fall into these categories are also described at the end of each section.

6.2   3D/3D Registration

Image-guided navigation systems utilize 3D/3D rigid registration for two purposes, alignment of complementary image data sets for planning and alignment of image data to the physical world for intraoperative navigation.

---

[1] By *sufficiently accurate* we mean that the registration error does not affect the procedure outcome. That is, the distance between correct and computed point locations is less than a pre-specified threshold as defined by a physician for a specific procedure (a subjective measure).

Definition 6.1: Given two data sets defined over the domains $\Omega_l \subset \Re^3$, $\Omega_r \subset \Re^3$:

$$F_l : \mathbf{x}_l \in \Omega_l \mapsto F_l(\mathbf{x}_l)$$
$$F_r : \mathbf{x}_r \in \Omega_r \mapsto F_r(\mathbf{x}_r) \tag{6.1}$$

with, possibly, additional side information (e.g., pairing between corresponding features) find the rigid transformation:

$$\Im : \mathbf{x}_l \mapsto \mathbf{x}_r \Leftrightarrow \Im(\mathbf{x}_l) = \mathbf{x}_r \tag{6.2}$$

where $\mathbf{x}_l \in \Omega_l$, $\mathbf{x}_r \in \Omega_r$.

Specific registration instances are defined by the mappings F_l and F_r. Two common mapping combinations are: (1) F_l and F_r are the identity map, i.e., point-set to point-set registration; and (2) F_l and F_r map locations to intensity values, i.e., image to image registration.

6.2.1 Geometry-Based Methods

Various geometric objects have been used for 3D/3D registration with point and surface data being the most popular, and thus are the focus of this section.

To understand why these are the geometric objects of choice, we evaluate them with regard to a set of desired characteristics:

1. Closed form solution: There is a registration algorithm on the basis of this geometric object that has a closed form solution
2. Number of detectable objects: The number of corresponding objects detectable across data sets is sufficient for registration
3. Localization: Accurate object localization in all data sets is simple and has a low computational cost
4. Correspondence: Establishing object correspondence across data sets is simple

Point data arise from two sources: anatomical structures and fiducial markers. In both cases, there are closed form solutions when correspondences between data sets are known [Arun et al. 1987; Faugeras and Hebert 1986; Horn 1987; Horn et al. 1988; Schönemann 1966; Umeyama 1991; Walker et al. 1991]. This is the primary reason for the popularity of point-based registration, which is one of the few registration tasks that have a closed form solution. On the one hand, the number of distinct anatomical points that can be detected per organ across modalities is usually small, and their accurate localization is a difficult task that is still the subject of research [Wörz and Rohr 2006]. On the other hand, fiducial points arise from markers that are designed to have the desired characteristics (see Fig. 6.1

for examples). The number of points is set by the user and the fiducial design is such that detecting and accurately localizing it across the relevant modalities can be done efficiently [Maurer et al. 1997; Wang et al. 1996]. Finally, for both point types, establishing correspondences can be done both automatically [Grimson and Lozano-Perez 1987] or manually, with the manual approach most often used when registering images to physical space.

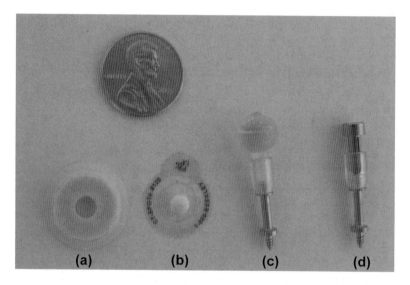

Fig. 6.1. Registration fiducials, from *left* to *right*: (**a**) CT/MR compatible adhesive skin marker from IZI Medical Products Corp., Baltimore MD, USA; (**b**) CT compatible adhesive skin marker from Beekley Corp., Bristol CT, USA; (**c, d**) Acustar II CT/MR compatible implantable markers with interchangeable caps from Z-kat, Hollywood Fla, USA, manufactured by Stryker, Kalamazoo MI, USA; (**c**) with imaging cap, and (**d**) with conical cap for pointer-based digitization (implantable markers courtesy of J. M. Fitzpatrick)

Surfaces arise from segmentation of anatomical structures in images and from dense point digitization of exposed anatomical structures. Unlike point data, there is no closed form solution to surface-based registration. In most cases, a single surface in each data set is used for registration, providing that the detected surfaces have sufficient overlapping regions. The ease of iso-surface segmentation in medical images is the primary reason for the widespread use of surface data for registration, most notably the marching-cubes algorithm [Lorensen and Cline 1987]. Finally, establishing correspondences between surfaces is usually not an issue, as in most cases only a single surface is involved.

6.2.1.1 Paired-Point Methods

Paired-point registration arises when the mappings F_l and F_r in Definition 6.1 are the identity mapping, and point correspondences are known. For a unique solution to exist, the data must include three or more noncollinear points. In general, we are given two sets of corresponding 3D points obtained in two Cartesian coordinate systems using a measurement process having additive noise:

$$\mathbf{x}_{li} = \hat{\mathbf{x}}_{li} + \mathbf{e}_{li}$$
$$\mathbf{x}_{ri} = \hat{\mathbf{x}}_{ri} + \mathbf{e}_{ri} \qquad (6.3)$$

where $\hat{\mathbf{x}}_{li}$, $\hat{\mathbf{x}}_{ri}$ are the true point coordinates that satisfy the constraint $\Im(\hat{\mathbf{x}}_{li}) = \hat{\mathbf{x}}_{ri}$, $\mathbf{x}_{li}$, $\mathbf{x}_{ri}$ are the observed coordinates, and $\mathbf{e}_{li}, \mathbf{e}_{ri}$ are the respective errors in the measurement process. The most common solution to this problem is based on a least-squares formulation:

$$\Im : \sum_{i=1}^{n} \left\| \mathbf{x}_{ri} - \Im(\mathbf{x}_{li}) \right\|^2 \rightarrow \min \qquad (6.4)$$

The transformation $\Im = [R, \mathbf{t}]$ is optimal when the errors, $R(\mathbf{e}_l) - \mathbf{e}_r$, are independent and have identical zero mean Gaussian distributions. This assumes that the original errors are isotropic, independent and identically distributed (IID) with a zero mean Gaussian distribution. In most cases, these assumptions do not hold (e.g., optical tracking where the uncertainty is greater along the viewing direction). Several algorithms that relax these assumptions have been published, including a generalized total least squares formulation [Ohta and Kanatani 1998], a heteroscedastic errors-in-variables regression formulation [Matei and Meer 1999], a method for dealing with anisotropy arising from the use of reference frames [Balachandran et al. 2005], an extended Kalman filter formulation [Pennec and Thirion 1997], and an unscented Kalman filter formulation [Moghari and Abolmaesumi 2005].

Currently, none of these methods is in widespread use. The continued use of least squares solutions can be attributed to their mathematical and implementational simplicity, and to the fact that for many procedures their accuracy is sufficient, although not optimal.

The primary difference between the various least squares solutions is in their representation of the transformation operator. These include the standard matrix representation [Arun et al. 1987; Horn et al. 1988; Schönemann 1966; Umeyama 1991], a unit quaternion-based rotation representation [Faugeras and Hebert 1986; Horn 1987], and a dual quaternion representation of the transformation [Walker et al. 1991]. While the mathematical derivation of the solution varies according to the transformation representation, the performance of all algorithms has been empirically found to be comparable [Eggert et al. 1997].

We now briefly describe the two most popular solutions, with the rotation operator represented as a matrix and unit quaternion. In both cases, the estimation of the rotation and translation is decoupled by replacing the original measurements with their demeaned versions:

$\mathbf{x}'_{li} = \mathbf{x}_{li} - \boldsymbol{\mu}_l$, $\mathbf{x}'_{ri} = \mathbf{x}_{ri} - \boldsymbol{\mu}_r$. The least squares formulation is then rewritten as:

$$[R,\mathbf{t}]: \sum_{i=1}^{n}\left\|\mathbf{x}'_{ri} - R(\mathbf{x}'_{li}) - \mathbf{t}'\right\| \rightarrow \min, \quad \mathbf{t}' = \mathbf{t} - \boldsymbol{\mu}_r + R(\boldsymbol{\mu}_l) \qquad (6.5)$$

with the optimal translation given by:

$$\mathbf{t} = \boldsymbol{\mu}_r - R(\boldsymbol{\mu}_l) \qquad (6.6)$$

In both cases, computation of the optimal rotation utilizes the following correlation matrix:

$$C = \sum_{i=1}^{n}\mathbf{x}'_{li}\mathbf{x}'^{\mathrm{T}}_{ri} = \begin{bmatrix} C_{xx} & C_{xy} & C_{xz} \\ C_{yx} & C_{yy} & C_{yz} \\ C_{zx} & C_{zy} & C_{zz} \end{bmatrix} \qquad (6.7)$$

with the matrix-based solution using the singular value decomposition (SVD), $\mathrm{SVD}(C) = U\Sigma V^{\mathrm{T}}$, yielding the optimal rotation matrix as:

$$R = U\begin{bmatrix} 1 & & \\ & 1 & \\ & & \det(UV^{\mathrm{T}}) \end{bmatrix}V^{\mathrm{T}} \qquad (6.8)$$

and the unit quaternion-based solution given by the eigenvector corresponding to the maximal eigenvalue of the matrix:

$$N = \begin{bmatrix} C_{xx}+C_{yy}+C_{zz} & C_{yz}-C_{zy} & C_{zx}-C_{xz} & C_{xy}-C_{yx} \\ C_{yz}-C_{zy} & C_{xx}-C_{yy}-C_{zz} & C_{xy}+C_{yx} & C_{zx}+C_{xz} \\ C_{zx}-C_{xz} & C_{xy}+C_{yx} & C_{yy}-C_{xx}-C_{zz} & C_{yz}+C_{zy} \\ C_{xy}-C_{yx} & C_{zx}+C_{xz} & C_{yz}+C_{zy} & C_{zz}-C_{xx}-C_{yy} \end{bmatrix} \qquad (6.9)$$

6.2.1.2 Surface-Based Methods

Surface registration arises when one or both of the mappings F_l and F_r in Definition 6.1 are indicator functions with a value of one at surface points, and zero otherwise. Although this description uses an implicit surface representation, in most cases surfaces are represented explicitly as triangular meshes, although other implicit (e.g., distance maps) and explicit (e.g., NURBS) representations are also possible.

We limit our description of surface-based registration methods to the case where one or both surfaces are represented as a set of points, as in the medical context this is the most ubiquitous instance of surface registration.

This is primarily because it is easy to reduce all surface registration tasks to this specific task via sampling. For descriptions of additional surface-based algorithms, including deformable registration see Audette et al. [2000].

One of the first successful surface-based registration algorithms is the head-and-hat algorithm of Pelizzari et al. [1989], which aligns two surface representations of the brain segmented from complementary imaging modalities. The surface extracted from the lower resolution data, the hat, is represented as a set of points, while the surface extracted from the higher resolution data, the head, is represented as a set of stacked 2D closed contours. The algorithm iteratively minimizes the sum of distances between the rays originating at "hat" points going through the head centroid, and the head surface using Powell's standard optimization method [Press et al. 1992]. Note that this algorithm is tailored for registration of images of the head, as the point matching strategy best suits spherical objects. In many ways, this algorithm is a precursor of what is currently the common approach to point set to surface registration, the iterative closest point (ICP) algorithm.

The ICP algorithm was independently introduced by [Besl and McKay 1992; Chen and Medioni 1992; Zhang 1994], with Besl and McKay coining the name ICP. In practice, the acronym ICP is now used to describe algorithms that follow an iterative corresponding point framework, rather than the original closest point approach. In essence, the ICP framework is an iterative two-step approach with the first step establishing point correspondences and the second computing a transformation, based on these matches, yielding incremental transformations whose composition is the registration result. Table 6.1 summarizes this general framework.

The popularity of the ICP framework is primarily due to its presentation by Besl and McKay. The algorithm is simple and a proof of

Table 6.1 Iterative Corresponding Point (ICP) Framework

Input: P_l – point set, S_r – surface, $\tau > 0$ improvement threshold, n – maximal number of iterations

0. Initialization:
   a. Set cumulative transformation and apply to points
   b. Find *corresponding* points and compute similarity (e.g., root mean square distance)
1. Iterate:
   a. Compute incremental transformation using the current correspondences (e.g., analytic least squares solution), update cumulative transformation and apply to points
   b. Find *corresponding* points and compute similarity
   c. If improvement in similarity is less than τ or number of iterations has reached n terminate

---

local convergence when correspondence based on the Euclidean distance is given. Additionally, the technique is shown to be versatile and successful, as the authors describe both closest point computations using several surface representations, and show successful registration results on a variety of geometric objects. In practice, the original framework suffers from several deficiencies:

1. Convergence is local, requiring an initial transformation near the global optimum
2. Point pairing is a computationally expensive operation
3. The framework uses a least squares method for computing the incremental transformations and is thus sensitive to outliers and makes the implicit assumption that noise is isotropic IID with a zero mean Gaussian distribution

These issues have been addressed by a large body of literature.

Methods for improving the probability of convergence to the global optimum include, initialization approaches such as manual alignment of the data, or initial registration using inaccurately localized paired points such as anatomical landmarks [Ma and Ellis 2003], multiple registration runs with different initial transformations [Besl and McKay 1992], and use of heuristic global optimization methods such as simulated annealing [Gong et al. 2006; Luck et al. 2000; Penney et al. 2001].

Methods for accelerating the running time include the use of the kd-tree spatial data structure [Besl and McKay 1992; Greenspan and Yurick 2003; Simon 1996], closest point caching [Simon 1996], extrapolation of the transformation parameters [Besl and McKay 1992; Simon 1996], approximate nearest neighbor searches [Greenspan and Yurick 2003], parallelized nearest neighbor searches [Langis et al. 2001], hierarchical coarse-to-fine data sampling approaches [Jost and Hugli 2003; Zhang 1994], and combinations of these methods.

Methods for dealing with the deficiencies of the least squares approach provide robustness by replacing the least squares formulation with methods based on M-estimators [Kaneko et al. 2003; Ma and Ellis 2003], least median of squares [Masuda and Yokoya 1995; Trucco et al. 1999], least trimmed squares [Chetverikov et al. 2005], and weighted least squares [Maurer et al. 1998; Turk and Levoy 1994; Zhang 1994]. To remove the assumption on the noise characteristics, the least squares approach can be replaced by the generalized total least squares [Estépar et al. 2004], the unscented Kalman filter [Moghari and Abolmaesumi 2005], or any of the other methods described in the previous section.

Finally, it should be noted that some researchers [Fitzgibbon 2003] advocate the use of classical optimization approaches instead of the two-step ICP framework, following the rationale that the large body of research on robust estimation using classical optimization tools can be brought to bear on the current task. The proposed algorithm replaces point pairing with a precomputed distance map and a liner interpolation approach to estimate point to surface distances. Optimization is then carried out using the Levenberg-Marquardt algorithm with M-estimators replacing the sum of squares objective function. Although this approach was not evaluated using medical data, a similar solution has been used successfully in the medical context [Barratt et al. 2006], registering point data extracted from ultrasound to a bone surface extracted from CT.

6.2.2 *Intensity-Based Methods*

Intensity-based registration arises when the mappings F_l and F_r in Definition 6.1 map locations to intensity values, as in image to image registration. These data are either the original images as acquired by the imaging apparatus or images derived from them.

Although most intensity-based registration algorithms utilize the original intensity values directly, some methods perform a "fuzzy segmentation," attempting to strike a balance between the geometric feature-based and purely intensity-based approaches. Images derived from the originals are created by mapping the original intensities to values that are loosely related to geometric structures found in the images. The new images are then used as input for the registration algorithm.

Examples of this approach include registration of CT/MR brain images [Maintz et al. 1996], registration of US/MR liver images [Penney et al. 2004], and registration of US/CT bone images [Penney et al. 2006]. In Maintz et al. [1996], the original intensities are replaced with values related to the likelihood of the spatial location being an edge or ridge, on the basis of gradient and Laplacian information. In Penney et al. [2004] and [2006], the original intensities are replaced with values representing the probability that the spatial location is part of a blood vessel in the former case, and a bone soft tissue interface in the latter. The mapping function is learned from a segmented training set using image features such as intensity values, gradient magnitude, and characteristics of intensity profiles along the beam direction in the case of US. In all cases, the derived images replace the originals as input for intensity-based registration.

Intensity-based registration is cast as an optimization task where the objective function is directly dependent on the image intensity values and the transformation parameters. Given that optimization is carried out over a continuous domain, and intensity values are only available on a discrete grid, the registration process invariably requires interpolation of intensity values at nongrid locations.

A registration algorithm is thus uniquely defined by the following components:

1. Similarity measure (objective function)
2. Optimization algorithm
3. Interpolation scheme

The first step when casting a problem as an optimization task is to define the objective function. Most research has focused on devising task-specific similarity measures, as this is the only component in the registration algorithm that is directly related to the data at hand.

Ideally, a similarity measure is continuous, strictly monotonic, and has a unique global optimum for the correct transformation parameters. In practice, the only requirement from a similarity measure is that it should have a local optimum for the correct parameters. Given this condition, it is not surprising that many similarity measures have been proposed. In general, similarity measures can be divided into two classes, measures that assume the existence of a deterministic functional relationship between intensities and measures that assume a stochastic relationship. Table 6.2 presents various image intensity relationships and appropriate similarity measures that are described in the following discussion.

The simplest intensity relationships arise in the context of intra-modality registration. Intensity values are assumed to be identical across images, or related via an affine transformation (often referred to as linear).

Two related similarity measures that assume intensities are only subject to zero mean Gaussian noise are the sum of squared differences (SSD), squared L_2 norm of the difference image, and sum of absolute differences (SAD), L_1 norm of the difference image. The primary distinction between them is that the L_1 norm degrades more gracefully in the presence of outliers, although it is not robust in the breakdown point sense. Another, more robust, measure that makes the same assumption is the entropy of the difference image, $H(F_l(\mathbf{x}) - F_r(\mathbf{x}))$ [Buzug et al. 1997], although it is less popular because of its greater computational complexity.

In practice, even when intensities are assumed to be identical, the noise does not necessarily follow a zero mean Gaussian distribution. This is why more often an affine intensity mapping is assumed and the normalized cross correlation (NCC), *Pearson's r* [Press et al. 1992], is used. This is probably the most popular similarity measure to assume a deterministic functional relationship between intensities. It should be noted that simple variations of the NCC, such as tessellating the images and using the sum of *local* NCC values as the similarity measure, can accommodate more general functional relationships, such as those relating MR and CT [Weese et al. 1999]. A mathematical model motivating such an approach can be derived if it is assumed that the intensity relationship between the images is characterized by a low frequency, spatially varying multiplicative and additive bias field:

$$F_r(\mathbf{x}) = f_1(\mathbf{x})F_l(\mathbf{x}) + f_2(\mathbf{x}) \tag{6.10}$$

Using the Taylor expansion and taking only the first terms we get:

$$
\begin{aligned}
F_r(\mathbf{x}_0 + \delta) &= [f_1(\mathbf{x}_0) + \nabla f_1(\mathbf{x}_0)\delta + O(\delta^2)]F_l(\mathbf{x}_0 + \delta) + \\
&\quad [f_2(\mathbf{x}_0) + \nabla f_2(\mathbf{x}_0)\delta + O(\delta^2)] \\
&\cong f_1(\mathbf{x}_0)F_l(\mathbf{x}_0 + \delta) + f_2(\mathbf{x}_0)
\end{aligned} \tag{6.11}
$$

The intensity relationship is locally affine to first order, making the sum of NCC values in a tessellated image a natural similarity measure.

The most generic similarity measure that assumes intensities are related via a deterministic functional is the correlation ratio [Roche et al. 1998]. Unlike the previous similarity measures, the correlation ratio does not require an explicit functional. This is an advantage, as explicit functionals are usually based on *approximations* of the physical imaging processes, which are often hard to model. Although the correlation ratio is not in widespread use, it has been successfully applied to rigid registration of PET/T1, CT/T1, and T1/T2 data sets [Roche et al. 1998].

More complex intensity relationships arise in the context of inter-modality registration, where the intensity relationships are stochastic and not deterministic. Similarity measures based on the information theoretic concept of entropy were introduced in the 1990s. These measures assume that intensities are related via a statistical process, and that the joint and marginal image entropies can be used to align the images. In most cases, the measures use Shannon's definition of entropy, $H = -\sum_i p_i \log p_i$, although other definitions exist [Jumarie 1997].

The two most widely used similarity measures in this category are mutual information (MI) and normalized mutual information (NMI). MI was independently proposed as a similarity measure by [Collignon et al. 1995; Maes et al. 1997] and [Viola and Wells- 1995; Viola and Wells- 1997]. It has been successfully applied to various inter and intramodality registrations, including CT/MR, PET/MR, MR/MR, and CT/CT. NMI was proposed by Studholme et al. [1999], as an overlap invariant version of MI. The normalization results in a measure that does not depend on the changes in the marginal entropy values because of the changes in the region of overlap.

An exhaustive survey of these similarity measures and their application to various registration tasks is given by Pluim et al. [2003]. This survey is perhaps one of the few papers to explicitly address the fact that implementation decisions can significantly influence registration performance. In the case of MI, its definition is unique, but its implementation relies on the estimation of the joint and marginal intensity probability distributions. Thus, the choice of estimation method and its parameters can influence the registration results. The two common estimation approaches are joint histogram computation and Parzen windowing [Duda et al. 2001]. Interestingly, the original MI papers also differ in their implementation choices with Collignon et al. [1995] using a histogram-based estimate and Viola and Wells [1995] using a Parzen windowing estimate.

Although MI is applicable in many registration tasks, it does not address all registration challenges. Most notably the correct transformation parameters often correspond to a local, rather than a global optimum. This requires either good initialization when using general purpose optimization techniques or caution when applying heuristic global search methods, such as simulated annealing. In addition, the computational cost of MI is higher than that of most deterministic functional similarity measures.

Currently, there is no universal similarity measure that is optimal for all registration tasks, although without problem-specific knowledge, MI is at least applicable. Incorporating problem specific knowledge when devising or choosing a similarity measure usually improves all aspects of registration performance.

In most cases, the best similarity measure is chosen from several applicable candidates on the basis of its computational complexity, robustness, accuracy, and convergence range. The first two criteria can be analyzed in a context-independent manner on the basis of the mathematical definition of the similarity measure. The remaining criteria, accuracy, and convergence range, do depend on the specific imaging modalities, and are most often evaluated in one of two ways: assessing registration performance as a function of the similarity measure, and by exploring the behavior of the similarity measure as a function of the transformation parameters. In the former case, the similarity measure is evaluated on the basis of its impact on the accuracy and convergence range of the registration by comparing registration results to a known gold standard transformation. In the latter case, 2D graphs of the similarity measure as a function of each of the transformation parameters are plotted. These are 2D, axis-aligned, orthogonal slices through the 6D parameter space, centered on the known parameter values obtained from a gold standard transformation.

Both approaches are lacking. The registration-based approach does not evaluate the similarity measure, but rather evaluates the combination of similarity measure and a specific optimization technique. The parameter space exploration approach is based on visual inspection and on the ability of the viewer to mentally reconstruct a six-dimensional terrain on the basis of six axis-aligned orthogonal slices, a task that is nearly impossible, and is thus qualitative rather than quantitative.

A quantitative parameter space exploration approach has been recently presented by Škerl et al. [2006]. This approach starts by exhaustively sampling the parameter space along diameters of a six-dimensional hypersphere centered on the gold standard parameter values. After evaluating the similarity measure at the sample points, several figures of merit are computed. These describe the function behavior on the basis of the extrema points along the diameters, and the similarity measures rate of change near these extrema.

The second component of iterative intensity-based registration is the optimization algorithm. The majority of algorithms utilize general purpose iterative optimization algorithms, unconstrained or constrained. Starting from an initial transformation $\Im^{(0)}$ in each iteration, a new transformation $\Im^{(i)}$ is estimated, based on the similarity measure and the previous estimate.

This sequence converges to a local optimum $\Im^{(*)}$, with the iterations terminated when a user specified convergence test is satisfied. For detailed descriptions of standard optimization methods, the reader is referred to [Fletcher 1987].

Table 6.2 Examples of intensity relationships and appropriate similarity measures. All similarity measures are defined over the domain $\Omega_{lr} = \Im(\Omega_l) \cap \Omega_r$, where $\Im$ is a rigid transformation and Ω_l, Ω_r are the original image domains. The MI and NMI similarity measures are expressed using the Shannon entropy, $H = -\sum_i p_i \log p_i$

Relationship between Intensity values	Similarity Measure	
Identity	Sum of Squared Differences (SSD)	$\dfrac{1}{n} \sum_{\mathbf{x} \in \Omega_{lr}} \lVert F_l(\mathbf{x}) - F_r(\mathbf{x}) \rVert^2$
Identity	Sum of Absolute Differences (SAD)	$\dfrac{1}{n} \sum_{\mathbf{x} \in \Omega_{lr}} \lvert F_l(\mathbf{x}) - F_r(\mathbf{x}) \rvert$
Affine	Normalized Cross Correlation (NCC)	$\dfrac{\sum\limits_{\mathbf{x} \in \Omega_{lr}} (F_l(\mathbf{x}) - \overline{F}_l(\mathbf{x}))(F_r(\mathbf{x}) - \overline{F}_r(\mathbf{x}))}{\sqrt{\sum\limits_{\mathbf{x} \in \Omega_{lr}} (F_l(\mathbf{x}) - \overline{F}_l(\mathbf{x}))^2 \sum\limits_{\mathbf{x} \in \Omega_{lr}} (F_r(\mathbf{x}) - \overline{F}_r(\mathbf{x}))^2}}$
General Functional	Correlation Ratio (CR)	$1 - \dfrac{\operatorname{var}[F_l(\mathbf{x}) - E[F_l(\mathbf{x}) \mid F_r(\mathbf{x})]}{\operatorname{var}[F_l(\mathbf{x})]}$
Stochastic	Mutual Information	$H(F_l(\mathbf{x})) + H(F_r(\mathbf{x})) - H(F_l(\mathbf{x}), F_r(\mathbf{x}))$
Stochastic	Normalized Mutual Information	$\dfrac{H(F_l(\mathbf{x})) + H(F_r(\mathbf{x}))}{H(F_l(\mathbf{x}), F_r(\mathbf{x}))}$

Although many general purpose optimization algorithms are available, the no-free-lunch theorem [Ho and Pepyne 2002] proves that without making prior assumptions on the objective function, there is no single algorithm that is superior to all others across all possible inputs. Thus, the choice of optimization algorithm cannot be separated from that of the similarity measure, as an algorithm will outperform all others only if it incorporates prior information on the objective function.

Finally, there is a plethora of heuristic strategies for improving the registration convergence range. These include multiresolution strategies, multistart strategies, and heuristic search algorithms such as simulated annealing and genetic algorithms. Again, we emphasize that while these strategies can improve the probability of convergence, they should be used with care, incorporating problem-specific constraints, as the correct transformation parameters often coincide with a local and not global extremum.

The third component required for iterative intensity-based registration is an interpolation scheme. The majority of algorithms use linear interpolation, usually viewed as a compromise between computational complexity and accuracy of the estimated intensity values. In some cases, this has an adverse effect on the similarity measure, for example MI and NMI estimates on the basis of linear interpolation exhibit additional local extrema when the images are translated to grid locations [Pluim et al. 2000], although this effect can be mitigated by blurring the images prior to registration [Hill et al. 2001].

Evaluation studies of various interpolation schemes using medical images [Lehmann et al. 1999; Meijering et al. 2001] have shown that barring nearest neighbor, linear interpolation is the fastest interpolation method, although its accuracy is lacking. Both studies show that the best tradeoff between accuracy and computational complexity is obtained for B-spline interpolation. Given these conclusions, it is surprising to find that most registration algorithms still use linear interpolation. This preference has to do with the effect of the interpolation scheme on the optimization process, primarily its running time and accuracy. The impact of the interpolation scheme on the total running time is considerable, as interpolation is performed many times during optimization. The impact it has on accuracy is usually not as great. Given that the necessary condition for accurate Registration is that the similarity measure have a local extremum for the correct transformation parameters, inaccurate interpolation may not be too detrimental as long as this condition is satisfied. Finally, as we are dealing with iterative optimization, interpolation schemes that introduce additional local extrema in the similarity measure reduce the convergence range, which can greatly impact automated registration algorithms, as is the case of linear interpolation and MI [Pluim et al. 2000].

6.3   2D/3D Registration

Image-guided navigation systems utilize 2D/3D rigid registration to align image data to the physical world for intraoperative navigation.

Definition 6.2: Given two data sets over the spatial domains $\Omega_l \subset \mathfrak{R}^3$, $\Omega_{ri} \subset \mathfrak{R}^2$ $(i = 1....n)$,

$$F_l : \mathbf{x}_l \in \Omega_l \mapsto F_l(\mathbf{x}_l)$$
$$F_r : \mathbf{x}_{ri} \in \Omega_{ri} \mapsto F_r(\mathbf{x}_{ri})$$
(6.12)

and camera matrices, $K_i = P_i T_i$, where T_i is a rigid transformation and P_i a perspective projection matrix, find the rigid transformation:

$$\Im : \mathbf{x}_l \mapsto \mathbf{x}_{ri} \Leftrightarrow K_i(\Im(\mathbf{x}_l)) = \mathbf{x}_{ri}$$
(6.13)

where $\mathbf{x}_l \in \Omega_l, \mathbf{x}_{ri} \in \Omega_{ri}$.

It should be noted that, in the medical context, the only modalities that are modeled as 2D perspective images are X-ray imaging and video images, such as those acquired by endoscopic systems. Although the pin-hole camera model is applicable to both modalities, they do differ in the location of the image plane relative to the imaged object. Figure 6.2 shows the relationships between camera, object, and image plane in both cases.

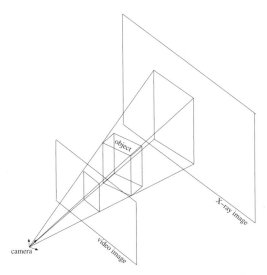

Fig. 6.2. Pinhole camera model for X-ray and video images. Location of the image plane is behind the imaged object in the former case and in front of the object in the latter case

Figure 6.3 describes the generic 2D/3D registration problem. One or more perspective images are acquired from known poses relative to a *world* (fixed) coordinate system W. Registration is then the task of estimating the transformation relating the volume coordinate system to the world co-ordinate system $\Im_V^W$. In general, 2D/3D registration is formulated as an optimization task where the objective function is a sum of objective functions computed individually for each image.

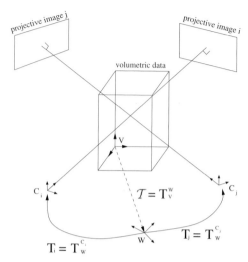

Fig. 6.3. Coordinate systems used in 2D/3D registration. One or more images are acquired with known camera poses relative to a fixed, world coordinate system. The estimated transformation relates the 3D volumetric coordinate system to the fixed coordinate system. Known transformations are marked by *solid lines* and the estimated transformation by a *dashed line*. The figure uses a X-ray image plane to object relationship

Note that 2D/3D registration as defined earlier is closely related to the extensively studied computer vision problem of pose estimation, where a single image is used as an input and the world and camera coordinate systems coincide. Corresponding features, usually points or lines, are extracted from a geometric 3D model and the 2D image, and are used to compute the camera to model transformation. Feature extraction is performed only once, and the accuracy of the whole approach is highly dependent on accurate feature extraction and pairing, tasks that are difficult to perform using images of anatomical structures, as the number of distinct features is usually small.

In the medical context, all 2D/3D rigid registration algorithms are iterative, requiring transformation initialization. Choice of an initialization approach depends both on the available data, and on the expected convergence range of the registration algorithm. Several common initialization schemes exist:

1. *Manual initialization*: The user interactively explores the transformation parameter space, visually comparing the medical images with computer-generated images created using the current parameter

values. The initial transformation parameters correspond to the most similar computer generated images, as visually assessed by the user.

2. *Clinical setup*: Knowledge of patient position (e.g., supine) and imaging apparatus poses define bounds on the transformation parameters. For example, in X-ray imaging, each camera pose defines a bounding pyramid for the imaged object, with the image extent serving as the pyramid base and the camera location, its apex. For improved object localization, it is possible to use the intersection of multiple pyramids as the bounding volume.

3. *Approximate paired point registration*: Using a paired point closed form solution with approximate point data. This approach can be used:

    a. when the locations of three or more anatomical landmarks are available. Anatomical landmark locations can be estimated in one of two ways: touching the landmark with a calibrated tracked probe, if the landmark is already exposed as part of the procedure, or by indicating the landmark location on multiple perspective images and using triangulation to localize it in physical space. In both cases, registration inaccuracy is primarily due to the difficulties in accurate identification of anatomical landmarks both on the patient anatomy [Robinson et al. 2006], and across multiple images; or

    b. when using skin adhesive fiducials. Fiducial locations are estimated by touching the fiducials with a calibrated tracked probe. In this case, registration inaccuracy is primarily due to fiducial motion between the imaging and digitization stages.

6.3.1 Geometry-Based Methods

In many ways, geometry-based 2D/3D registration algorithms are very similar to their 3D/3D counterparts. The geometric objects are 3D surfaces, 2D image points corresponding to feature locations, and 3D rays emanating from the camera location and going through the spatial locations that correspond to the 2D features (back-projected rays). Figure 6.4 shows these geometric entities in the context of CT/X-ray registration.

In Bijhold [1993], known 2D/3D paired points are used to align CT and portal images for patient positioning in radiotherapy. The 3D points are projected onto the portal image, and the distances between their projection and the known point locations are minimized in the image plane. Two closed form solutions are presented with the first assuming that the 3D points are approximately planar allowing for a weak perspective projection model, and the second assuming small rotations allowing for rotation.

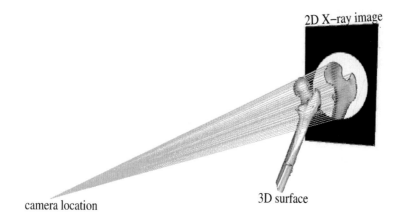

2D X–ray image

camera location

3D surface

Fig. 6.4. Geometric entities used in 2D/3D (CT/X-ray) geometry-based registration of a femur bone. These include the 3D bone surface extracted from CT, the spatial locations of the 2D bone contour points on the X-ray image and the corresponding back-projected rays. Bone model is displayed in its correct position with back-projected rays tangent to the model surface

linearization. This is in practice a simplified version of the classical computer vision task of pose estimation.

A registration algorithm for aligning X-ray and CT images of the head described in [Murphy 1997] can be viewed as a variant of the head-and-hat algorithm [Pelizzari et al. 1989] with optimization carried out in 2D instead of 3D. In each iteration, a digitally reconstructed radiograph (DRR), a simulated X-ray image derived from CT, is generated. A set of 2D rays emanating from the center of the X-ray image (*head* centroid) and going toward the image boundary at regular angular intervals is defined. An edge detector is then used to determine the skull edge location along the ray direction in the DRR and X-ray images and this distance is minimized, along with the mean grey level value along the ray. Optimization is performed with an algorithm that initially performs gradient descent, and then switches to an approximation of the function using the first terms of the Taylor expansion.

A straightforward extension of the ICP algorithm to 2D/3D registration is described in [Wunsch and Hirzinger 1996]. In this case, instead of matching two sets of 3D points, back-projected rays are matched to the closest 3D model points. Once the pairs of ray-model points are established, the incremental transformation is computed using the SVD-based analytic solution for 3D/3D paired-point rigid registration. To improve robustness, the sum of squares objective function is replaced with its weighted version using the Huber M-estimator.

A similar ICP-like approach is described in [Gueziec et al. 1998]. Incremental transformations are computed with a weighted version of the sum of squares objective function using the Tukey M-estimator, and an analytic solution of the 3D/3D paired point based on the Cayley rotation representation is derived. In addition, only a small subset of model points is used in the closest point computation stage. The authors observe that at the correct position, all back-projected rays are tangent to the model surface defining a 3D space curve on the surface of the model. As the rays are defined by the object's 2D boundary, its apparent contour, they should only match points on the 3D space curve that separates front-facing from back-facing regions, the contour generator. At each iteration, the contour generator is computed on the basis of the object's current pose. The closest points are then constrained to lie on this 3D curve.

A feature-based two stage algorithm for registering endoscopic video images to CT is described in Burschka et al. [2005]. In the first stage, the endoscopic camera motion and a scaled 3D model are estimated. The estimate is based on the identification of three or more corresponding points across multiple video images. In the second stage, the scaled 3D model is registered to a surface derived from the CT. Initially, the scale of the reconstructed model is estimated using principle component analysis (PCA) of the model and a roughly corresponding local CT surface patch. Once the model's scale is known, the problem is reduced to 3D/3D point to surface registration, and the transformation is estimated using the ICP algorithm.

Lavallée and Szeliski [1995] register X-ray images to CT data, using back-projected rays corresponding to object contours in the X-ray image and an implicit surface representation. Observing that for the correct registration parameters the back-projected rays are tangent to the object surface, the sum of squared distances between the rays and surface is used as an objective function. Minimization is then performed with the Levenberg-Marquardt method. The novel aspect of this approach is in the use of an adaptive, octree-based, distance map to represent the surface. Figure 6.5 visually illustrates this spatial data structure. It should be noted that the algorithm assumes that *all* image contour points arise from projections of the object's surface points, an assumption that is rarely valid because of the presence of multiple objects in an image. In Hamadeh et al. [1998], this restriction is mitigated by using a cooperative registration–segmentation approach. Instead of using all contour points to generate the back-projected rays, the surface model is projected onto the image, using the initial registration estimate, and only contour points that are within a specified distance from the projected surface are utilized. This in turn implies that the initial registration estimate is close to the correct one. Interestingly, the basic algorithm can be viewed as the 2D/3D equivalent of the 3D/3D registration approach proposed by Fitzgibbon [2003] and described in section 6.2.1. The primary difference between these methods is in the implementation of the distance map. In the 3D/3D case, the distance map is unsigned and spatially uniform, while in the 2D/3D case it represents a signed distance and is spatially adaptive.

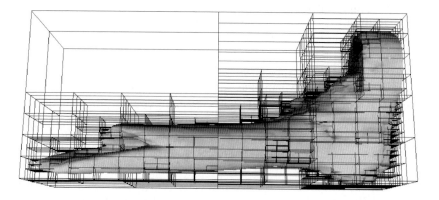

Fig. 6.5. Surface of femur embedded inside an octree spatial data structure, providing an adaptive distance map. The distance to the object surface is computed for all vertices of the octree's terminal nodes (leaves). Given a query point its distance is computed using linear interpolation of the vertex distances for the terminal node that contains it

6.3.2 Intensity-Based Methods

Intensity-based 2D/3D registration methods use the same iterative optimization framework as their 3D/3D counterparts with a slight modification because of the dimensionality difference between data sets. As direct comparison of the 2D and 3D images is not possible, an intermediate step is introduced in which 2D simulated images are generated using the 3D image and the current transformation parameters. These simulated images are then compared with the actual ones using a similarity measure as in the 3D/3D case. It should be noted that image interpolation is performed during the 2D image generation stage, and no interpolation is required as part of the similarity measure computation.

Although this approach is the rule, there is an exception as described by Tomaževič et al. [2006]. Instead of simulating 2D X-ray images from the 3D data, in this approach the 2D images are used to reconstruct a low quality 3D volume. This reduces the task of 2D/3D registration to 3D/3D registration, which is then solved using a multifeature mutual information-based similarity measure.

The task of generating a 2D perspective image from a 3D image, direct or indirect volume rendering, has been studied extensively in the computer graphics domain [Foley et al. 1996]. In computer graphics, the end result is the image, and the goal is to achieve visual realism. That is, the result of the simulation should be as similar as possible to an actual 2D image as obtained with an imaging apparatus. Luckily, for the purpose of 2D/3D registration a perfect simulation is not necessary, and interestingly, it is not sufficient. In most cases, even a perfect simulation will not provide an exact match with the 2D images, as the 3D data do not represent the same physical reality as the 2D images. These two physical situations most often differ by the presence of tools and shift of soft tissue structures. Thus, the quality of the simulation primarily impacts the choice of the similarity measure and does not directly determine the quality of the registration.

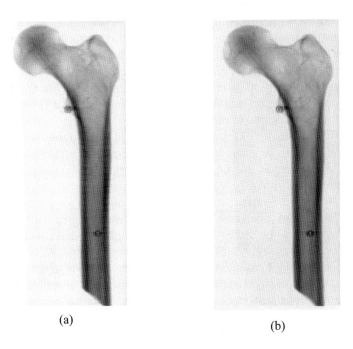

(a)   (b)

Fig. 6.6. Digitally reconstructed radiograph of dry femur from CT using a ray casting approach with (**a**) nearest neighbor and (**b**) linear interpolation of the intensity values. The interval between consecutive samples is 1 mm. Note the visible discontinuities corresponding to CT slice locations when using the nearest neighbor interpolator

Most of the research to date has focused on registration of various types of X-ray images to volumetric, primarily CT, data. In this context, a digitally reconstructed radiograph (DRR) is most often generated by casting rays from the known camera position toward the image plane and summing the volume intensity values found along each ray's path. In practice, the ray segment contained within the volume is sampled at regular intervals and the intensity values at these spatial locations are estimated via interpolation.

Figure 6.6 illustrates this approach and the effect of the interpolation on the quality of the simulated image.

Other direct volume rendering methods are also applicable but are less common. One such method is the splatting technique, which was used for DRR generation in Birkfellner et al. [2005]. This is an object-order, direct volume rendering method, where the voxels, or more often a kernel function that is placed at the voxel locations, are projected onto the image plane. A DRR is created by summing the intensity values of the projected voxels at each pixel location.

One of the first papers describing intensity-based registration of X-ray and CT was the work of Lemieux et al. [1994]. They generated DRR's using the ray casting rendering method with registration performed using the NCC similarity measure and Powell's standard optimization technique. This work identified the main limitation of intensity-based methods, the high computational complexity associated with DRR rendering. This is perhaps the primary factor that has delayed the introduction of intensity-based 2D/3D registration methods into clinical use.

In Hipwell et al. [2003], digital subtraction angiography images (X-ray angiography) were registered to a magnetic resonance (MR) angiography image. To enable the use of DRR image generation via ray casting, the MR angiography intensity values were mapped to new values, resulting in a CT-like angiographic image. Intensity mapping is performed using various hard, zero one, and fuzzy, probabilistic, segmentation methods. This is similar to the fuzzy segmentation approach described for 3D/3D registration. Interestingly, a decade after the initial work on intensity-based registration, the high computational complexity of DRR generation via ray casting was still identified as the limiting factor of this registration approach.

The high computational cost of rendering volumetric images has long been a subject of research in the computer graphics community. A more recent development on the border of computer graphics and computer vision is the subject of image-based rendering. This subject covers all methods that use a set of images to render novel views from camera poses not included in the original set of images. A prime example of this approach is the data structure known as the Lumigraph [Gortler et al. 1996] or light field [Levoy and Hanrahan 1996]. This is a 4D parameterized representation of the flow of light through space in a static scene, as computed from a set of images of the scene.

This approach was first adopted for fast DRR generation for X-ray CT registration in LaRose [2001] under the name Transgraph, with a reported hundred fold improvement in the rendering time. In this context, the images used to construct the light field are DRR's rendered prior to the registration process, transferring the bulk of the work to the data structure construction phase. This approach was used later on by Knaan and Joskowicz [2003] and more recently by Russakoff et al. [2005].

Although the light field does improve the rendering speed, it has two limitations. The size of the data structure is large, because of the amount of information required for rendering novel views, and the novel views are limited to camera poses that are close to those used to generate the images in the data structure construction phase. This second limitation is the more constrictive as it requires that the pose of the 2D X-ray imaging apparatus be roughly known in advance. In clinical practice, this is an assumption that can often be accommodated as there are standard viewing poses (e.g., anterior–posterior). An approach that mitigates the camera pose limitation at the cost of a smaller improvement in DRR rendering speed was presented by Rohlfing et al. [2005]. Instead of constructing the light field in advance, it is constructed progressively during the registration process when the pose is roughly known.

Another approach to reducing the rendering speed, is based on the use of the graphics processing unit (GPU). DRR's are generated by loading the CT volume into texture memory, rasterizing parallel polygonal slices that are perpendicular to the viewing direction and blending them using a transparency value [Cabral et al. 1994]. In LaRose [2001], this approach enabled the generation of 200×200 DRR images from CT volumes of up to $256 \times 256 \times 256$ voxels in approximately 25 ms. In Khamene et al. [2006], a similar approach enabled the generation of 256×256 DRR images from CT volumes of up to $256 \times 256 \times 216$ voxels in approximately 60 ms.

Although the majority of algorithms deal with 2D X-ray images, intensity-based registration of 2D video images from bronchoscopy to CT data has also been studied in Mori et al. [2002]. The registration framework remains the same, with the only difference being the rendering method. DRR generation is replaced by a standard surface rendering of a polygonal model extracted from the CT data. A similar approach is described by Turgeon et al. [2005] for registering coronary angiograms. In this case, rendered images of a 3D polygonal model of the coronaries are compared with segmented 2D X-ray images.

6.3.3 Gradient-Based Methods

Gradient-based methods cast registration as an optimization task where the objective function is directly dependent on image or surface gradients. This approach has been applied to registration of X-ray images to CT [Livyatan et al. 2003; Tomažević et al. 2003], X-ray images to MR [Tomazevic et al. 2003], and bronchoscopic video images to CT [Deligianni et al. 2004].

Livyatan et al. [2003] and Tomažević et al. [2003] show that there is a direct relationship between the 3D gradient vectors computed from CT intensity values and the 2D gradient vectors computed from an X-ray image of the same physical object. The relationship is derived using the physical model of X-ray propagation through material and assumes a logarithmic sensor response, as follows. The 2D image gradient is proportional to the projection onto the image plane of the weighted sum of 3D gradient vectors along the ray:

$$\nabla \operatorname{Im}(\tilde{\mathbf{p}}) \propto \begin{pmatrix} \mathbf{x}^{\mathrm{T}} \\ \mathbf{y}^{\mathrm{T}} \end{pmatrix} r(\tilde{\mathbf{p}}) \int_{\lambda} \lambda \nabla V(\mathbf{p}(\lambda)) d\lambda \tag{6.14}$$

where $\mathbf{x}$ and $\mathbf{y}$ are the camera coordinate system's axis with the viewing direction $\mathbf{z}$, $\tilde{\mathbf{p}}$ is a point on the image plane, $\mathbf{p}(\lambda)$ is a point on the ray connecting the camera location and $\tilde{\mathbf{p}}$, and $r(\tilde{\mathbf{p}})$ is the distance between the camera location and $\tilde{\mathbf{p}}$. Figure 6.7 illustrates these relationships.

Livyatan et al. [2003] use this observation to register X-ray images to CT in the following manner. For each X-ray image, a set of back-projected rays is defined via edge detection. The gradient of the CT volume is computed and the objective function is defined as a function of the magnitude of the volumetric gradient vectors projected onto the image plane along the back-projected rays. The optimal transformation is that which maximizes the magnitude of these projections, which means that the rays are close to the 3D surface in the volume.

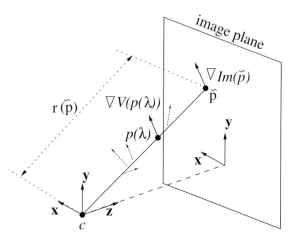

Fig. 6.7. Relationship between 3D gradient vectors, $\nabla V(\mathbf{p}(\lambda))$ along the ray connecting camera location $\mathbf{c}$ and image point $\tilde{\mathbf{p}}$, and the corresponding 2D gradient vector $\nabla \operatorname{Im}(\tilde{\mathbf{p}})$

In Tomaževič et al. [2003], the outlook is reversed. Surface points and their normals are obtained via edge detection from CT or MR. These points define a set of rays that emanate from the camera location. The gradient of each of the X-ray images is computed, and the objective function is defined as a function of the magnitudes of the 3D point normals and back-projections of the 2D gradients at the locations where the rays intersect the image plane, and the angular deviation between these two vectors. The optimal transformation maximizes the magnitude of the 2D back-projected gradients and the 3D normals, while at the same time minimizing their angular deviation.

Interestingly, this latter approach utilizes the rate of change in depth along the $\mathbf{x}$ and $\mathbf{y}$ camera axes at a specific surface point, which is known in the shape from shading literature as the surface gradient, $(p,q)= (\partial z/\partial x, \partial z/\partial y)$ [Zhang et al. 1999]. The use of the surface gradient for registration of bronchoscopic video images to CT is described by Deligianni et al. [2004]. In this case, a 3D model is extracted from the CT, and its surface gradient from the current estimated viewpoint is computed. An estimate of the surface gradient at each video pixel location is obtained using a shape from shading technique. The objective function is then defined as a function of the angular deviation between the two estimates of the surface gradient. The optimal transformation is the one that minimizes this deviation.

6.4   Registration Evaluation

To evaluate registration, we start by defining the characteristics of an ideal registration algorithm and then describe the criteria for evaluating Registration as they relate to these characteristics. An ideal registration algorithm is:

1. Fast: The result is obtained in real time
2. Accurate: After successful registration, the distance between corresponding points in the region of interest is less than 0.1 mm. This is the well-known target registration error (TRE) introduced in Maurer et al. [1997]
3. Robust: Has a breakdown point of $N/2$, more than half of the data elements must be outliers in order to throw the registration outside of reasonable bounds
4. Automatic: No user interaction is required
5. Reliable: Given the expected clinical input the registration always succeeds

Given these characteristics, registration is evaluated using the following criteria: (1) execution time, theoretical analysis, and performance on in vivo or in vitro data sets; (2) accuracy in the region of interest, a theoretical analysis, and performance on in vivo or in vitro data sets with a known *gold standard*; (3) breakdown point, a theoretical analysis; (4) automation, a binary classification of algorithms as either semiautomatic or automatic; (5) reliability of the algorithm, if iterative, provide proof of global convergence, and an estimate of the convergence range using *in vitro* or *in vivo* data sets with a known gold standard transformation. These are the maximal parameter deviations from the gold standard that result in a 95% success rate as judged by the accuracy in the region of interest and the limits imposed by the specific clinical application.

Given these evaluation criteria, it is clear that evaluation necessitates data sets with a known gold standard. Preferably these are *in vivo*, reflecting a clinical situation. In practice, most evaluation studies use in vitro data, as the common approach to obtaining a gold standard is based on implanting fiducials, which is not possible in most *in vivo* situations. More importantly, these data sets are usually not publicly available, precluding comparative algorithm evaluations.

The Retrospective Image Registration Evaluation project [Fitzpatrick 2007] addresses this issue for 3D/3D registration, by providing CT/MR and PET/MR in vivo data sets with known *gold standard* transformations. This is a well-established database that has been used to evaluate a wide variety of algorithms from more than 20 research groups [Fitzpatrick 2007; West et al. 1997].

The Standardized Evaluaton Methodology for 2D/3D Registration database [Van De Kraats 2007] is a more recent effort, providing in vitro data sets with known gold standards for evaluation of 2D/3D registration. The database includes pairs of 2D X-ray images and MR/CT/3DRX (cone beam CT) data sets. As this is a rather recent effort, it has only been used to evaluate a small number of algorithms [Van De Kraats et al. 2005].

Returning to our evaluation criteria, we divide them into two categories, those that are directly observable and those that are not. The former include the algorithm's execution time, its breakdown point, and its degree of automation. The latter include algorithm accuracy and reliability.

An algorithm's execution time is directly observable. In some cases theoretical analysis of the algorithm's computational complexity is also possible, although most evaluation studies only report empirical results. For most clinical procedures, real time performance is ideal but not necessary. Rather, a maximal execution time is defined and all algorithms whose execution time is below this threshold can be considered equivalent. It should be emphasized that the execution time criterion includes the total running time. It is often the case that iterative algorithms do not report the running time of their initialization phase. This is somewhat misleading as it is the total running time required to obtain the registration result that ascertains its applicability.

An algorithm's breakdown point, its robustness to outlying data, is analyzed in a theoretical manner. Interestingly, even a low breakdown point does not imply that an algorithm is not useful, only that a prior outlier rejection phase is required if the algorithm is used. This is clearly the case with the analytic paired-point registration algorithms whose breakdown point is one, yet are in widespread use.

We classify registration algorithms as either automatic or semiautomatic, requiring some form of user interaction. On the one hand, analytic algorithms are automatic. On the other hand, iterative algorithms may require user interaction as part of their initialization. In most cases, this fact is downplayed with emphasis placed on the automatic nature of the main body of the algorithm. To gauge an algorithm's applicability for a specific procedure, the whole framework should be classified, and not just the main body of the algorithm.

Algorithm accuracy is the single most important evaluation criterion, as it directly addresses the goal of registration, alignment of corresponding points. Two aspects of this criterion should be noted; accuracy is spatially variant, and it cannot be directly inferred from the optimal value of the objective function. Very few analytic estimates of accuracy have been developed. Currently, these are limited to paired-point registration algorithms. The seminal work on this subject was presented in Fitzpatrick et al. [1998]. This work established the relationship between the expected squared values of the error measures associated with paired-point registration: (1) fiducial localization error (*FLE*) – error in fiducial localization in both data sets; (2) fiducial registration error (*FRE*) – error in corresponding fiducial locations after registration; and (3) target registration error (*TRE*) – error in corresponding nonfiducial point locations after registration.

Prior to this work, *FRE* was used in many navigation systems as an indicator of registration accuracy, leading, in some cases, to over or under estimation of the registration accuracy at the target. Note that the derivation by Fitzpatrick et al. assumes that fiducial localization errors are isotropic, and IID with a zero mean Gaussian distribution. Under this assumption, the relationship between FLE and FRE is given as:

$$\mathrm{E}\left(FRE^2\right) \approx \frac{(n-2)\,\mathrm{E}\left(FLE^2\right)}{\mathrm{n}} \qquad (6.15)$$

where n is the number of fiducials. The expected squared *TRE* was then derived as:

$$\mathrm{E}\left(TRE^2(\mathbf{p})\right) \approx \frac{\mathrm{E}\left(FRE^2\right)}{(n-2)}\left(1+\frac{1}{3}\sum_{i=1}^{3}\frac{d_k^2}{f_k^2}\right) \qquad (6.16)$$

where $\mathbf{p}$ is the target point, d_k^2 is the squared distance between the target point and the kth principle axis of the fiducial configuration, and f_k^2 is the mean squared distance between the fiducial points and the same axis.

Later on, Fitzpatrick and West [2001] introduced a first order approximation of the distribution of the *TRE*. More recently, Moghari and Abolmaesumi [2006] introduced a second order approximation of the distribution of the *TRE* on the basis of the Unscented Kalman Filter.

For all other registration algorithms, accuracy is evaluated empirically. That is, evaluation studies are carried out in one of two ways, with or without a known *gold standard* transformation. When a *gold standard* is available, accuracy is readily quantified across the region of interest. This approach provides insight into an algorithm's behavior, but it cannot be used to estimate the accuracy that is obtained on data sets not included in the study. When a *gold standard* is not available, accuracy is often assessed qualitatively by visual inspection, and quantitatively by manually identifying corresponding points. Although this approach does provide accuracy information at specific point-locations, it depends on the accuracy of manual localization and the information is limited to the specific spatial locations.

Finally, the reliability of iterative algorithms is most often evaluated empirically using data sets that have a *gold standard* transformation. By initializing the registration with parameter values sampled in the region of the *gold standard* values the convergence range can be estimated. As this is an empirical approach, its conclusions are only valid if the input data represent the distribution of the general data set population. Ensuring this requires the use of a large number of data sets.

6.5   Conclusions

Rigid registration, whether as an end in itself, or as a precursor to a nonrigid registration procedure, remains a fundamental component of all image-guided surgical applications. Most problems in rigid registration have been addressed, with research focus shifting to nonrigid registration, although there is still work to be done in evaluation and validation.

Currently, only the paired-point registration algorithms are truly complete. They have analytic solutions, their computational complexity is known, and most importantly, the expected *TRE* and its distribution can be computed. That is, we are guaranteed to find the optimum, we know how long it will take, and once we have the transformation we can estimate the error at our target. This is not the case with all other registration algorithms. The probability to find the optimum subject to certain constraints is high, the computational complexity is known, but we do not have methods for estimating the *TRE*.

Interestingly, for 2D/3D registration of bronchoscopic/endoscopic video images to CT, it is still not clear how well the existing algorithms deal with clinical data, as most of the reported evaluation studies have been done on phantoms. It is still also not clear if rigid registration is sufficiently accurate for these types of procedures as it is an approximation of the true physical reality.

Finally, we still need to establish standard in vivo data sets with known gold standard transformations for evaluating registration of US data to 3D images, 2D/3D registration of X-ray images to 3D images, and bronchoscopic/endoscopic images to 3D images.

References

Arun KS, Huang TS, and Blostein SD. (1987). "Least-squares fitting of two 3D point sets." *IEEE Transact Pattern Anal Machine Intell*, 9(5), 698–700.

Audette MA, Ferrie FP, and Peters TM. (2000). "An algorithmic overview of surface registration techniques for medical imaging." *Med Image Anal*, 4(3), 201–217.

Balachandran R, Fitzpatrick JM, and Labadie RF. (2005). "Fiducial registration for tracking systems that employ coordinate reference frames." *SPIE Med Imaging: Visualization, Image-guided Procedures, Display*, 5744, 134–145.

Barratt DC, Penney GP, Chan CS, Slomczykowski M, Carter TJ, Edwards PJ, and Hawkes DJ. (2006). "Self-calibrating 3D-ultrasound based bone registration for minimally invasive orthopedic surgery." *IEEE Trans Med Imaging*, 25(3), 312–323.

Besl PJ and McKay ND. (1992). "A method for registration of 3D shapes." *IEEE Transact Pattern Anal Machine Intell*, 14(2), 239–255.

Bijhold J. (1993). "Three-dimensional verification of patient placement during radiotherapy using portal images." *Med Phys*, 20(2), 347–356.

Birkfellner W, Seemann R, Figl M, Hummel J, Ede C, Homolka P, Yang X, Niederer P, and Bergmann H. (2005). "Wobbled splatting–a fast perspective volume rendering method for simulation of X-ray images from CT." *Phys Med Biol*, 50(9), N73–84.

Burschka D, Li M, Ishii M, Taylor RH, and Hager GD. (2005). "Scale-invariant registration of monocular endoscopic images to CT-scans for sinus surgery." *Med Image Anal*, 9(5), 413–426.

Buzug TM, Weese J, Fassnacht C, and Lorenz C. (1997). "Image registration: convex weighting functions for histogram-based similarity measures." *CVRMed-MRCAS 1997*, Springer, Berlin Heidelberg New York, 203–212.

Cabral B, Cam N, and Foran J. (1994). "Accelerated volume rendering and tomographic reconstruction using texture mapping hardware." *Proceedings of the 1994 Symposium on Volume Visualization*, ACM Press, New York, USA, 91–98.

Chen Y and Medioni G. (1992). "Object modeling by registration of multiple range images." *Image Vis Comput*, 10(3), 145–155.

Chetverikov D, Stepanov D, and Krsek P. (2005). "Robust Euclidean alignment of 3D point sets: the trimmed iterative closest point algorithm." *Image Vis Comput*, 23(3), 299–309.

Collignon A, Vandermeulen D, Suetans P, and Marchal G. (1995). "3D multi modality medical image registration using feature space clustering." *Computer Vision, Virtual Reality and Robotics in Medicine*, Springer, Berlin Heidelberg New York, 195–204.

Deligianni F, Chung A, and Yang GZ. (2004). "Patient-specific bronchoscope simulation with pq-space-based 2D/3D registration." *Comput Aided Surg*, 9(5), 215–226.

Duda RO, Hart PE, and Stork DG. (2001). *Pattern Classification*, 2nd Ed., Wiley, New York.

Eggert DW, Lorusso A, and Fisher RB. (1997). "Estimating 3-D rigid body transformations: a comparison of four major algorithms." *Machine Vis Appl*, 9(5–6), 272–290.

Estépar RSJ, Brun A, and Westin C-F. (2004). "Robust generalized total least squares iterative closest point registration." *Seventh International Conference on Medical Image Computing and Computer-Assisted Intervention (MICCAI'04)*, Springer-Verlag, St. Malo, France, 234–241.

Faugeras OD and Hebert M. (1986). "The representation, recognition, and locating of 3-D objects." *Int J Robotics Res*, 5(3), 27–52.

Fitzgibbon AW. (2003). "Robust registration of 2D and 3D point sets." *Image Vis Comput*, 21(13–14), 1145–1153.

Fitzpatrick JM. (2007). "Retrospective image registration evaluation project." http://www.insight-journal.org/rire/index.html, accessed February 2007.

Fitzpatrick JM and West JB. (2001). "The distribution of target registration error in rigid-body point-based registration." *IEEE Trans Med Imaging*, 20(9), 917–927.

Fitzpatrick JM, West JB, and Maurer CR, Jr. (1998). "Predicting error in rigid-body point-based registration." *IEEE Trans Med Imaging*, 17(5), 694–702.

Fletcher R. (1987). *Practical Methods of Optimization*, 2nd Ed., Wiley-Interscience, New York.

Foley JD, van Dam A, Feiner SK, and Hughes JF. (1996). *Computer graphics: Principles and practice*, 2nd Ed., Addison-Wesley Longman, Boston, MA.

Gong RH, Stewart AJ, and Abolmaesumi P. (2006). "A new method for CT to fluoroscope registration based on unscented Kalman filter." *Ninth International Conference on Medical Image Computing and Computer-Assisted Intervention (MICCAI'06)*, Springer-Verlag, Copenhagen, Denmark. (Pt 1), 891–898.

Gortler S, Grzeszczuk R, Szeliski R, and Cohen M. (1996). "The Lumigraph." Proceedings of the 23rd Annual Conference on *Computer Graphics, Annual Conference Series 1996 (SIGGRAPH '96)*, ACM press, New York, USA, 43–54.

Goshtasby A. (2005). *2-D and 3-D Image Registration*, Wiley, New York.

Greenspan M and Yurick M. (2003). "Approximate K-D tree search for efficient ICP." *Proceedings of the Fourth International. Conference on 3-D Digital Imaging and Modeling*, 442–448.

Grimson WEL and Lozano-Perez T. (1987). "Localizing overlapping parts by searching the interpretation tree." *IEEE Transact Pattern Anal Machine Intell*, 9(4), 469–482.

Gueziec A, Kazanzides P, Williamson B, and Taylor RH. (1998). "Anatomy-based registration of CT-scan and intraoperative X-ray images for guiding a surgical robot." *IEEE Trans Med Imaging*, 17(5), 715–728.

Hajnal JV, Hill DLG, and Hawkes DJ. (2001). *Medical Image Registration*, CRC Press.

Hamadeh A, Lavallée S, and Cinquin P. (1998). "Automated 3-dimensional computed tomographic and fluoroscopic image registration." *Comput Aided Surg*, 3(1), 11–19.

Hill DL, Batchelor PG, Holden M, and Hawkes DJ. (2001). "Medical image registration." *Phys Med Biol*, 46(3), R1–R45.

Hipwell JH, Penney GP, McLaughlin RA, Rhode K, Summers P, Cox TC, Byrne JV, Noble JA, and Hawkes DJ. (2003). "Intensity-based 2-D-3-D registration of cerebral angiograms." *IEEE Trans Med Imaging*, 22(11), 1417–1426.

Ho YC and Pepyne DL. (2002). "Simple explanation of the no-free-lunch theorem and its implications." *J Optimization Theor Appl*, 115(3), 549–570.

Horn BKP. (1987). "Closed-form solution of absolute orientation using unit quaternions." *J Opt Soc Am A*, 4(4), 629–642.

Horn BKP, Hilden HM, and Negahdaripour S. (1988). "Closed-form solution of absolute orientation using orthonormal matrices." *J Opt Soc Am A*, 5(7), 1127–1135.

Jost T and Hugli H. (2003). "A multi-resolution ICP with heuristic closest point search for fast and robust 3D registration of range images." *Proceedings of the Fourth International Conference on 3-D Digital Imaging and Modeling (3DIM 2003)*, 427–433.

Jumarie G. (1997). "A new information theoretic approach to the entropy of non-random discrete maps relation to fractal dimension and temperature of curves." *Chaos, Solitons and Fractals*, 8(6), 953–970.

Kaneko S, Kondo T, and Miyamoto A. (2003). "Robust matching of 3D contours using iterative closest point algorithm improved by M-estimation." *Pattern Recognition*, 36(9), 2041–2047.

Khamene A, Bloch P, Wein W, Svatos M, and Saur F. (2006). "Automatic registration of portal images and volumetric CT for patient positioning in radiation therapy." *Med Image Anal*, 10(1), 96–112.

Knaan D and Joskowicz L. (2003). "Effective intensity-based 2D/3D rigid registration between fluoroscopic X-ray and CT." *Medical Image Computing and Computer-Assisted Intervention (MICCAI 2003)*, Springer-Verlag, Montreal, Canada, 351–358.

Langis C, Greenspan M, and Godin G. (2001). "The parallel iterative closest point algorithm." *Proceedings of the Third International Conference on 3-D Digital Imaging and Modeling (3DIM 2001)*, 195–204.

LaRose DA. (2001). "Iterative X-ray/CT Registration Using Accelerated Volume Rendering," PhD, Carnegie Mellon University, Pittsburgh, PA.

Lavallée S and Szeliski R. (1995). "Recovering the position and orientation of free-form objects from image contours using 3D distance maps." *IEEE Transact Pattern Anal Machine Intell*, 17(4), 378–390.

Lehmann TM, Gonner C, and Spitzer K. (1999). "Survey: Interpolation methods in medical image processing." *IEEE Trans Med Imaging*, 18(11), 1049–1075.

Lemieux L, Jagoe R, Fish DR, Kitchen ND, and Thomas GT. (1994). "A patient-to-computed-tomography image registration method based on digitally reconstructed radiographs." *Med Phys*, 21(11), 1749–1760.

Levoy M and Hanrahan P. (1996). "Light field rendering." *Proceedings of the 23rd Annual Conference on Computer graphics and interactive techniques (SIGGRAPH 1996)*, ACM Press, New York, USA, 31–42.

Livyatan H, Yaniv Z, and Joskowicz L. (2003). "Gradient-based 2D/3D rigid registration of fluoroscopic X-ray to CT." *IEEE Trans Med Imaging*, 22(11), 1395–1406.

Lorensen WE and Cline HE. (1987). "Marching cubes: A high resolution 3D surface construction algorithm." *Comput Graphics*, 21(4), 163–169.

Luck JP, Little CQ, and Hoff W. (2000). "Registration of range data using a hybrid simulated annealing and iterative closest point algorithm." *Proceedings of the IEEE International Conference on Robotics and Automation (ICRA 2000)*, 4, 3739–3744.

Ma B and Ellis R. (2006). "Analytic expressions for fiducial and surface target registration error." *Medical Image Computing and Computer-Assisted*

Intervention (MICCAI 2006), Springer-Verlag, Copenhagen, Denmark, 637–644.

Ma B and Ellis RE. (2003). "Robust registration for computer-integrated orthopedic surgery: laboratory validation and clinical experience." *Med Image Anal*, 7(3), 237–250.

Maes F, Collignon A, Vandermeulen D, Marchal G, and Suetens P. (1997). "Multimodality image registration by maximization of mutual information." *IEEE Trans Med Imaging*, 16(2), 187–198.

Maintz JB, van den Elsen PA, and Viergever MA. (1996). "Comparison of edge-based and ridge-based registration of CT and MR brain images." *Med Image Anal*, 1(2), 151–161.

Maintz JB and Viergever MA. (1998). "A survey of medical image registration." *Med Image Anal*, 2(1), 1–36.

Masuda T and Yokoya N. (1995). "A robust method for registration and segmentation of multiple range images." *Comput Vis Image Understanding*, 61(3), 295–307.

Matei B and Meer P. (1999). "Optimal rigid motion estimation and performance evaluation with bootstrap." *IEEE Computer Society conference on Computer ision and Pattern Recognition (CVPR 1999)*, 1339–1347.

Maurer CR, Jr., Fitzpatrick JM, Wang MY, Galloway RL, Jr., Maciunas RJ, and Allen GS. (1997). "Registration of head volume images using implantable fiducial markers." *IEEE Trans Med Imaging*, 16(4), 447–462.

Maurer CR, Jr., Maciunas RJ, and Fitzpatrick JM. (1998). "Registration of head CT images to physical space using a weighted combination of points and surfaces." *IEEE Trans Med Imaging*, 17(5), 753–761.

Meijering EH, Niessen WJ, and Viergever MA. (2001). "Quantitative evaluation of convolution-based methods for medical image interpolation." *Med Image Anal*, 5(2), 111–126.

Moghari MH and Abolmaesumi P. (2005). "A novel incremental technique for ultrasound to CT bone surface registration using Unscented Kalman Filtering." *Eighth International Conference on Medical Image Computing and Computer-Assisted Intervention (MICCAI 2005)*, Springer-Verlag, Palm Springs, 8(Pt 2), 197–204.

Moghari MH and Abolmaesumi P. (2006). "A high-order solution for the distribution of target registration error in rigid-body point-based registration." *Ninth International Conference on Medical Image Computing and Computer-Assisted Intervention (MICCAI 2006)*, Springer-Verlag, Copenhagen, Denmark, 603–611.

Mori K, Deguchi D, Sugiyama J, Suenaga Y, Toriwaki J, Maurer CR, Jr., Takabatake H, and Natori H. (2002). "Tracking of a bronchoscope using epipolar geometry analysis and intensity-based image registration of real and virtual endoscopic images." *Med Image Anal*, 6(3), 321–336.

Murphy MJ. (1997). "An automatic six-degree-of-freedom image registration algorithm for image-guided frameless stereotaxic radiosurgery." *Med Phys*, 24(6), 857–866.

Ohta N and Kanatani K. (1998). "Optimal estimation of three-dimensional rotation and reliability evaluation." *Computer Vision – ECCV 1998*, Springer, Heidelberg, Germany, 175–187.

Pelizzari CA, Chen GT, Spelbring DR, Weichselbaum RR, and Chen CT. (1989). "Accurate three-dimensional registration of CT, PET, and/or MR images of the brain." *J Comput Assist Tomogr*, 13(1), 20–26.

Pennec X and Thirion J-P. (1997). "A framework for uncertainty and validation of 3-D registration methods based on points and frames." *Int J Comput Vision*, 25(3), 203–229.

Penney GP, Barratt DC, Chan CS, Slomczykowski M, Carter TJ, Edwards PJ, and Hawkes DJ. (2006). "Cadaver validation of intensity-based ultrasound to CT registration." *Med Image Anal*, 10(3), 385–395.

Penney GP, Blackall JM, Hamady MS, Sabharwal T, Adam A, and Hawkes DJ. (2004). "Registration of freehand 3D ultrasound and magnetic resonance liver images." *Med Image Anal*, 8(1), 81–91.

Penney GP, Edwards PJ, JKing AP, Blackall JM, Batchelor PG, and Hawkes DJ. (2001). "A stochastic iterative closest point algorithm (stochastICP)." *Medical Image Computing and Computer-Assisted Intervention – MICCAI 2001*, Springer-Verlag, Heidelberg, Germany, 762–769.

Pluim JP, Maintz JB, and Viergever MA. (2003). "Mutual-information-based registration of medical images: a survey." *IEEE Trans Med Imaging*, 22(8), 986–1004.

Pluim JPW, Maintz JBA, and Viergever MA. (2000). "Interpolation artefacts in mutual information-based image registration." *Computer Vision and Image Understanding*, 77(2), 211–223.

Press WH, Flannery BP, Teukolsky SA, and Vetterling WT. (1992). *Numerical Recipes: The Art of Scientific Computing*, 2nd Ed., Cambridge University Press, Cambridge.

Robinson M, Eckhoff DG, Reinig KD, Bagur MM, and Bach JM. (2006). "Variability of landmark identification in total knee arthroplasty." *Clin Orthop Relat Res*, 442, 57–62.

Roche A, Malandain G, Pennec X, and Ayache N. (1998). "The correlation ratio as a new similarity measure for multimodal image registration." *Medical Image Computing and Computer-Assisted Intervention – MICCAI 1998*, Springer-Verlag, Heidelberg, Germany, 1115–1124.

Rohlfing T, Russakoff DB, Denzler J, Mori K, and Maurer CR, Jr. (2005). "Progressive attenuation fields: fast 2D-3D image registration without precomputation." *Med Phys*, 32(9), 2870–2880.

Russakoff DB, Rohlfing T, Mori K, Rueckert D, Ho A, Adler JR, Jr., and Maurer CR, Jr. (2005). "Fast generation of digitally reconstructed radiographs using attenuation fields with application to 2D-3D image registration." *IEEE Trans Med Imaging*, 24(11), 1441–1454.

Schönemann PH. (1966). "A generalized solution of the orthogonal procrustes problem." *Psychometrika*, 31, 1–10.

Simon D. (1996). "Fast and Accurate Shape-Based Registration," PhD, Carnegie Mellon University. Pittsburgh, PA.

Škerl D, Likar B, and Pernus F. (2006). "A protocol for evaluation of similarity measures for rigid registration." *IEEE Trans Med Imaging*, 25(6), 779–791.

Studholme C, Hill DLG, and Hawkes DJ. (1999). "An overlap invariant entropy measure of 3D medical image alignment." *Pattern Recognition*, 32(1), 71–86.

Tomaževič D, Likar B, and Pernus F. (2006). "3-D/2-D registration by integrating 2-D information in 3-D." *IEEE Trans Med Imaging*, 25(1), 17–27.

Tomazežič D, Likar B, Slivnik T, and Pernus F. (2003). "3-D/2-D registration of CT and MR to X-ray images." *IEEE Trans Med Imaging*, 22(11), 1407–1416.

Trucco E, Fusiello A, and Roberto V. (1999). "Robust motion and correspondence of noisy 3-D point sets with missing data." *Pattern Recognition Lett*, 20(9), 889–898.

Turk G and Levoy M. (1994). "Zippered polygon meshes from range images." *Proceedings of the 21st Annual Conference on Computer graphics and interactive techniques (SIGGRAPH 1994)*, ACM Press, New York, USA, 311–318.

Umeyama S. (1991). "Least-squares estimation of transformation parameters between two point patterns." *IEEE Transact Pattern Anal Machine Intell*, 13(4), 376–380.

van de Kraats EB. (2007). "Standardized evaluation methodology for 2D-3D registration." http://www.isi.uu.nl/Research/Databases/GS/, accessed February 2007.

van de Kraats EB, Penney GP, Tomazevic D, van Walsum T, and Niessen WJ. (2005). "Standardized evaluation methodology for 2-D-3-D registration." *IEEE Trans Med Imaging*, 24(9), 1177–1189.

Viola P and Wells III WM. (1995). "Alignment by maximization of mutual information." *IEEE International Conference on Computer Vision*, 16–23.

Viola P and Wells III WM. (1997). "Alignment by maximization of mutual information." *Int J Comput Vision*, 24(2), 137–154.

Walker MW, Shao L, and Volz RA. (1991). "Estimating 3-D location parameters using dual number quaternions." *CVGIP: Image Understanding*, 54(3), 358–367.

Wang MY, Maurer CR, Jr., Fitzpatrick JM, and Maciunas RJ. (1996). "An automatic technique for finding and localizing externally attached markers in CT and MR volume images of the head." *IEEE Trans Biomed Eng*, 43(6), 627–637.

Weese J, Rosch P, Netsch T, Blaffert T, and Quist M. (1999). "Gray-value based registration of CT and MR images by maximization of local correlation." *Medical Image Computing and Computer-Assisted Intervention (MICCAI 1999)*, Springer-Verlag, Heidelberg, Germany, 656–663.

West J, Fitzpatrick JM, Wang MY, Dawant BM, Maurer CR, Jr., Kessler RM, Maciunas RJ, Barillot C, Lemoine D, Collignon A, Maes F, Suetens P, Vandermeulen D, van den Elsen PA, Napel S, Sumanaweera TS, Harkness B, Hemler PF, Hill DL, Hawkes DJ, Studholme C, Maintz JB, Viergever MA, Malandain G, Woods RP, et al. (1997). "Comparison and evaluation of retrospective intermodality brain image registration techniques." *J Comput Assist Tomogr*, 21(4), 554–566.

Wörz S and Rohr K. (2006). "Localization of anatomical point landmarks in 3D medical images by fitting 3D parametric intensity models." *Med Image Anal*, 10(1), 41–58.

Wunsch P and Hirzinger G. (1996). "Registration of CAD-models to images by iterative inverse perspective matching." *Proceedings of the 13th International Conference on Pattern Recognition (ICPR 1996)*, Vienna, Austria, 78–83.

Zhang R, Tsai P-S, Cryer JE, and Shah M. (1999). "Shape from shading: A survey." *IEEE Transact Pattern Anal Machine Intell*, 21(2), 690–706.

Zhang Z. (1994). "Iterative point matching for registration of free-form curves and surfaces." *Int J Comput Vision*, 13(2), 119–152.

Chapter 7

Nonrigid Registration

David Hawkes, Dean Barratt, Tim Carter, Jamie McClelland,
and Bill Crum

Abstract

This chapter describes the convergence of technologies between interventional
radiology, image-guided surgery, and image-directed therapy. Nonrigid registration has an important part to play in this trend and different approaches to nonrigid
registration are summarized. The role of nonrigid registration for image-guided
procedures in the building and instantiation of anatomical atlases, modeling large
deformations of soft tissues by incorporating biomechanical models, and modeling
cyclic respiratory and cardiac motion for image guidance is described. These
concepts are illustrated with descriptions of prototype systems with applications in
the brain, breast, lung, liver, and orthopaedics.

7.1   Introduction

Conventional image-guided intervention (IGI) uses rigid body registration
between the plan and the operative scene as described in Chap. 6: Rigid
Registration. These methods are generally limited to structures such as the
components of the skeleton that are inherently rigid, or to structures for which
a rigid transformation is sufficiently accurate. Computer-assisted orthopaedic surgery is an example of the former, while image-guided surgery of the
brain and other intracranial structures are examples of the latter, where prior
to osteotomy, anatomy is encased by the skull and experiences only small
deformations. Conventional IGI does not provide direct feedback of any
change in the interrelationship between anatomical structures. This can only
be provided by intraoperative sensing and imaging coupled either with the
means to compare with the surgical plan, using, for example, augmented
reality displays, or with some means of establishing correspondence between
intra and preoperative data, such as by nonrigid registration.

Similar principles are used in image-directed therapy and, in particular, image-directed radiotherapy. A plan of treatment and the dose to be

delivered is created from preoperative imaging, and *in-room* imaging is used to position the patient and register the plan. *In-room* imaging can include optical camera systems, megavoltage CT incorporated within the linear accelerator (linac), kilovoltage CT attached to the linac gantry, and even interventional MR or ultrasound sensors. In the future, these will be used to compensate for any patient motion or change in patient anatomy between fractions of therapy.

Interventional radiology relies entirely on real-time imaging to provide feedback between the interventional device, such as the catheter or needle, and related radiological anatomy. If other 3D information is required to guide the procedure, then registration is required to establish spatial correspondence between this 3D preoperative information and the interventional image coordinates. This can be used to localize structures not visible in the interventional image, but visible in preprocedure images and plans generated from them.

Each paradigm may make use of information derived from anatomical and functional computer models or atlases. Atlas generation and the establishment of spatial correspondence between the atlas and the preoperative image coordinates during planning and guidance will generally require nonrigid registration.

This leads to a generalized paradigm of spatial support for image-guided interventions as described in Fig. 7.1. Although this paradigm is generalizable to almost any intervention that uses imaging for guidance, nonrigid registration technologies that are currently available lack the robustness required for clinical practice. Currently, there are few reports of the clinical validation of an image guidance system that makes use of a deformable computational model, motion model, or deformable atlas. However, it is clear that such technology could have a major impact on some of the most common life-threatening conditions for which surgery provides the best option for the patient [Hawkes et al. 2005]. Recent examples of experimental procedures that have been reported include the use of statistical atlases to assist in electrode placement in deep brain stimulation described in Chap. 11: Neurosurgical Applications [Guo et al. 2006, 2007; D'Haese et al. 2005] and the use of deformable atlases of bony anatomy in orthopaedic surgery in the spine [Lavallee et al. 2004] or hip [Yao and Taylor 2003; Chan et al. 2004]. Motion models are being developed in image-directed radiotherapy of the lung [McClelland et al. 2006], interventions in the liver [Blackall et al. 2005; Penney et al. 2004; Coolens et al. 2007], and in interventional cardiac applications using a combined X-ray and MR system where an affine model is used [Rhode et al. 2005]. Looking ahead, examples where deformable models might assist include a wide range of interventions and targeted therapies that will have significant clinical impact in the brain, head and neck region, lung, heart, breast, liver, pancreas, prostate, and colon.

Planning the Intervention

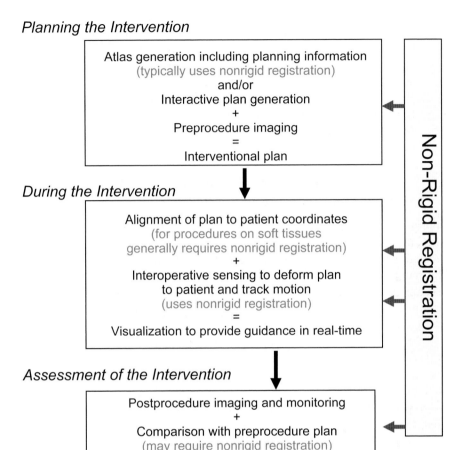

Fig. 7.1. Input of nonrigid registration to the three stages of planning, guidance, and postprocedure assessment

As we will show, there is a convergence of technologies driven by clinical requirements and methodological developments between image-guided interventional radiology and image-guided surgery. A core technology required for these developments is robust and accurate nonrigid registration.

This chapter describes the various nonrigid registration technologies that have been proposed for atlas generation, intraoperative guidance, and treatment monitoring. We describe the most promising technologies, and approaches to their validation in specific application areas. The structure of the chapter is as follows:

1. Introduction to nonrigid registration technologies
2. Applications to atlas building and subsequent patient-specific instantiation
3. Nonrigid registration coupled with biomechanical models to compensate for tissue deformation between plan and intervention
4. How nonrigid registration is used to derive models of cyclic motion because of cardiac or respiratory motion
5. A brief description of applications in the brain, breast, lung, liver, and in orthopaedics.

7.2   Nonrigid Registration Technologies Potentially Applicable to Image-Guided Interventions

Nonrigid registration is most well-developed in 3D-to-3D applications in atlas building; otherwise 3D-to-3D registration is only used in rather specialized guidance applications using interventional MRI, CT, or 3D ultrasound. The temporal and spatial resolutions of 3D ultrasound, in particular, are developing very rapidly and are quite likely to have a major impact in interventional work, with a concomitant demand for fast, robust, and accurate nonrigid registration.

Most rigid body techniques can be extended relatively straightforwardly from the six degrees-of-freedom of rigid body motion (translations along and rotations around the three ordinates) to affine by including scaling in each ordinate (three degrees-of-freedom) and shearing (an extra two degrees of freedom). Affine transformations are useful for compensating for global changes in size and scanner calibration errors that can cause images to shear and image scaling errors. In some circumstances, local rigid registration can be used effectively to correct for nonrigid transformations, as described in the neuron example given below. As rigid body algorithms are considered in Chap. 6: Rigid Registration, they will not be considered further here.

A basic nonmathematical review of nonrigid registration is provided in Crum et al. [2004], while more thorough reviews are provided in Hajnal et al. [2001], Hill et al. [2001], and Modersitzki [2004]. Generally, nonrigid registration algorithms have three components:

1. A transformation model that defines the class of possible transformations
2. A measure of alignment of corresponding structures for feature-based registration, or a voxel similarity measure for intensity-based registration
3. A means of optimizing the transformation, including regularization, that produced a best fit of one image to the other

There are two main categories of methods used to register 3D image pairs, those based on establishing correspondence between extracted features (points, lines, surfaces, and even volumes), so called *feature-based,* and those in which a measure of similarity is computed directly from the voxel intensities, often termed *intensity-based.*

A key issue with all registration methods is the definition of correspondence. Registration establishes the relationship between points in images that correspond to the same anatomical or tissue location in each image. When aligning a preoperative image (or plan derived from it) with an intraoperative image, then the definition of correspondence is relatively straightforward. Although structure may not be visible in both sets of images, their presence can be inferred. Exceptions occur when new tissue is formed, such as occurs with tumor growth, or disappear, due to necrosis, tissue resorption, or tissue resection by the intervention itself. In some cases of tumor resection, alignment of the plan may provide information on tumor extent at the beginning of the procedure, and this can be useful information when checking that the resection is complete. The definition of correspondence is less straightforward when aligning a statistical shape model with the intraoperative data. For example, this might be used to infer the location of structure that is not visible in the intraoperative image, removing the need for preoperative imaging entirely. Whether this is done correctly will depend on correspondence between model and patient and the accuracy of the instantiation of the model. The validity of this process is a key requirement of system validation.

7.2.1 Feature-Based Algorithms

Feature-based algorithms rely on the accurate extraction of corresponding or adjacent features. Examples include those based on identification of corresponding points and contour orientation at these points [Rohr et al. 2001, 2003], identification of corresponding ridges and crest lines [Monga and Benayoun 1995] and even tubes (e.g., vascular trees) [Aylward et al. 2003] and the matching of surfaces. An example of the latter is the matching of brain and skin surfaces from MR and CT to intraoperative brain surfaces from cortical range imaging [Audette et al. 1999]. On the one hand, feature-based algorithms usually operate by minimizing a distance metric between corresponding features. These algorithms tend to be faster and therefore more suited to real-time application than intensity-based algorithms. On the other hand, corresponding features need to be identified as a preprocessing step and this might introduce inaccuracies. Also, robustness of the algorithm may be limited as there is unlikely to be sufficient information (i.e., corresponding points) to derive a nonrigid transformation that has many degrees of freedom. An approach to better regularization of the problem is to incorporate other information. An early example of this approach was the embedding of rigid structures within a deforming matrix defined by a radial basis function [Little et al. 1997].

7.2.2 Intensity-Based Algorithms

Intensity-based algorithms operate directly on voxel intensities and do not require any prior object identification, except in certain circumstances to delineate a region of interest over which the transformation is to be computed. Transformation models can be based on spline functions decomposed into the principle warps of a thin plate [Bookstein et al. 1989], a free form deformation given by approximating B-splines defined by a rectangular array of node points [Rueckert et al. 1999], the deformation of a linear elastic material [Bajscy and Kovacic 1989; Gee et al. 1993], or the motion of a viscous fluid [Christensen et al. 1996]. The demons algorithm, on the basis of optical flow, can be thought of as an approximation to fluid-based registration [Bro-Nielsen and Grankow 1996; Thirion 1998].

The nonrigid registration algorithm that uses free-form deformations defined by approximating B-splines has found very wide application and is inherently multiscale, with scale defined by the node point spacing [Rueckert et al. 1999]. It also has local rather than global support, and thus is well-suited to computing a local deformation, for example from a focal intervention. The resulting deformation field can fold and so extra precautions are required to avoid this [Rueckert et al. 2006]. Unfortunately, running the algorithm at high resolution (and hence higher accuracy) can be very computationally expensive, and so it is not so well-suited to real-time image guidance applications. Recently, multiscale versions of the viscous fluid algorithm have been reported [Crum et al. 2005], and these now have a competitive computational cost when compared with the B-spline algorithm. The deformation field produced is diffeomorphic (i.e., it does not fold).

7.2.2.1 Similarity Measures

The intensity-based algorithms are all based on an optimization process that assesses the *fitness* of trial deformations on the basis of some measure of *similarity* of the corresponding intensity distributions. If the same modality is used pre and intraoperatively then the optimal measure for images that have a Gaussian noise distribution is the sum of squares of intensity differences (SSD). If there is a linear scaling of intensities, then the correlation coefficient is the measure of choice. If there is a statistical dependence between the two intensity distributions at alignment, then mutual information and its normalized form [Wells 1996; Viola and Wells 2005; Maes et al. 1997; Studholme et al. 1996, 1997, 1999] or the correlation ratio [Roche et al.

1998] are the methods of choice. The merits of the different measures are discussed in detail in Hajnal et al. [2001].

7.2.3 Optimization

None of the nonrigid registration algorithms described earlier provides direct analytic solutions, and so optimization is required. Various optimization strategies have been proposed, but the most popular remain the most simple on the basis on a multiresolution search. Methods used include Downhill Simplex, Powell's Method, Steepest Gradient, Conjugate Gradient [Press et al. 1992]. Fourier methods have recently been shown to solve the linear partial differential equations (PDEs) inherent in nonparametric nonrigid registration for all combinations of standard regularisers and boundary conditions [Cahill et al. 2007].

These algorithms have been fine-tuned for three main application areas:

1. Building shape models from structures that show relatively little changes in shape between subjects
2. Compensating for the relatively small changes in shape and size that may occur during dynamic imaging sequences
3. Using motion models to provide estimates of the location of structures that move with respiratory or cardiac motion.

Unfortunately, the deformations that occur during many interventions are large, and standard algorithms have an insufficient capture range to converge to the correct solution. A promising solution is to link feature or intensity-based registration with a biomechanical model.

7.2.4 Nonrigid 2D-3D Registration

Frequently, intraoperative sensors provide data of lower dimensionality, typically as 2D slices (e.g., ultrasound), as projection images (e.g., X-ray or video projections), or as extracted or measured features such as points, lines, or surfaces. As in the 3D-to-3D case, this leads to two classes of algorithm, those that optimize similarity computed directly from the image intensities, termed *intensity-based*, and those that compute transformations directly from the location of extracted or measured features, called *feature-based*. For more details of these algorithms see Chap. 6: Rigid Registration. Although reasonably robust and validated, 3D-to-2D rigid registration algorithms now exist for many applications (e.g., spinal surgery, hip surgery, and radiotherapy set-up), their extension to include nonrigid transformations remains a research area.

7.2.5 *Incorporation of Biomechanical Models*

The sparse nature of intraoperative measurements means that additional information is required to constrain the registration to deformations that are physically plausible, and using a biomechanical model is one approach to this problem. Early work attempted to model tissue as a network of springs [Bucholz et al. 1997; Edwards et al. 1997] but assigning realistic material parameters to such models proved challenging. Continuum mechanics techniques (where mass and energy are distributed throughout the body) in general, and the finite element method in particular, have therefore become predominant.

The theory of elasticity provides a set of partial differential equations that describe the equilibrium conditions for a body in terms of the external loads, the stresses (internal pressure), and the strain (a measure of the deformation) within the body. For an arbitrarily shaped body, this will not be analytically soluble, and so in the finite element method the body is *meshed* into a set of elements with simple topology (usually tetrahedrals or hexahedrals) connected at node points. Displacements are defined at the nodes but are interpolated within each element, which allows the behavior of the body to be described using a finite number of variables. More details on the finite element method are available in many textbooks, such as Bathe [1996].

Making the assumption that the change in strain is infinitesimal, and therefore neglecting the stress contribution due to changing geometry usually allows the problem to be solved rapidly. Larger deformations more properly require finite strain theory to be used, which requires Newton-type iterations to be performed, so the systems of equations can take much longer to solve and convergence is not guaranteed. Therefore, infinitesimal strain is frequently assumed even for large displacements when modeling for IGI, balancing the surgical requirements of speed and accuracy.

The relationship between the stress and the strain for a tissue is given by the constitutive equation for that material, and a wide range of constitutive laws have been proposed. The majority of IGI technology that incorporates biomechanical models is around the head. Constitutive models of the brain used for IGI have included linear elasticity [Ferrant et al. 2001; Skrinjar et al. 2001; Warfield et al. 2002; Clatz et al. 2003], a coupled fluid-elastic model in which white and grey matter is considered as an elastic solid, while cerebral spinal fluid is modeled as a fluid [Hagemann et al. 1999] and a porous media model in which the brain is considered as a solid matrix saturated by a fluid [Lunn et al. 2003; Paulsen et al. 1999]. Deformations of the brain have been found to be strain-rate dependent and to have differing properties in extension and compression, and this behavior can be included within the model [Miller and Chinzei 2002]. Biological tissues are typically modeled as being incompressible [Fung 1993].

Two types of boundary conditions can be imposed on the nodes of a model – force and displacement. With the exception of gravity, the forces usually are not known but the displacements can be extracted from intra-operative images. Typically, it will be the completeness of the displacement boundary conditions, rather than factors such as the material properties that will be the over-riding factor determining the accuracy of a biomechanically-based registration.

7.2.6 Statistical Shape Models

Another approach to the interpolation or extrapolation of incomplete inter-operative data is to incorporate additional anatomical information from a statistical shape model. Statistical shape models encode the mean shape and size of a particular structure and its relationship to adjacent structures, together with statistical information gathered from a population of examples on the variation in size and shape. The most common representation is based on principle component analysis (PCA) of the distribution of corresponding points to form an active shape model [Cootes et al. 1995]. Many adaptations of this basic concept have been reported, including active appearance models (AAM) that incorporate intensity information [Cootes et al. 2001] and the statistical deformation model (SDM) that builds the shape model directly from a deformation field produced by nonrigid registration. In an example of the latter, the node points that control the approximating B-splines that define the deformation field are used directly to build the model [Rueckert et al. 2003]. Spatial correspondence is established by the registration algorithm and is only as good as that process [Crum et al. 2003].

Applications of the use of statistical shape models in image-guided interventions include building shape models of the vertebrae, pelvis, and bones of the lower limbs in orthopaedic surgery [Lavallee et al. 2004; Yao et al. 2003; Chan et al. 2004] and building atlases of the deep brain structures in image-guided functional neurosurgery [Guo et al. 2006; D'Haese et al. 2005], Chap. 11: Neurosurgical Applications.

7.2.7 Real-Time Requirements

Real-time processing is a requirement at the navigation and tracking stage of image-guided interventions. "Real-time" means "sufficiently fast for the application". This clearly depends on the precise stage in each application that the information is required and is a key issue in system design and integration. Certain tasks need to be computable in a few minutes, such as during patient set-up and preparation on the operating table. At certain stages in the procedure, a processing delay of a few tens of seconds may be tolerated, for example while checking plan alignment after tumor resection.

At other critical stages of the procedure, information may be needed sufficiently fast to guide physical manipulation and intervention. This raises complex issues of human factors and human–computer interface, but time delays of no less than one video frame rate (30–40 ms) may be required. This, in general, will mean that processing must be fast and some form of predictive tracking will be required. There is usually scope to precompute data such as the meshing of a finite element model and transformations, which make information in the preoperative plan easier to register to intra-operative data. Nevertheless, to have this operate in a nonrigid framework pushes current technologies to the limit of what is feasible. The rapid development of the new generation of graphics processing units (GPUs) and implementation on them of the PDE solvers for nonrigid registration, to-gether with predictive tracking, is showing promise that some of these algorithms may be able to operate in "real-time" in the next 3–5 years.

7.3   Validation

Validation of any of these algorithms for interventional use is very difficult. Any of these nonrigid registration algorithms can produce a plausible morphing of one dataset to another, but as there will generally be a very large set of possible deformations that produce images of rather similar appearance, there is no guarantee that the solution produced will be the correct one. This is particularly important in interventional work, where the image quality and field of view is likely to be compromised by patient motion and the need for rapid image acquisition. In particular, B-spline and fluid-based algorithms can become unstable and produce bizarre deforma-tions outside their volume of support from interoperative data. They are reasonably good at interpolating missing data, but very poor at extrapola-tion. The large number of degrees of freedom, which is a requirement of a flexible transformation, means that the solution is significantly under-determined and other constraints are quite likely to be required to produce accurate and robust methods. Incorporation of plausible deformations via a biomechanical model, motion model, or statistical shape atlas are likely to provide robust and accurate solutions, but these technologies impose even more challenging issues of validation and robustness assessment.

Validation methodology for nonrigid registration in image-guided interventions is being developed, but there is a real shortage of accepted techniques, and this is an impediment to more widespread adoption of this technology. Methods will evolve that use computer simulation [Schnabel et al. 2003; Tanner et al. 2007], identification of anatomical point land-marks, and implanted fiducials. The latter are the preferred option, and methods based on implanted radiofrequency tracking devices will become more widespread. By their nature, these will be invasive and so an evolving strategy through physical phantoms, animal models, and *in vivo* studies will be required. Within the radiotherapy physics community, we are beginning to see sharing of data to test nonrigid registration algorithms. For more information on validation, please see Chap. 18: Assessment of Image-Guided Interventions.

7.4   Applications of Image-Guided Applications to Soft Deforming Tissue

7.4.1   *Locally Rigid Transformations*

An approximation to nonrigid transformations can be achieved by transforming small regions of the image using a local rigid body transformation. This has been used with some success to correct for brain shift in image-guided neurosurgery using intraoperative tracked 2D (B-mode) ultrasound. Figure 7.2 shows a slice through a preoperatively acquired MR volume, orientated to the plane of an ultrasound image acquired through the dura after craniotomy. The ultrasound image clearly shows a bifurcation of a significant vascular structure that is not seen on the corresponding MR slice. After rigid registration to the vascular structure, which was clearly visible on the MRA sequence, the images are brought back into alignment allowing image guidance to proceed with confidence.

7.4.2   *Biomechanical Models*

7.4.2.1   Biomechanical Modeling of the Brain for IGI

Although accurate spatial information about the brain is available preoperatively, the brain deforms by around 5–10 mm [Hartkens et al. 2003] during surgery. The principle causes of this brain shift are the release of cerebral-spinal fluid when the dura mater is opened, physiological responses to anaesthesia, and the manipulation and excision of brain tissue by the surgeon. Effective modeling of the brain, constrained using (relatively) low resolution intraoperative imaging could mitigate for this deformation when performing navigation tasks.

Ferrant et al. [2001] used surfaces extracted from a sequence of MR images acquired during neurosurgery to deform a linear elastic FEM of the brain. The mean distance between the measured and computed position of 400 landmarks within the brain was 0.9 mm.

An extensive series of papers modeling the deformation of the brain as it undergoes surgical-type deformations have been published by the group at Dartmouth College (e.g., Lunn et al. [2003] and Paulsen et al. [1999]). In these papers, the authors represent the brain as a porous media model. By adjusting the level of the cerebrospinal fluid, or by imposing displacements upon nodes, the effects of gravity-induced deformation, balloon inflation, piston indentation, and hemisphere retraction can be modeled. This group performed porcine brain validations using intraoperative CT and implanted landmarks. The intraoperative images allowed boundary conditions to be imposed; typically, the cortical surface away from the region of interest was required to remain fixed, while appropriate displacement boundary conditions were imposed where the brain was in contact with the device causing the deformation. These validations showed that the deformation predictions are able to recover approximately 80% of the tissue motion, measured using intraoperative CT and implanted landmarks. When the model was applied to clinical data, it was found the model could recover the mean brain shift occurring when the dura was opened to 1.2 mm (compared with a total displacement of 5.7 mm).

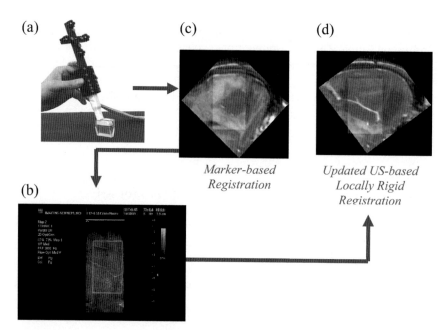

Fig. 7.2. A system for correcting for brain shift using tracked B-mode ultrasound: A tracked B-mode ultrasound probe (**a**) is used to collect soft tissue images after craniotomy (**b**). This is aligned with a preoperative MR image (**c**) demonstrating that there has been *brain shift*. Locally rigid registration re-registers the vascular structures bringing the preoperative images back into alignment (**d**)

One of the greatest challenges is to establish the best way to incorporate boundary conditions into the model for real patient data where the intraoperative data are much sparser, as intraoperative CT would not be available. One approach to this is to use data assimilation techniques, which (for a nonperfect model and noisy parameters) attempt to estimate the most likely state of the model while simultaneously estimating the parameters of the model. These techniques have been used by Lunn et al. [2003] in a porcine test system.

7.4.2.2 Biomechanical Modeling of the Breast for IGI

An example of tissue that undergoes a large deformation between imaging and surgery is the breast. During breast-conserving surgery, the surgeon attempts to remove the lesion, while minimizing the amount of healthy tissue removed, to improve the cosmetic result. A significant proportion of these procedures requires a repeat operation because of incomplete excision of cancerous tissue. Incorporating spatial information about the lesion from a dynamic contrast enhanced magnetic resonance (DCE-MR) image might help reduce this reexcision rate. DCE-MR of the breast must be performed with the patient lying prone with her breasts pendulant in a breast coil to minimize the breathing motion between images in the sequence. Breast surgery is performed with the patient lying supine and the significant deformation that occurs between these two positions means that rigid-body IGI techniques cannot be applied.

Carter et al. [2006] have adopted a two-stage approach to this registration problem. In the preoperative stage, the preenhancement image from the DCE sequence is registered to an unenhanced supine image so that the cancer can be located in the supine image, and then in the intraoperative stage, this supine image is registered to the patient. The deformation in the preoperative step is so large that there is insufficient overlap between corresponding anatomies in the two images to enable conventional intensity-based registration techniques to converge. Therefore, a biomechanical model of the breast is used to model the deformation due to gravity between prone and supine, and these displacements are used to initialize an intensity-based registration technique [Crum et al. 2005].

Immediately prior to surgery, a stereo camera is used to record the surface of the breast, including an aligned texture map. After rigid alignment of the fiducial marker locations, the model of the breast (in the supine position) is deformed using displacement boundary conditions so that it aligns with this surface. The biomechanical basis of the model constrains it sufficiently so that the surface displacements can be extrapolated by the model to localize the lesion. Initial results [Carter et al. 2006] indicate that using a biomechanical model to initialize the prone-supine registration improves the registration accuracy from ~8 mm to ~3 mm, and that the biomechanical model can predict the location of a lesion accurately identified in a supine MR image to about 2 mm. The system accuracy is estimated to be around 4mm. This is less than the 5–10mm margins around the cancer currently used by surgeons.

The process of registration of prone and supine MR images followed by alignment to the position of the patient's breast in the operating room, as recorded by a stereo camera system, is illustrated in Fig. 7.3.

7.4.3 Motion Models

7.4.3.1 Lung

Lung tumors can move significantly with the respiratory cycle, and this creates problems when planning and delivering high precision, conformal, and intensity-modulated radiotherapy. The current solutions involve setting wide margins to compensate for motion, but this unnecessarily irradiates large volumes of normal lung tissue, which in turn limits the total dose that can be delivered. If the trajectory of the tumor over the breathing cycle is known, then either targeted radiotherapy can be delivered during a part of the breathing cycle (gating) or the beam can be directed to follow the trajectory of the tumor (tracking). It has been proposed that high resolution 4D (3D + time) imaging can be used to determine trajectories of the target and adjacent tissues *at risk*. 4DCT has been used together with nonrigid registration to estimate tumor motion over the respiratory cycle. See also Chap. 16: Radiosurgery, and Chap 17: Radiation Oncology.

We have used cine 4DCT combined with nonrigid registration to generate motion models that are continuous in space and time [McClelland et al. 2006]. In this method, motion models are constructed from CT data acquired in cine mode, while the patient is free breathing. Contiguous slabs of such data are each acquired over 20 s, resulting in about 30 volumes covering 5–8 respiratory cycles. The slab thickness corresponds to the axial extent of the multislice CT acquisition. In addition, a high resolution breath-hold scan is taken over the whole lung field. This breath-hold scan is then registered to each slab of data using the free-form deformation-based algorithm described earlier. The free-form deformation is computed using a set of approximating B-splines defined by the displacement of the node points. The position of each image in the respiratory cycle is estimated by the displacement of an optically tracked point fixed to the skin surface of the abdomen. Each ordinate of the displacement of each node point is fitted to a cyclic B-spline over the breathing cycle.

The resulting model is described by the set of these cyclic B-splines for each model. This results in a continuous model of lung density (Hounsfield number) for each position in the lung at any arbitrary position in the respiratory cycle, i.e., the model is continuous in space and time. The Jacobian of the displacement field also gives an estimate of local density change with the breathing cycle.

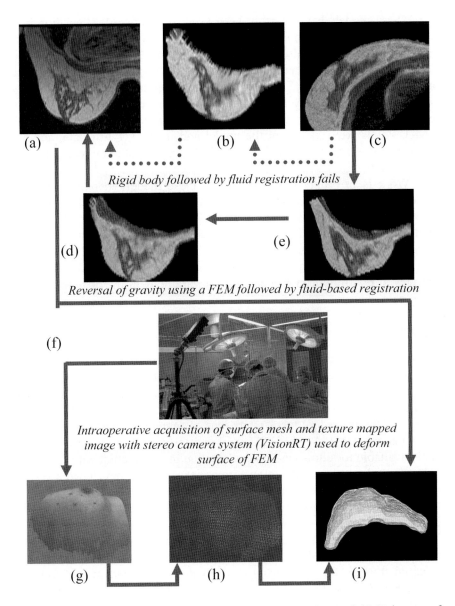

Fig. 7.3. Demonstration for image-guided breast surgery: Transaxial MR images of the breast of a volunteer in the supine (**a**) and prone position (**c**). Nonrigid transformation of supine image to prone image: initial rigid body registration followed by fluid registration fails (**b**); using the rigid body plus FEM-based transformation as a starting estimate (**e**) to 3D fluid registration [Crum et al. 2005] (**d**) gives reasonable correspondence with (**a**). VisionRT Camera system in the operating room (**f**), texture map (**g**) and surface mesh (**h**) and finally (**i**) meshed FEM from (**e**) aligned with (**h**) [Carter et al. 2006]

These models have recently been used to optimize leaf position in a simulation of intensity-modulated lung radiotherapy with a moving multileaf collimator synchronised to the breathing cycle [McClelland et al. 2007]. Figure 7.4 shows a schematic of how the motion model is formed from the original slab data. Figure 7.4d shows a typical reconstruction at an arbitrary point in the respiratory cycle. Validation of the model has been achieved by testing the model against cine CT data that were not used to generate the model. Points were picked in the model and in the CT test data, and the mean error was 1.6 mm while the mean TRE of the registration was estimated to be 1.3 mm.

Work is in progress to synchronise these models in real-time to an external breathing monitoring device, and to extend the models to encode variation in breathing. We have recently shown how these models can be used in a simulation to optimize the motion of multileaf collimator positions when tracking tumor motion due to breathing [McClelland et al. 2007]. The next step will be to implement a practical system for dose delivery that operates in real time, can compensate for variations in the breathing cycle, and is safe.

7.4.3.2 Liver

Radiofrequency ablation and other focal therapies are a promising way to treat liver metastases e.g., Solbiati et al. [2001]. Therapy is usually planned on a breath-hold CT scan that is acquired after administration of iodinated contrast material. Treatment is usually guided by ultrasound or CT fluoroscopy. As the procedure takes many tens of minutes to perform, breathing motion is inevitable. A simple 2D rigid registration system is now commercially available for ultrasound-guided ablation in conjunction with CT, but it only operates with rigid body transformations. We have developed a system that builds a 4D motion model of the liver as described earlier. Guidance is then a two stage process in which the 4D model is registered rigidly to the patient coordinates.

A fixed part of the breathing cycle is selected (usually gentle exhale) and a series (3–10) of slices of tracked B-mode ultrasound images are acquired through the liver, using a calibrated ultrasound probe [Blackall et al. 2005; Penney et al. 2004; Barratt et al. 2001]. These are rigidly aligned to the 4D model at the same stage of the breathing cycle. During the intervention, while the patient is gently breathing, the real-time ultrasound is used to determine the position in the breathing cycle for each ultrasound image [Blackall et al. 2005]. A novel, fast ultrasound to MR or CT volume registration algorithms was developed for this purpose. The system was demonstrated off-line and a real-time system is being developed [Penney et al. 2004]. The operation of the system is shown schematically in Fig. 7.5.

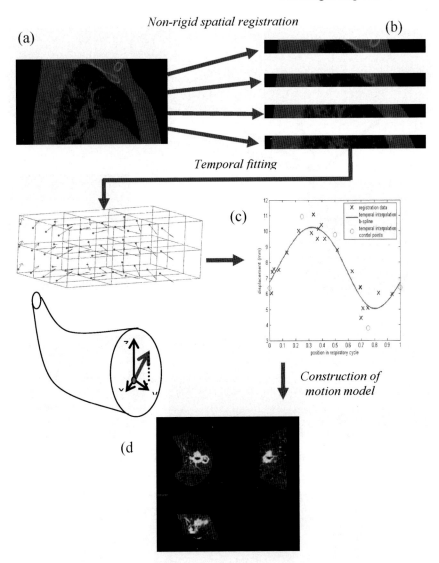

Fig. 7.4. Construction of motion models for lung radiotherapy: a high quality breath-hold volume of the whole lung, sagittal view (**a**) is registered to each slab of a high frame rate (0.5 fps) cine CT sequence (**b**) using the B-spline FFD nonrigid registration algorithm. (**c**) This shows how the displacement of the node points (*left*) that define the nonrigid transformation are synchronized to the position in the respiratory cycle (*right*) and fitted to a cyclic B-spline. (**d**) A still from the continuous motion model showing transaxial (*top left*), sagittal (*top right*), and coronal views (*bottom left*) at a particular instance of the breathing cycle but at the quality of the breath-hold scan [McClelland et al. 2006]

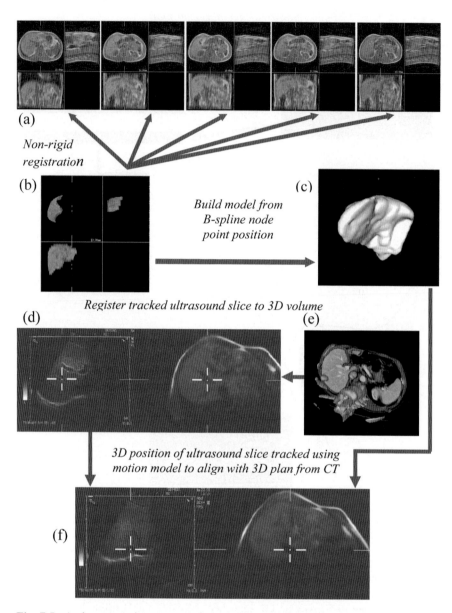

(a)

Non-rigid registration

(b)   (c)

Build model from B-spline node point position

Register tracked ultrasound slice to 3D volume

(d)   (e)

3D position of ultrasound slice tracked using motion model to align with 3D plan from CT

(f)

Fig. 7.5. A demonstration system for tracking breathing motion in percutaneous focal ablation: An MR EPI sequence (**a**) is acquired covering the liver while the patient is freely breathing, at a frame rate of ~0.5 s per volume. The individual images of this sequence are registered to a breath-hold scan (**b**). The nodal displacements are used to generate a continuous motion model, a surface shaded representation of which is shown (**c**). This is registered to the breath-hold CT scan showing the target lesion (**d, e**) and synchronized with real-time tracked ultrasound (**f**) [Penney et al. 2004; Blackall et al. 2005]

7.4.4 Application of Statistical Shape Models

7.4.4.1 Orthopaedics

Shape models of bony anatomy can be generated from example CT scans of a representative population and these models can then be aligned to a specific patient's anatomy to help plan and guided surgical interventions. Fleute and Lavallee [1998] proposed a statistical shape model (SSM) for image-guided anterior cruciate ligament reconstruction. Surface points from ten dry femurs were digitized and registered to a *template* femur using the ICP algorithm [Besl and MacKay 1992] and PCA was used to generate an SSM. Tests using ~100 points acquired on two surgically exposed femoral notch surfaces resulted in RMS values between the instantiated model and the intraoperative data between 1.6 and 1.9 mm [Fleute and Lavallée 1999]. This group also showed how a statistical shape model of vertebrae could be build from 450 manually identified points of the exposed vertebrae. They showed how the model could be instantiated using two X-ray views with an RMS error of 0.62 mm. When tested against a CT scan of a cadaver, the average RMS error was 0.68 mm. The results were promising, but a shape model built from a larger database is required.

Yao and Taylor [2003] showed how a shape model could be generated from CT scans of hemi-pelves. The bone surface was represented as a hierarchical tetrahedral mesh incorporating both shape and density information. They reported how they could use two or three X-ray views to instantiate and register a *virtual CT* scan of the patient's hemi-pelvis.

Chan et al. [2004] constructed a statistical deformation model (SDM) by aligning a set of 16 CT scans of the femur and 10 CT scans of the pelvis. The method was close to that described by Rueckert et al. [2003] in which alignment of MR scans of the brain was done using the B-spline FFD algorithm described earlier [Rueckert et al. 1999]. The displacement of the node points is used as input to the PCA to produce the SDM. The novelty in Chan's approach was the use of percutaneous ultrasound to instantiate the shape model. This would allow the bony anatomy to be reconstructed without recourse to CT from a sweep of tracked and calibrated ultrasound data over the femur, and ultrasound accessible features such as the pubis, ilium, and iliac crest. Testing on three cadavers that were scanned with both CT and ultrasound showed that the bony surfaces could be reconstructed with an RMS error of between 1.1 and 2.0 mm for the six femurs and 2.3 and 4.2 mm for the three pelves. Work is in progress to build the SDMs from a much larger database of CT scans. An outline of the prototype system is shown in Fig. 7.6.

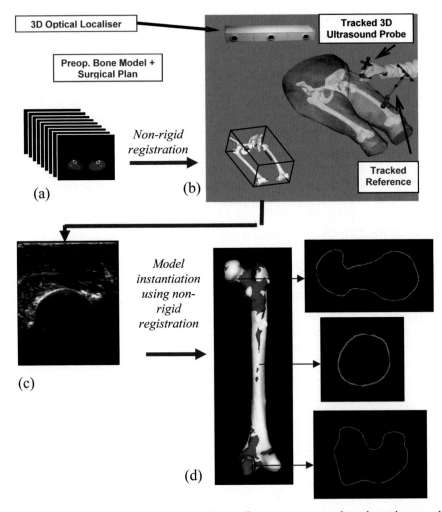

(a)

(b)

(c)

(d)

Fig. 7.6. A prototype image-guided orthopaedic surgery system based on ultrasound instantiation and alignment of a shape model: A set of CT scans (**a**) are registered to form a 3D statistical deformation model. A set of tracked ultrasound images (**c**) are used to instantiate a 3D model of the bone (**d**) from this statistical deformation model. The integrity of the model is shown on the *right*. The *grey-scale image* and contour is that of a CT scan of a cadaver femur and the *purple image* and contour shows the instantiated femur from ultrasound [Chan et al. 2004; Barratt et al. 2006]

7.4.4.2 Neurosurgery

Other examples of the use of shape models in image-guided surgery include models of the brain and, in particular, models of the deep brain structures, which is covered in more detail in Chap. 11: Neurosurgical Applications.

Models are generated by nonrigid registration of MR images of the brain into a common coordinate system. Shape models of deep brain structures can be augmented by information collected during deep brain stimulation [Guo et al. 2006, 2007; D'Haese et al. 2005].

7.5   Conclusion

This chapter has summarized our view of the role of nonrigid registration in image-guided interventions. As the component processes in image-guided surgery, image-directed therapy, and interventional radiology converge, we are likely to see a much more widespread use of nonrigid registration. We have outlined the key technologies on the basis of nonrigid registration that are currently available and under development in this fast moving area. Future prediction is always risky but we predict that nonrigid registration technologies in planning, image guidance, and treatment monitoring will only progress beyond purely experimental environments if they make full use of other spatial information. This might be provided by biomechanical modeling, learning repetitive motion due to respiration and cardiac pulsatility, or by using information learnt from statistical atlases of anatomy.

This chapter has summarized how each of these technologies might be incorporated into image guidance systems and provided practical examples in the head, breast, lung, liver, and orthopaedics.

We anticipate that these technologies will be introduced into image-directed endoscopic procedures and that fusion of preoperative models with intraoperative optical imaging will significantly widen the scope of image-directed minimally invasive methods. Intraoperative imaging will include endoscopic and microscopic imaging, and other novel optical-based technologies such as fluorescent imaging, optical coherence tomography, and hybrid technologies such as opto-acoustic imaging.

As of August 2007, there are no commercial systems that use nonrigid registration in any system licensed for use on patients. For the technologies outlined in this chapter to become widely available, there is a need for appropriately rigorous validation strategies that are recognized by the regulatory bodies and accepted by interventionists, therapists, surgeons, and their patients. Validation of nonrigid registration technologies is very difficult and to date, with very few exceptions, has been inadequately done, despite the fact that it is a prerequisite for translation of this technology to the clinic.

With the advent of appropriate validated methodology, we foresee a significant expansion of these technologies into areas of therapy and intervention in the soft tissues of the head, neck, chest, and abdomen. The potential benefit is enormous, as this will improve safety and efficacy and reduce invasiveness of treatment of many of the most common life threatening conditions for which surgery or other image-directed therapeutic interventions are likely to provide the best option for the patient.

References

Audette, M.A., Siddiqi, K., Peters, T.M. (1999) "Level-set surface segmentation and fast cortical range image tracking for computing intrasurgical deformations". *Proc. MICCAI'99, Lect Notes Comput Sci*; 1679:788–97.

Aylward, S.R., Jomier, J., Weeks, S., Bullitt, E. (2003) "Registration and analysis of vascular images". *Int J Comput Vision*; 55:123–38.

Bajcsy, R., Kovacic, S. (1989) "Multiresolution elastic matching". *Comp Vision Graphi Image Process*; 46:1–21.

Barratt, D.C., Davies, A.H., Hughes, A.D., Thom, S.A., Humphries, K.N. (2001) "Optimisation and evaluation of an electromagnetic tracking device for high-accuracy three-dimensional ultrasound imaging of the carotid arteries". *Ultrasound Med Biol*; 27:957–968.

Barratt, D.C., Penney, G.P., Chan, C.S.K., Slomczykowski, M., Carter, T.J., Edwards, P.J., Hawkes, D.J. (2006) "Self-calibrating 3D-ultrasound-based bone registration for minimally-invasive orthopaedic surgery". *IEEE Trans Med Imag*; 25:312–323.

Bathe, K.-J. (1996) *Finite element procedures*. Prentice Hall: Englewood cliffs, NJ.

Besl, P.J. and McKay, N.D. (1992) "A method for registration of 3D shapes". *IEEE Trans PAMI*; 14:239–256.

Blackall, J.M., Penney, G.P., King, A.P., Hawkes, D.J. (2005) "Alignment of sparse freehand 3D ultrasound with preoperative images of the liver and an interventional plan using models of respiratory motion and deformation". *IEEE Trans Med Imag*; 24:1405–1416.

Bookstein F.L. (1989) "Principal warps – thin-plate splines and the decomposition of deformations". *IEEE Trans Pattern Anal*; 11:567–85.

Bro-Nielsen, M. and Gramkow, C. (1996) "Fast fluid registration of medical images". *Proc Visual Biomed Comput Lect Notes Comput Sci*; 1131:267–76.

Bucholz, R.D., Yeh, D.D., Trobaugh, J., McDurmont, L.L., Sturm, C.D., Baumann, C., Henderson, J.M., Levy, A., Kessman, P. (1997) "The correction of stereotactic inaccuracy caused by brain shift using an intraoperative ultrasound device". *Proc CVRMed-MRCAS'97, Lect Notes Comput Sci*; 1205:459–466.

Cahill, N.D., Noble, J.A., Hawkes, D.J. (2007) "Fourier methods for nonparametric image registration". *Proc CVPR 2007.* Minneapolis, MN, USA.

Carter, T.J., Tanner, C., Crum, W.R., Beechey-Newman, N, Hawkes, D.J. (2006) "A framework for image-guided breast surgery". *Med Imag Augmented Reality, LNCS*; 4091:203–210.

Chan, C.S.K., Barratt, D.C., Edwards, P.J., Penney, G.P., Slomczykowski, M., Carter, T.J., Hawkes, D.J. (2004) "Cadaver validation of the use of ultrasound for 3D model instantiation of bony anatomy in image guided orthopaedic surgery". *Proc MICCAI, Lect Notes Comput Sci*; 3216:397–404.

Christensen, G., Joshi, S., Miller, M. (1996) "Volumetric transformation of brain anatomy". *IEEE Trans Med Imag*; 16:864–877.

Clatz, O., Delingette, H., Bardinet, E., Dormont, D., Ayache N. (2003) "Patient-specific biomechanical model of the brain: Application to Parkinson's disease procedure, in surgery simulation and soft tissue modeling". *Proc Lecture Notes Comput Sci*; 2673:321–331.

Coolens, C., White, M., et al. (2007) "Free breathing gated radiotherapy with external markers using MRI derived models of hepatic motion". *Proc XVth International Conference on the use of Computers in Radiation Therapy,* Toronto Canada, June 4–7, 2007.

Cootes, T.F., Taylor, C.J., Cooper, D.H., Graham, J. (1995) "Active shape models – Their training and application". *Comput Vision Image Understanding*; 61(1): 38–59.

Cootes, T.F., Edwards, G.J., Taylor, C.J. (2001) "Active Appearance Models", *IEEE Pattern Anal Mach Intell*, 23, 6, 681–685.

Crum, W.R., Griffin, L.D., Hill, D.L.G., Hawkes, D.J. (2003) "Zen and the art of medical image registration: Correspondence, homology and quality". *NeuroImage*; 20:1425–1437.

Crum, W.R., Hartkens, T., Hill, D.L.G. (2004) "Non-rigid image registration: Theory and practice". *Br J Radiol*; 77:S140–153.

Crum, W.R., Tanner, C., Hawkes, D.J. (2005) "Anisotropic multiscale fluid registration: evaluation in magnetic resonance breast imaging". *Phys Med Biol*; 50:5153–5174.

D'Haese, P.F., Cetinkaya, E., Konrad, P.E., Kao, C., Dawant, B.M. (2005) "Computer-aided placement of deep brain stimulators: from planning to intraoperative guidance". *IEEE Trans Med Imag*; 24(11):1469–78.

Edwards, P.J., Hill, D.L.G., Little, J.A., Hawkes D.J. (1997) "Deformation for image guided interventions using a three component tissue model". *Proc Inform Processing Med Imag Lect Notes Comput Sci*; 1230:218–231.

Ferrant, M., Nabavi, A., Macq, B., Jolesz, F.A., Kikinis, R., Warfield, S.K. (2001) "Registration of 3-D intraoperative MR images of the brain using a finite-element biomechanical model". *IEEE Trans Med Imag*; 20:1384–1397.

Fleute M., Lavallée S. (1999) "Nonrigid 3-D/2-D Registration of Images Using Statistical Models". *Proc MICCAI-2*, LNCS 1679, 138–147.

Fleute M., Lavallée S. (1998). "Building a Complete Surface Model from Sparse Data Using Statistical Shape Models: Application to Computer Assisted Knee Surgery System". *Proc MICCAI-1*, LNCS 1496, 879–887.

Fung, YC. (1993) *Biomechanics: Mechanical Properties of Living Tissues*. 2nd Ed. Springer-Verlag: NY.

Gee, J.C., Reivich, M., Bajcsy, R. (1993) "Elastically deforming 3D atlas to match anatomical brain images". *J Comp Assis t Tomogr*; 17:225–236.

Guo, T., Finnis, K.W.P.A.G., Peters, T.M. (2006) "Visualization and navigation system development and application for stereotactic deep-brain neurosurgeries". *Comput Aided Surg*; 11(5):231–239.

Guo T., Parrent A.G., Peters T.M. (2007). "Surgical targeting accuracy analysis of six methods for subthalamic nucleus deep brain stimulation". *Computer Assisted Surgery*. 12(6): 325–334.

Hagemann, A., Rohr, K., Stiehl, H.S., Spetzger, U., Gilsbach, J.M. (1999) "Biomechanical modeling of the human head for physically based, nonrigid image registration" *IEEE Trans Med Imag*; 18:875–884.

Hajnal, J.V., Hill, D.L.G., Hawkes, D.J. (eds) (2001) *Medical Image Registration*. CRC Press: West Palm Beach, FL. ISBN 0-8493-0064-9.

Hartkens, T., Hill, D.L.G., Castellano-Smith, A.D., Hawkes, D.J., Maurer, C.R., Jr., Martin, A.J., Hall, W.A., Liu, H., Truwitt, C.L. (2003) "Measurement and analysis of brain deformation during neurosurgery". *IEEE Trans Med Imag*; 22(1):82–92.

Hawkes, D.J., Barratt, D., Blackall, J.M., Chan, C., Edwards, P.J., Rhode, K., Penney, G.P., Hill, D.L.G. (2005) "Tissue deformation and shape models in image-guided interventions: A discussion paper". *Med Image Anal*; 8(2):163–175.

Hill, D.L.G., Batchelor, P.G., Holden, M., Hawkes, D.J. (2001) "Medical image registration." *Phys Med Bio*; l46(3):R1–R45.

Lavallée, S., Merloz, P., Stindel, E., Kilian, P., Troccaz, J., Cinquin, P., Langlotz, F., Nolte, L.P. (2004) "Echomorphing: introducing an intraoperative imaging modality to reconstruct 3D bone surfaces for minimally-invasive surgery". *Proc CAOS*; 38–39.

Little, J., Hill, D.L.G., Hawkes, D.J. (1997) "Deformation incorporating rigid structures". *Comput Vision Image Understanding*; 66:223–32.

Lunn, K.E., Paulsen, K.D., Roberts, D.W., Kennedy, F.E., Hartov, A., Platenik, L.A. (2003) "Nonrigid brain registration: synthesizing full volume deformation fields from model basis solutions constrained by partial volume intraoperative data". *Comp Vision Image Understanding*; 89:299–317.

Maes, F., Collignon, A., Vandermeulen, D., Marchal, G., Suetens, P. (1997) "Multimodality image registration by maximization of mutual information". *IEEE Trans Med Imag*; 16:187–198.

McClelland, J.M., Blackall, J.M., Tarte, S., Chandler, A., Hughes, S., Ahmad, S., Landau, D.B., Hawkes, D.J. (2006) "A continuous 4D motion model from multiple respiratory cycles for use in lung radiotherapy". *Med Phys*; 33(9): 3348–58.

McClelland, J.R., Webb, S., McQuaid, D., Binnie, D.M., Hawkes, D.J. (2007) "Tracking "differential organ motion" with a "breathing" multileaf collimator: Magnitude of problem assessed using 4D CT data and a motion-compensation strategy". *Phys Med Biol* 52, 16, 4805–4826.

Miller, K. and Chinzei, K. (2002) "Mechanical properties of brain tissue in tension". *J Biomech*; 35:483–490.

Modersitzki, J. (2004) *Numerical Methods for Image Registration.* Oxford University Press: NY.

Monga, O. and Benayoun, S. (1995) "Using partial derivatives of 3D images to extract typical surface features". *Comput Vision Image Understanding*; 61: 171–89.

Paulsen, K.D., Miga, M.I., Kennedy, F.E., Hoopes, P.J., Hartov, A., Roberts, D.W. (1999) "A computational model for tracking subsurface tissue deformation during stereotactic neurosurgery". *IEEE Trans Biomed Eng*; 46:213–225.

Penney, G.P., Blackall, J.M., Hamady, M., Sabharwal, T., Adam, A., Hawkes, D.J. (2004) "Registration of freehand 3D ultrasound and magnetic resonance liver images". *Med Image Anal*; 8:81–91.

Press, W.H., Teukolsky, S.A., Vetterling, W.T., Flannery, B.P. (1992) *Numerical recipes in C: The art of scientific computing.* Cambridge University Press: Cambridge, UK.

Rhode, K., Sermesant, M., Brogan, D., Hegde, S., Hipwell, J., Lambiase, P., Rosenthal, E., Bucknall, C., Qureshi, S.A., Gill, J.S., Razavi, R., Hill, D.L.G. (2005) "A system for real-time XMR guided cardiovascular intervention". *IEEETrans Med Imag*; 24:1428–1440.

Roche, A., Malandain, G., Pennec, X., Ayache, N. (1998) "The correlation ratio as a new similarity measure for multimodal image registration". *Proc MICCAI'98, Lect Notes Comput Sci*; 1496:1115–1124.

Rohr, K., Fornefett, M., Stiehl, H.S. (2003) "Spline-based elastic image registration: Integration of landmark errors and orientation attributes". *Comput Vision Image Understanding*; 90:153–68.

Rohr, K., Stiehl, H.S., Sprengel, R., Buzug, T.M., Weese, J., Kuhn, M.H. (2001) "Landmark-based elastic registration using approximating thin-plate splines". *IEEE Trans Med Imaging*; 20:526–34.

Rueckert, D., Sonoda, L.I., Hayes, C., Hill, D.L.G., Leach, M.O., Hawkes, D.J. (1999) "Non-rigid registration using free-form deformations: Application to breast MR images". *IEEE Trans Med Imag*; 18:712–721.

Rueckert, D., Frangi, A.F., Schnabel, J.A. (2003) "Automatic construction of 3-D statistical deformation models of the brain using non-rigid registration". *IEEE Trans Med Imag*; 22:1014–1025.

Rueckert, D., Aljabar, P., Heckemann, R.A., Hajnal, J.V., Hammers, A. (2006) "Diffeomorphic registration using B-splines". *Proc MICCAI 2006, Lect Notes Comput Sci*; 4191:702–709.

Schnabel, J.A., Tanner, C., Castellano-Smith, A.D., Degenhard, A., Leach, M.O., Hose, D.R., Hill, D.L.G., Hawkes, D.J. (2003) "Validation of non-rigid image registration using finite element methods: Application to breast MR images". *IEEE Trans Med Imag*; 22(2):238–247.

Skrinjar, O.M., Studholme, C., Nabavi, A., Duncan J. (2001) "Steps toward a stereo-camera-guided biomechanical model for brain shift compensation". *Proc IPMI, Davis CA, June 18-22, 2001 Lecture Notes in Computer Science* 2082, 863–866.

Solbiati, L., Livraghi, T., Goldberg, S., Ierace, T., Meloni, F., Dellanoce, M., Cova, L., Halpern, E., Gazelle, G. (2001) "Percutaneous radiofrequency ablation of hepatic metastases from colorectal cancer: long term results in 117 patients". *Radiology*; 221:159–166.

Studholme, C., Hill, D.L.G., Hawkes, D.J. (1999) "An overlap invariant entropy measure of 3D medical image alignment". *Pattern Recognition*; 32:71–86.

Studholme, C., Hill, D.L.G., Hawkes, D.J. (1996) "Automated 3D registration of MR and CT images of the head". *Med Image Anal*; 1:163–75.

Studholme, C., Hill, D.L.G., Hawkes, D.J. (1997) "Automated 3D registration of MR and PET brain images by multi-resolution optimisation of voxel similarity measures". *Med Phys*; 24:25–36.

Tanner, C., Schnabel, J.A., Hill, D.L., Hawkes, D.J. et al. (2007). "Quantitative evaluation of free-form deformation registration for dynamic contrast-enhanced MR mam-mography". *Med Phys* 34(4): 1221–1233.

Thirion, J-P. (1998) "Image matching as a diffusion process: An analogy with Maxwell's demons". *Med Image Anal*; 2:243–260.

Viola, P., Wells, W.M. (2005) "Alignment by maximization of mutual information". *Int J Comput Vision*; 24:137–154.

Warfield, S.K., Talos, F., Tei, A., Bharatha, A., Nabavi, A., Ferrant, M., Black, P.M., Jolesz, F.A., Kikinis, R. (2002) "Real-time registration of volumetric brain MRI by biomechanical simulation of deformation during image guided neurosurgery". *Comput Visual Sci*; 5:3–11.

Yao, J. and Taylor, R. (2003) "A multiple-layer flexible mesh template matching method for nonrigid registration between a pelvis model and CT images". *Proc SPIE*; 1117–1124.

Chapter 8

Model-Based Image Segmentation for Image-Guided Interventions

Wiro Niessen

Abstract

Medical image segmentation plays an important role in the field of image-guided surgery and minimally invasive interventions. By creating three-dimensional anatomical models from individual patients, training, planning, and computer guidance during surgery can be improved. This chapter briefly describes the most frequently used image segmentation techniques, shows examples of their application and potential in the field of image-guided surgery and interventions, and discusses future trends.

8.1   Introduction

Image segmentation is one of the central research themes in biomedical image analysis, and with the increasing number of imaging studies, both in biomedical research and clinical practice, the necessity for automated biomedical image segmentation methods is expanding.

In medical imaging, the extraction of three-dimensional static or dynamic models of patient anatomy or pathology is of particular interest. These models facilitate visualization that is tailored to the diagnostic task, quantification for diagnostic purposes, or therapy planning, monitoring, and guidance of interventions or surgery.

The increasing relevance of biomedical imaging only partially explains why medical image segmentation continues to be an active research field; the major reason is that the field poses substantial difficulties. The variability in patient anatomy and pathology, the complexity and sheer size of state-of-the-art medical imaging data, with the requirements of accuracy, reproducibility, and robustness imposed by the application domain, make medical image segmentation a very challenging task.

T. Peters and K. Cleary (eds.), *Image-Guided Interventions.*
© Springer Science + Business Media, LLC 2008

When using image segmentation in the field of image-guided surgery and minimally invasive interventions, additional challenges are faced, including time constraints, compromised intraoperative image quality, and deforming anatomy. Despite these challenges, image segmentation is increasingly used as an invaluable tool for training, preoperative planning, and image guidance during surgery and interventions, and its role is expected to increase.

A large body of literature has been devoted to medical image segmentation. These different approaches can roughly be categorized into two classes. The first class, low-level image segmentation, uses image features to define regions or to classify voxels into tissue types. Thresholding, region growing, clustering methods, (trained) classifiers, and morphology-based segmentation fall within this category. The second class consists of model-based approaches, which aim to fit models to the image data. Examples are the classical deformable models (e.g., snakes), level sets, active shape and appearance models, and atlas- (registration-) based approaches. However, this distinction is somewhat artificial, as the interest in hybrid approaches that combine both aspects is increasing. Model-based and hybrid methods probably are most popular and promising in the field of image-guided interventions. Owing to the large number of segmentation methods addressed in this chapter, we will only briefly discuss the underlying methodology and provide references to other papers for more in depth treatment of specific approaches.

This chapter is organized as follows; the next two sections review the basics of low-level-based segmentation and a number of 3D model-based image segmentation techniques, including tissue classification, deformable model-based segmentation, level set-based segmentation, active shape and appearance models, and registration-based segmentation. We then describe how these methods can be applied to assist in the preoperative situation in image-guided surgery and minimally invasive intervention, and we will discuss future developments.

8.2   Low-Level Image Segmentation

The most widely used low-level image segmentation techniques, such as thresholding and region growing, are addressed in standard image processing text books and so are not discussed here. This section is limited to a brief discussion of tissue classification techniques, as they are increasingly used in combination with model-based image segmentation.

Classification is a pattern recognition technique, the aim of which is to partition the image into classes, on the basis of such characteristics as image intensity and/or features derived from the images. In classification techniques, a feature space is constructed, whose dimensionality is determined by the number of features (or in case of multisequence MRI, by the number of images multiplied by the number of features per image). Features may include both the image appearance and spatial (location) information. This feature space subsequently is used to partition the image voxels into differrent classes.

Both supervised and unsupervised classification techniques can be distinguished. In supervised classification, a training stage precedes the classification. In this training stage, labeled imaging data are used to learn the distribution of the different classes in feature space. This information is subsequently used in the classification of image voxels of a new image to be segmented. In unsupervised classification, such a training stage is absent. Unsupervised classification techniques group image voxels in a (mostly predetermined) number of classes by analyzing the distribution of the voxels in feature space. Clusters of voxels can be found by minimizing intraclass distances and maximizing interclass distances.

Supervised techniques have the important advantage that prior information specific to a certain segmentation task can be incorporated. However, the eventual segmentation depends on the quality of the training set (i.e., to what extent are the training data representative for the medical image segmentation task). Furthermore, the training stage may be laborious, and it may be necessary to repeat this step if, for example, the image acquisition protocol has changed. This situation frequently occurs in biomedical applications in view of the rapid developments in medical imaging technology.

Classification methods can further be subdivided into parametric and nonparametric. Parametric techniques model the feature space by parameterized probability density functions (pdf) of the different classes. A frequently used model is the Gaussian mixture model, which assumes that the classes are normally distributed in feature space. The parameters describing the Gaussian mixture model can be obtained in a training phase (supervised) or can be estimated from the image to be segmented (unsupervised). An example of a nonparametric supervised classifier is the k nearest neighbors method (kNN). In the kNN method, voxels in the image are classified by determining their position in feature space, and locating the k nearest neighbors using an appropriately chosen metric. Typically, the voxel is then assigned to the most frequently occurring label among the neighbors, although the approach also naturally lends itself for probabilistic image segmentation. Fig. 8.1 gives an example of kNN-based segmentation of multisequence MRI brain data into grey matter, white matter, and cerebrospinal fluid.

To improve the performance of voxel classification, important issues are feature extraction, feature selection, and the choice of classifier, which are all active areas of research in pattern recognition and (medical) image

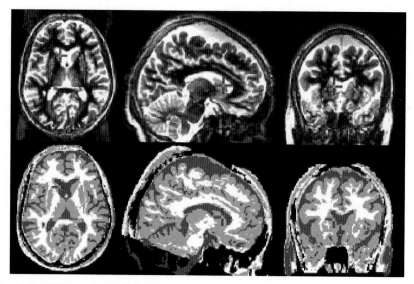

Fig. 8.1. kNN-based segmentation of grey matter, white matter, and cerebrospinal fluid. The top row shows original data, while the lower row demonstrates the segmented regions.

segmentation. Examples are the use of filter banks, different approaches to feature selection, and the combination of different classifiers (boosting). A good overview of relevant developments in the field of pattern recognition and machine learning is given in a number of text books [Bishop 2006; Duda et al. 2000].

8.3   Model-Based Image Segmentation

8.3.1 Introduction

Model-based segmentation techniques have become very popular in medical image analysis. By incorporating prior information into the segmentation approach, the accuracy and robustness of the segmentation procedure can be improved greatly. Different types of prior knowledge can be distinguished, e.g., prior information on object shape and topology, prior information on object appearance and image formation, and prior information from expert observers. The different model-based image segmentation approaches mainly differ in the extent, and in the way this prior information is incorporated. In this section, classical deformable models and level sets are discussed, in which prior information is mainly restricted to smoothness constraints, although some authors have incorporated prior knowledge in these models. We then discuss statistical shape modeling, in which prior information is incorporated increasingly in the image segmentation problem. In this section registration- (or atlas-based) segmentation is also briefly addressed.

8.3.2 Classical Parametric Deformable Models or Snakes

Deformable model-based segmentation was introduced in computer vision by Kass et al. [1987]. A deformable model is a contour or surface, which after initialization deforms as a function of local image properties such as intensity or edge strength, intrinsic constraints such as the length or curvedness, and a priori knowledge of the object to be segmented. Most initial research focused on two-dimensional deformable models, most notably snakes. Classical snakes [Kass et al. 1987] are contours that deform to reach a state of minimal (local) energy. The energy of a snake $C(\vec{x})(s)$, parameterized by $s \in [0,1]$, is defined as:

$$E(C) = \int_0^1 E_{int} + E_{im} + E_{user} ds, \qquad (8.1)$$

where E_{int} represents the internal energy, typically containing an elasticity term and a rigidity term:

$$E_{int} = c_1 |C_s|^2 + c_2 |C_{ss}|^2. \qquad (8.2)$$

Here the subscript s denotes differentiation with respect to the curve parameter, and c_1 and c_2 are constants. E_{im} is the image energy term, which attracts the contour to edges. Mostly the image gradient magnitude has been used. Finally, E_{user} consists of user-supplied constraints such as the initialization, a priori knowledge, and possible interventions during the segmentation (in a correction stage in an interactive segmentation approach).

A local minimum can be found by solving the Euler Lagrange equation of (8.2):

$$-\frac{\partial}{\partial s}(c_1 |C_s|^2) + \frac{\partial^2}{\partial s^2}(c_2 |C_{ss}|^2) + \nabla(E_{im} + E_{ext}) = 0 \qquad (8.3)$$

Classical snakes perform well if the initialization is close to the desired object. To make snakes less sensitive to initialization, inflation or deflation forces were introduced by Cohen et al. [1992], which aim to make the contour less sensitive to spurious edges. Still, in most medical image applications the issue of a proper initialization of a snake-based approach remains an important issue, as there are often multiple surrounding anatomical structures, to which the contour can be attracted.

The use of parameterized deformable models in medical image analysis has been (and continues to be) a very active field of research (for examples, see a number of books and review papers on this subject [Metaxas 1996; Singh et al. 1998; Suri and Farag 2007]). A large number of extensions and improvements to the classical framework have been proposed. First, the approach has been extended to 3D and 4D to deal with (deforming) 3D objects. The theoretical extension of the snake framework to three dimensions is rather straightforward, by considering surfaces rather than contours, and by imposing shape constraints on the basis of the surface curvatures. Second, alternative parameterizations have been proposed, such as generic low degree of freedom parameterizations such as Fourier descriptors [Staib and Duncan 1996] and superquadrics [Terzopoulos and Metaxas 1991] or application specific shape templates, e.g., based on medial representations [Pizer et al., 1999, 2003]. These latter approaches are better suited for incorporating prior shape information by using a training set to learn the distribution of the parameters describing the shape, examples of which may be seen in the following references [Pizer et al. 2005; Staib and Duncan 1996]. Third, considerable research has focused on the development of improved, application specific image energy terms E_{im}, as the image intensity gradient is not always the most informative feature for detecting the boundary of anatomical objects. As an example, local appearance models may be trained from examples, and used in the segmentation stage [Pizer et al. 2005]. Fourth, an important issue in deformable model-based image analysis is full automation vs. the exploitation of user knowledge through effective user interaction [De Bruijne et al. 2004; Olabarriaga and Smeulders 2001] or user correction [Kang et al. 2004].

8.3.3 *Level Set Segmentation*

8.3.3.1 Conventional Level Set Segmentation

Level set based segmentation was introduced independently by Caselles et al. [1997] and Malladi et al. [1995], on the basis of the work of Osher and Sethian [1988]. In level set based segmentation, rather than having an explicit parameterization (as in snake-based segmentation), the evolving contour is defined as the zero level set of a higher dimensional function. This approach has a number of advantageous properties. The most important is that the level set can change topology (split, merge), while the evolution of the embedding level function remains well defined. Furthermore, level sets are easily implemented on a discrete grid and can readily be applied in arbitrary dimensions.

Let $I(\vec{x})$ denote the function that embeds the zero level set. The zero level set should be a Jordan curve, i.e., the gradient of I should be nonzero at $I = 0$. Given a contour $C(\vec{x})$ in 2D or a surface $S(\vec{x})$ in 3D, $I(\vec{x})$ can (e.g.,) be constructed by computing the distance transform to the contour or surface.

The underlying idea of level set-based segmentation is to evolve the embedding function I such that its zero level set captures the object of interest. We proceed by considering the following evolution of the function I, which embeds the zero level set:

$$\frac{\partial I}{\partial t} = g(\vec{x})(\alpha I_w + I_{vv}),$$

(8.4)

where v and w denote the tangential and normal direction to the isophotes of I, α is a constant, and $g(\vec{x})$ is a function that steers the evolution of the zero level set of I based on the image to be segmented (we will discuss different choices for $g(\vec{x})$ later).

Using the fact that I is a Jordan curve, and setting the total derivative of I to zero, it is easy to show that when evolving I according to (4), its zero level set evolves as follows:

$$\frac{\partial C}{\partial t} = g(\vec{x})(\alpha + \kappa)\vec{N},$$

(8.5)

where κ denotes isophote curvature:

$$\kappa = -\frac{I_{vv}}{I_w},$$

(8.6)

and $\vec{N}$ denotes the unit vector normal to the curve. This evolution can be interpreted as a geometric flow of the zero level set, which is controlled by the speed function $g(\vec{x})$. The α-term is equivalent to an erosion or dilation (depending on the sign) of the zero level contour with a disc as structuring element (Fig. 8.2). This term can be interpreted as pushing the level set inwards or outwards, depending on the sign of g. The second term is a curvature motion term that results in a geometric smoothing of the zero level set; for $g = 1$ and $\alpha = 0$, we obtain the Euclidean shortening flow (with the normal vector $\vec{N}$ pointing inward:

$$\frac{\partial C}{\partial t} = \kappa\vec{N},$$

(8.7)

which is the geometric flow that reduces the arc length of C as quickly as possible. The geometric smoothing behavior of this equation can easily be understood by considering the sign of the curvature (Fig. 8.2); in convex (concave) regions κ is positive (negative) and the curve moves inwards (outwards).

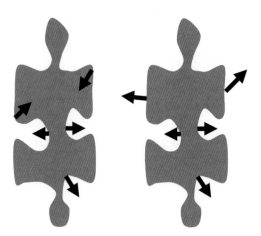

Fig. 8.2. The effect of the Euclidean shortening flow (ESF) and normal motion illustrated. ESF achieves a geometric smoothing; in convex regions, the *curve* moves inwards under the ESF, in concave regions, outwards (*left*). In normal motion (*right*), the *curve* moves inwards or outwards, depending on the sign, resulting in an erosion or dilation with a disc as structuring element

The function $g(\vec{x})$ at $I = 0$ is selected such that the level set contour evolves toward the edges of interest. In many applications, a decreasing function of the image gradient is selected:

$$g(\vec{x}) = e^{-\frac{|\nabla L|^2}{k^2}}. \tag{8.8}$$

To update (8.4), the function $g(\vec{x})$ should be extended to the entire image domain in such a way to prevent crossing of level sets. Updating the embedding function I over the entire image domain is a costly procedure. A speed up of the algorithm can be obtained by using a narrow band implementation, in which I is only updated in a small region around the zero level set. This narrow band needs to be reinitialized if the level set approaches the boundaries of the narrow band.

8.3.3.2 Geodesic Level Sets

The model as presented in (8.4) and (8.5) constitutes the original formulation of implicit deformable models. One of the limitations of this formulation is that, in contrast to the classical snake approach, there is no energy term to minimize in the evolution process. The implicit deformable model can also be derived using an energy minimization approach, by evolving the zero level set such that a geodesic curve or surface in image space is found, where distances in image space are defined on the basis of image content in the image to be segmented [Caselles et al. 1997].

Here, a modified metric is introduced, such that the state of minimal energy corresponds to the desired object segmentation.

We will review here a two-dimensional example. Consider a two-dimensional contour $C(\vec{x}(s))$ parameterized by s. Let dp_g denote the modified Euclidean arc-length dp, obtained by multiplying dp with an image dependent function $g(\vec{x})$, which serves the same purpose as in (8.4) and (8.5).

$$dp_g = gdp = \left|\vec{x}_s\right|^2 gds \qquad (8.9)$$

If $g(\vec{x})$ is a decreasing function of the gradient magnitude, distances along the zero level sets decrease at higher gradient magnitude, so that states of minimum energy (i.e., states of minimal modified length) occur at high values of the gradient. The flow that decreases the modified length L of $C_g(\vec{x}(s))$ most rapidly is given by Kichenassamy et al. [1995]:

$$\frac{\partial C}{\partial t} = g\kappa\vec{N} - \nabla g . \qquad (8.10)$$

Note that if $g = 1$ (Euclidean arc-length) this reduces to the Euclidean shortening flow (which indeed decreases the Euclidean length as fast as possible).

The evolution of the embedding function corresponding to this curve evolution is given by:

$$\frac{\partial I}{\partial t} = gI_{vv} + \nabla g \cdot \nabla I \qquad (8.11)$$

The inner product term in (8.11) attracts contours to the boundaries of objects. Note that this term changes direction at the edge, such that it prevents curves from crossing over edges.

8.3.3.3 Extensions and Applications of Level Sets

On the basis of the conventional level-set-based segmentation and its geodesic version, a number of extensions have been proposed, which have expanded the application area of level-set-based segmentation and have improved their performance. Lorigo et al. [2001] introduced a framework for the segmentation of vasculature structures. Owing to the varying shape and topology of vascular structures, the level set approach has proven to be very powerful for many vascular image processing problems [Manniesing et al. 2006; Van Bemmel et al. 2004] (Figs. 8.3 and 8.4).

Other authors have considered the segmentation of multiple objects simultaneously, by considering the evolution of multiple level sets [Brox and Weickert 2004; Brox and Weickert 2006] and coupled level sets [Yang et al. 2004]. Coupled level sets have effectively been used to determine the cortical thickness in MR brain images [Zeng et al. 1999].

Another direction toward the improvement of level set approaches is by improving the image-derived speed function. Chan and Vese [2001] introduced a framework to evolve the zero level on the basis of statistics of the inner and outer region of the zero level set.

Owing to their implicit representation, level sets do not lend themselves very well to the incorporation of prior shape information. Some authors have explored the use of such information by performing statistical analysis on distance functions [Tsai et al. 2003], or by using a Bayesian approach incorporating prior knowledge on object shape and grey values [Yang and Duncan 2004]. Whereas these approaches have shown to improve performance, explicit shape models, as discussed in the next section, are more suitable to encode prior information on shape and appearance.

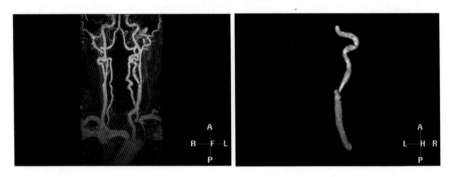

Fig. 8.3. MR dataset of the carotid arteries (*left*) and segmentation, which was obtained using a level-set technique (*right*). On the basis of the segmentation, the diameter of stenosis can accurately be determined, which can be used for clinical decision making

8.3.4 Statistical Shape Models

In the last decade, model-based segmentation techniques that incorporate prior statistical information on shape, appearance, motion, and deformation have received considerable attention. This *a priori* knowledge is learned from a set of examples and is typically expressed as an average and a set of characteristic variations. These models greatly improve robustness to noise, artifacts, and missing data, and hence improve the reliability of image segmentation.

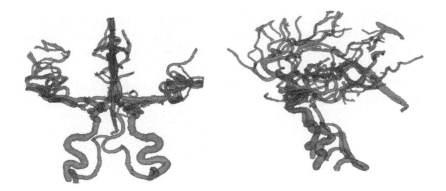

Fig. 8.4. Fully automatically segmented cerebral vasculature from CTA data

Several different types of statistical shape models have been developed. Some of the most popular are active shape models (ASM) [Cootes et al. 1994; Cootes et al. 1995], active appearance models (AAM) [Cootes et al. 2001; Mitchell et al. 2001], models based on Fourier or M-rep parameterization [Pizer et al. 2003], and statistical deformation models (SDM) [Rueckert et al. 2003]. We will describe the ASM, AAM, and SDM here, and provide a brief review and references to literature for the other models.

8.3.4.1 Active Shape, Appearance, and Deformation Models

In ASMs, shapes are presented by a set of landmarks. If we consider ASMs in 3D, a shape is thus described by a $3n$-dimensional vector $\vec{x}$, where n is the number of landmarks. To model shape statistics, a number of training shapes is required in which the same landmarks have been annotated. This set of training shapes is mapped in some common coordinate system, as we are only interested in the shape variation, and not in differences in pose. From the set of training data, it is now possible to construct the mean shape:

$$\bar{x} = \frac{1}{n}\sum_{i=1}^{n}\vec{x}. \qquad (8.12)$$

Furthermore, shape variation can be modeled by studying the covariance matrix:

$$S = \frac{1}{N}\sum_{i=1}^{N}(x_i - \bar{x})(x_i - \bar{x})^T. \qquad (8.13)$$

By performing a principal components analysis (PCA) of S, a matrix ψ can be constructed, which contains the t eigenvectors corresponding to the largest eigenvalues of the covariance matrix. The value of t is typically chosen such that a predefined proportion of the variance present in the training data can be described by the model.

Any shape in the training set can now be approximated by the mean shape and this matrix, i.e.:

$$\vec{x} \approx \bar{x} + \psi \vec{b} , \tag{8.14}$$

where

$$\vec{b} = \psi^T (\vec{x} - \bar{x}) . \tag{8.15}$$

Shapes similar to those seen in the training set can be generated by varying $\vec{x}$ according to (14) while applying limits to the parameters b_i, e.g.,

$$-3\sqrt{\lambda_i} \le b_i \le 3\sqrt{\lambda_i} .$$

In this way, a set of plausible shapes is described (under the assumption of a Gaussian distribution).

Figure 8.5 shows an example of a heart model built out of fourteen segmented datasets.

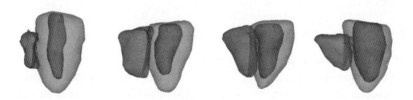

Fig. 8.5. Four instances of a shape model, which have been constructed by varying the four most significant modes of deformation

Image segmentation with the constructed statistical shape model is now achieved by finding the pose (typically a rigid registration to bring the model into object-centered space) and shape (i.e., the parameter vector $\vec{b}$) that best matches the image data. This is typically achieved in an iterative fashion. For all model points, a profile perpendicular to the shape is searched for the most likely edge position. This results in a vector of candidate points $\vec{x}$. Subsequently, the parameter vector $\vec{b}$ is determined, which minimizes the sum of square distances between the model points and the candidate points. This procedure is repeated until convergence.

A major advantage of ASMs, in contrast to more generic deformable models, is that the segmentation outcome is limited to plausible shapes, i.e., shapes that are similar to those that are observed in the dataset. The performance of ASMs is dependent on the accuracy with which the candidate edge points are extracted. The straightforward approach would be to consider the location of maximal gradient. A more commonly used approach is to exploit the imaging data in the training set of the ASM. For example, in the original ASM approach as proposed by Cootes et al. [1994], a statistical model of the grey value profile at correct boundary positions is constructed during the training phase. In the different iterations of model fitting, the most likely edge position is found by comparing the profiles at candidate edge points with the trained profile model, and selecting the best fit. Van Ginneken et al. [2002] approached the estimation of the most likely edge point as a classification task, by selecting features both at the correct boundary position and in the background. This is an example of a hybrid approach, combining concepts of statistical shape modeling, with pattern recognition-based classification.

One of the serious drawbacks of ASMs, which has been a limitation toward a wider use of ASMs for 3D biomedical image segmentation, is that establishing correspondence between landmarks is a time-consuming and tedious task, especially in 3D. Several authors have proposed automatic procedures for finding corresponding landmark points on the basis of segmented images, e.g., using nonrigid image registration [Frangi et al. 2002].

An important extension of the ASM is the so-called active appearance model (AAM). These models not only describe statistics on shape, but also on appearance. An AAM is built in a two-step approach. First, image data are warped to the mean shape, to remove texture variation owing to differences in shape. Subsequently, in *shape normalized space*, a statistical model of image appearance is constructed. The iterative segmentation procedure of the AAM approach differs from ASM in the sense that now a model vector $\vec{b}$ is optimized containing both a shape ($\vec{b}_s$) and appearance component ($\vec{b}_g$). The optimal model vector is found by minimizing the difference between the model image, parameterized by $\vec{b}$, with the actual image.

Statistical deformation models (SDMs) are another important extension of the ASM approach [Rueckert et al. 2003]. The underlying idea of statistical deformation models is inspired by atlas-based segmentation. Atlas-based segmentation is essentially a means to solve a segmentation task via registration. If a labeled dataset (the atlas) is available, segmentation can be achieved by registering the labeled data with the image to be segmented. This registration step is usually carried out using a nonrigid registration technique, to account for differences between the atlas and the object to be segmented. The idea of SDMs is not to use a single atlas, but to build a statistical model of the nonrigid transformations necessary to map a (training) set of image data to each other. In contrast to a PCA on the landmark vectors, a PCA is performed on the deformation fields, and the mean deformation and main modes of deformation are established. In the initial approach, as proposed by Rueckert et al. [2003], this is achieved by performing a PCA on the control points of a cubic b-spline representation of the deformation field.

8.4   Applications

8.4.1 Segmentation in Image-Guided Interventions

Medical image segmentation in the field of image-guided surgery and minimally invasive image-guided intervention consists mostly of the prior extraction of 3D anatomical models, which is useful for planning and guiding interventions [Pommert et al. 2006; Sierra et al. 2006].

In image-guided surgery, there are many examples, including planning and guidance in neurosurgery [Letteboer et al. 2004; Prastawa et al. 2004], liver surgery [Soler et al. 2001], orthopedics [Hoad and Martel 2002], and head and neck surgery [Descoteaux et al. 2006]. In minimally invasive interventions, segmentation is used for the planning and guidance of cardiac ablation [De Buck et al. 2005; Sra et al. 2006], and in radiotherapy for planning and guiding prostate brachytherapy [Ghanei et al. 2001; Wei et al. 2005], prostate radiotherapy planning [Freedman et al. 2005; Hodge et al. 2006; Mazonakis et al. 2001], and radiation therapy treatment planning for brain tumors [Mazzara et al. 2004; Popple et al. 2006].

Image segmentation is also frequently employed for the construction of surgical simulators or training devices for minimally invasive interventions. Examples include hip surgery simulators [Ehrhardt et al. 2001; Pettersson et al. 2006], minimally invasive interventions for beating heart surgery [Wierzbicki et al. 2004], simulation for cardiac ablation [Sermesant et al. 2006], and simulation systems for training in intravascular interventions [Alderliesten et al. 2006]. The above list is far from complete, but indicates the wide range of applications of image segmentation in treatment planning and guidance.

Owing to the larger challenges that are associated with the analysis of intraoperative imaging data, most notably time constraints and compromised image quality, intraoperative segmentation has been less widely adopted. For neurosurgery, a method for the measurement of brain tumor resection via segmentation has been developed [Hata et al. 2005]. Also for neurosurgery, [Wu et al. 2005] focused on the development of a fast segmentation technique for MR brain images to facilitate the construction of finite elements in the operating room. Other authors have reported intraoperative lesion segmentation for guidance in interventional MR

RF treatment [Lazebnik et al. 2005]. A considerable amount of work has focused on the extraction (or segmentation) of devices from intraoperative images, including needle and seed segmentation in brachytherapy in the prostate [Ding and Fenster 2004; Ding et al. 2006], instrument segmentation in abdominal surgery [Doignon et al. 2005], needle extraction from ultrasound [Okazawa et al. 2006], and extraction of guide wires and catheters in intravascular interventions [Baert et al. 2003].

In Figs. 8.6 and 8.7, two examples of the additional value of image segmentation in image-guided surgery and interventions are given. Figure 8.6 shows a preoperative MR image, which is used for planning and guiding in brain tumor resections.

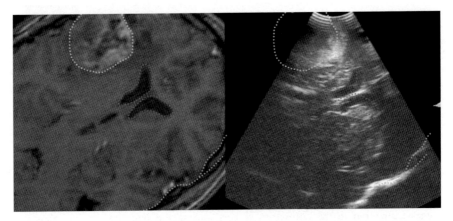

Fig. 8.6. Example of the additional value of segmented MR brain structures for image-guided neurosurgery. By superimposing these structures on intraoperative US data, which have been registered to the MR brain data using an image-guided surgery system, the intraoperative brain shift can effectively be visualized

During surgery, an intraoperative ultrasound dataset is acquired with a calibrated ultrasound system. Using the image-guided surgery system, the relation between the MR image and ultrasound image can be obtained, such that an integrated display of the MR and ultrasound image is facilitated. However, owing to imperfections in the registration, and deformations during surgery (*brain shift*), the match between the data is imperfect. To appreciate the magnitude and direction of brain shift, it is very useful to overlay structures segmented on the MR brain image (in this case, the tumor outline, ventricles, and cortex) onto the ultrasound image.

Figure 8.7 shows a potential application of coronary segmentation for improving guidance in interventional cardiology. Modern CTA data provide a detailed visualization of the coronary arteries, which can be useful for the planning and guidance of interventional cardiology. For example, for treatment of total chronic coronary artery occlusions, intraoperative coronary angiography is unable to visualize the occluded segment, whereas CTA can. To provide preoperative CTA data during the intervention, the relation between pre and intraoperative data needs to be established. Intensity-based 2D-3D registration, in which simulated projection X-ray images are compared with actual X-ray images to estimate the geometric relation between CTA and X-ray data, is a promising approach to achieve this. However, in intraoperative X-ray angiography a selective contrast injection is used, the coronaries should be extracted from the CTA data prior to generating a simulated projection image.

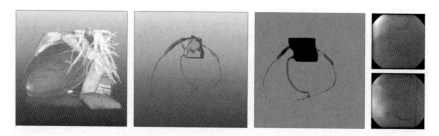

Fig. 8.7. Coronary segmentation as a preprocessing step for registering preoperative CTA data to intraoperative coronary angiograms. Intensity-based 2D-3D registration, in which simulated projection images are compared with actual projection images, is a powerful technique to determine the geometric relation between preoperative CTA data and intraoperative angiography data. However, a selective contrast injection in the coronaries is used during the intervention, and thus the coronaries should be extracted from the CTA data prior to generating simulated projection X-ray images

8.5   Future Directions

Research in recent years has shown that the incorporation of prior information can considerably improve robustness and accuracy of image segmentation. It is therefore expected that the trend toward introducing more and more informative prior knowledge in model-based image segmentation will continue. Until very recently, most methods focused on including statistics on shape, but increasingly the image appearance also is taken into account. The appearance models that are being used are becoming more sophisticated; locally optimized models of image appearance have been proposed, and it is expected that such approaches will outperform global appearance models in most applications. In addition, techniques for multiple object segmentation will become more widespread, as the interrelation between objects contains valuable information for image segmentation. The trend to incorporate more a priori information can be observed in almost all deformable model-based approaches [Kaus et al. 2004; Pizer et al. 2003, 2005; Van Ginneken et al. 2002; Yang and Duncan 2004]. An important research issue over the next few years will be which frameworks can most effectively incorporate this prior information.

Another trend that can be observed is the increased interest in spatio-temporal segmentation, which is mainly due to the increased capabilities of modern imaging modalities, most notably MRI, CT, and ultrasound. Addressing image segmentation as an optimization in space-time has the potential to improve the accuracy and robustness of the segmentation, for example, by yielding segmentation results that are consistent over time. Moreover, spatiotemporal models of anatomy may be used for providing preoperative information to the surgeon even in case of preoperative motion, which is due to cardiac or breathing motion [Hawkes et al. 2005]. This is just one of the examples how advanced shape and appearance models will not only improve the performance of image segmentation for preoperative planning and guidance, but will also pave the way for updating preoperative models during surgery.

Acknowledgements

The author acknowledges Henri Vrooman, Coert Metz, Michiel Schaap, Kees van Bemmel, Rashindra Manniesing, and Marloes Letteboer for the figures used in this chapter.

References

Alderliesten T, Konings MK, and Niessen WJ. (2006). "Robustness and complexity of a minimally invasive vascular intervention simulation system." *Med Phys*, 33(12), 4758–4769.

Baert SAM, Viergever MA, and Niessen WJ. (2003). "Guide-wire tracking during endovascular interventions." *IEEE Trans Med Imaging*, 22(8), 965–972.

Bishop CM. (2006). *Pattern Recognition and Machine Learning*, Springer, Berlin Heidelberg New York.

Brox T and Weickert J. (2004). "Level set based image segmentation with multiple regions." *Pattern Recognit*, 3175, 415–423.

Brox T and Weickert J. (2006). "Level set segmentation with multiple regions." *IEEE Trans Image Process*, 15(10), 3213–3218.

Caselles V, Kimmel R, and Sapiro G. (1997). "Geodesic active contours." *Int J Comput Vis*, 22(1), 61–79.

Chan TF and Vese LA. (2001). "Active contours without edges." *IEEE Trans Image Process*, 10(2), 266–277.

Cohen I, Cohen LD, and Ayache N. (1992). "Using deformable surfaces to segment 3-D images and infer differential structures." *Cvgip-Image Understanding*, 56(2), 242–263.

Cootes TF, Edwards GJ, and Taylor CJ. (2001). "Active appearance models." *IEEE Trans Pattern Anal Machine Intell*, 23(6), 681–685.

Cootes TF, Hill A, Taylor CJ, and Haslam J. (1994). "Use of active shape models for locating structure in medical images." *Image Vis Comput*, 12(6), 355–365.

Cootes TF, Taylor CJ, Cooper DH, and Graham J. (1995). "Active shape models – Their training and application." *Comput Vis Image Understanding*, 61(1), 38–59.

de Bruijne M, van Ginneken B, Viergever MA, and Niessen WJ. (2004). "Interactive segmentation of abdominal aortic aneurysms in CTA images." *Med Image Anal*, 8(2), 127–138.

De Buck S, Maes F, Ector J, Bogaert J, Dymarkowski S, Heidbuchel H, and Suetens P. (2005). "An augmented reality system for patient-specific guidance of cardiac catheter ablation procedures." *IEEE Trans Med Imaging*, 24(11), 1512–1524.

Descoteaux M, Audette M, Chinzei K, and Siddiqi K. (2006). "Bone enhancement filtering: Application to sinus bone segmentation and simulation of pituitary surgery." *Comput Aided Surg*, 11(5), 247–255.

Ding M and Fenster A. (2004). "Projection-based needle segmentation in 3D ultrasound images." *Comput Aided Surg*, 9(5), 193–201.

Ding M, Wei Z, Gardi L, Downey DB, and Fenster A. (2006). "Needle and seed segmentation in intra-operative 3D ultrasound-guided prostate brachytherapy." *Ultrasonics*, 44(Suppl 1), e331–e336.

Doignon C, Graebling P, and de Mathelin M. (2005). "Real-time segmentation of surgical instruments inside the abdominal cavity using a joint hue saturation color feature." *Real-Time Imaging*, 11(5–6), 429–442.

Duda RO, Hart PE, and Stork DG. (2000). *Pattern Classification*, Second Edition, ISBN: 987-0-471-05669-0, Wiley Interscience.

Ehrhardt J, Handels H, Malina T, Strathmann B, Plotz W, and Poppl SJ. (2001). "Atlas-based segmentation of bone structures to support the virtual planning of hip operations." *Int J Med Inf*, 64(2–3), 439–447.

Frangi AF, Rueckert D, Schnabel JA, and Niessen WJ. (2002). "Automatic construction of multiple-object three-dimensional statistical shape models: Application to cardiac modeling." *IEEE Trans Med Imaging*, 21(9), 1151–1166.

Freedman D, Radke RJ, Zhang T, Jeong Y, Lovelock DM, and Chen GT. (2005). "Model-based segmentation of medical imagery by matching distributions." *IEEE Trans Med Imaging*, 24(3), 281–292.

Ghanei A, Soltanian-Zadeh H, Ratkewicz A, and Yin FF. (2001). "A three-dimensional deformable model for segmentation of human prostate from ultrasound images." *Med Phys*, 28(10), 2147–2153.

Hata N, Muragaki Y, Inomata T, Maruyama T, Iseki H, Hori T, and Dohi T. (2005). "Intraoperative tumor segmentation and volume measurement in MRI-guided glioma surgery for tumor resection rate control." *Acad Radiol*, 12(1), 116–122.

Hawkes DJ, Barratt D, Blackall JM, Chan C, Edwards PJ, Rhode K, Penney GP, McClelland J, and Hill DL. (2005). "Tissue deformation and shape models in image-guided interventions: A discussion paper." *Med Image Anal*, 9(2), 163–175.

Hoad CL and Martel AL. (2002). "Segmentation of MR images for computer-assisted surgery of the lumbar spine." *Phys Med Biol*, 47(19), 3503–3517.

Hodge AC, Fenster A, Downey DB, and Ladak HM. (2006). "Prostate boundary segmentation from ultrasound images using 2D active shape models: Optimisation and extension to 3D." *Comput Methods Programs Biomed*, 84(2–3), 99–113.

Kang Y, Engelke K, and Kalender WA. (2004). "Interactive 3D editing tools for image segmentation." *Med Image Anal*, 8(1), 35–46.

Kass M, Witkin A, and Terzopoulos D. (1987). "Snakes – active contour models." *Int J Comput Vis*, 1(4), 321–331.

Kaus MR, von Berg J, Weese J, Niessen W, and Pekar V. (2004). "Automated segmentation of the left ventricle in cardiac MRI." *Med Image Anal*, 8(3), 245–254.

Kichenassamy S, Kuma A, Olver PJ, Tannenbaum A, and Yezzi AJ. (1995). "Gradient flows and geometric active contour models." *Proceedings of the Fifth International Conference on Computer Vision*, IEEE Computer Society Press, Washington DC, USA, 810–815.

Lazebnik RS, Weinberg BD, Breen MS, Lewin JS, and Wilson DL. (2005). "Semi-automatic parametric model-based 3D lesion segmentation for evaluation of MR-guided radiofrequency ablation therapy." *Acad Radiol*, 12(12), 1491–1501.

Letteboer MM, Olsen OF, Dam EB, Willems PW, Viergever MA, and Niessen WJ. (2004). "Segmentation of tumors in magnetic resonance brain images using an interactive multiscale watershed algorithm." *Acad Radiol*, 11(10), 1125–1138.

Lorigo LM, Faugeras OD, Grimson WEL, Keriven R, Kikinis R, Nabavi A, and Westin CF. (2001). "CURVES: Curve evolution for vessel segmentation." *Med Image Anal*, 5(3), 195–206.

Malladi R, Sethian JA, and Vemuri BC. (1995). "Shape modeling with front propagation – A level set approach." *IEEE Trans Pattern Anal Machine Intell*, 17(2), 158–175.

Manniesing R, Velthuis BK, van Leeuwen MS, van der Schaaf IC, van Laar PJ, and Niessen WJ. (2006). "Level set based cerebral vasculature segmentation and diameter quantification in CT angiography." *Med Image Anal*, 10(2), 200–214.

Mazonakis M, Damilakis J, Varveris H, Prassopoulos P, and Gourtsoyiannis N. (2001). "Image segmentation in treatment planning for prostate cancer using the region growing technique." *Br J Radiol*, 74(879), 243–248.

Mazzara GP, Velthuizen RP, Pearlman JL, Greenberg HM, and Wagner H. (2004). "Brain tumor target volume determination for radiation treatment planning through automated MRI segmentation." *Int J Radiat Oncol Biol Phys*, 59(1), 300–312.

Metaxas DN. (1996). *Physics-Based Deformable Models: Applications to Computer Vision, Graphics, and Medical Imaging*, Kluwer Academic, Boston, MA.

Mitchell SC, Lelieveldt BPF, van der Geest RJ, Bosch HG, Reiber JHC, and Sonka M. (2001). "Multistage hybrid active appearance model matching: Segmentation of left and right ventricles in cardiac MR images." *IEEE Trans Med Imaging*, 20(5), 415–423.

Okazawa SH, Ebrahimi R, Chuang J, Rohling RN, and Salcudean SE. (2006). "Methods for segmenting curved needles in ultrasound images." *Med Image Anal*, 10(3), 330–342.

Olabarriaga SD and Smeulders AWM. (2001). "Interaction in the segmentation of medical images: A survey." *Med Image Anal*, 5(2), 127–142.

Osher S and Sethian JA. (1988). "Fronts propagating with curvature-dependent speed – Algorithms based on Hamilton-Jacobi formulations." *J Comput Phys*, 79(1), 12–49.

Pettersson J, Knutsson H, Nordqvist P, and Borga M. (2006). "A hip surgery simulator based on patient specific models generated by automatic segmentation." *Stud Health Technol Inf*, 119, 431–436.

Pizer SM, Fletcher PT, Joshi S, Gash AG, Stough J, Thall A, Tracton G, and Chaney EL. (2005). "A method and software for segmentation of anatomic object ensembles by deformable m-reps." *Med Phys*, 32(5), 1335–1345.

Pizer SM, Fletcher PT, Joshi S, Thall A, Chen JZ, Fridman Y, Fritsch DS, Gash AG, Glotzer JM, Jirousek MR, Lu CL, Muller KE, Tracton G, Yushkevich P, and Chaney EL. (2003). "Deformable M-reps for 3D medical image segmentation." *Int J Comput Vis*, 55(2–3), 85–106.

Pizer SM, Fritsch DS, Yushkevich PA, Johnson VE, and Chaney EL. (1999). "Segmentation, registration, and measurement of shape variation via image object shape." *IEEE Trans Med Imaging*, 18(10), 851–865.

Pommert A, Hohne KH, Burmester E, Gehrmann S, Leuwer R, Petersik A, Pflesser B, and Tiede U. (2006). "Computer-based anatomy a prerequisite for computer-assisted radiology and surgery." *Acad Radiol*, 13(1), 104–112.

Popple RA, Griffith HR, Sawrie SM, Fiveash JB, and Brezovich IA. (2006). "Implementation of talairach atlas based automated brain segmentation for radiation therapy dosimetry." *Technol Cancer Res Treat*, 5(1), 15–21.

Prastawa M, Bullitt E, Ho S, and Gerig G. (2004). "A brain tumor segmentation framework based on outlier detection." *Med Image Anal*, 8(3), 275–283.

Rueckert D, Frangi AF, and Schnabel JA. (2003). "Automatic construction of 3-D statistical deformation models of the brain using nonrigid registration." *IEEE Trans Med Imaging*, 22(8), 1014–1025.

Sermesant M, Delingette H, and Ayache N. (2006). "An electromechanical model of the heart for image analysis and simulation." *IEEE Trans Med Imaging*, 25(5), 612–625.

Sierra R, Zsemlye G, Szekely G, and Bajka M. (2006). "Generation of variable anatomical models for surgical training simulators." *Med Image Anal*, 10(2), 275–285.

Singh A, Goldgof D, and Terzopoulos D (Eds.). (1998). *Deformable Models in Medical Image Analysis*, IEEE Computer Society Press, Los Alamitos, CA.

Soler L, Delingette H, Malandain G, Montagnat J, Ayache N, Koehl C, Dourthe O, Malassagne B, Smith M, Mutter D, and Marescaux J. (2001). "Fully automatic anatomical, pathological, and functional segmentation from CT scans for hepatic surgery." *Comput Aided Surg*, 6(3), 131–142.

Sra J, Narayan G, Krum D, and Akhtar M. (2006). "Registration of 3D computed tomographic images with interventional systems: Implications for catheter ablation of atrial fibrillation." *J Interv Card Electrophysiol*, 16, 141–148.

Staib LH and Duncan JS. (1996). "Model-based deformable surface finding for medical images." *IEEE Trans Med Imaging*, 15(5), 720–731.

Suri JS and Farag A (Eds.). (2007). *Deformable Models: Biomedical and Clinical Applications*, Springer-Verlag, New York.

Terzopoulos D and Metaxas D. (1991). "Dynamic 3d Models with Local and Global Deformations – Deformable Superquadrics." *IEEE Trans Pattern Anal Mach Intell*, 13(7), 703–714.

Tsai A, Yezzi A, Jr., Wells W, Tempany C, Tucker D, Fan A, Grimson WE, and Willsky A. (2003). "A shape-based approach to the segmentation of medical imagery using level sets." *IEEE Trans Med Imaging*, 22(2), 137–154.

van Bemmel CM, Viergever MA, and Niessen WJ. (2004). "Semiautomatic segmentation of 3D contrast-enhanced MR and stenosis quantification angiograms of the internal carotid artery." *Magn Resonance Med*, 51(4), 753–760.

van Ginneken B, Frangi AF, Staal JJ, Romeny BMT, and Viergever MA. (2002). "Active shape model segmentation with optimal features." *IEEE Trans Med Imaging*, 21(8), 924–933.

Wei Z, Ding M, Downey D, and Fenster A. (2005). "3D TRUS guided robot assisted prostate brachytherapy." *Proc MICCAI 8, Part II, Lecture Notes in Computer Science* 3750, 17–24.

Wierzbicki M, Drangova M, Guiraudon G, and Peters T. (2004). "Validation of dynamic heart models obtained using non-linear registration for virtual reality training, planning, and guidance of minimally invasive cardiac surgeries." *Med Image Anal*, 8(3), 387–401.

Wu Z, Paulsen KD, and Sullivan JM, Jr. (2005). "Adaptive model initialization and deformation for automatic segmentation of T1-weighted brain MRI data." *IEEE Trans Biomed Eng*, 52(6), 1128–1131.

Yang J and Duncan JS. (2004). "3D image segmentation of deformable objects with joint shape-intensity prior models using level sets." *Med Image Anal*, 8(3), 285–294.

Yang J, Staib LH, and Duncan JS. (2004). "Neighbor-constrained segmentation with level set based 3-D deformable models." *IEEE Trans Med Imaging*, 23(8), 940–948.

Zeng XL, Staib LH, Schultz RT, and Duncan JS. (1999). "Segmentation and measurement of the cortex from 3-D MR images using coupled-surfaces propagation." *IEEE Trans Med Imaging*, 18(10), 927–937.

Chapter 9

Imaging Modalities

Kenneth H. Wong

Abstract

This chapter provides an overview of the different imaging modalities used for image-guided interventions, including x-ray computed tomography (CT) and fluoroscopy, nuclear medicine, magnetic resonance imaging (MRI), and ultrasound. The emphasis is on the distinguishing physical and engineering properties of each modality and how these characteristics translate into strengths and weaknesses for the end user. Because the imaging methods are very different, there is no single ideal modality for image-guided interventions; rather, they are largely complementary and can all provide valuable information about the patient. The chapter also covers current research topics in medical imaging relating to image-guided interventions and how these trends could potentially improve image-guided interventions in the future.

9.1   Introduction

A wide array of medical imaging modalities is in use currently, and almost all of them have been integrated into some form of image-guidance system. An exhaustive treatment of these different modalities is far beyond the scope of this chapter, but many excellent reference textbooks are available [Bushberg et al. 2002; McRobbie et al. 2003; Webb 2002]. The goal of this chapter is to provide an introductory level overview and comparison of these modalities in the context of image-guided intervention systems, addressing the perspective of both the system designer and the practitioner. Some knowledge of basic physics, engineering, and anatomy is assumed. The information in this chapter should help the reader to:

1. understand basic physical and engineering principles of each imaging modality, including key limitations, such as spatial resolution, temporal resolution, and field of view;

T. Peters and K. Cleary (eds.), *Image-Guided Interventions.*
© Springer Science + Business Media, LLC 2008

2. understand the types of biological and physiologic information that can be obtained from the different modalities; and
3. compare the advantages and disadvantages of different imaging modalities for image-guided intervention applications.

The following modalities are covered in this chapter: x-ray fluoroscopy, x-ray computed tomography (CT), nuclear medicine, magnetic resonance imaging (MRI), and ultrasound. These five are the most commonly used modalities for image-guided interventions.

9.2   X-Ray Fluoroscopy and CT

9.2.1 Basic Physics Concepts

Both fluoroscopy and CT utilize x-rays to form images and so there are some common features that will help us to understand the performance of these systems. X-rays are generated by accelerating electrons and directing them toward a metal target, as shown in Fig. 9.1.

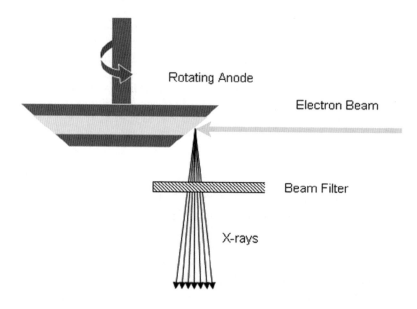

Fig. 9.1. Schematic of a simple x-ray generator. The electron beam impacts the anode and creates x-rays via bremsstrahlung (braking radiation). The anode rotates to dissipate heat from the electron beam, and in many cases is also liquid cooled. A filter removes low-energy x-rays from the beam, since these would only be absorbed in the patient and would not contribute to the formation of the image

The electrons rapidly decelerate upon encountering this material, dissipating their energy as heat and bremsstrahlung (braking radiation) x-rays. The electron source is focused so that the x-rays are emitted from what is essentially a small point source, resulting in a divergent cone beam of x-rays.

Typical x-ray generators have a maximum electron acceleration voltage between 70 and 300 kV, so the maximum energy of the emitted x-rays ranges from 70 to 300 keV. However, the peak of the resulting x-ray spectrum is at approximately one third of the maximum energy. Furthermore, thin metal transmission filters remove lower energy x-rays from the spectrum, so the final spectrum reaching the patient is similar to the one shown in Fig. 9.2.

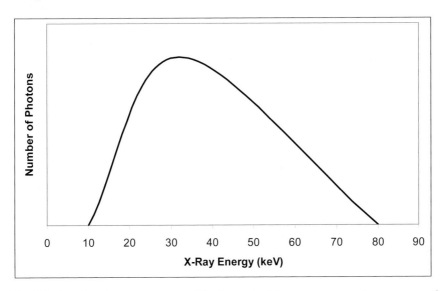

Fig. 9.2. Simulated x-ray spectrum. The bremsstrahlung process produces x-rays of all possible energies up to the maximum energy of the electron beam, but low-energy x-rays are removed from the beam by self-filtering in the anode and external beam filters. Depending on the application, the beam filters can be changed to allow more or less of the low-energy photons to reach the patient

The x-ray photons travel in straight lines from the source. Given the typical x-ray energies involved in fluoroscopy and CT, the x-ray photons interact with the patient through the photoelectric effect and Compton scattering. These mechanisms are dependent on the x-ray energy, elemental composition of the tissue, and tissue density. In the human body, this means that structures with a higher content of calcium and phosphorous (such as bones) will be more attenuating than soft tissues. Similarly, tissues with low density (such as the lungs) will be less attenuating than fat or muscle.

Photons interacting through the photoelectric effect are essentially absorbed in the patient and do not reach the detector. Compton scattered photons may be scattered in any direction, so a significant number of these photons could potentially reach the detector. However, since the location of the scattering cannot be determined, these scattered photons do not carry any useful imaging information. Thus, a grid of small metal vanes is placed in front of the detector so that the scattered photons will be absorbed in the grid rather than detected.

The net result of this imaging approach is that the detected x-rays are considered to have traveled in a straight line from the source to the detector, and the number of photons reaching the detector (typically expressed as I/I_0, where I is the intensity at the detector and I_0 is the initial beam intensity) is based on the density and elemental composition of the tissue along that line. X-ray images are often described as shadowgrams or projection images.

Since both fluoroscopy and CT use x-rays for image formation, image-guided procedures using these modalities expose the patient, physician, nurses, technologists, and other staff to potentially hazardous radiation. When considering risk from x-ray exposure during a procedure, it is important to remember that the medical personnel using the equipment are most affected, since they work with the equipment on a daily basis, whereas patients usually are exposed only during a few visits. To mitigate these risks, x-ray imaging systems have several common safeguards. First, many x-ray sources are designed with feedback systems that regulate the tube output. These systems try to maintain a constant flux on the detector, and will lower the tube output in areas of the body, such as the lungs, where organs are less dense. This approach minimizes the dose while maintaining a constant level of image quality. Second, manually operated sources, such as those in fluoroscopy, have dose counters and timers to prevent inadvertent overexposure. Third, advances in detector sensitivity have enabled significant dose reduction, and this trend is likely to continue. Finally, professional and regulatory agencies such as the International Commission on Radiation Protection (ICRP) and the Food and Drug Administration (FDA) have promulgated guidelines for fluoroscopy training and credentialing, which help to ensure proper training and awareness of risks related to x-ray image guidance [Valentin 2000; Archer 2006].

9.2.2 Fluoroscopy

9.2.2.1 System Components

An example of a fluoroscopy system is shown in Fig. 9.3. The x-ray generator and the detector are mounted facing each other on a curved arm (commonly referred to as a C-arm). The patient table lies between the

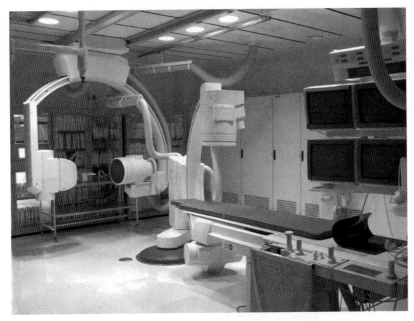

Fig. 9.3. Fluoroscopy system. The patient table is shown in the foreground, and viewing monitors for the fluoroscopy images are visible in the upper right of the photo. One C-arm is mounted on a rotating floor plate that allows it to move in and out from the patient table, and the other is mounted on rails in the ceiling that allow it to move around the room. The C-arm closest to the table is oriented so that the x-ray generator is below the table and the image intensifier is above the table

generator and the detector, and the arm can be rotated around the patient so that the fluoroscope image can be acquired from any angle.

The traditional fluoroscopy detector is an image intensifier that uses a scintillator to convert the x-rays into visible light. The visible light is then converted to an electronic signal, amplified, and then converted back into a video image that can be displayed on a monitor and/or recorded on video tape. Recently, digital detectors have been developed to replace the image intensifier. In addition to being more compact, the digital detectors have far less image distortion and greater dynamic range, so it is likely that digital detectors will eventually supplant the image intensifier, much as flat-panel monitors have replaced cathode ray tubes (CRTs) in personal computers.

9.2.2.2 Image Characteristics

An example of a fluoroscopy image is shown in Fig. 9.4. The spatial resolution of fluoroscopy is high so that submillimeter-sized objects can be resolved. This 2D image clearly shows the contrast between different materials (such as bone and liver) and different tissue densities (such as the heart and lungs). However, this does not apply to soft tissue structures, such as the heart chambers or the lung airways, which cannot be resolved. The image also reveals a key limitation of 2D imaging, which is that overlying structures are all reduced to a single imaging plane. This overlap is an unavoidable consequence of projection imaging.

One advantage of a pure projection imaging technique is that no post-processing or reconstruction is required, so fluoroscopy is a real-time,

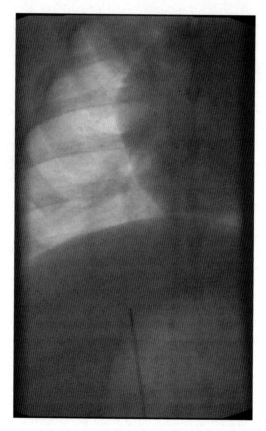

Fig. 9.4. Fluoroscopy image of a swine chest. The ribs, heart, lungs, and diaphragm are clearly visible because of their large variance in contrast. A metal needle implanted into the liver is also easy to see. However, internal soft tissue structures such as vessels in the liver or airways in the lungs cannot be seen. The projection image covers a large region of the body, but does not provide any depth information; for example, the barrel shape of the ribcage is flattened into a single plane

imaging method.[1] Fluoroscopy users can immediately observe changes in the patient or the transit of tools and catheters inserted into the patient. For these reasons, fluoroscopy is used extensively in interventional radiology cardiology, and electrophysiology, and is seeing increasing use for image-guided oncology therapies such as radiofrequency ablation (RFA).

9.2.2.3 Patient Access and Work Environment

Fluoroscopy is the workhorse modality for interventional radiology, and thus systems for fluoroscopy are designed with patient access as a primary goal. The x-ray generator and the detector are relatively small and do not create much of an obstruction for the physician. The C-arm gantry also can be rotated to move the components somewhere more unobtrusive. Furthermore, both the C-arm gantry and the patient table can be translated apart from each other or close together to modify the workspace for the physician. Some C-arm systems are even designed to be portable, so that they can be easily moved in and out of operating rooms or other locations in the hospital where x-ray imaging is needed.

9.2.3 Computed Tomography

9.2.3.1 System Components

In CT, the x-ray generator and detector are mounted on a gantry that rotates around the patient as he or she lies on a movable bed. An example photograph of a CT scanner is shown in Fig. 9.5.

The majority of current CT systems are based on fan-beam geometry, where the x-ray beam is collimated to match an arc-shaped detector on the opposite side of the gantry. The minimal configuration of detectors in this geometry is a single row, but as detector design and electronics speed have improved, multiple rows of detectors or large detector panels are used, as illustrated in Fig. 9.6. By increasing the detector area, the system can image a larger area of the body in a single exposure, which allows for faster scanning. Modern multidetector CT systems can acquire an entire image of the torso in just a few seconds.

---

[1] There are different definitions of "real-time," but in this chapter we will define the term from an imaging perspective, where real time means that images are obtained at video rates (30 Hz) so that there is no perception of individual image frames.

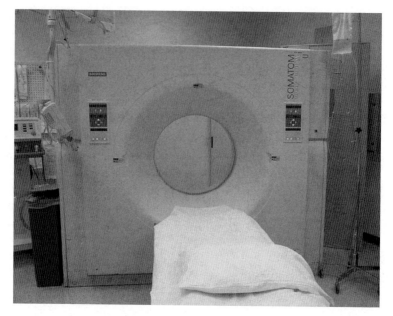

Fig. 9.5. Photograph of a CT scanner used for image-guided interventions. This scanner has a CT fluoroscopy mode for acquiring images in near real time (approximately 6 frames/s), which enables CT-guided interventions

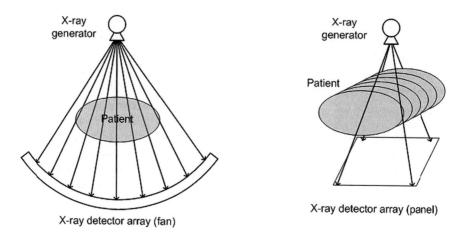

Fig. 9.6. CT system schematics showing fan beam geometry (*left*) and cone-beam geometry (*right*)

The detector usually is made from a solid scintillator or high-pressure xenon gas and is pixellated (typically on the order of 700–1000 elements), so the x-ray fan beam can be spatially sampled by individual elements, each having submillimeter width. When x-rays are absorbed in a detector element, the detector generates an electrical current that is then read by an amplifier to form the detector signal. Because the source and the detector are in constant motion and it is necessary to acquire a number of angular samples comparable to the number of detectors, x-ray detectors in CT scanners operate at much higher sampling rates (several kilohertz) than those in fluoroscopy systems.

As the gantry rotates, projection images of the patient are acquired at fixed angular intervals. Once a sufficient number of angular samples have been obtained, the projection images are then mathematically reconstructed into 3D axial slices through the patient. Although the reconstruction process requires a fast or parallelized computer, x-ray CT reconstruction can be performed analytically using backprojection methods [Herman and Liu 1977; Lakshminarayanan 1975; Scudder 1978], and thus can be performed in almost real time.

9.2.3.2 Image Characteristics

Due to the excellent image quality of CT images, they are used extensively for pretreatment imaging and treatment planning, as discussed in Chapter 3: Visualization in Image-Guided Interventions. Using CT for direct guidance has some benefits over fluoroscopy, due to the ability to see structures in

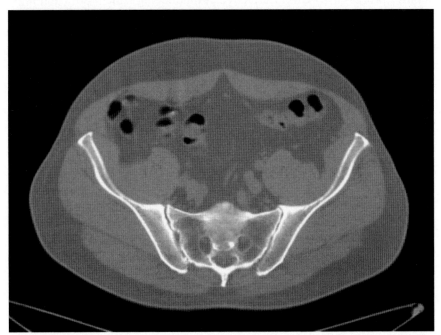

Fig. 9.7. This CT image is an axial slice through the patient's pelvis. As with the fluoroscopy image, bones and air spaces are readily visible against the soft tissue background. The soft tissue, especially the boundaries, can be visualized more clearly than with fluoroscopy because overlapping structures are not compressed into a single plane

three dimensions, but the real-time performance is not as high as with fluoroscopy. To acquire sufficient projections for a CT image, the x-ray generator and detector must rotate at least 180° around the patient. The rotation speed of the gantry is limited to roughly 0.4 s per revolution for physical reasons, which corresponds to about 2 images per s, assuming an instantaneous reconstruction. Figure 9.7 shows an example of a CT image.

9.2.3.3 Patient Access and Work Environment

The CT scanner environment offers less work area than fluoroscopy because of the large gantry. Although the patient bed can be translated in and out of the scanner for positioning and setup, the field of view of the CT scanner is limited to the portion of the patient that is inside the gantry. Accordingly, physicians must typically stand beside the gantry and lean over the patient, or extend their hands into the imaging region if the CT is used for direct guidance. An alternative strategy is to use an "advance and check" approach, where the interventional tool is moved a small distance with the scanner off, and then the patient is imaged again to determine magnitude and direction of the next move. In the hands of an experienced operator this iterative process can be very effective at minimizing patient dose and localizing a target, but such expertise is uncommon.

One limitation to the CT imaging approach is that the natural image plane of the CT system is axial, with the image plane running from left to right and anterior to posterior. This means it is difficult to track an object such as a catheter that is moving in a superior–inferior direction, because the object is only within the field of view of the scanner for a short time. For this reason, CT is used more for percutaneous procedures where the movement of the interventional tool is mostly within the axial plane, as opposed to intravascular procedures where the major vessels run perpendicular to the axial plane.

9.2.4 Current Research and Development Areas

Given the different capabilities of CT and fluoroscopy, it is only natural that efforts are being made to combine the systems and provide dual-use capability for image-guided interventions. A handful of CT scanners now offer a CT-fluoroscopy mode where images can be generated at 4–6 frames per s. To accomplish this speed, the systems generate a reconstructed image from a full rotation, and then update that image using projection data from a partial gantry rotation. With this scheme, even if the gantry only rotates twice per second, new images can be generated at higher rates and still provide salient information, such as the location of an interventional probe.

The reverse approach is to provide CT-like capabilities in the fluoroscopy environment. Since the x-ray source and detector of a fluoroscopy system are already mounted on an arm that can rotate around the patient, it is possible to acquire multiple projections with the fluoroscopy system and use these projections to reconstruct a 3D image of the patient. In this approach, the detector is an area detector, and the x-ray beam is collimated into a cone rather than a fan (as shown on the right side of Fig. 9.6), and so the technique is generically referred to as cone-beam CT (CBCT).

Although this concept has always been theoretically possible with fluoroscopy systems, limitations of the image intensifiers used in fluoroscopy prevented it from being used on a widespread basis, although prototype systems were successfully demonstrated [Endo et al. 1998]. With the advent of fully digital x-ray detectors and improved mechanical control of the fluoroscopy system, tomographic imaging options for fluoroscopy are now being offered by all major medical imaging equipment vendors. Similar systems are also being used in radiation medicine applications to provide setup and or intra-treatment imaging [Jaffray et al. 2002].

9.3   Nuclear Medicine

9.3.1 Basic Physics Concepts

Nuclear medicine encompasses two different imaging techniques: positron emission tomography (PET) and single photon emission tomography (SPET), which is also commonly referred to as single photon emission computed tomography (SPECT). In nuclear medicine, the patient is injected with a radioactive tracer that has some useful biochemical properties. For example, the tracer may distribute in proportion to glucose metabolism, or bind to a particular molecule preferentially expressed on cancer cells. Upon decay of the radioactive atom attached to the tracer, either a positron or gamma ray is emitted. In the case where a positron is emitted, the positron quickly encounters an electron in the body and the two annihilate each other, creating a pair of gamma rays.

The gamma rays are high-energy photons and are considered to move in straight lines from the source. As with x-ray imaging, the gamma rays are attenuated by the photoelectric effect and Compton scattering. However, the detectors used in nuclear medicine have important differences from those in x-ray imaging. First, unlike in x-ray systems, the precise source location is not known in advance, but the photon energy is known because the emissions from radioactive nuclei are monoenergetic. A nuclear medicine detector rejects scattered radiation by determining the energy of each detected photon; if the original photon scatters in the body before reaching the detector, its energy will have been reduced by the scattering event. Second, because the source location is not known in advance, the nuclear medicine detector must have some other way of determining where the photon originated. The means of accomplishing this is different for PET and SPET, and will be discussed in more detail in the following sections.

Finally, the number of photons used to form a nuclear medicine image is typically orders of magnitude lesser than the number required to form an x-ray image. The detectors in nuclear medicine are therefore specifically designed to operate at these much lower event rates. This low event rate also means that nuclear medicine images require a longer time to acquire (tens of minutes) and also contain more noise.

9.3.2 Positron Emission Tomography

9.3.2.1 System Components

A system for PET is illustrated in Figs. 9.8 and 9.9.

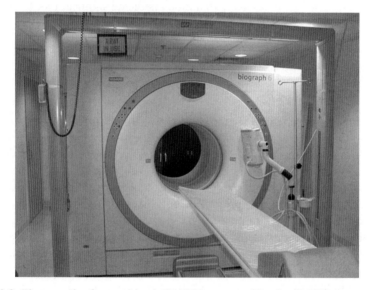

Fig. 9.8. Photograph of a combined CT/PET scanner. Nearly all PET scanners sold today are this type of combined unit. The scanners are arranged in tandem inside a single housing, so that the patient bed can easily move the patient from one scanner to the other. In this case, the CT scanner is on the proximal end of the gantry, and the PET scanner is on the distal end of the gantry

When the positron and the electron annihilate, the gamma rays are emitted in opposite directions. The typical PET detector setup is therefore a ring or cylinder of detectors around the patient, so that both of these photons can be detected. Since both emitted photons have the same speed, they will both reach the detector at almost exactly the same time.[2] If the PET system detects two photons within a short time window, these photons must have come from the same position, and that position lies somewhere along the line connecting the two detectors.

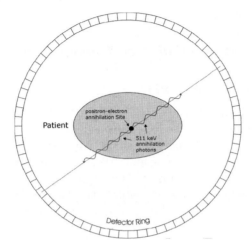

Fig. 9.9. Schematic for a PET scanner. The patient is surrounded by a ring or cylinder of detectors so that photons emitted in all directions can be captured

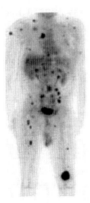

Fig. 9.10. Example of a PET image. This is a coronal view covering a region from the neck to the lower legs. Darker regions correspond to areas of increased radiotracer concentration, and therefore regions of suspected cancer involvement

---

[2] The gamma ray photons travel at the speed of light, so if the photons were emitted from the exact center of a typical PET system, they would reach the detectors approximately 1 ns later. If the photons were emitted close to the edge of the patient, there would be roughly a 0.5 ns difference between the detection times of the two photons. As long as two photons are detected within a few nanoseconds of each other, they are considered to have come from the same positron decay.

9.3.2.2 Image Characteristics

An example PET image is shown in Fig. 9.10. Although some anatomical structures can be discerned, the more salient features of the image are the numerous dark spots throughout the body, which correspond to metastatic cancer in those locations.

9.3.3 Single Photon Emission Tomography

9.3.3.1 System Components

A SPET system is illustrated in Figs. 9.11 and 9.12. SPET cameras localize the emissions coming from the patient by using a collimator, which contains thousands of thin channels that only admit radiation on a path perpendicular to the detector face. Photons reaching the detector are converted to visible light by a large scintillator crystal. This crystal is read out by an array of photomultiplier tubes, which determine the location where the photon entered the crystal by finding the centroid of the light recorded in all of the photomultipliers.

9.3.3.2 Image Characteristic

An example of a SPET image is shown in Fig. 9.13. As with the PET image, the image is more blurry and noisy than a CT image, and identification of structures is more difficult. Spatial resolution in SPET images is slightly worse than those of PET images, because the collimator imposes a distance-dependent blurring on the reconstructed image. Typical SPET systems have a resolution in the order of 6–9 mm.

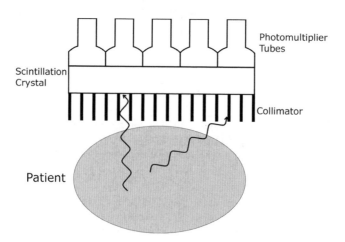

Fig. 9.11. Schematic of a single-head SPET scanner

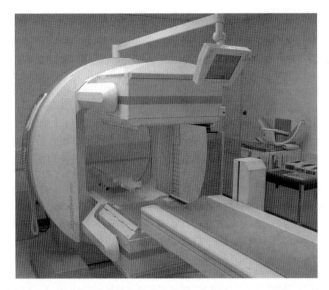

Fig. 9.12. Photograph of a SPET scanner. This SPET scanner shown in the photograph has two imaging cameras, one above the patient bed and one below the patient. The cameras are mounted on a gantry that allows them to rotate around the patient in order to collect projection data from multiple angles

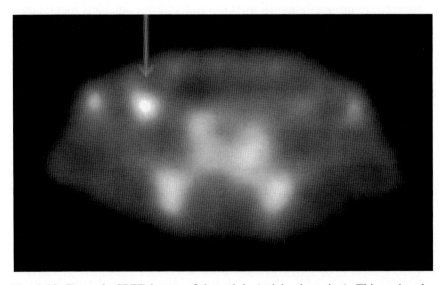

Fig. 9.13. Example SPET image of the pelvis (axial orientation). This patient has been injected with a radiotracer that binds to prostate cancer cells. Bright areas in the image correspond to areas of increased radioactivity concentration. The arrow on the top of the image indicates a potential area of disease, although other areas of the image are equally bright, reflecting nonspecific uptake of the tracer in the digestive and skeletal systems

9.3.4 *Patient Access and Work Environment*

Both PET and SPET are designed as diagnostic imaging systems and are rarely used for direct image guidance. As with a CT system, the patient can be moved in and out of the gantry by translating the patient table, and for SPET the detectors can be rotated around the patient, so that access to the patient is similar to that available in a CT system. However, the major limitation for using PET and SPET for image guidance is that neither of them is a real-time imaging modality. Because the number of photons being emitted from the patient per second is significantly lower than the number of photons used to form an x-ray image, it is necessary to image the patient for longer periods of time. Even in the last decade, scan times in excess of an hour were not uncommon for whole-body imaging. Although the acquisition times have been much reduced by advancements in scanner technology and are currently on the order of a few to tens of minutes, the images still cannot be obtained in real time. Furthermore, PET and SPET reconstruction must be done using iterative methods that require significantly more computation time or power than the reconstruction methods used in x-ray CT, which further limits the speed at which images can be acquired and displayed to a physician.

Because radioactive materials are used in PET and SPET, these procedures carry some of the same risks that occur with x-ray imaging. However, because the number of photons used to form an x-ray image is much larger than the number of photons used to form a nuclear medicine image, the risk of overdose, acute radiation injuries, or long-term side effects is much lower in nuclear medicine than in x-ray imaging.

9.3.5 *Current Research and Development Areas*

PET and SPET provide unique biological information about the patient, and could potentially be ideal for oncologic interventions where a critical question is to determine whether or not a particular region of the body contains cancer cells. As such, there are numerous emerging research efforts designed to overcome the limitations of nuclear medicine imaging and to make it more compatible with image-guided interventions.

One approach is to combine the biochemical imaging data from PET/SPET with an anatomical imaging modality such as CT or MRI. In this scheme, the anatomical image provides a structural road map of the body, and the nuclear medicine image provides the functional status of locations within the anatomy. The fusion of these two types of modalities has been widely accepted in diagnostic imaging since the first systems were proposed for CT/SPECT [Hasegawa et al. 1990] and CT/PET [Beyer et al. 2000], and in the current medical imaging marketplace the stand-alone full-body PET scanner has been wholly replaced with combined PET/CT systems.

Since, for example, a CT image can be obtained much more quickly than nuclear medicine images, the nuclear medicine data can be registered in advance to a planning CT image. These registered data sets can then be used for image guidance by registering the planning CT to a CT or fluoroscopy data set acquired during an intervention. Once one has obtained the mapping between the planning CT and the current x-ray image of the patient, it is then possible to use a similar function to map the preregistered nuclear medicine data into the current x-ray image.

An alternative approach is to redesign the nuclear medicine detection systems for real-time use. In most cases, this involves replacing the large nuclear medicine camera or gantry with compact detectors. In some cases, these detectors are no longer imaging systems, but instead are directional probes that provide an audio feedback based on the rate of detected photons. Although these devices do not provide true image guidance, they provide information about the patient which could not be obtained through other means and thus have found an important niche role in certain procedures, such as sentinel lymph node biopsy for breast cancer [Gulec et al. 2002] and prostate cancer [Wawroschek et al. 1999]. More recently, small handheld detectors have been developed that can provide in situ imaging compatible with surgical and interventional environments. Although these systems cannot provide large field of view images, they may be very useful in tumor resections and image-guided biopsy procedures [Wernick et al. 2004].

9.4   Magnetic Resonance Imaging

9.4.1 Basic Physics Concepts

MRI is based on the phenomenon of nuclear magnetic resonance (NMR). Certain atomic nuclei have inherent magnetic moments, and when these nuclei are placed into a magnetic field, they have a resonant frequency that scales linearly with the magnetic field strength. If these nuclei are subjected to radiofrequency waves at the resonant frequency, they absorb this energy and transition to a higher energy state. These excited nuclei then relax back to their ground state and accordingly emit radiofrequency waves. The relaxation of these nuclei depends strongly on their surroundings, so contrast in the MRI image is based on both the density of nuclei and their chemical environment. For this reason, MRI has much better soft tissue contrast than x-ray-based techniques, since the biochemical properties of soft tissue vary much more than their density or elemental composition. By varying the radiofrequency pulses used to interrogate the tissue, it is also possible to highlight different types of tissue or materials. Thus, contrast mechanisms in the MRI image can be tuned to specific image detection and identification tasks.

9.4.2 System Components

An example of MRI scanner is shown in Fig. 9.14. There are three major hardware components to the scanner. The first component is the main magnet that produces the large static magnetic field. This magnetic field is typically 1.5T or greater, which is roughly 30,000 times stronger than the earth's magnetic field. The second component is a series of coils that transmit and receive radio waves from the part of the patient being imaged. The third component is a set of gradient coils, which allows the system to dynamically and spatially vary the magnetic field. Since the resonant frequency of the nuclei is dependent on the magnetic field strength, the gradients allow the system to spatially encode location through frequency and phase variations.

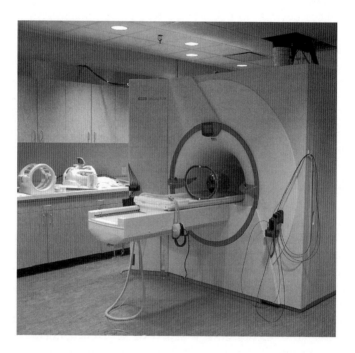

Fig. 9.14. Typical MRI scanner. This scanner has a "closed-bore" design, meaning that the patient lies on a bed within a cylindrical bore. The tank on the bed is a test pattern used for calibration of the scanner during maintenance. This particular scanner is used extensively for functional brain imaging, so there are many cables and sensors for providing audiovisual stimulation and feedback to the patient during imaging. Specialty coils for head imaging are seen on the shelf to the left of the scanner

9.4.3 Image Characteristics

It is somewhat difficult to describe a "typical" MRI image, because by varying the parameters of the image acquisition it is possible to create a vast array of possible images from a given region of the body. However, MRI images typically have excellent soft tissue contrast and good spatial resolution, so they are ideal for identifying structures and boundaries.

Image distortion is a potential complicating factor with MRI imaging. Because spatial information is encoded using magnetic field strength, inhomogeneities in the field can cause erroneous shifts in the image data. These inhomogeneities can be caused by the patient, objects worn by the patient, prosthetics/implants, or surgical devices such as frames. Such irregularities in the image pose a particular challenge in image-guided interventions, because they are not easy to characterize in advance (and therefore be corrected).

9.4.4 Patient Access and Work Environment

MRI-based image-guided procedures pose unique challenges. The first challenge is that the high magnetic field creates a very hazardous work environment. The field strength rises rapidly as one approaches the center of the magnet and is strong enough to pull in large, heavy objects such as chairs, gurneys, and oxygen tanks, with potentially fatal results. Small ferromagnetic objects such as scalpels, probes, and paperclips can similarly be turned into dangerous missiles. For this reason, it is critical that every object be evaluated for compatibility before it is brought into the MRI suite. In most cases, this requires investing in a completely separate set of procedural tools and equipment that are dedicated solely to MRI-based interventions.

The second challenge is that the high magnetic fields and radiofrequency radiation can adversely affect electronic devices such as cameras, position trackers, and computers. Some of these devices will completely fail, while others will operate incorrectly or generate artifacts. In most cases, these problems can be mitigated by redesigning the instrument, but again this requires a separate set of devices for the MRI environment.

The third challenge is the amount of available workspace. To create a homogeneous main magnetic field, the bore of the MRI system is long and only slightly wider than the patient, leaving very little room for instruments or even the physician's hands and arms. Different technical solutions to the limited workspace have been proposed, such as the "double-donut" magnet design, open MRI designs using large flat pole magnets rather than a cylinder, and MRI systems specifically designed with larger bores. However, none of these designs are in widespread use, and the vast majority of MRI systems are not designed with interventions in mind.

9.4.5 *Current Research and Development Areas*

Despite the many challenges involved with interventional and intraoperative MRI, the superb visualization capabilities and the capacity for functional imaging have led to many innovative solutions for MRI-guided interventions.

9.4.5.1 MRI-Based Neurosurgery

MRI has proven particularly useful, and therefore achieved the most widespread use in intraoperative brain imaging [Albayrak et al. 2004; Jolesz et al. 2002; Mittal and Black 2006; Yrjana et al. 2007]. Brain MRI provides superior soft tissue detail for visualization of the anatomy. Furthermore, functional brain imaging using MRI can determine which regions of the brain are involved in speech, sensory, and motor tasks. Such information is vital during tumor removal since it enables the surgeon to more accurately avoid those important regions. Similarly, the placement of brain stimulators or other assistive devices can benefit from intraprocedure MRI mapping of critical structures.

Methods for intraoperative brain MRI are often classified into low-field, mid-field, and high-field approaches, depending on the type of MRI system used for imaging.

Low-field imaging systems [Lewin and Metzger 2001] (approximately 0.1T main magnet field strength) tend to have limited imaging capabilities and almost no capacity for functional imaging; however, the low-field strength enables them to be very compact and movable, and requires less modification to the operating room environment. These systems can be thought of as MR-based surgical microscopes, in that they can be added to an existing operating room. Although such systems could, in principle, make intraoperative MRI guidance a more widely available technology, many practitioners feel that the poor image quality severely hampers the clinical utility of these systems.

Mid-field systems [Schwartz et al. 2001] (approximately 0.5T main magnet field strength) are something of a compromise between imaging capability and the restrictions of the operating room, although chronologically these were actually the first systems to be developed. In these systems the main magnet can be more open than that on a conventional scanner, which allows the physician to stand right beside the patient, although the available space is still quite limited. Specialized MRI-compatible equipment and rooms are still required, but a key advantage is that the patient does not have to be moved to acquire images.

High-field systems [Truwit and Hall 2001] (1.5T main magnet field strength and higher) are typically implemented as a multiroom operating suite, where a patient is in one location for the surgery, but can be moved or rotated into an MRI scanner for imaging. The MRI scanner may be behind a door or other form of shielding, but the operating suite still must maintain a very high level of MRI compatibility. The main advantage of this approach is that it produces very high quality images and functional data, since the scanner is on par with normal diagnostic MRI devices. However, the time required to move the patient between the operating area and the imaging area limits the number of images that can be practically acquired. This type of system is also generally the most expensive and complex to implement because of the large physical space requirements.

9.4.5.2 MRI-Based Interventional Radiology

Interventional radiology makes use of natural pathways in the body, primarily the circulatory system, to deliver therapy. Catheters and probes are inserted into large vessels and then navigated through the vasculature to the intended target. Although interventional radiology has traditionally been performed with x-ray-based methods such as fluoroscopy, MRI is an attractive image guidance method for several reasons. First, the space requirements for an interventional radiology procedure are relatively low, and it is possible to perform these procedures without having the physician standing directly next to the patient. Thus, the confined quarters of the MRI scanner represent less of a challenge. Second, fluoroscopy exposes both patients and staff to ionizing radiation, which can be especially harmful during long procedures or in sensitive populations such as children. Third, MRI offers potentially significant improvements in visualization over fluoroscopy, including identification of vessels without using contrast and full 3D image acquisition.

Interventional MRI has shown encouraging successes in its early trials, especially in the arena of cardiovascular procedures. In cases of abdominal aortic aneurysm or thoracic aortic dissection, where flow and vessel structure are complex, the visualization benefits of 3D MRI can be advantageous. MRI also can provide improved visualization of the myocardium for many procedures, including delivery of therapeutic materials, placement of prosthetic devices, and electrophysiological corrections [Ozturk et al. 2005].

Naturally, as with MRI-based neurosurgery, there are significant equipment and facilities costs associated with construction of an MRI-based interventional radiology suite, and only a handful of hospitals have access to this level of technology. Furthermore, most commercial MRI scanners are optimized for the diagnostic imaging process (where image quality is paramount) rather than interventional techniques (where some image quality may be sacrificed for real-time performance), so interventional MRI requires a high level of engineering expertise. Finally, the ongoing financial costs of interventional MRI are expected to be higher than that with conventional interventional radiology, because the cost of consumables will likely be larger, although it is too early to tell if the same economies of scale will apply once interventional MRI becomes more prevalent. For these reasons,

MRI-based interventional radiology is still primarily a research area and has not yet achieved widespread clinical use.

9.4.5.3 MRI-Based Prostate Therapy and Robotics

MRI offers several advantages for prostate imaging, including excellent definition of anatomical boundaries, improved visualization of tumor extension and invasion, and the capacity for spectroscopic analysis of tissue. Thus, localized prostate therapies such as brachytherapy could benefit from MRI-based guidance as they would enable improved targeting. However, the standard lithotomy positioning/peritoneal access used for prostate therapies has the patient lying on their back with their legs and feet suspended in stirrups, a position that would be impossible to achieve in a conventional MRI scanner. Thus, investigators have developed specialized MRI scanners to allow prostate brachytherapy to be done inside the imager itself, along with a host of associated technologies for real-time imaging and treatment planning [D'Amico et al. 1998; Haker et al. 2005]. This approach to prostate therapy has demonstrated encouraging clinical results, but has not been adopted at many other sites, in part because of its cost and complexity versus ultrasound, which is used for the majority of prostate brachytherapy implants.

Because the typical MRI scanner is such a cramped work environment, MRI-based interventions benefit from remotely controlled robots that can operate inside the scanner, providing dexterous manipulation in spaces where a person could not work. With robotics, the physician or operator can be outside the scanner or even in another room. Although robots typically have extensive metal and electronic components that would be incompatible with the MRI environment, innovative technologies using pneumatics and plastics have been used to create robots that are compatible with most types of imaging modalities, including MRI [Stoianovici 2005]. These components have been used to develop robotic systems for brachytherapy seed placement or other needle-based therapies in the prostate, and can be deployed in conventional diagnostic MRI scanners [Stoianovici et al. 2007].

9.5   Ultrasound

9.5.1 Basic Physics Concepts

For ultrasound imaging, sound waves in the frequency range of 5–10 MHz are transmitted into the body by a handheld transducer. These waves readily penetrate into soft tissue, but are reflected at tissue boundaries because of the mismatch between the speed of sound in the different tissues. Ultrasound waves used in medicine are stopped by air (because the density of air is too low) and bone (because the density and stiffness of bone is too high). This means that the transducer must be aimed to avoid these structures, and that overlying bones or air masses will block the imaging of objects deeper in the body. This has several important implications for image-guided interventions. In the thorax, the ultrasound transducer must be placed in the intercostal space between the ribs in order to image organs such as the liver, but the lungs cannot be imaged at all. In the abdomen and pelvis, ultrasound excels because the ribs do not present a barrier, but digestive system gas can potentially be a problem. In the brain, the skull represents a solid bone barrier, effectively precluding ultrasound imaging.[3]

Ultrasound at diagnostic wavelengths and power levels poses no risk to either the operator or the patient, which is one of the reasons why ultrasound is the dominant modality for fetal imaging. This property is also a significant benefit to researchers working in image-guided interventions, since it means that ultrasound systems can be easily used in the lab or office environment.

Because ultrasound works with reflected sound waves, the Doppler effect enables straightforward imaging and quantification of motion within the body. Ultrasound is therefore used extensively in cardiac and vascular imaging, where dynamic features such as flow, turbulence, ventricle wall motion, and valve opening/closing can readily be observed.

9.5.2 System Components

Figure 9.15 shows a typical medical ultrasound imaging system. The computer system and display are mounted on a small wheeled cart that allows the system to be easily moved from room to room. Several different probes can be attached to the computer system; each probe has a specific frequency range and shape designed to match a particular imaging task.

The ultrasound transducer can take on many forms. A single element transducer interrogates a line of tissue in front of it, so the simplest possible system would be a single element that was moved over the organ of interest. In practice, however, this method provides too little information to the physician and is also too slow to be clinically useful. The most common system approach is to have either a single element that is mechanically oscillated across the imaging area or a linear array of elements. These are referred to as 2D transducers since their field of view is a single slice. Recently, some system vendors have developed 3D transducers, where a linear array of elements is oscillated across the field, or the transducer has a multi-row array of elements.

---

[3] There is a notable exception to this statement. Because the skull is relatively thin, low-frequency ultrasound waves are able to pass through the skull and image the brain. However, this is a very atypical application for ultrasound, although it is an active and intriguing area of research.

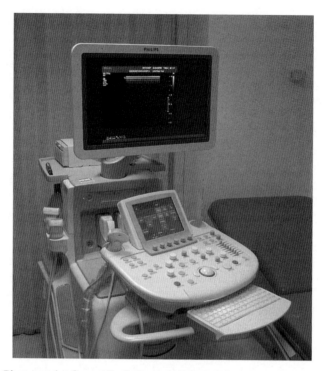

Fig. 9.15. Photograph of a medical ultrasound imaging system. As with most ultrasound units, the entire system is on a wheeled cart, so it can easily be moved around the hospital. The integrated system includes a keyboard, additional imaging controls, a monitor for viewing the images, and a small printer for hardcopy output. Different ultrasound probes and other supplies for imaging can also be stored on the cart

Since ultrasound is inherently a real-time modality, some ultrasound scanners offer a 4D imaging mode that allows for visualization of dynamic processes. This scanning mode is essentially 3D imaging at video rates. Because these images contain a large amount of data, they are often presented as a rendered and lighted 3D surface that changes with time. This method is especially useful in cardiac and fetal imaging where there is a clear and easily identifiable structure of interest.

9.5.3 Image Characteristics

Some representative ultrasound images are shown in Fig. 9.16. Several particular characteristics of these images are immediately apparent. The first is that the image is grainy; this appearance is the result of speckle, a non-coherent reflection phenomenon that is endemic to any form of reflection imaging. The second is that the field of view of the image is limited to a 2D wedge-shaped area emerging from end of the probe. The effective viewing depth of a typical medical ultrasound system is about 20 cm, so unlike other

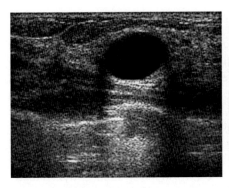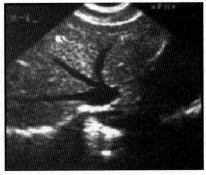

Fig. 9.16 Ultrasound images of a cyst in the breast (*left image*) and vascular structure in the liver (*right*)

modalities, ultrasound is a regional imaging modality and cannot provide full cross-sectional slices of the body.

9.5.4 Patient Access and Work Environment

Because ultrasound probes are small enough to be handheld, patient access is unsurpassed. Subject to the constraints of overlying bone and air structures, the probe can be easily repositioned to change the field of view or clear the way of a surgical instrument. Probes also can be inserted into body cavities or surgical fields for close access to the object being imaged. Furthermore, even though most ultrasound systems are already on a small, wheeled computer cart, complete imaging systems have been miniaturized to work with portable computers so that the entire system can fit into an even smaller footprint.

The use of a handheld probe poses some interesting problems for ultrasound guidance systems. Because the probe must be pressed tightly against the skin, either the physician or an assistant must be holding the probe at all times, which leaves only one hand for other tasks. A more subtle problem is that the arbitrary orientation of the ultrasound probe can present images that are quite different from conventional cross-sectional imaging (e.g., CT, MRI) to the physician. The physician must therefore mentally integrate the oblique ultrasound view into their reference frame, and this can be a challenging task for new practitioners.

9.5.5 Current Research and Development Areas

9.5.5.1 Ultrasound Registration to Other Modalities

Because ultrasound provides real-time imaging capabilities in a small form factor without the use of ionizing radiation, there is great interest in combining ultrasound with other imaging modalities. In these approaches, cross-sectional images of the patient and fiducial markers are first obtained using

MRI or CT. The fiducial markers or anatomic landmarks are used to establish a coordinate reference frame for cross-sectional images. A tracked ultrasound probe (typically using optical or electromagnetic tracking; see Chapter 2 for more information) is then registered to the reference frame. As the ultrasound probe is moved around the patient, its position and pose in the tracker frame can be transformed to a position and pose in the reference frame. By resampling and reslicing the cross-sectional image data, a CT or MRI image corresponding to the "live" ultrasound image can be generated and displayed, either as an overlay or a side-by-side image. Image processing techniques, where the view seen by the ultrasound system is dynamically matched to cross-sectional image views obtained in another modality, may also be utilized. This approach has the advantage of not strictly requiring a position tracking system, although it is also more susceptible to variations and artifacts in the images themselves.

Prostate brachytherapy is a good candidate for image fusion; ultrasound is used to guide the implantation of the radioactive seeds, but the ultrasound images may not show as much tissue detail or define the anatomy as well as other modalities. Furthermore, the combination of imaging modalities can provide better postimplant dosimetry by improving visualization of critical structures in combination with the seeds themselves. Ultrasound fusion with both MRI [Daanen et al. 2006; Kaplan et al. 2002; Reynier et al. 2004] and CT/fluoroscopy [French et al. 2005; Fuller et al. 2005; Rubens et al. 2006; Su et al. 2007] has been used in prostate brachytherapy.

Ultrasound registration to CT and MRI is also of great benefit during procedures in the abdomen and thorax. In these regions of the body, involuntary motions such as respiration, peristalsis, and heartbeat can create significant displacements and deformation of organs, and the real-time imaging capabilities of ultrasound provide a great benefit to the physician. By being able to overlay the cross-sectional imaging data on the ultrasound, diagnostic capabilities can be much enhanced [Huang et al. 2005] and intra-procedure navigation can be improved [Beller et al. 2007]. Although motion and deformation of organs is clearly a major challenge in these procedures, as the CT or MRI are most often acquired during a breath hold, the use of landmarks such as vessels [Lange et al. 2003] and mathematical modeling of respiration [Blackall et al. 2005] are being used to address these challenges.

Ultrasound-to-CT registration also has become of great interest in external beam radiation therapy, where it is used to determine the location of the target organ prior to delivery of therapy. Radiation therapy plans are usually derived from a single CT volume acquired before the start of treatment, but anatomical changes in the patient can cause the target organ to shift within the body, so that the pretreatment CT is no longer an accurate image of the patient. The prostate, in particular, can move several millimeters from day to day because of differences in bowel and bladder filling.

To mitigate these anatomical variations, an ultrasound unit referenced to the coordinate frame of the linear accelerator or the treatment room is used to image the patient immediately before the delivery of therapy. The ultrasound is compared to the planning CT and the therapist then moves the patient table to compensate for any changes. This process helps to ensure that the target organ is once again in the proper location for treatment.

9.5.5.2 Ultrasound Contrast Agents

Ultrasound contrast agents are similar to those used in x-ray imaging and MRI, in that they provide information about the patient that would not normally be obtainable with that modality. For example, an x-ray contrast agent is a dense material, usually iodine or barium, introduced into a body compartment (such as the vasculature) to change the x-ray attenuation of that structure and increase its conspicuity. Gadolinium and superparamagnetic iron oxide (SPIO) are used as MRI contrast agents because they affect the local magnetic field experienced by the tissue, and therefore the relaxation times of the nuclei. Contrast agents in the blood are often used to identify tumors, since most tumors have an excessively fenestrated capillary bed, which allows the contrast agent to preferentially leak out into the surrounding tissue.

The predominant type of ultrasound contrast agent is the microbubble, a tiny sphere (1–5 μm diameter) that can easily pass through the entire circulatory system. These microbubbles have a polymer shell and an internal core filled with a biologically innocuous gas. The materials and size are chosen so that the microbubbles will strongly reflect the incident ultrasound waves. Because the microbubble is a tuned mechanical system, it also resonates at harmonic frequencies of the input sound wave, enabling the ultrasound system to specifically detect the presence of the contrast agent due to its characteristic resonance.

There are two broad classes of ultrasound contrast agents. The first is the untargeted contrast agent, which travels through the circulatory system much like iodinated CT contrast agents or gadolinium-based MRI agents. Since these agents are designed to remain in the blood pool, they are used primarily in cardiography studies to increase the visibility of the structures in the heart. A handful of these types of agents are FDA approved for regular clinical use. The second class of ultrasound contrast agent is the targeted contrast agent. These agents have a physical structure similar to the untargeted agents, but the shell includes chemicals that allow the microbubble to preferentially bind to biomarkers of disease. Thus, these agents could preferentially define the borders of tumors or allow confirmation of inflammation in important blood vessels. Although initial research in this area has been promising, technology is still developing and none of the targeted ultrasound contrast agents have moved from research into regular clinical use.

9.5.5.3   High-Intensity Focused Ultrasound

Although ultrasound in medicine is primarily used for diagnostic imaging, it also can be used therapeutically by increasing the intensity of the trans-mitted waves. This increased intensity can cause localized heating effects (hyperthermia) or ablate the tissue outright, depending on the energy and the length of time that it is applied. Another important design difference between diagnostic and therapeutic systems is that diagnostic ultrasound typically uses a diverging beam to produce a cone-shaped field of view, whereas therapeutic ultrasound uses a concave transducer or transducer array, which focuses the ultrasound energy onto a point within the body. By moving either the body or the transducer, the focal point can be moved, enabling the treatment of larger body regions.

High-intensity focused ultrasound (HIFU) covers a broad range of transducers and applications. In the prostate, the HIFU transducer is placed in a transrectal probe that also contains an ultrasound imaging system. The ultrasound images provide guidance for positioning of the probe, since prostate anatomy is often imaged using ultrasound. Some studies of the prostate-specific HIFU systems recently have been reported in the literature. According to Murat et al. [2007], results suggest that the technique could be an effective alternative to radiation therapy in certain patient populations.

HIFU is also being used for treatment of breast tumors [Wu et al. 2007], liver and kidney tumors, and uterine fibroids [Leslie and Kennedy 2007]. In these treatments, the ultrasound source is located outside the body and usually integrated with a larger imaging system. Image guidance is provided by either ultrasound imaging or MRI. As these imaging methods are both potentially sensitive to the temperature of the local tissue, imaging can be used to guide and monitor the progress of the therapy, enabling the therapy to be adjusted during treatment to achieve the desired effects.

An important non-oncologic use of HIFU is in the creation of hemo-stasis following trauma. In many trauma patients, internal bleeding can have severe consequences and is difficult to address without invasive surgery, which naturally carries its own risks and is difficult to perform in the field. HIFU can enable cauterization of vessels and tissue deep inside the body. The principal challenges of this technique are preservation of nearby critical structures and accurate assessment of the bleeding locations, since in most field trauma cases specialized imaging equipment is not readily available [Vaezy et al. 2007].

9.6   Summary and Discussion

A summary of the different imaging systems' properties is provided in Table 9.1. There are some notable themes which emerge from this com-parison chart:

1. It is clear that no single modality is superior in all areas, and in fact, the modalities are often complementary to each other. For example, some modalities have excellent real-time capability (ultrasound and fluoroscopy), whereas others are more suited to pretreatment imaging, but have better soft tissue visualization, such as MRI and CT. Thus, bridging these gaps (e.g., by combining ultrasound and CT) is a common theme in image-guided interventions research and in image registration in general (this topic is covered more fully in Chapter 6: Rigid Registration and Chapter 7: Nonrigid Registration for Image-Guided Interventions) and is a critical support technology for these efforts.

Table 9.1. Summary chart of imaging modalities and their relative strengths and limitations in the context of image-guided interventions

Modality	Strengths	Limitations
Fluoroscopy	▪ Sub-millimeter spatial resolution ▪ Real-time imaging ▪ Good patient access	▪ Limited to 2D projections ▪ Requires ionizing radiation ▪ Poor soft tissue contrast
CT	▪ Sub-millimeter spatial resolution ▪ Fast coverage of large volumes ▪ Generates 3D volumes ▪ Moderate patient access	▪ Small number of systems with CT fluoro option ▪ Requires ionizing radiation
PET/SPET	▪ Provides unique biochemical and functional information ▪ Sensitive to nanomolar amounts of tracer	▪ Image formation requires several minutes ▪ Requires ionizing radiation ▪ Spatial resolution ~ 2–3 mm
MRI	▪ Millimeter spatial resolution ▪ Excellent soft tissue contrast ▪ Can also image functional information ▪ No ionizing radiation	▪ Magnetic field creates potential hazards ▪ Specialized MRI-compatible equipment needed ▪ Limited real-time capabilities
Ultrasound	▪ Real-time imaging ▪ Excellent imaging of flow and motion ▪ No ionizing radiation ▪ Handheld probes with excellent patient access	▪ Limited, wedge-shaped field of view ▪ Images contaminated by speckle ▪ Most systems limited to 2D imaging

2. Many researchers are also attempting to expand the capabilities of a particular modality to make it more compatible with image-guided interventions. For example, more CT scanners are capable of fluoroscopic acquisition, and frame rates are now as high as 8 Hz. Likewise, many ultrasound systems are incorporating array transducers that allow acquisition of a 3D volume image rather than a single 2D slice. With sufficient acquisition speed, the 3D volume can be acquired rapidly, allowing excellent visualization of moving structures such as heart valves.

3. Since image-guided interventions are usually performed using physical tools, such as forceps, the ideal would be for the imaging system to clearly and accurately image those tools as they move inside the patient. Ultrasound and fluoroscopy are, for the most part, capable of this task, but other modalities with poor real-time imaging are not as effective. Therefore, technologies for instrument tracking within the imaging space and inside the patient are an active development area, and registration is essential for ensuring that the image coordinates match those of the tracking system.

Acknowledgments

The author wishes to thank the faculty and staff of the Department of Radiology at Georgetown University Hospital, the Center for Functional and Molecular Imaging at Georgetown University, and the Department of Radiology at the University of California, San Francisco, for assistance with images gathered for this chapter.

References

Albayrak B, Samdani AF, and Black PM. (2004). "Intra-operative magnetic resonance imaging in neurosurgery." *Acta Neurochir (Wien)*, 146(6), 543–556; discussion 557.

Archer BR. (2006). "Radiation management and credentialing of fluoroscopy users." *Pediatr Radiol*, 36(Suppl 14), 182–184.

Beller S, Hunerbein M, Lange T, Eulenstein S, Gebauer B, and Schlag PM. (2007). "Image-guided surgery of liver metastases by three-dimensional ultrasound-based optoelectronic navigation." *Br J Surg*, 94(7), 866–875.

Beyer T, Townsend DW, Brun T, Kinahan PE, Charron M, Roddy R, Jerin J, Young J, Byars L, and Nutt R. (2000). "A combined PET/CT scanner for clinical oncology." *J Nucl Med*, 41(8), 1369–1379.

Blackall JM, Penney GP, King AP, and Hawkes DJ. (2005). "Alignment of sparse freehand 3-D ultrasound with preoperative images of the liver using models of respiratory motion and deformation." *IEEE Trans Med Imaging*, 24(11), 1405–1416.

Bushberg J, Seibert J, Leidholdt E, and Boone J. (2002). *The Essential Physics of Medical Imaging, 2nd edition*, Lippincott Williams & Wilkins, Baltimore.

D'Amico AV, Cormack R, Tempany CM, Kumar S, Topulos G, Kooy HM, and Coleman CN. (1998). "Real-time magnetic resonance image-guided interstitial brachytherapy in the treatment of select patients with clinically localized prostate cancer." *Int J Radiat Oncol Biol Phys*, 42(3), 507–515.

Daanen V, Gastaldo J, Giraud JY, Fourneret P, Descotes JL, Bolla M, Collomb D, and Troccaz J. (2006). "MRI/TRUS data fusion for brachytherapy." *Int J Med Robot*, 2(3), 256–261.

Endo M, Yoshida K, Kamagata N, Satoh K, Okazaki T, Hattori Y, Kobayashi S, Jimbo M, Kusakabe M, and Tateno Y. (1998). "Development of a 3D CT-scanner using a cone beam and video-fluoroscopic system." *Radiat Med*, 16(1), 7–12.

French D, Morris J, Keyes M, Goksel O, and Salcudean S. (2005). "Computing intraoperative dosimetry for prostate brachytherapy using TRUS and fluoroscopy." *Acad Radiol*, 12(10), 1262–1272.

Fuller DB, Jin H, Koziol JA, and Feng AC. (2005). "CT-ultrasound fusion prostate brachytherapy: a dynamic dosimetry feedback and improvement method. A report of 54 consecutive cases." *Brachytherapy*, 4(3), 207–216.

Gulec SA, Eckert M, and Woltering EA. (2002). "Gamma probe-guided lymph node dissection ('gamma picking') in differentiated thyroid carcinoma." *Clin Nucl Med*, 27(12), 859–861.

Haker SJ, Mulkern RV, Roebuck JR, Barnes AS, Dimaio S, Hata N, and Tempany CM. (2005). "Magnetic resonance-guided prostate interventions." *Top Magn Reson Imaging*, 16(5), 355–368.

Hasegawa B, Gingold E, Reilly S, Liew S, and Cann C. (1990). "Description of a simultaneous emission-transmission CT system." *Proc Soc Photo Opt Instrum Eng*, 1231, 50–60.

Herman GT, and Liu HK. (1977). "Display of three-dimensional information in computed tomography." *J Comput Assist Tomogr*, 1(1), 155–160.

Huang X, Hill NA, Ren J, Guiraudon G, Boughner D, and Peters TM. (2005). "Dynamic 3D ultrasound and MR image registration of the beating heart." *Med Image Comput Comput Assist Interv Int Conf Med Image Comput Comput Assist Interv*, 8(Pt 2), 171–178.

Jaffray DA, Siewerdsen JH, Wong JW, and Martinez AA. (2002). "Flat-panel cone-beam computed tomography for image-guided radiation therapy." *Int J Radiat Oncol Biol Phys*, 53(5), 1337–1349.

Jolesz FA, Talos IF, Schwartz RB, Mamata H, Kacher DF, Hynynen K, McDannold N, Saivironporn P, and Zao L. (2002). "Intraoperative magnetic resonance imaging and magnetic resonance imaging-guided therapy for brain tumors." *Neuroimaging Clin N Am*, 12(4), 665–683.

Kaplan I, Oldenburg NE, Meskell P, Blake M, Church P, and Holupka EJ. (2002). "Real time MRI-ultrasound image guided stereotactic prostate biopsy." *Magn Reson Imaging*, 20(3), 295–299.

Lakshminarayanan AV. (1975). *Reconstruction from divergent x-ray data*, State University of New York, Buffalo NY.

Lange T, Eulenstein S, Hunerbein M, and Schlag PM. (2003). "Vessel-based non-rigid registration of MR/CT and 3D ultrasound for navigation in liver surgery." *Comput Aided Surg*, 8(5), 228–240.

Leslie TA, and Kennedy JE. (2007). "High intensity focused ultrasound in the treatment of abdominal and gynaecological diseases." *Int J Hyperthermia*, 23(2), 173–182.

Lewin JS, and Metzger AK. (2001). "Intraoperative MR systems. Low-field approaches." *Neuroimaging Clin N Am*, 11(4), 611–628.

McRobbie DW, Pritchard S, and Quest RA. (2003). "Studies of the human oropharyngeal airspaces using magnetic resonance imaging. I. Validation of a three-dimensional MRI method for producing *ex vivo* virtual and physical casts of the oropharyngeal airways during inspiration." *J Aerosol Med*, 16(4), 401–415.

Mittal S, and Black PM. (2006). "Intraoperative magnetic resonance imaging in neurosurgery: the Brigham concept." *Acta Neurochir Suppl*, 98, 77–86.

Murat FJ, Poissonnier L, Pasticier G, and Gelet A. (2007). "High-intensity focused ultrasound (HIFU) for prostate cancer." *Cancer Control*, 14(3), 244–249.

Ozturk C, Guttman M, McVeigh ER, and Lederman RJ. (2005). "Magnetic resonance imaging-guided vascular interventions." *Top Magn Reson Imaging*, 16(5), 369–381.

Reynier C, Troccaz J, Fourneret P, Dusserre A, Gay-Jeune C, Descotes JL, Bolla M, and Giraud JY. (2004). "MRI/TRUS data fusion for prostate brachytherapy. Preliminary results." *Med Phys*, 31(6), 1568–1575.

Rubens DJ, Yu Y, Barnes AS, Strang JG, and Brasacchio R. (2006). "Image-guided brachytherapy for prostate cancer." *Radiol Clin North Am*, 44(5), 735–748, viii–ix.

Schwartz RB, Kacher DF, Pergolizzi RS, and Jolesz FA. (2001). "Intraoperative MR systems. Midfield approaches." *Neuroimaging Clin N Am*, 11(4), 629–644.

Scudder H. (1978). "Introduction to computer aided tomography." *Proc IEEE*, 66, 628.

Stoianovici D. (2005). "Multi-imager compatible actuation principles in surgical robotics." *Int J Med Robot*, 1(2), 86–100.

Stoianovici D, Song D, Petrisor D, Ursu D, Mazilu D, Mutener M, Schar M, and Patriciu A. (2007). "MRI Stealth" robot for prostate interventions." *Minim Invasive Ther Allied Technol*, 16(4), 241–248.

Su Y, Davis BJ, Furutani KM, Herman MG, and Robb RA. (2007). "Seed localization and TRUS-fluoroscopy fusion for intraoperative prostate brachytherapy dosimetry." *Comput Aided Surg*, 12(1), 25–34.

Truwit CL, and Hall WA. (2001). "Intraoperative MR systems. High-field approaches." *Neuroimaging Clin N Am*, 11(4), 645–650, viii.

Vaezy S, Zderic V, Karmy-Jones R, Jurkovich GJ, Cornejo C, and Martin RW. (2007). "Hemostasis and sealing of air leaks in the lung using high-intensity focused ultrasound." *J Trauma*, 62(6), 1390–1395.

Valentin J. (2000). "Avoidance of radiation injuries from medical interventional procedures." *Ann ICRP*, 30(2), 7–67.

Wawroschek F, Vogt H, Weckermann D, Wagner T, and Harzmann R. (1999). "The sentinel lymph node concept in prostate cancer – first results of gamma probe-guided sentinel lymph node identification." *Eur Urol*, 36(6), 595–600.

Webb A. (2002). *Introduction to Biomedical Imaging, 1st edition,* Wiley-IEEE Press, Hoboken, NJ.

Wernick M, Brankov J, Chapman D, Anastasio M, Zhong Z, Muehleman C, and Li J. (2004). "Multiple-image Computed Tomography." *IEEE International Symposium on Biomedical Imaging: From Nano to Macro*, Arlington, VA.

Wu F, ter Haar G, and Chen WR. (2007). "High-intensity focused ultrasound ablation of breast cancer." *Expert Rev Anticancer Ther*, 7(6), 823–831.

Yrjana SK, Tuominen J, and Koivukangas J. (2007). "Intraoperative magnetic resonance imaging in neurosurgery." *Acta Radiol*, 48(5), 540–549.

Chapter 10

MRI-Guided FUS and its Clinical Applications

Ferenc Jolesz, Nathan McDannold, Greg Clement, Manabu Kinoshita, Fiona Fennessy, and Clare Tempany

Abstract

Focused ultrasound offers a completely noninvasive means to deliver energy to targeted locations deep within the body. It is actively being investigated for thermal ablation to offer a noninvasive alternative to surgical resection, and for altering tissue or cell membrane properties as a means to enhance or enable the delivery of drugs at targeted locations. Although focused ultrasound technology has been investigated for more than 60 years, it has not found widespread use because of the difficulty of guiding and monitoring the procedure. One needs to accurately identify the target tissue, confirm that the focal point is correctly targeted before high energies are employed, ensure that sufficient energy is delivered safely to the entire target, and evaluate the outcome after the treatment. Combining focused ultrasound with MRI overcomes all of these problems through MRI's abilities to create high quality anatomical images and to quantify temperature changes. This chapter provides an overview of the marriage of these two technologies. We describe the basics of focused ultrasound technology and MRI methods to guide thermal therapies. This chapter also describes how this technology is currently being used in the clinic, and overviews some new opportunities that are being developed, such as targeted drug delivery in the brain.

10.1 Introduction

First proposed for noninvasively producing lesions in the brain in 1942 [Lynn et al. 1942], therapeutic ultrasound or high intensity focused ultrasound (HIFU) is more than a half a century old. Since then, many investigators have recognized the potential of acoustic energy deposition for noninvasive surgery using HIFU's thermal coagulative effect at a focal spot location. Specifically, HIFU's potential for treating deep lying tumors without damaging surrounding normal tissue has been studied, particularly in applications involving the central nervous system [Fry et al. 1955]. It has also been

T. Peters and K. Cleary (eds.), *Image-Guided Interventions.*
© Springer Science + Business Media, LLC 2008

extensively tested for the so-called *trackless* surgery of the brain both in animals and humans [Fry and Fry 1960; Lele 1962]. Outside the brain, the method has also been developed for many other clinical applications, including the treatment of benign and malignant prostate disease and diseases of the liver, kidney, breast, bone, uterus, and pancreas. These clinical investigations and their related extensive literature have been described in several review papers [Kennedy 2005; Kennedy et al. 2003; Kennedy et al. 2004; Madersbacher and Marberger 2003; Ter Haar 2001].

When HIFU is used surgically, the term often used is *focused ultrasound surgery* (FUS). FUS has still not been fully acknowledged as a bona fide substitute to invasive surgery because of the belief that ultrasound still has poor image quality and a lack of energy deposition control when used as an image guidance method.

When FUS was integrated with magnetic resonance imaging (MRI), a major step was taken toward a fully controlled noninvasive image-guided therapy alternative to traditional tumor surgery. MRI-guided FUS (MRgFUS) has developed over the last decade [Jolesz and Hynynen 2002; Jolesz et al. 2004; Jolesz et al. 2005; Moonen et al. 2001] and combines MRI-based tumor localization with temperature monitoring, and the real-time, closed-loop control of energy deposition. Using this combination, the system can ablate targeted tissue without damaging surrounding normal tissue.

In fact, MRgFUS is a noninvasive, bloodless, incisionless, and scarless method, making it arguably an *ideal surgery*. The concept of ideal surgery is in essence a technical solution that allows for the removal or destruction of tumor tissue without injuring adjacent normal tissue. The surgery requires no invasive trajectory to the target, which means no incision or probe insertion is necessary. Early on in HIFU's history, it was acknowledged before the introduction of MRI that it could be an ideal surgery once image guidance provided tumor localization and targeting. To be a truly noninvasive and clinically effective image-guided therapy delivery system capable of ideal surgery, the system should be able to correctly localize tumor margins, find acoustic windows and localize focal spots, and monitor energy deposition in real time. This last feature is important not only for safety, but also for effectiveness and, specifically, for the control of the deposited thermal dose within the entire targeted tumor volume.

10.2   MRgFUS Technology

One issue with FUS, as with all thermal therapies, is the difficulty in accurately predicting temperature rise, because of the natural tissue variations that occur between patients and even between tissue regions in a single patient. These variations can make thermal therapy procedures difficult to control, especially for long-heating durations (more than a few seconds) in which perfusion and blood flow effects dominate [Billard et al. 1990].

Because of these difficulties, intense interest has arisen in using different medical imaging methods to map temperature changes.

Currently, only one technique is available with a temperature sensitivity ability that is not tissue-specific, and which does not change when the tissue is coagulated: the water proton resonant frequency (PRF) shift measured with MRI. The temperature sensitivity of the water PRF stems from heat-induced alterations in hydrogen bonds that change the amount of electron screening and the magnitude of the local magnetic field at the nucleus [Hindman 1966]. As the magnetic field in a MRI scanner is not perfectly homogeneous, only changes in water PRF can typically be used to detect temperature changes.

Changes in water PRF, and thus temperature, are estimated from phase-difference images [Ishihara et al. 1995], using the following relationship:

$$\Delta T \cong \frac{\Delta f}{B\alpha(T)\gamma} = \frac{\Delta\phi}{2\pi TE \cdot B\alpha(T)\gamma} \tag{10.1}$$

where B is the magnetic field strength in Tesla, γ is the gyromagnetic ratio of the proton (42.58 MHz/T), α is the water PRF temperature sensitivity (−0.01 ppm/°C in pure water [Hindman 1966] and linear in the range of thermal therapies [Kuroda et al. 1998], Δf is the temperature-induced change in PRF in hertz, $\Delta\phi$ is the corresponding phase change in radians, and TE is the echo time of the MR pulse sequence – the time that the phase is allowed to develop during the image acquisition. Examples of temperature mapping during a clinical focused ultrasound treatment are shown in Fig. 10.1.

Although the temperature dependence of the water PRF is relatively small, it is sensitive enough to detect a small temperature rise that allows one to localize the heating before thermal damage occurs with clinical MRI scanners [Hynynen et al. 1997]. This ability is especially important for focused ultrasound heating in which the energy source is located outside the body. Being able to measure temperature changes below the damage threshold can also be helpful in determining optimal exposure parameters for the subsequent thermal ablation [McDannold et al. 2002].

During ablation, temperature mapping can be used to guide the procedure, as it allows one to confirm that the exposure levels are sufficient to induce a lethal thermal exposure, but are not so high as to induce boiling. One can also use these maps to establish that the entire tumor volume is sufficiently heated, and to protect surrounding critical structures.

An important advantage of the water PRF shift is that it can be employed using standard MRI pulse sequences and hardware. Its disadvantages (sufficient to limit the method's use in some clinical targets) are its lack of sensitivity in fat [De Poorter 1995] and bone, and its motion sensitivity.

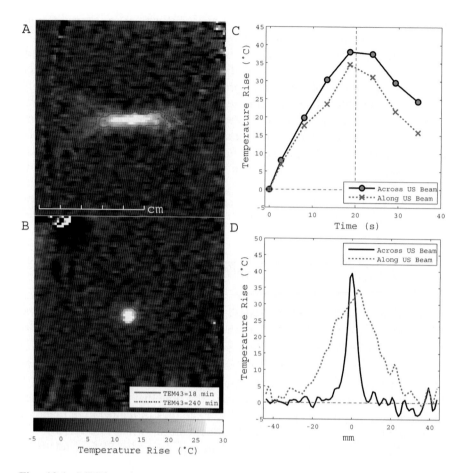

Fig. 10.1. MRI-based temperature image acquired during a focused ultrasound sonication during thermal ablation of a uterine fibroid. (**a**) Coronal image in the focal plane; (**b**) Sagittal image acquired along the direction of the ultrasound beam; (**c, d**) Plots showing the temperature rise as a function of time and the spatial temperature distribution in the focal plane at peak temperature rise. Contours in (**a, b**) indicate regions that reached a thermal dose of at least 240 equivalent min at 43°C

Still other sources of error exist for this method [Peters and Henkelman 2000; Peters et al. 1999; Stollberger et al. 1998], but they are typically small and usually ignored.

Although the water PRF shift has proven useful in numerous animal and clinical studies [McDannold 2005], it can be improved further. Perhaps most pressing is the need to reduce or eliminate the technique's motion sensitivity that hampers its use with moving organs. Although several promising methods for reducing motion effects [De Zwart et al. 2001; Kuroda et al. 2003; Rieke et al. 2004; Vigen et al. 2003] exist, they have not been extensively validated. Another need is to reduce image acquisition time so that multiple image planes can be sampled rapidly. Echo planar [Stafford et al. 2004], spiral [Stafford et al. 2000], echo-shifted [De Zwart et al. 1999], and parallel imaging [Bankson et al. 2005; Guo et al. 2006] techniques have each been tested for temperature imaging, but clinical feasibility has not been validated. The added signal-to-noise ratio and increased temperature sensitivity provided by higher field strengths may also allow for faster or multiplane imaging. The need for faster imaging is of particular importance for focused ultrasound heating, which is typically delivered with shorter exposure times than are used for interstitial devices such as laser and RF probes.

10.2.1 Acoustic Components

Focusing ultrasound for treatment requires skillful systems design. Over time, ultrasound has moved from a single-focused applicator, or planar applicator with a focused lens, to a phased array design. With a single-focused applicator, an ultrasound beam is steered in the body by mechanically moving the applicator. Phased-arrays reduce or even eliminate the need for mechanical movement by increasing the range of the applicator and dividing the surface of a transducer into many elements, thereby, using a larger area of the transducer's field. These features are particularly important in using ultrasound with MRI, because of the tendency of mechanical devices to cause imaging artifacts.

Ultrasound phased arrays also have the potential to correct distorted ultrasound beams, but this process requires certain knowledge of the field a priori [Clement and Hynynen 2002], including the type of tissue and its location relative to the phased array. Given this data, an ultrasound field model predicts the path of the beam into the tissue. In practice, this may be performed by numerically propagating elements forward toward the intended focus, and by providing amplitude and phase at the target. Alternatively, an idealized point-like focal source may be assumed, and the wavefront propagated numerically backward in time through the tissue to the transducer array [Thomas and Fink 1996]. In either case, a driving phase and amplitude is selected that provides the optimal focus on the basis of the simulations. One such approach has been implemented in MRgFUS to restore the focus through the intact human skull [Hynynen et al. 2004].

An additional and perhaps surprising benefit to the use of phased arrays is a potential cost reduction in driving electronics, because of the significant discrepancy between high-power and low-power radiofrequency driving electronics. Although more elements must be powered, the total power required by each element reduces inversely with the number of elements. For example, a single-channel, high-power radiofrequency amplifier can typically exceed $5,000, while designs for lower-power (1 W/channel) array driving systems have been described with a cost as low as $20 per channel [Sokka et al. 1999].

Phased-array systems are not without their challenges, given the potential for the array to distort the MRI images in the presence of a high magnetic field. Despite this, there has been significant success in creating MRI-compatible arrays, with transducers of at least 500 elements [Hynynen et al. 2004] tested in the clinic.

The most well known, and accordingly most utilized use of phased array systems is for phase-controlled beam steering [Fjield et al. 1996]. This process is analogous to beam focusing in diagnostic ultrasound, in which a focus is defined as the point where the waves emitting from the individual elements of the array arrive in phase. To achieve a focus, the phase of each element is generally predetermined with a straightforward geometric calculation. At this focus, constructive interference of the waves is maximized, providing the highest possible amplitude at that point for a given power level. The focus may be easily and rapidly moved in three dimensions by recalculating the phasing for a new location [Daum and Hynynen 1999]. It is also possible to create multiple foci simultaneously [Cain and Umemura 1986].

Individual phased array transducers can loosely be categorized into head, body, and intercavitary arrays. The typical body array design (Fig. 10.2a) is a spherically-focused transducer sectioned into any of a variety of array element configurations. Individual geometries vary but generally range from 10–15 cm in diameter, with radii of curvature ranging from 8–16 cm, and operating frequencies of 1–2 MHz. Randomized geometries have been suggested to reduce ultrasound grating lobes [Sokka et al. 1999]; however, most geometries consist of more symmetric layouts, typically dividing the spherical section first into rings for axial focusing. These rings may then be further subdivided into smaller elements for off-axis steering.

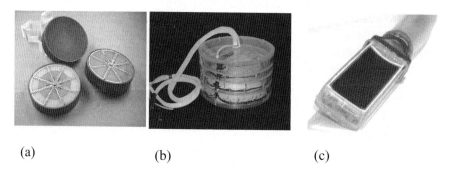

(a)   (b)   (c)

Fig. 10.2. (a) Frontal and rear views of a 104-element extracorporeal array. **(b)** A 64-element 30-cm diameter array designed for transcranial focusing. **(c)** An intracavitary 128-element linear array

Both lead-zirconate-titanate and piezocomposite arrays are used for body transducers, but piezocomposite transducers (PZT) have allowed for significant flexibility in geometry. For the brain, a full hemispherical array design has been utilized, with a lower operating frequency than body arrays (<1 MHz) to penetrate through the skull (Fig. 10.2b). The hemisphere is filled with water and surrounds the cranium to evenly distribute power over the skull surface, with capabilities of beam steering and aberration correction. A variety of MRI-compatible linear and 2D arrays have also been developed for intercavity use [Hutchinson and Hynynen 1998] (Fig. 10.2c).

10.2.2 Closed-Loop Control

The ability to quantify temperature changes with MRI allows for closed-loop feedback control over thermal ablation procedures such as focused ultrasound. To use the imaging in this way, it is essential to know the threshold for tissue damage and how well one can predict which regions will be thermally coagulated on the basis of MRI-based thermometry. This knowledge ensures that the temperature rise produced during the thermal ablation procedure is sufficient for tumor destruction, to protect neighboring tissues from being heated excessively, and to optimize therapy delivery.

The temperature threshold for thermal damage depends on the heating time. Although one could use a single temperature value to monitor the treatment progression for a given exposure time, the effects of multiple exposures will not be taken into account. As focused ultrasound treatments often consist of sonications at multiple overlapping locations, the effects of multiple low-level heating sessions must be accounted for to protect critical structures.

The thermal dose, a nonlinear function of the temperature and time that relates an arbitrary temperature–time profile to that of a constant temperature at 43°C, was proposed for taking into account the temperature history during hyperthermia [Sapareto and Dewey 1984], and later for guiding higher temperature thermal ablation techniques, such as focused ultrasound [Chung et al. 1999]. The thermal dose is defined by the following equation:

$$t_{43} = \sum_{t=0}^{t=final} R^{43-T} dt , \qquad (10.2)$$

where t_{43} is the *thermal isoeffective dose* (in equivalent minutes at 43°C), T is the average temperature during time dt, and R is a constant that compensates for a temperature change of ±1°C. Typically, R is taken to be 0.5 for temperatures greater than 43°C and 0.25 for temperatures less than 43°C, which fits most experimental data [Dewhirst et al. 2003]. The thermal dose equation was based on an Arrhenius model and was developed as a simplification of experimental data.

As currently implemented clinically, tissue volumes are ablated with focused ultrasound by employing short (<20 s) sonications targeted at multiple overlapping locations. During sonication, one can observe the heating in the images as they are acquired, and abort the sonication if it is not correctly targeted. After each sonication, the tissue is allowed to cool back to its baseline value to avoid the build-up of heat in the ultrasound beam path [Damianou and Hynynen 1993; Fan and Hynynen 1996a]. During this cooling period, the temperature and thermal dose maps created from MR images acquired during sonication can be inspected, and the ultrasound exposure parameters can be adjusted if necessary. On the basis of these dose maps, one can also choose the next sonication target to optimize treatment. This control strategy is fairly conservative in that it does not demand continuous temperature monitoring for extended periods of time, and it keeps the thermal deposition well controlled. Because of the delay needed between sonications, however, this feedback control method can result in long treatment times. If multiple tumors or one very large tumor is being treated, areas that are sufficiently far away can be targeted, so as not to overlap with the previous sonication during the cool-down procedure, as shown in Fig. 10.3. Another strategy is to use inertial cavitation [Holt and Roy 2001; Sokka et al. 2003] or nonlinear ultrasound absorption [Hynynen 1991] to increase the focal heating at the same time-averaged power without increasing the temperature in the beam path.

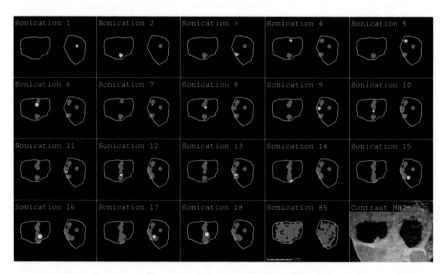

Fig. 10.3. MR imaging acquired during the thermal ablation of two uterine fibroids with focused ultrasound. To decrease the treatment time, the order of the sonications was alternated between the two fibroids. By sonicating in this pattern, one can decrease the amount of time required between sonications, which allows the tissue to cool back to baseline

It also may be possible to automate the feedback control as studies have demonstrated in animal experiments. The first demonstration was shown using a fairly simple PID (proportional integral and derivative) controller that forces the temperature at a single point to follow a predetermined trajectory [Hynynen 1991; Smith et al. 2001] similar to what was described earlier using invasive temperature measurements [Lin et al. 1990]. Because of the relatively low temporal resolution of MRI, this method has only been demonstrated during long-duration heating with ultrasound. Others have suggested methods for automatic control of MRI-based temperature measurements during short-duration focused ultrasound exposures [Vanne and Hynynen 2003], but this has not been shown experimentally. Still other researchers have used a physical model of the energy deposition and taken thermal conduction into account to improve the controller [Salomir et al. 2000b]. Methods have been developed to control the thermal dose deposition directly instead of the temperature rise [Arora et al. 2006a; Arora et al. 2005]. MRI-based automated closed-loop feedback has also been used to control thermal ablation with interstitial laser probes [McNichols et al. 2004] and in hyperthermia treatments using a microwave phased array [Behnia et al. 2002; Kowalski et al. 2002].

Methods to control two-dimensional heating patterns have also been suggested [Hutchinson et al. 1998], such as the mechanically scanned focused ultrasound transducer for long-duration heating. A spiral pattern scanning has been used to control the heating produced by the ultrasound focus [Mougenot et al. 2004; Palussiere et al. 2003; Salomir et al. 2000a]. With this method, the ultrasound transducer is moved, or the focal region scanned electronically with a phased array so that the focal coordinate travels in a double spiral trajectory. Temperature measurements acquired during the first spiral are used to modify the velocity of the transducer during the second spiral to achieve uniform heating over the target volume. The technique has been feasible in in vivo animal experiments with implanted tumors.

Alternative sonication trajectories for use in automated MRI-based temperature feedback control have been proposed by Malinen et al. for the treatment of breast tumors with a phased array transducer [Malinen et al. 2005]. Others have investigated different ultrasound trajectories to control the thermal dose deposition [Arora et al. 2006b].

Another approach that uses MRI-based closed loop feedback has been described for planar transurethral ultrasound probes designed for the treatment of prostate cancer [Chopra et al. 2005; Chopra et al. 2006]. These probes are inserted into the urethra and the ultrasound beam propagates radially outwards, ablating a neighboring strip of tissue. By rotating the probe, one can ablate the entire prostate. During the treatment, the system chooses the acoustic parameters and rotation rate that should ablate out to the desired depth. Although this system uses an one-dimensional proportional-gain algorithm to control a temperature point at the edge of the prostate, this control point is updated as the probe is rotated, resulting in control of a two-dimensional treatment. An advantage of this method is that one can update the baseline images as the probe is rotated and potentially reduce artifacts induced by small patient or tissue motions.

Most of these automated feedback methods use the thermal build-up acquired by previous sonications to decrease the heating duration. Depending on the geometry of the ultrasound source and the shape of the tumor target, the actual improvement in treatment time may be limited. For example, if one is using a spherically-curved transducer located outside the body, the thermal build-up occurs in a direction along the beam path. For tumors that are relatively long in the direction of the ultrasound beam, one may be able to significantly decrease the treatment time by taking advantage of the thermal build-up. However, if the tumor is short in that direction, one may have to wait for the tissue in the ultrasound beam path to cool to avoid damage outside of the target zone, thus limiting the treatment time improvement. Approaches that use a long-heating duration may also be limited because of the effects of perfusion and blood flow, which will not be known with precision for a given tissue type, and that can change in response to heating [Song 1984]. Clinical implantation of these strategies may also be challenging because of issues related to the MRI-based thermometry. Continuous temperature monitoring with MRI-based thermometry can be difficult, as it is susceptible to errors due to small patient motion, magnetic field drift [De Poorter 1995], and tissue swelling [Daniel and Butts 2000; McDannold et al. 2001].

10.3   Planning and Execution

The primary function of focused ultrasound is relatively simple: to focus a beam into a target region causing localized heating by acoustic absorption and other mechanisms. However, clinical execution requires careful and precise planning. The focus must be designed to thermally ablate the target tissue, while leaving surrounding tissues unharmed. Therefore, the desired intensity at the focus varies with the procedure. In general, however, the intensity is 103–104 W/cm^2 applied for a period of 1–20 s. Shorter times are generally preferred as perfusion cooling effects become increasingly important over time. Tissue complexities cause rises in temperature and can sometimes make the focal location difficult to predict. With such variation inherent to focused ultrasound planning and execution, MR targeting and monitoring becomes a critical step during procedures.

Focused ultrasound treatments are planned on the basis of the size of the ultrasound focus and the volume to be treated. Tumors are localized and the patient's position in orientation to the ultrasound transducer is registered [Jolesz and Hynynen 2002]. MRI's high sensitivity not only detects tumors excellently, but also delineates the target volume to be ablated very well.

In fact, a series of overlapping focal volumes can be planned so that the target volume is completely filled (Fig. 10.3). In practice, this can be performed over a series of stacked planes perpendicular to the ultrasound beam if needed [McDannold et al. 1998] to fill the entire treatment volume if it is large.

Once planned, treatment time can be estimated and the projected ultrasound path through the body may be evaluated to assure that no critical structures are traversed. This process also confirms an acoustic window between the transducer and the target. Computer algorithms indicate the volume of tissue that will potentially be exposed to ultrasound radiation during treatment. The actual treatment volume and the size of the ablated area is dependent on several controlled parameters, including sonication time, focal depth, transducer geometry, transducer efficiency, and element configuration. They also depend on the lesser-known acoustic properties of the tissues within the ultrasound beam. An overview of how preplanning relates to the entire focused ultrasound procedure is illustrated below (Fig. 10.4).

Despite the encouraging clinical results of MRI-based thermometry to guide FUS, large variations in focal temperature distribution can exist [McDannold et al. 2002]. Treatment planning has the potential to reduce this variation by the addition of advanced techniques for predicting ultrasound beams and their resulting temperature rises. The observed variations are the result of a number of factors, including tissue composition and heterogeneity as well as the size and shape of the ultrasound beam. Significant tissue inhomogeneity leads to focal beam distortion that can restrict the ability to focus energy in deep-seated tissues. It is, however, possible to restore a distorted focus by means of planning algorithms specifically tailored to ultrasound propagation [Clement and Hynynen 2003].

10.4   The Commercial Therapy Delivery System

The first commercially available, FDA-approved, MRI-guided, focused ultrasound surgery device is the ExAblate 2000, developed by InSightec of Haifa, Israel. Concepts for this system and validation studies were performed in collaboration with investigators at the Brigham and Women's Hospital in Boston, MA.

On the basis of previous work with a prototype clinical system developed by General Electric Medical Systems (now GE Healthcare of Milwaukee, WI) in collaboration with the same researchers [Gianfelice et al. 2003c; Hynynen et al. 1996b; Hynynen et al. 2001b], it represents the commercial application of extensive preclinical studies that have been performed over the past decade [Chung et al. 1996; Chung et al. 1999; Cline et al. 1993; Damianou et al. 1993; Daum et al. 1998; Daum and Hynynen 1998; Daum et al. 1999; Fan and Hynynen 1996a; Fan and Hynynen 1996b;

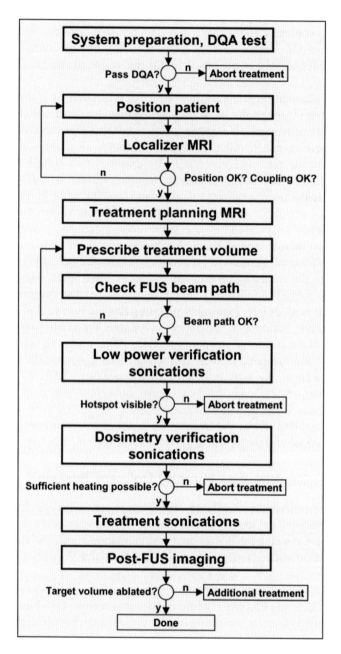

Fig. 10.4. Flowchart describing the steps taken before, during, and after a clinical focused ultrasound treatment

Hynynen et al. 1996a; Hynynen et al. 1993a; Hynynen et al. 1993b; Hynynen et al. 1996b; Hynynen et al. 1997; McDannold et al. 1998]. To the authors' knowledge, the ExAblate is not only one of the earliest commercially available robotic devices that operates within an MRI, but is also the first approved application of MRI-based thermometry.

This system utilizes a 208-element phased array transducer to generate the ultrasound beam. This 12-cm diameter transducer is spherically focused with a focal length of 16 cm. The array can steer the beam to different depths between 5 and 20 cm by changing the phases for each array element electronically. It can also be used to increase the focal volume per sonication by changing the phasing pattern during sonication. The frequency can also be set by the user (range: approximately 0.9–1.3 MHz) if desired.

The transducer is attached to a robotic positioning system that can move in two lateral directions, and be tilted ±20° in two directions. It is mounted in a sealed tank filled with degassed water with a thin plastic membrane at the top that allows for ultrasound propagation vertically out of the system into the patient. This tank, together with MRI-compatible motors and position encoders and the RF driving system for the 208 element array are built into a standard clinical MRI table. The table is attached via the penetration panel to driving hardware and controller computers located outside of the MRI room. The focused ultrasound treatment table can be undocked from the MRI scanner when it is not being used, to easily allow for routine clinical scanning when patients are not being treated.

The procedure used with this system is outlined in Fig. 10.4. The patient is positioned on the device with a gel pad and degassed water placed between the patient and the system to ensure acoustic coupling. MR images are acquired, and the treatment plan is prescribed. The sequence of events that occur during each sonication is outlined in Fig. 10.5.

During sonication, the system automatically prescribes and triggers the MRI to acquire temperature maps in the correct imaging plane. The user can choose to have these images acquired either in the focal plane or along the direction of the ultrasound beam.

After sonication, the system displays temperature maps acquired during the procedure. Regions that reached a thermal dose threshold of 240 equivalent minutes at 43°C are superimposed on these images. This threshold was based on previous animal studies [Meshorer et al. 1983] and is a conservative threshold for thermal coagulation. All the regions from previous sonication are superimposed on the treatment planning images to allow the user to ensure that the entire target volume reaches this thermal dose value. If there are any regions within the target zone that did not reach this threshold, additional sonications can be added. One can also reposition future sonications if necessary so that regions are not treated twice.

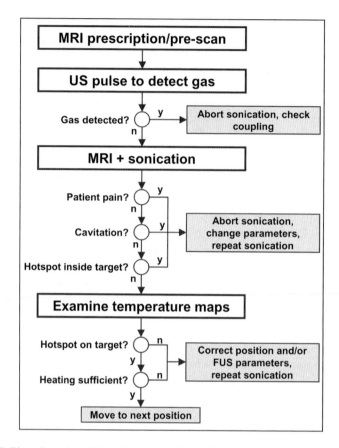

Fig. 10.5. Flowchart describing the steps taken before, during, and after a sonication during a clinical focused ultrasound treatment

The system has many features to ensure patient safety. Before treatment, a quality assurance test is performed in an ultrasound/MRI phantom to ensure that the system is operating within specifications [McDannold and Hynynen 2006; Wu and Felmlee 2002]. During treatment planning, the system superimposes the ultrasound beam path on top of the planning images to ensure that the beam does not traverse critical structures. One can also inspect these images to detect gas bubbles at skin level.

Before the treatment starts, the exact position of the ultrasound focus is determined before any ablation occurs, first roughly using the wide field of view MRI scans, and next in temperature maps acquired during low-power sonications that produce heating below the thermal threshold for damage. Also, during any sonication, the user can watch the raw MR images as they are acquired to allow for localized heating within the target tissue. Future versions of this system will have the ability to display the temperature maps as the sonication is delivered.

Immediately before the start of the procedure, a short burst sonication is performed and the acoustic signal is received from one of the transducer elements displayed for the user. If gas is present in the beam, it can be detected and the sonication aborted by the operator using a panic button at the console.

During sonication, the acoustic emission is detected by an array element that is not used for the sonication, and the frequency response is displayed in real time. If inertial cavitation occurs – evident in this frequency spectrum as a wideband signal – the user can abort the sonication using a panic button. Additional buttons are also available to the nurse in the room and to the patient.

In these authors' experience, feedback from the patient has been critical in providing a safe treatment. The physician and treatment team are in constant contact with the patient who can notify them in event of heating or pain in the skin or in surrounding (nontargeted) structures before irreversible damage occurs. This feedback allows the treatment team to adjust the ultrasound parameters in subsequent sonications. At the end of the treatment, MR imaging is acquired that allows the team to immediately detect any unwanted thermal damage.

10.5   Clinical Applications

The first clinical application of MrgFUS was in the breast, with its feasibility established by treating benign fibroadenoma [Hynynen et al. 2001b]. The first clinical trial was then aimed at locally ablating breast cancer [Furusawa et al. 2006; Gianfelice et al. 2003a; Gianfelice et al. 2003b].

The standard treatment for breast cancer is usually surgery followed by radiation therapy. Depending on the tumor location and size, different types of surgery may be performed, ranging from lumpectomy to mastectomy. Management of early breast cancer also may include the option of breast conservation in conjunction with a variety of minimally invasive techniques to induce tumor cell death. MRgFUS is one such option currently being investigated.

The feasibility of treating small breast cancers with MRgFUS was first evaluated with a small group of 12 patients [Gianfelice et al. 2003a; Gianfelice et al. 2003b]. While residual tumor was identified at the periphery of the tumor on pathological analysis, MRgFUS was shown to be promising. Another group reported on a treatment in a single patient, also with promising findings [Huber et al. 2001].

Early clinical trials subsequent to this with a larger patient population have confirmed the efficacy and safety of MRgFUS in the treatment of breast cancer [Gombos et al. 2006]. These tumors were early stage (T1-2, N0-2, M0), less than 3.5 cm in size, with a biopsy-proven pathology. Viable tumor was identified at pathology in less than 1% of original tumor volume. Phase two of this study is currently underway to evaluate the safety and effectiveness of MRgFUS in the ablation of early breast tumors, without excision. The efficacy goal is to demonstrate low level of local recurrence following MRgFUS treatment and MRI-based follow-up. Eligible patients with early stage single tumor of less than 1.5 cm will be treated with MRgFUS as a replacement for lumpectomy, and will be closely followed for 5 years.

Investigation into the use of dynamic MR imaging to correlate with histopathological findings post-MRgFUS has also been undertaken. Results suggest that dynamic MR posttreatment is a reliable way to assess for residual tumor following MRgFUS treatment of breast tumors [Gianfelice et al. 2003c]. A post-treatment delay of 7 days is best for the accurate assessment of the presence of residual tumor by dynamic MRI imaging [Khiat et al. 2006].

The largest clinical experience with MRgFUS has been in the treatment of uterine fibroids, with more than 2,000 patients treated to date worldwide [Fennessy and Tempany 2005; Fennessy et al. 2007; Hindley et al. 2004; Hindley et al. 2002; Stewart et al. 2003; Tempany et al. 2003]. This work has led to expanding treatment guidelines that, in turn, increase the procedure's efficacy and safety. Although options such as uterine artery embolization, laparoscopic and hysteroscopic myomectomy, or cryoablation are less invasive than hysterectomy, these options could be considered semi-invasive or minimally invasive, and may be restricted to women with fibroids in certain locations. MRgFUS provides an attractive, totally non-invasive option. Also, compared with other therapies, MRgFUS allows more fibroid volume to be treated, and results in a greater early symptom decrease, fewer adverse events reported, and a decrease in number of patients seeking alternative treatment. Additionally patients have experienced significant symptomatic improvement at 3 and 6 months, sustained at 1 year post-treatment [Fennessy et al. 2007].

The FDA has approved this procedure for premenopausal females with symptomatic uterine fibroids, who have no desire for future pregnancy. It is not indicated for pregnant women, postmenopausal women, or those with contrast-enhanced MR imaging contraindications. Extensive anterior abdominal wall scarring is evaluated prior to treatment, as these women are at risk of skin burns [Leon-Villapalos et al. 2005]. Less extensive scarring can usually be negotiated through beam angulation.

Coursing bowel loops lying anterior to the uterus at the level of the uterine fibroid may also cause planning difficulties. Conscious sedation is used during treatment to minimize patient motion and decrease discomfort. It also allows the patient to remain awake to allow for continuous feedback between the operator and the patient about any sensation or pain she may feel during the procedure.

In addition to its many other applications, FUS has great potential in the treatment of liver cancer [Jolesz et al. 2004] as well as for skeletal metastases, particularly in the palliation of pain [Catane et al. 2007]. Today, a major effort is underway to develop FUS for prostate and brain tumor treatment.

In a population of potentially curable patients, for example, several studies are investigating the feasibility of FUS for the treatment of localized prostate cancer [Gianduzzo et al. 2006; Poissonnier et al. 2007]. The first human studies in this area were published by Madersbacher et al. [1995]. Current results with ultrasound-guided systems show that FUS is a treatment option achieving similar results to those of other nonsurgical treatments for prostate cancer [Poissonnier et al. 2003].

The potential of using MRgFUS has a significant advantage in several aspects, namely the improved imaging of the prostate to define the extent and type of local prostate cancer, coupled with the critical ability to monitor thermal energy deposition in real time; this approach seems to offer an important opportunity.

As the aging baby boomers move into their 60s and 70s, we anticipate a very significant rise in the number of men diagnosed with prostate cancer per year in US, with some estimates as high as 450,000 annually. This situation will place enormous pressure on the health care system and the patients themselves, as they will begin to seek out alternatives to today's treatments.

The opportunity to perform focal tumor ablation on these patients using MRgFUS is very appealing, although several important issues need to be resolved if this opportunity is to be realized. First, patients for focal therapy must be appropriately selected, and second, the specificity of current imaging techniques must be improved to define the focal prostate lesion that would be the MRgFUS treatment target. After all, the effectiveness of MRgFUS for local therapy will only be as good as the feedback during pretreatment planning, energy delivery, and after ablation allows.

10.5.1 Commercial Brain Treatment System: ExAblate

In terms of brain surgery, MRgFUS as a treatment alternative cannot come too soon. Traditional neurosurgical approaches to deep seated tumors usually result in more or less brain damage due to the dissection of the normal brain. FUS, being noninvasive, can destroy targeted tissue without injuring the normal brain. With that known, research to develop FUS as an *ideal* neurosurgical method has continued since the mid-twentieth century [Fry et al. 1955; Fry and Fry 1960; Lele 1962; Lele 1967].

Most of that research involved craniotomies in which the ultrasound beam propagated into the brain without going through the skull. Nevertheless, it is known that it is possible to direct the ultrasound beam transcranially to make the entire procedure noninvasive [Aubry et al. 2003; Hynynen and

Jolesz 1998]. In this procedure, ultrasound exposure is accomplished using phased array transducers surrounding the skull. The phase shifts caused by the irregular skull bone can be compensated for by the thickness measurements generated from X-ray computed tomography (CT) data. The phase corrections permit focusing at relatively lower frequencies. A prototype focused ultrasound phased-array research system for trans-skull brain tissue ablation using 500-element ultrasound phased array operating at frequencies of 700–800 kHz was developed by Insightec and the Brigham and Women's Hospital FUS Laboratory [Hynynen et al. 2004].

A clinical system designed for the MRgFUS thermal surgery of the brain through the intact skull was developed by Insightec, and tested in rhesus monkeys [Hynynen et al. 2006] and in three patients at the Brigham and Women's Hospital. The ultrasound beam is generated by a 512-channel phased array system (ExAblate (®) 3000, InSightec, Haifa, Israel).

In early 2007, the FDA IDE approved a Phase I clinical trial for using the device to treat brain tumors through the intact skull. This research is currently being conducted exclusively at the Brigham and Women's Hospital in Boston, but the brain system will be installed in multiple US sites eventually. Initial cases involve inoperable malignant brain tumors, but in the future benign tumors may also be treated.

FUS can be used to treat various CNS diseases, including lesions associated with epilepsy, pain, or Parkinson disease, and by noncoagulative effects on preformed bubbles circulating within the vasculature to target drug delivery via the selective opening of the blood–brain barrier (BBB) as described later. In fact, throughout the entire body, cavitation-related effects can deliver drugs and gene therapy to targets [Bednarski et al. 1997; Greenleaf et al. 1998; Price et al. 1998; Shohet et al. 2001; Unger et al. 2001; Unger et al. 2002; Unger et al. 1997; Unger et al. 2004; Vannan et al. 2002].

10.6   Targeted Drug Delivery and Gene Therapy

As the previous descriptions of focused ultrasound demonstrate, the technology, along with its associated contrast agents, has broadened into a versatile diagnostic and treatment modality. Ultrasound has dimensions beyond thermal therapy, and ultrasound's progress with the use of microbubbles is a case in point. The scattering of gas-filled microbubbles by ultrasound's sound waves can be made visible using contrast agent, so that once the microbubbles localize a strong contrast, enhancement of the image results [Klibanov 2006; Miller and Nanda 2004]. It can then highlight hyper-vascular tissues in vivo [Gwyther 2005].

Ultrasound's use incorporating microbubbles has even greater potential in a process known as *sonoporation*, in which the collapse of microbubbles triggered by ultrasound causes transient enhancement of cell membrane permeability, enabling the delivery of extracellular molecules into the cell [Deng et al. 2004]. These molecules might be DNA, peptides, and RNA, and all of which have been witnessed moving into intracellular compartments [Kinoshita and Hynynen 2005a; Kinoshita and Hynynen 2005b; Li et al. 2003; Taniyama et al. 2002a; Taniyama et al. 2002b] in both in vitro and in vivo. As a result, sonoporation is considered as a promising tool for future gene therapy treatment, making unnecessary the use of harmful agents such as viruses to make these deliveries.

Sonoporation is powerful. It has been able to push dyes that usually do not cross the blood vessel walls into the tissue through cell membranes [Miller and Quddus 2000; Skyba et al. 1998] as well as the transdermal delivery of large molecular proteins, including insulin [Mitragotri et al. 1995; Tachibana 1992; Tachibana and Tachibana 1991] and even the enhancement of the delivery of systemic chemotherapeutic agent into solid tumors [Yuh et al. 2005]. These facts seem astounding considering that skin is impermeable to various substances, and to accomplish delivery of molecules, ultrasound has to actually reorganize the skin's outer layer [Mitragotri et al. 1995].

However, sonoporation is not without its downside. Its major problems in vitro are its low efficiency and high toxicity. Although the efficiency can be improved by the use of ultrasound contrast agents, the overall outcome of sonoporation is still inferior to those by other transfection methods, such as electroporation and lipofection. Factors such as the center frequency of ultrasound exposure, duty cycle, and pulse repetition frequency can affect the overall efficiency of sonoporation. There are reports suggesting that the presence of standing waves a can be an important factor for improving sonoporation efficiency [Kinoshita and Hynynen 2007]. The experimental settings, however, differ from one report to another and the most important factor is not yet determined. Toxicity from sonoporation can also destroy cells through lysis. According to 2005 data, more than 50% of a whole cell population has been destroyed by sonoporation, while only less than 10% of the cells experience the effect suitably [Guzman et al. 2003; Guzman et al. 2002; Kinoshita and Hynynen 2005a; Zarnitsyn and Prausnitz 2004].

10.6.1 BBB Disruption

One potentially revolutionary use of focused ultrasound is the ability to target the delivery of drugs to the brain by disruption of the BBB. This barrier is a specialized structure in the wall of blood vessels in the central nervous system, which effectively limits the transport and diffusion of many substances from the vasculature [Abbott and Romero 1996; Kroll and Neuwelt 1998; Pardridge 2002a]. It is composed of a functional and structural barrier at the level of the basal lamina, and intercellular attachments of the endothelial cells known as *tight junctions*. This inability to get drugs past the BBB significantly limits the development of therapeutic or imaging agents for the central nervous system. Current strategies to deliver large-molecule agents to the brain include the design of special drugs or drug carriers, which allow transport across the BBB [Pardridge 2002a; Pardridge 2002b; Pardridge 2003] local injections of hyperosmotic solutions, or other substances that diffusely induce temporary BBB disruption [Doolittle et al. 2000], bypassing the vasculature completely by directly infusing agents [Bobo et al. 1994] or using implanted delivery systems [Guerin et al. 2004]. These strategies are either invasive, nonlocalized, or require the need to develop new drugs or drug carriers.

Ultrasound has the unique capability of noninvasively disrupting the BBB to allow even large molecular size agents such as antibodies to reach the brain [Kinoshita et al. 2006b]. If proven successful in patients it would represent a huge advance in neurosurgery, since, today the most advanced antibody-based chemotherapeutic agents cannot be used effectively in the central nervous system because of the BBB. This hurdle has been crossed in animal studies, potentially opening the door to completely new treatment strategies for diseases that currently have no options.

With this ultrasound method, very low-power short focused ultrasound pulses follow an injection of an ultrasound contrast agent, such as Optison (GE Healthcare, Milwaukee, WI, USA) or Definity (Bristol-Myers Squibb Medical Imaging, N. Billerica, MA, USA) [Hynynen et al. 2005; Hynynen et al. 2001a; Hynynen et al. 2006; Kinoshita and Hynynen 2005a; Kinoshita et al. 2006a; McDannold et al. 2005a; McDannold et al. 2005b; Sheikov et al. 2006; Sheikov et al. 2004; Treat et al. 2007]. These contrast agents consist of preformed gas bubbles (diameter ~1–5 μm) that circulate in the vasculature for a few minutes after a bolus injection. They serve to concentrate the effects of the ultrasound beam to the blood vessel walls to induce BBB disruption.

The mechanisms for the BBB disruption are currently unknown. When microbubbles interact with an ultrasound beam, a range of biological effects has been observed or proposed, including those related to bubble oscillation, violent collapse (inertial cavitation), acoustic streaming of the fluid surrounding the bubbles, and effects related to radiation force [Leighton 1994; Miller 1988; Nyborg et al. 2002].

The preformed microbubbles that make up the ultrasound contrast agents presumably can exhibit these behaviors either with or without the shells being broken apart by the ultrasound beam. Tests where the acoustic emission produced during sonication was monitored indicate that the BBB disruption can occur without inertial cavitation [McDannold and Hynynen 2006]. When such cavitation does occur, it may be responsible for the extravasated erythrocytes that are sometimes observed in histology. Examination of the brain samples under electron microscopy indicates that the BBB disruption is an active transport mechanism (transcellular passage via caveolae and cytoplasmic vacuolar structures) in addition to some paracellular passage via widened tight junctions [Hynynen et al. 2005; Hynynen et al. 2006; Sheikov et al. 2004]. Observation of the blood vessels in vivo in mice suggests that the sonications are associated with temporary vaso-constriction [Raymond et al. 2007].

This ultrasonic method offers several advantages over existing strategies to bypass the BBB. Applied at frequencies suited for transcranial sonication [Hynynen et al. 2005; Hynynen et al. 2006], the ultrasonic method can be completely noninvasive. It is also inherently targeted to allow one to tailor the delivery and potentially avoid dose-limiting side effects in other parts of the brain. One can also focus at multiple locations and disrupt a large area, even the whole brain if desired. As short pulses (~10 ms) and low-duty cycles (~1%) are employed, this steering of the ultrasound focal point can potentially be done rapidly during a single injection of ultrasound contrast agent by using a phased array. Finally, this method has an advantage over some of the other strategies in that it can be used with existing agents, avoiding the expense and time needed to develop new drugs or to develop drug carriers for old drugs. This feature may be especially useful for the delivery of chemotherapy agents for brain metastases when effective agents are already available for treating the primary tumor and extracranial metastases.

A range of particle sizes have been shown in animal studies to cross the BBB after sonication: MRI contrast agents (molecular weight: 938 (Magnevist; Berlex Laboratories, Wayne, NJ) and 10,000 (monocrystalline iron oxide nanoparticles (MION)) [Hynynen et al. 2006] trypan blue (molecular weight: 961, larger when bound to albumin) [Hynynen et al. 2005], horseradish peroxidase (molecular weight: 40,000) [Hynynen et al. 2005], and antibodies (molecular weight 150,000) [Kinoshita et al. 2006b]. An example demonstrating BBB disruption at four targeted locations in a rabbit brain is shown in Fig. 10.6. Recent tests have investigated the delivery of therapeutic agents. In one study, the concentration of liposomal doxorubicin (Doxil, Ben Venue Laboratories, Bedford, OH) in the rat brain was investigated using fluorometry after ultrasound-induced BBB disruption [Treat et al. 2007]. These tests found it was possible to produce drug concentrations of 886 ± 327 ng/g tissue that are within the therapeutic range of 819 ± 482 ng/g tumor in vivo and that are reported to correlate with a 39% clinical response rate in patients with breast carcinoma [Cummings and McArdle 1986]. Higher concentrations were possible for exposure conditions that produced some damage to the brain, which may be acceptable for a cancer treatment.

Other tests have shown that Herceptin (Trastuzumab, Genentech), an antibody-based agent that works on the HER2/neu (erbB2) receptor can be delivered past the BBB in mice [Kinoshita et al. 2006a]. Although this agent has been shown to be effective for the treatment of breast cancer for patients with tumors that overexpress this receptor, it is less effective in patients where the tumor has metastasized to the CNS, presumably because of the BBB [Bendell et al. 2003].

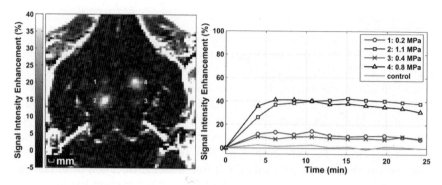

Fig. 10.6. BBB disruption with focused ultrasound. *Left*: Image showing the signal intensity enhancement after four focused ultrasound sonications in a rabbit brain as measured with contrast-enhanced T1-weighted MRI. The enhancing spots at the focal targets confirm the leakage of the MRI contrast agent (Magnevist; Berlex Laboratories, Wayne, NJ) through the BBB at the targeted regions. The image was acquired in the focal plane of the ultrasound tranducer. *Right*: Signal enhancement in the focal zone as a function of time for the four locations and a control region that did not receive sonication.

Histological examination of the brains has found only small effects on the brain tissue caused by the ultrasound-induced BBB disruption. Most of the effects appear related to the presence of small regions with a few extra-vasated erythrocytes that sometimes accompany the BBB disruption. The presence of these erythrocytes indicates that sometimes the sonication causes temporary damage to some of the blood vessels. However, neuronal damage appears to be negligible, and long-term studies have not found any damage to the sonicated regions. Investigation of ischemic neurons (using VAF-toluidine blue) or DNA strand breaks as an indicator of apoptosis (using TUNEL staining) has not found brain regions that are ischemic or apoptotic, as one might expect if the vessel damage was severe. These effects are clearly much less than would result from direct infusion of agents into the brain. The most recent studies have also indicated that when the ultrasound frequency is low (~250 kHz), low-level BBB disruption is possible without any extravasation [Hynynen et al. 2006].

Although ultrasound-induced BBB disruption has only been tested to date in animals, it shows great promise and could offer the possibility of delivering agents that are currently limited by the BBB. Future work is needed to investigate the effects of multiple sessions of BBB disruption to accompany the treatment schedule for chemotherapy agents. A method to monitor the procedure online should also be determined, as it is difficult to predict with precision the ultrasound exposure in the brain, especially when the ultrasound is applied transcranially.

10.7   Conclusion

In this discussion of ultrasound and its many advances therapeutically, MRI's involvement should be underlined as being significant to its therapeutic path forward. Indeed, the most important feature of MRgFUS is MRI. On the basis of our experience, we can conclude that without MRI's ability to define correct tumor margins and without MRI thermometry, the method is inadequate for tumor treatment. FUS requires accurate targeting and real time control of the energy deposition. Today this is not possible with any other guidance method. We believe that FUS can compete with other surgical or ablation methods, but only when it is integrated with MRI.

MRgFUS with closed-loop control is a safe and effective substitute for invasive thermal ablations and for traditional excisional surgery. It uses no toxic ionizing radiation, such as radiosurgery, and can be repeated indefinitely. In fact, as a directly monitored and controlled repeatable treatment approach, FUS will likely prove safer than radiation therapy, even as its costs are comparable.

MR-guided FUS is the only disruptive technology in the field of image-guided therapy today and, as such, will change the surgical specialty and radiation therapy field. It will be preferable to surgery for treating benign tumors (e.g., uterine fibroid and breast fibroadenoma) and will replace and/or substitute for surgery or radiation therapy in the treatment of malignant tumors. It will also offer new therapeutic solutions such as targeted drug delivery and gene therapy, and, with these advancements, may generate a paradigm shift in the entire field of oncology as well.

Future progress in MRI research will most likely result in better target definition and more accurate tumor ablation. With further advances in phased array technology, treatment times may be reduced and the number of anatomic locations applicable to FUS treatment will expand.

References

Abbott NJ and Romero IA. (1996). "Transporting therapeutics across the blood-brain barrier." *Mol Med Today*, 2(3), 106–113.

Arora D, Cooley D, Perry T, Guo J, Richardson A, Moellmer J, Hadley R, Parker D, Skliar M, and Roemer RB. (2006a). "MR thermometry-based feedback control of efficacy and safety in minimum-time thermal therapies: Phantom and in vivo evaluations." *Int J Hyperthermia*, 22(1), 29–42.

Arora D, Cooley D, Perry T, Skliar M, and Roemer RB. (2005). "Direct thermal dose control of constrained focused ultrasound treatments: Phantom and in vivo evaluation." *Phys Med Biol*, 50(8), 1919–1935.

Arora D, Minor MA, Skliar M, and Roemer RB. (2006b). "Control of thermal therapies with moving power deposition field." *Phys Med Biol*, 51(5).

Aubry JF, Tanter M, Pernot M, Thomas JL, and Fink M. (2003). "Experimental demonstration of noninvasive transskull adaptive focusing based on prior computed tomography scans." *J Acoust Soc Am*, 113(1), 84–93.

Bankson JA, Stafford RJ, and Hazle JD. (2005). "Partially parallel imaging with phase-sensitive data: Increased temporal resolution for magnetic resonance temperature imaging." *Magn Reson Med*, 53(3), 658–665.

Bednarski MD, Lee JW, Callstrom MR, and Li KC. (1997). "In vivo target-specific delivery of macromolecular agents with MR-guided focused ultrasound." *Radiology*, 204(1), 263–268.

Behnia B, Suthar M, and Webb A. (2002). "Closed-loop feedback control of phased-array microwave heating using thermal measurements from magnetic resonance imaging." *Concepts Magn Reson*, 15(1), 101–110.

Bendell JC, Domchek SM, Burstein HJ, Harris L, Younger J, Kuter I, Bunnell C, Rue M, Gelman R, and Winer E. (2003). "Central nervous system metastases in women who receive trastuzumab-based therapy for metastatic breast carcinoma." *Cancer*, 97(12), 2972–2977.

Billard BE, Hynynen K, and Roemer RB. (1990). "Effects of physical parameters on high temperature ultrasound hyperthermia." *Ultrasound Med Biol*, 16(4), 409–420.

Bobo RH, Laske DW, Akbasak A, Morrison PF, Dedrick RL, and Oldfield EH. (1994). "Convection-enhanced delivery of macromolecules in the brain." *Proc Natl Acad Sci USA*, 91(6), 2076–2080.

Cain C and Umemura S. (1986). "Concentricring and sector-vortex phased-array applicators for ultrasound hyperthermia." *IEEE Trans Microw Theory Tech*, 34(5), 542–551.

Catane R, Beck A, Inbar Y, Rabin T, Shabshin N, Hengst S, Pfeffer RM, Hanannel A, Dogadkin O, Liberman B, and Kopelman D. (2007). "MR-guided focused ultrasound surgery (MRgFUS) for the palliation of pain in patients with bone metastases – preliminary clinical experience." *Ann Oncol*, 18(1), 163–167.

Chopra R, Burtnyk M, Haider MA, and Bronskill MJ. (2005). "Method for MRI-guided conformal thermal therapy of prostate with planar transurethral ultrasound heating applicators." *Phys Med Biol*, 50(21), 4957–4975.

Chopra R, Wachsmuth J, Burtnyk M, Haider MA, and Bronskill MJ. (2006). "Analysis of factors important for transurethral ultrasound prostate heating using MR temperature feedback." *Phys Med Biol*, 51(4), 827–844.

Chung AH, Hynynen K, Colucci V, Oshio K, Cline HE, and Jolesz FA. (1996). "Optimization of spoiled gradient-echo phase imaging for in vivo localization of a focused ultrasound beam." *Magn Reson Med*, 36(5), 745–752.

Chung AH, Jolesz FA, and Hynynen K. (1999). "Thermal dosimetry of a focused ultrasound beam in vivo by magnetic resonance imaging." *Med Phys*, 26(9), 2017–2026.

Clement GT and Hynynen K. (2002). "A non-invasive method for focusing ultrasound through the human skull." *Phys Med Biol*, 47(8), 1219–1236.

Clement GT and Hynynen K. (2003). "Forward planar projection through layered media." *IEEE Trans Ultrason Ferroelectr Freq Control*, 50(12), 1689–1698.

Cline HE, Schenck JF, Watkins RD, Hynynen K, and Jolesz FA. (1993). "Magnetic resonance-guided thermal surgery." *Magn Reson Med*, 30(1), 98–106.

Cummings J and McArdle CS. (1986). "Studies on the in vivo disposition of adriamycin in human tumours which exhibit different responses to the drug." *Br J Cancer*, 53(6), 835–838.

Damianou C and Hynynen K. (1993). "Focal spacing and near-field heating during pulsed high temperature ultrasound therapy." *Ultrasound Med Biol*, 19(9), 777–787.

Damianou C, Hynynen K, and Fan X. (1993). "Application of the thermal dose concept for predicting the necrosed tissue volume during ultrasound surgery." *Proc Ultrason Symp*, 2, 1199–1202.

Daniel B and Butts K. (2000). "Deformation of breast tissue during heating; MRI observations of ex vivo radio frequency ablation." *Proceedings of the Eighth Meeting of the International Society for Magnetic Resonance in Medicine*, 1341.

Daum DR, Buchanan M, Fjield T, and Hynynen K. (1998). "Design and evaluation of a feedback based phased array system for ultrasound surgery." *IEEE Trans Ultrason Ferroelectr Freq Contr*, 45(2), 431–438.

Daum DR and Hynynen K. (1998). "Thermal dose optimization via temporal switching in ultrasound surgery." *IEEE Trans Ultrason Ferroelectr Freq Control*, 45(1), 208–215.

Daum DR and Hynynen K. (1999). "A 256 element ultrasonic phased array system for treatment of large volumes of deep seated tissue." *IEEE Trans Ultrason Ferroelectr Freq Control*, 46(5), 1254–1268.

Daum DR, Smith NB, King R, and Hynynen K. (1999). "In vivo demonstration of noninvasive thermal surgery of the liver and kidney using an ultrasonic phased array." *Ultrasound Med Biol*, 25(7), 1087–1098.

De Poorter J. (1995). "Non-invasive MRI thermometry with the proton resonance frequency method: Study of susceptibility effects." *Magn Reson Med*, 34(3), 359–367.

de Zwart J, Vimeux F, Palussiere J, Salomir R, Quesson B, Delalande C, and Moonen C. (2001). "On-line correction and visualization of motion during MRI-controlled hyperthermia." *Magn Reson Med*, 45(1), 128–137.

de Zwart JA, Vimeux FC, Delalande C, Canioni P, and Moonen CT. (1999). "Fast lipid-suppressed MR temperature mapping with echo-shifted gradient-echo imaging and spectral-spatial excitation." *Magn Reson Med*, 42(1), 53–59.

Deng CX, Sieling F, Pan H, and Cui J. (2004). "Ultrasound-induced cell membrane porosity." *Ultrasound Med Biol*, 30(4), 519–526.

Dewhirst MW, Viglianti BL, Lora-Michiels M, Hanson M, and Hoopes PJ. (2003). "Basic principles of thermal dosimetry and thermal thresholds for tissue damage from hyperthermia." *Int J Hyperthermia*, 19(3), 267–294.

Doolittle ND, Miner ME, Hall WA, Siegal T, Jerome E, Osztie E, McAllister LD, Bubalo JS, Kraemer DF, Fortin D, Nixon R, Muldoon LL, and Neuwelt EA. (2000). "Safety and efficacy of a multicenter study using intraarterial chemotherapy in conjunction with osmotic opening of the blood-brain barrier for the treatment of patients with malignant brain tumors." *Cancer*, 88(3), 637–647.

Fan X and Hynynen K. (1996a). "A study of various parameters of spherically curved phased arrays for noninvasive ultrasound surgery." *Phys Med Biol*, 41(4), 591–608.

Fan X and Hynynen K. (1996b). "Ultrasound surgery using multiple sonications – treatment time considerations." *Ultrasound Med Biol*, 22(4), 471–482.

Fennessy FM and Tempany CM. (2005). "MRI-guided focused ultrasound surgery of uterine leiomyomas." *Acad Radiol*, 12(9), 1158–1166.

Fennessy FM, Tempany CM, McDannold NJ, So MJ, Hesley G, Gostout B, Kim HS, Holland GA, Sarti DA, Hynynen K, Jolesz FA, and Stewart EA. (2007). "Uterine leiomyomas: MR imaging-guided focused ultrasound surgery–results of different treatment protocols." *Radiology*, 243(3), 885–893.

Fjield T, Fan X, and Hynynen K. (1996). "A parametric study of the concentric-ring transducer design for MRI guided ultrasound surgery." *J Acoust Soc Am*, 100(2 Pt 1), 1220–1230.

Fry WJ, Barnard JW, Fry EJ, Krumins RF, and Brennan JF. (1955). "Ultrasonic lesions in the mammalian central nervous system." *Science*, 122(3168), 517–518.

Fry WJ and Fry FJ. (1960). "Fundamental neurological research and human neuro-surgery using intense ultrasound." *IRE Trans Med Electron*, ME-7, 166–181.

Furusawa H, Namba K, Thomsen S, Akiyama F, Bendet A, Tanaka C, Yasuda Y, and Nakahara H. (2006). "Magnetic resonance-guided focused ultrasound surgery of breast cancer: Reliability and effectiveness." *J Am Coll Surg*, 203(1), 54–63.

Gianduzzo TR, Eden CG, and Moon DA. (2006). "Treatment of localised prostate cancer using high-intensity focused ultrasound." *BJU Int*, 97(4), 867–868.

Gianfelice D, Khiat A, Amara M, Belblidia A, and Boulanger Y. (2003a). "MR imaging-guided focused ultrasound surgery of breast cancer: Correlation of dynamic contrast-enhanced MRI with histopathologic findings." *Breast Cancer Res Treat*, 82(2), 93–101.

Gianfelice D, Khiat A, Amara M, Belblidia A, and Boulanger Y. (2003b). "MR imaging-guided focused US ablation of breast cancer: Histopathologic assessment of effectiveness – initial experience." *Radiology*, 227(3), 849–855.

Gianfelice D, Khiat A, Boulanger Y, Amara M, and Belblidia A. (2003c). "Feasibility of magnetic resonance imaging-guided focused ultrasound surgery as an adjunct to tamoxifen therapy in high-risk surgical patients with breast carcinoma." *J Vasc Interv Radiol*, 14(10), 1275–1282.

Gombos EC, Kacher DF, Furusawa H, Namba K. (2006). "Breast focused ultrasound surgery with magnetic resonance guidance." *Top Magn Reson Imaging*, 17(3), 181–8.

Greenleaf WJ, Bolander ME, Sarkar G, Goldring MB, and Greenleaf JF. (1998). "Artificial cavitation nuclei significantly enhance acoustically induced cell transfection." *Ultrasound Med Biol*, 24(4), 587–595.

Guerin C, Olivi A, Weingart JD, Lawson HC, and Brem H. (2004). "Recent advances in brain tumor therapy: Local intracerebral drug delivery by polymers." *Invest New Drugs*, 22(1), 27–37.

Guo JY, Kholmovski EG, Zhang L, Jeong EK, and Parker DL. (2006). "k-space inherited parallel acquisition (KIPA): Application on dynamic magnetic resonance imaging thermometry." *Magn Reson Imaging*, 24(7), 903–915.

Guzman HR, McNamara AJ, Nguyen DX, and Prausnitz MR. (2003). "Bioeffects caused by changes in acoustic cavitation bubble density and cell concentration: A unified explanation based on cell-to-bubble ratio and blast radius." *Ultrasound Med Biol*, 29(8), 1211–1222.

Guzman HR, Nguyen DX, McNamara AJ, and Prausnitz MR. (2002). "Equilibrium loading of cells with macromolecules by ultrasound: effects of molecular size and acoustic energy." *J Pharm Sci*, 91(7), 1693–1701.

Gwyther SJ. (2005). "New imaging techniques in cancer management." *Ann Oncol,* 16(Suppl 2), ii63–70.

Hindley J, Gedroyc W, Regan L, Stewart EA, Tempany CM, Hynynen K, McDannold NJ, Inbar Y, Itzchak Y, Rabinovici J, Kim K, Geschwind J, Hesley G, Giostout B, Ehrenstein T, Hengst S, Sklair-Levy M, Shushan A, and Jolesz FA. (2004). "MRI guidance of focused ultrasound therapy of uterine fibroids: Early results." *AJR Am J Roentgenol,* 183(6), 1713–1719.

Hindley J, Law P, Hickey M, Smith S, Lamping D, Gedroyc W, and Regan L. (2002). "Clinical outcomes following percutaneous magnetic resonance image guided laser ablation of symptomatic uterine fibroids." *Human Reproduction,* 17(10), 2737–2741.

Hindman J. (1966). "Proton resonance shift of water in the gas and liquid states." *J Chem Phys,* 44(12), 4582–4592.

Holt RG and Roy RA. (2001). "Measurements of bubble-enhanced heating from focused, MHz-frequency ultrasound in a tissue-mimicking material." *Ultrasound Med Biol,* 27(10), 1399–1412.

Huber PE, Jenne JW, Rastert R, Simiantonakis I, Sinn HP, Strittmatter HJ, von Fournier D, Wannenmacher MF, and Debus J. (2001). "A new noninvasive approach in breast cancer therapy using magnetic resonance imaging-guided focused ultrasound surgery." *Cancer Res,* 61(23), 8441–8447.

Hutchinson E, Dahleh M, and Hynynen K. (1998). "The feasibility of MRI feedback control for intracavitary phased array hyperthermia treatments." *Int J Hyperthermia,* 14(1), 39–56.

Hutchinson EB and Hynynen K. (1998). "Intracavitary ultrasound phased arrays for prostate thermal therapies: MRI compatibility and in vivo testing." *Med Phys,* 25(12), 2392–2399.

Hynynen K. (1991). "The role of nonlinear ultrasound propagation during hyperthermia treatments." *Med Phys,* 18(6), 1156–1163.

Hynynen K, Chung AH, Fjield T, Buchanan M, Daum DR, Colucci V, Lopath P, and Jolesz FA. (1996a). "Feasibility of using ultrasound phased arrays for MRI monitored noninvasive surgery." *IEEE Trans Ultrason Ferroelectr Freq Contr,* 43(6), 1043.

Hynynen K, Clement GT, McDannold N, Vykhodtseva N, King R, White PJ, Vitek S, and Jolesz FA. (2004). "500-element ultrasound phased array system for noninvasive focal surgery of the brain: A preliminary rabbit study with ex vivo human skulls." *Magn Reson Med,* 52(1), 100–107.

Hynynen K, Damianou C, Darkazanli A, Unger E, and Schenck JF. (1993a). "The feasibility of using MRI to monitor and guide noninvasive ultrasound surgery." *Ultrasound Med Biol,* 19(1), 91–92.

Hynynen K, Darkazanli A, Unger E, and Schenck JF. (1993b). "MRI-guided noninvasive ultrasound surgery." *Med Phys,* 20(1), 107–115.

Hynynen K, Freund WR, Cline HE, Chung AH, Watkins RD, Vetro JP, and Jolesz FA. (1996b). "A clinical, noninvasive, MR imaging-monitored ultrasound surgery method." *Radiographics,* 16(1), 185–195.

Hynynen K and Jolesz FA. (1998). "Demonstration of potential noninvasive ultrasound brain therapy through an intact skull." *Ultrasound Med Biol,* 24(2), 275–283.

Hynynen K, McDannold N, Sheikov NA, Jolesz FA, and Vykhodtseva N. (2005). "Local and reversible blood-brain barrier disruption by noninvasive focused ultrasound at frequencies suitable for trans-skull sonications." *Neuroimage*, 24(1), 12–20.

Hynynen K, McDannold N, Vykhodtseva N, and Jolesz FA. (2001a). "Noninvasive MR imaging-guided focal opening of the blood-brain barrier in rabbits." *Radiology*, 220(3), 640–646.

Hynynen K, McDannold N, Vykhodtseva N, Raymond S, Weissleder R, Jolesz FA, and Sheikov N. (2006). "Focal disruption of the blood-brain barrier due to 260-kHz ultrasound bursts: A method for molecular imaging and targeted drug delivery." *J Neurosurg*, 105(3), 445–454.

Hynynen K, Pomeroy O, Smith DN, Huber PE, McDannold NJ, Kettenbach J, Baum J, Singer S, and Jolesz FA. (2001b). "MR imaging-guided focused ultrasound surgery of fibroadenomas in the breast: A feasibility study." *Radiology*, 219(1), 176–185.

Hynynen K, Vykhodtseva NI, Chung AH, Sorrentino V, Colucci V, and Jolesz FA. (1997). "Thermal effects of focused ultrasound on the brain: Determination with MR imaging." *Radiology*, 204(1), 247–253.

Ishihara Y, Calderon A, Watanabe H, Okamoto K, Suzuki Y, Kuroda K, and Suzuki Y. (1995). "A precise and fast temperature mapping using water proton chemical shift." *Magn Reson Med*, 34(6), 814–823.

Jolesz FA and Hynynen K. (2002). "Magnetic resonance image-guided focused ultrasound surgery." *Cancer J*, 8(Suppl 1), S100–112.

Jolesz FA, Hynynen K, McDannold N, Freundlich D, and Kopelman D. (2004). "Non-invasive thermal ablation of hepatocellular carcinoma by using magnetic resonance imaging-guided focused ultrasound." *Gastroenterology*, 127(5, Suppl 1), S242–247.

Jolesz FA, Hynynen K, McDannold N, and Tempany C. (2005). "MR imaging-controlled focused ultrasound ablation: A noninvasive image-guided surgery." *Magn Reson Imaging Clin N Am*, 13(3), 545–560.

Kennedy JE. (2005). "High-intensity focused ultrasound in the treatment of solid tumours." *Nat Rev Cancer*, 5(4), 321–327.

Kennedy JE, Ter Haar GR, and Cranston D. (2003). "High intensity focused ultrasound: Surgery of the future?" *Br J Radiol*, 76(909), 590–599.

Kennedy JE, Wu F, ter Haar GR, Gleeson FV, Phillips RR, Middleton MR, and Cranston D. (2004). "High-intensity focused ultrasound for the treatment of liver tumours." *Ultrasonics*, 42(1–9), 931–935.

Khiat A, Gianfelice D, Amara M, and Boulanger Y. (2006). "Influence of post-treatment delay on the evaluation of the response to focused ultrasound surgery of breast cancer by dynamic contrast enhanced MRI." *Br J Radiol*, 79(940), 308–314.

Kinoshita M and Hynynen K. (2005a). "Intracellular delivery of Bak BH3 peptide by microbubble-enhanced ultrasound." *Pharm Res*, 22(5), 716–720.

Kinoshita M and Hynynen K. (2005b). "A novel method for the intracellular delivery of siRNA using microbubble-enhanced focused ultrasound." *Biochem Biophys Res Commun*, 335(2), 393–399.

Kinoshita M, McDannold N, Jolesz FA, and Hynynen K. (2006a). "Noninvasive localized delivery of Herceptin to the mouse brain by MRI-guided focused ultrasound-induced blood-brain barrier disruption." *Proc Natl Acad Sci USA*, 103(31), 11719–11723.

Kinoshita M, McDannold N, Jolesz FA, and Hynynen K. (2006b). "Targeted delivery of antibodies through the blood-brain barrier by MRI-guided focused ultrasound." *Biochem Biophys Res Commun*, 340(4), 1085–1090.

Kinoshita M and Hynynen K. (2007). "Key factors that affect sonoporation efficiency in in vitro settings: The importance of standing wave in sonoporation." *Biochem Biophys Res Commun*, 359(4), 860–865.

Klibanov AL. (2006). "Microbubble contrast agents: Targeted ultrasound imaging and ultrasound-assisted drug-delivery applications." *Invest Radiol*, 41(3), 354–362.

Kowalski ME, Behnia B, Webb AG, and Jin JM. (2002). "Optimization of electromagnetic phased-arrays for hyperthermia via magnetic resonance temperature estimation." *IEEE Trans Biomed Eng*, 49(11), 1229–1241.

Kroll RA and Neuwelt EA. (1998). "Outwitting the blood-brain barrier for therapeutic purposes: Osmotic opening and other means." *Neurosurgery*, 42(5), 1083–1099, Discussion 1099–1100.

Kuroda K, Chung AH, Hynynen K, and Jolesz FA. (1998). "Calibration of water proton chemical shift with temperature for noninvasive temperature imaging during focused ultrasound surgery." *J Magn Reson Imaging*, 8(1), 175–181.

Kuroda K, Takei N, Mulkern RV, Oshio K, Nakai T, Okada T, Matsumura A, Yanaka K, Hynynen K, and Jolesz FA. (2003). "Feasibility of internally referenced brain temperature imaging with a metabolite signal." *Magn Reson Med Sci*, 2(1), 17–22.

Leighton T. (1994). *The Acoustic Bubble*, Academic Press, San Diego, USA.

Lele PP. (1962). "A simple method for production of trackless focal lesions with focused ultrasound: Physical factors." *J Physiol*, 160, 494–512.

Lele PP. (1967). "Production of deep focal lesions by focused ultrasound–current status." *Ultrasonics*, 5, 105–112.

Leon-Villapalos J, Kaniorou-Larai M, and Dziewulski P. (2005). "Full thickness abdominal burn following magnetic resonance guided focused ultrasound therapy." *Burns*, 31(8), 1054–1055.

Li T, Tachibana K, Kuroki M, and Kuroki M. (2003). "Gene transfer with echo-enhanced contrast agents: Comparison between Albunex, Optison, and Levovist in mice – initial results." *Radiology*, 229(2), 423–428.

Lin WL, Roemer RB, and Hynynen K. (1990). "Theoretical and experimental evaluation of a temperature controller for scanned focused ultrasound hyperthermia." *Med Phys*, 17(4), 615–625.

Lynn JG, Zwemer RL, and Chick AJ. (1942). "New method for the generation and use of focused ultrasound in experimental biology." *J Gen Physiology*, 26, 179–193.

Madersbacher S and Marberger M. (2003). "High-energy shockwaves and extracorporeal high-intensity focused ultrasound." *J Endourol*, 17(8), 667–672.

Madersbacher S, Pedevilla M, Vingers L, Susani M, and Marberger M. (1995). "Effect of high-intensity focused ultrasound on human prostate cancer in vivo." *Cancer Res*, 55(15), 3346–3351.

Malinen M, Huttunen T, Kaipio JP, and Hynynen K. (2005). "Scanning path optimization for ultrasound surgery." *Phys Med Biol*, 50(15), 3473–3490.

McDannold, Hynynen K, Wolf D, Wolf G, and Jolesz F. (1998). "MRI evaluation of thermal ablation of tumors with focused ultrasound." *J Magn Reson Imaging*, 8(1), 91–100.

McDannold N. (2005). "Quantitative MRI-based temperature mapping based on the proton resonant frequency shift: review of validation studies." *Int J Hyperthermia*, 21(6), 533–546.

McDannold N and Hynynen K. (2006). "Quality assurance and system stability of a clinical MRI-guided focused ultrasound system: Four-year experience." *Med Phys*, 33(11), 4307–4313.

McDannold N, Hynynen K, and Jolesz F. (2001). "MRI monitoring of the thermal ablation of tissue: Effects of long exposure times." *J Magn Reson Imaging*, 13(3), 421–427.

McDannold N, King RL, Jolesz FA, and Hynynen K. (2002). "The use of quantitative temperature images to predict the optimal power for focused ultrasound surgery: In vivo verification in rabbit muscle and brain." *Med Phys*, 29(3), 356–365.

McDannold N, Vykhodtseva N, and Hynynen K. (2005a). "Targeted disruption of the blood-brain barrier with focused ultrasound: Association with Inertial Cavitation." *Proc Ultrason Symp*, 2, 1249–1252.

McDannold N, Vykhodtseva N, Raymond S, Jolesz FA, and Hynynen K. (2005b). "MRI-guided targeted blood-brain barrier disruption with focused ultrasound: histological findings in rabbits." *Ultrasound Med Biol*, 31(11), 1527–1537.

McNichols RJ, Gowda A, Kangasniemi M, Bankson JA, Price RE, and Hazle JD. (2004). "MR thermometry-based feedback control of laser interstitial thermal therapy at 980 nm." *Lasers Surg Med*, 34(1), 48–55.

Meshorer A, Prionas SD, Fajardo LF, Meyer JL, Hahn GM, and Martinez AA. (1983). "The effects of hyperthermia on normal mesenchymal tissues. Application of a histologic grading system." *Arch Pathol Lab Med*, 107(6), 328–334.

Miller AP and Nanda NC. (2004). "Contrast echocardiography: New agents." *Ultrasound Med Biol*, 30(4), 425–434.

Miller DL. (1988). "Particle gathering and microstreaming near ultrasonically activated gas-filled micropores." *J Acoust Soc Am*, 84(4), 1378–1387.

Miller DL and Quddus J. (2000). "Diagnostic ultrasound activation of contrast agent gas bodies induces capillary rupture in mice." *Proc Natl Acad Sci USA*, 97(18), 10179–10184.

Mitragotri S, Blankschtein D, and Langer R. (1995). "Ultrasound-mediated transdermal protein delivery." *Science*, 269(5225), 850–853.

Moonen CT, Quesson B, Salomir R, Vimeux FC, de Zwart JA, van Vaals JJ, Grenier N, and Palussiere J. (2001). "Thermal therapies in interventional MR imaging. focused ultrasound." *Neuroimaging Clin N Am*, 11(4), 737–747.

Mougenot C, Salomir R, Palussiere J, Grenier N, and Moonen CT. (2004). "Automatic spatial and temporal temperature control for MR-guided focused ultrasound using fast 3D MR thermometry and multispiral trajectory of the focal point." *Magn Reson Med*, 52(5), 1005–1015.

Nyborg W, Carson P, Carstensen E, Dunn F, Miller DL, and Miller M. (2002). "Exposure criteria for medical diagnostic ultrasound: II. Criteria based on all known mechanisms." NCRP Report No. 140, National Council on Radiation Protection and Measurements, Bethesda, Maryland, USA.

Palussiere J, Salomir R, Le Bail B, Fawaz R, Quesson B, Grenier N, and Moonen CT. (2003). "Feasibility of MR-guided focused ultrasound with real-time temperature mapping and continuous sonication for ablation of VX2 carcinoma in rabbit thigh." *Magn Reson Med*, 49(1), 89–98.

Pardridge WM. (2002a). "Drug and gene delivery to the brain: The vascular route." *Neuron*, 36(4), 555–558.

Pardridge WM. (2002b). "Drug and gene targeting to the brain with molecular Trojan horses." *Nat Rev Drug Discov*, 1(2), 131–139.

Pardridge WM. (2003). "Blood-brain barrier genomics and the use of endogenous transporters to cause drug penetration into the brain." *Curr Opin Drug Discov Devel*, 6(5), 683–691.

Peters RD and Henkelman RM. (2000). "Proton-resonance frequency shift MR thermometry is affected by changes in the electrical conductivity of tissue." *Magn Reson Med*, 43(1), 62–71.

Peters RD, Hinks RS, and Henkelman RM. (1999). "Heat-source orientation and geometry dependence in proton-resonance frequency shift magnetic resonance thermometry." *Magn Reson Med*, 41(5), 909–918.

Poissonnier L, Chapelon JY, Rouviere O, Curiel L, Bouvier R, Martin X, Dubernard JM, and Gelet A. (2007). "Control of prostate cancer by transrectal HIFU in 227 patients." *Eur Urol*, 51(2), 381–387.

Poissonnier L, Gelet A, Chapelon JY, Bouvier R, Rouviere O, Pangaud C, Lyonnet D, and Dubernard JM. (2003). "[Results of transrectal focused ultrasound for the treatment of localized prostate cancer (120 patients with PSA < or + 10 ng/ml)]." *Prog Urol*, 13(1), 60–72.

Price RJ, Skyba D, Kaul S, and Skalak T. (1998). "Delivery of colloidal particles and red blood cells to tissue through microvessel ruptures created by targeted microbubble destruction with ultrasound." *Circulation*, 98, 1264–1267.

Raymond SB, Skoch J, Hynynen K, and Bacskai BJ. (2007). "Multiphoton imaging of ultrasound/optison mediated cerebrovascular effects in vivo." *J Cereb Blood Flow Metab*, 27(2), 393–403.

Rieke V, Vigen KK, Sommer G, Daniel BL, Pauly JM, and Butts K. (2004). "Referenceless PRF shift thermometry." *Magn Reson Med*, 51(6), 1223–1231.

Salomir R, Palussiere J, Vimeux FC, de Zwart JA, Quesson B, Gauchet M, Lelong P, Pergrale J, Grenier N, and Moonen CT. (2000a). "Local hyperthermia with MR-guided focused ultrasound: spiral trajectory of the focal point optimized for temperature uniformity in the target region." *J Magn Reson Imaging*, 12(4), 571–583.

Salomir R, Vimeux FC, de Zwart JA, Grenier N, and Moonen CT. (2000b). "Hyperthermia by MR-guided focused ultrasound: Accurate temperature control based on fast MRI and a physical model of local energy deposition and heat conduction." *Magn Reson Med*, 43(3), 342–347.

Sapareto SA and Dewey WC. (1984). "Thermal dose determination in cancer therapy." *Int J Radiat Oncol Biol Phys*, 10(6), 787–800.

Sheikov N, McDannold N, Jolesz F, Zhang YZ, Tam K, and Hynynen K. (2006). "Brain arterioles show more active vesicular transport of blood-borne tracer molecules than capillaries and venules after focused ultrasound-evoked opening of the blood-brain barrier." *Ultrasound Med Biol*, 32(9), 1399–1409.

Sheikov N, McDannold N, Vykhodtseva N, Jolesz F, and Hynynen K. (2004). "Cellular mechanisms of the blood-brain barrier opening induced by ultrasound in presence of microbubbles." *Ultrasound Med Biol*, 30(7), 979–989.

Shohet R, Chen S, Zhou Y-T, Wang Z, Meidell R, Unger R, and Grayburn P. (2001). "Echocardiographic destruction of albumin microbubbles directs gene delivery to the myocardium." *Circulation*, 101, 2554.

Skyba D, Price RJ, Linka A, Skalak T, and Kaul S. (1998). "Direct in vivo visualization of intravascular destruction of microbubbles by ultrasound and its local effects on tissue." *Circulation*, 98(4), 290–293.

Smith NB, Merrilees NK, Dahleh M, and Hynynen K. (2001). "Control system for an MRI compatible intracavitary ultrasound array for thermal treatment of prostate disease." *Int J Hyperthermia*, 17(3), 271–282.

Sokka SD, King R, and Hynynen K. (2003). "MRI-guided gas bubble enhanced ultrasound heating in in vivo rabbit thigh." *Phys Med Biol*, 48(2), 223–241.

Sokka SD, King R, McDannold N, and Hynynen K. (1999). "Design and evaluation of a linear intracavitary ultrasound phased array for MRI-guided prostate ablative therapies." *IEEE Ultrason Symp*, 1435–1438.

Song CW. (1984). "Effect of local hyperthermia on blood flow and microenvironment: A review." *Cancer Res*, 44(10, Suppl), S4721–S4730.

Stafford RJ, Hazle JD, and Glover GH. (2000). "Monitoring of high-intensity focused ultrasound-induced temperature changes in vitro using an interleaved spiral acquisition." *Magn Reson Med*, 43(6), 909–912.

Stafford RJ, Price RE, Diederich C, Kangasniemi M, Olsson L, and Hazle JD. (2004). "Interleaved echo-planar imaging for fast multiplanar magnetic resonance temperature imaging of ultrasound thermal ablation therapy. " *J Magn Reson Imaging*, 20(4), 706–714.

Stewart EA, Gedroyc WM, Tempany CM, Quade BJ, Inbar Y, Ehrenstein T, Shushan A, Hindley JT, Goldin RD, David M, Sklair M, and Rabinovici J. (2003). "Focused ultrasound treatment of uterine fibroid tumors: Safety and feasibility of a noninvasive thermoablative technique." *Am J Obstet Gynecol*, 189(1), 48–54.

Stollberger R, Ascher PW, Huber D, Renhart W, Radner H, and Ebner F. (1998). "Temperature monitoring of interstitial thermal tissue coagulation using MR phase images." *J Magn Reson Imaging*, 8(1), 188–196.

Tachibana K. (1992). "Transdermal delivery of insulin to alloxan-diabetic rabbits by ultrasound exposure." *Pharm Res*, 9(7), 952–954.

Tachibana K and Tachibana S. (1991). "Transdermal delivery of insulin by ultrasonic vibration." *J Pharm Pharmacol*, 43(4), 270–271.

Taniyama Y, Tachibana K, Hiraoka K, Aoki M, Yamamoto S, Matsumoto K, Nakamura T, Ogihara T, Kaneda Y, and Morishita R. (2002a). "Development of safe and efficient novel nonviral gene transfer using ultrasound: Enhancement of transfection efficiency of naked plasmid DNA in skeletal muscle." *Gene Ther*, 9(6), 372–380.

Taniyama Y, Tachibana K, Hiraoka K, Namba T, Yamasaki K, Hashiya N, Aoki M, Ogihara T, Yasufumi K, and Morishita R. (2002b). "Local delivery of plasmid DNA into rat carotid artery using ultrasound." *Circulation*, 105(10), 1233–1239.

Tempany CM, Stewart EA, McDannold N, Quade BJ, Jolesz FA, and Hynynen K. (2003). "MR imaging-guided focused ultrasound surgery of uterine leiomyomas: A feasibility study." *Radiology*, 226(3), 897–905.

Ter Haar GR. (2001). "High intensity focused ultrasound for the treatment of tumors." *Echocardiography*, 18(4), 317–322.

Thomas JL and Fink M. (1996). "Ultrasonic beam focusing through tissue inhomogeneities with a time reversal mirror: Application to transskull therapy." *IEEE Trans Ultrason Ferroelectr Freq Control*, 43(6), 1122–1129.

Treat LH, McDannold N, Vykhodtseva N, Zhang Y, Tam K, and Hynynen K. (2007). "Targeted delivery of doxorubicin to the rat brain at therapeutic levels using MRI-guided focused ultrasound." *Int J Cancer*, 121(4), 901–907.

Unger EC, Hersh E, Vannan M, and McCreery T. (2001). "Gene delivery using ultrasound contrast agents." *Echocardiography*, 18(4), 355–361.

Unger EC, Matsunaga TO, McCreery T, Schumann P, Sweitzer R, and Quigley R. (2002). "Therapeutic applications of microbubbles." *Eur J Radiol*, 42(2), 160–168.

Unger EC, McCreery TP, and Sweitzer RH. (1997). "Ultrasound enhances gene expression of liposomal transfection." *Invest Radiol*, 32(12), 723–727.

Unger EC, Porter T, Culp W, Labell R, Matsunaga T, and Zutshi R. (2004). "Therapeutic applications of lipid-coated microbubbles." *Adv Drug Deliv Rev*, 56(9), 1291–1314.

Vannan M, McCreery T, Li P, Han Z, Unger E, Kuersten B, Nabel E, and Rajagopalan S. (2002). "Ultrasound-mediated transfection of canine myocardium by intravenous administration of cationic microbubble-linked plasmid DNA." *J Am Soc Echocardiogr*, 15(3), 214–218.

Vanne A and Hynynen K. (2003). "MRI feedback temperature control for focused ultrasound surgery." *Phys Med Biol*, 48(1), 31–43.

Vigen KK, Daniel BL, Pauly JM, and Butts K. (2003). "Triggered, navigated, multibaseline method for proton resonance frequency temperature mapping with respiratory motion." *Magn Reson Med*, 50(5), 1003–1010.

Wu T and Felmlee JP. (2002). "A quality control program for MR-guided focused ultrasound ablation therapy." *J Appl Clin Med Phys*, 3(2), 162–167.

Yuh EL, Shulman SG, Mehta SA, Xie J, Chen L, Frenkel V, Bednarski MD, and Li KC. (2005). "Delivery of systemic chemotherapeutic agent to tumors by using focused ultrasound: study in a murine model." *Radiology*, 234(2), 431–437.

Zarnitsyn VG and Prausnitz MR. (2004). "Physical parameters influencing optimization of ultrasound-mediated DNA transfection." *Ultrasound Med Biol*, 30(4), 527–538.

Chapter 11

Neurosurgical Applications

Terry Peters, Kirk Finnis, Ting Guo, and Andrew Parrent

Abstract

This chapter demonstrates a particular application of stereotactic neurosurgery, used in conjunction with deep brain atlases and an electrophysiological database, to guide the implantation of lesioning devices and stimulation electrodes to alleviate the symptoms of Parkinson's disease and other diseases of the motor system. Central to this work is the nonrigid mapping of individual patients' brains to a standard anatomical brain template. This operation not only maps the structure in the deep brain of individual patients to match the template, but also creates a warping matrix that allows the location of data collected from individual patients to be mapped to the database. This database may in turn be mapped to new patients to indicate the probable locations of stimuli and responses. This information can be employed to assist the surgeon in making an initial estimate of the electrode positioning, and reduce the exploration needed to finalize the target position in which to create a lesion or place a stimulator.

11.1   Introduction

As indicated in Chap. 1, neurosurgery was the first surgical discipline to adopt image guidance in any concerted manner, and the first application was for minimally invasive procedures. The stereotactic frame affixed to the patients' skull has been the key to these techniques for the dual purpose of both supporting the surgical instruments and establishing a coordinate system for navigating within the brain. This chapter describes the application of stereotactic neurosurgery in conjunction with atlases and electrophysiologic databases, to guide deep-brain electrode placement for the treatment of Parkinson's and other diseases related to impaired motor-function.

11.2   Stereotactic Neurosurgery

Over the past 30 years, image-guided neurosurgery has matured into a procedure that is now in regular use in the operating room. Although some

T. Peters and K. Cleary (eds.), *Image-Guided Interventions.*
© Springer Science + Business Media, LLC 2008

neurosurgical procedures can be performed solely on the basis of information in anatomical magnetic resonance imaging (MRI) or computed tomography (CT) images alone, others require the incorporation of additional physiological and functional information that must be obtained from other sources. These additional data generally can be acquired from functional MRI (fMRI), positron emission tomography (PET), single photon emission computed tomography (SPECT), diffusion and perfusion imaging, optical techniques, magneto- and electro-encephalography (MEG/EEG), or some other electrophysiological measurements. For example, the surgical treatment of Parkinson's disease (PD), essential tremor, and chronic pain entails either creating lesions, or placing chronic stimulators in precise locations relative to certain electrophysiologically defined regions, deep within the brain. Planning this type of surgery involves approximate localization of surgical targets on preoperative MRI or CT images. However, neither of these modalities can allow direct visualization and accurate delineation of thalamic nuclei or functional subregions within the subthalamus or globus pallidus internus (the targets for these procedures) with sufficient contrast. To facilitate localization of these structures, printed anatomical atlases [Schaltenbrand and Wahren 1977; Talairach and Tourneau 1988; Van Buren and Borke 1972] or digitized versions of them [Bertrand et al. 1973; Ganser et al. 2004; Nowinski et al. 1997], may be scaled to align with visible anatomical landmarks in the preoperative patient image and then displayed as an overlay.

The use of individualized and population-based atlases is a major field of research in the neurosciences, and a comprehensive treatment of this field is given by [Thompson et al. 2000]. Integrating digitized atlases into computer guidance for functional neurosurgery has proven to facilitate surgical planning and, as a result, several independently developed [Dawant et al. 2002; Finnis et al. 2003; Ganser et al. 2004; Kall et al. 1985; St-Jean et al. 1998] and commercially available surgical planning systems have incorporated anatomical atlas-based planning modules. Registration of the atlas to the patient is typically achieved using linear scaling techniques, based primarily on the length of the anterior commissural-posterior commissural (AC-PC) line and the width of the third ventricle [Finnis et al. 2003; Kall et al. 1985; Lehman et al. 2000]. Some research oriented systems also incorporate automatic nonrigid registration algorithms for this task [Collins et al. 1995; St-Jean et al. 1998]. When single or triplanar views of a digitized atlas registered to a patient image are displayed within a surgical planning system, virtual probe trajectories that directly intersect an atlas-predicted target may be modeled prior to surgery and the stereotactic coordinates of the target region provided to the surgeon. However, there are several limitations with existing anatomical atlases and atlas-based planning that need to be addressed.

11.3 Atlases

Classical atlases of the human brain used in stereotactic guidance are typically derived from either one whole-brain specimen [Talairach and Tourneau 1988] or multiple hemispheres [Schaltenbrand and Wahren 1977] from different individuals. Unfortunately, morphometric data relating to normal variations in shape, size, and position of subcortical anatomy within three dimensions as a function of age, sex, disease status, or other factors are not available with either type of atlas. This means the displayed anatomy is only representative of the cadaver brains from which it was made rather than the general population. The effects of normal anatomical variability are quite clearly demonstrated by the considerable mismatch that exists when digitized versions of these atlases are registered to patient images using the standard intercommissural AC-PC reference system. Therefore, the quality of the registration within homogeneous-appearing anatomy such as the thalamus, which is devoid of internal anatomical landmarks, should be questioned if other discernable anatomical borders are obviously misregistered.

An additional problem with stereotactic atlases is that some cadaver tissue sections may have been damaged in the slicing process, sectioned unevenly, or rendered unusable by excessive or uneven shrinkage during histological processing [Mark and Yakovlev 1995]. Accordingly, the available atlas slices may not correspond exactly to the slice containing the target. This problem is of particular relevance in the most popular of all the stereotactic atlases, the Schaltenbrand Wahren atlas [Schaltenbrand and Wahren 1977], where the interslice distances vary between 1 and 4 mm. To overcome this difficulty, various investigators have scanned and interpolated one of the Schaltenbrand atlas slice series into a three-dimensional volume for static display [Nowinski et al. 1998], or have resliced it at regular intervals [Yoshida 1987]. However, the irregular interslice distances make extensive manipulation of the data necessary to fill in the missing slices in the serial two-diemensional volume. As a result, anatomy contained within the volumetric atlas no longer reflects the original data.

To address the limitations of previous anatomical brain atlases, researchers recently have developed new atlases [Chakravarty et al. 2006; Nowinski et al. 2003; Toga et al. 2006; Yelnick et al. 2007] that integrate data representing both structural and functional aspects of the human brain from multiple subjects. The three-dimensional deformable atlas with a histological level of anatomical definition of the human basal ganglia [Yelnick et al. 2007] enables the delineation of fine deep brain structures of individual patients. Functional information derived from immuno-histochemical studies is also available in this atlas.

11.4   Intraoperative Electrophysiological Confirmation

The superposition of digitized anatomical atlases onto patient brain images can only provide an approximation of target loci, because of the limitations described earlier, regardless of the atlas-to-patient registration technique employed. Nevertheless, accurate identification of the surgical target is critical to achieve the optimal surgical outcome, as small deviations in the positioning may cause severe side effects brought about by the complexity and delicateness of deep brain structures. In actual clinical practice, to localize the final target to that approximated by the atlas, electrophysiological exploration must be performed intraoperatively within, and adjacent to the intended target to characterize tissue function and to map somatotopy. Somatotopy is the topography of the spatial relationships between the receptors in the body via their nerve fibers to where they terminate in the cerebral cortex. Their terminations form a spatial pattern of the different body parts in functional units.

Electrophysiological exploration is performed using multiple invasive exploratory trajectories with a recording and/or stimulating electrode, mounted in a holder fastened to the stereotactic frame (Fig. 11.1). Using this information, the surgeon can then mentally reconstruct the somatotopic organization contained in the vicinity of the target structure, and establish functional borders on the basis of the physical responses elicited by the patient, verbal descriptions of stimulation-induced sensory and motor phenomena, and microelectrode recording data obtained during exploration.

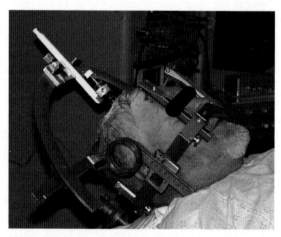

Fig. 11.1. Stereotactic frame with probe holder attached

Comparison of the patient somatotopic organization with that presented in the literature allows the probe tip position within a certain functional subdivision of the target to be estimated, and used to plan subsequent trajectories, until the ideal target foci and probe trajectories are determined.

The electrophysiologically refined target, as shown in studies focusing on pallidotomy (lesioning of the globus pallidus internus) [Alterman et al. 1999; Guridi et al. 1999] and chronic subthalamic stimulation [Cuny et al. 2002; Hamani et al. 2005; Starr et al. 1999; Zonenshayn et al. 2000], can be shifted dramatically from the original atlas-derived or visually identified stereotactic target, once electrophysiological exploration has been performed. These studies demonstrate that targeting using standard techniques often results in poor initial targeting accuracy, whereas the use of atlases, complemented by the use of EP exploration, greatly facilitates the process of minimally-invasive treatment of movement disorders.

11.5   Electrophysiological Databases

Several groups of researchers have compiled and analyzed functional information from subcortical structures acquired from patient populations [Giorgi et al. 1985; Tasker et al. 1982; Thompson et al. 1977; Yoshida et al. 1982]. These data were typically registered to a common coordinate space to facilitate examination of functional organization in relation to anatomic structures.

Previous electrophysiological atlases approximate the functional organization within some subcortical structures, but are of limited use in surgical guidance. The poor clustering of population data results primarily from the use of rigid, rather than nonrigid, image registration to accommodate inter-patient anatomical variability. In addition, their typically employed coding schemes are not sufficiently flexible to describe all aspects of an observed response in relation to the parameters that evoked it, or of the characteristics of the patient from whom the data originated.

More recent computerized atlases [Chakravarty et al. 2006; D'Haese et al. 2005a; D'Haese et al. 2005b; Nowinski et al. 2005a; Nowinski et al. 2005b] and a three-dimensional database [Finnis et al. 2003; Guo et al. 2006, 2007] of deep-brain electrophysiology have been implemented with more accurate nonrigid registration approaches, and more sophisticated coding schemes. An example is that developed by Finnis et al. [2003] and Guo et al. [2006]. This approach adds electrophysiological data to the database without relying on AC-PC based global or piecewise linear registration, or the need to manually identify anatomical landmarks. It accommodates for anatomical variability using a high performance, nonrigid registration algorithm that *warps* the deep brain anatomy in a patient MRI to that of the reference MR image volume [Finnis et al. 2003]. It also employs a high signal-to-noise (SNR) reference MR image – the "Colin27" template [Holmes et al. 1998] as the common coordinate system for the database, rather than a series of digitized anatomical atlas slices. User interaction is facilitated by an inter-active GUI that interfaces to a comprehensive standardized coding protocol for describing observed responses. These database codes are readily acces-sible via a flexible search engine that allows searches of various specificity, and whose results may be displayed as autonomous three-dimensional objects, or as cluster probability maps that can be nonrigidly registered to the MR images of individual patients. These features are integrated into a visuali-zation and navigation system that supports the comprehensive planning and guidance of functional stereotactic procedures.

To populate this particular database, data were acquired from 146 patients who had undergone a total of 199 surgeries (54 thalamotomy, 58 pallido-tomy, 23 thalamic deep brain stimulation (DBS), 6 pallidus DBS, and 58 STN DBS) for symptomatic treatment of Parkinson's disease, chronic pain, essential tremor, and other neurological disorders at London Health Sciences Centre (LHSC), London, Ontario, Canada. Of these patients, 107 had been diagnosed with Parkinson's disease, 23 with essential tremor, 6 with chronic pain, 5 with dystonias, 1 with torticollis, and 4 with tremor.

For each of these patients, preoperative T_1-weighted MR images were acquired using a 1.5T GE Signa scanner with a 3D SPGR sequence (TR/TE 8.9/1.9 ms, flip angle 20°, NEX 2, voxel size $1.17 \times 1.17 \times 1$ mm^3, dimen-sion $256 \times 256 \times 248$) and T_2-weighted MR images were also obtained on the same scanner using 2D fast spin-echo sequence (TR/TE 2800/110 ms, flip angle 90°, NEX 4, voxel size $1.0 \times 1.0 \times 1.5$ mm^3, spacing 0, coronal acquisition dimension $256 \times 256 \times 21$, axial acquisition dimension $256 \times 256 \times 20$) for STN DBS procedures. The Leksell G stereotactic frame (Elekta Instruments AB, Stockholm, Sweden) with an attached MR com-patible localizer was fixed to each patient immediately prior to imaging.

Electrophysiological data from each patient were recorded in the co-ordinate system of the preoperative MR image space and coded using a comprehensive scheme to further organize them into different groups accor-ding to specific parameters, such as intraoperative microelectrode-recording (MER), microstimulation, and macrostimulation groups.

11.6   Standard Brain Space

The electrophysiological data acquired from each individual surgical procedure are registered to a standard brain template (Colin27) [Holmes et al. 1998], using a high performance, rapid, nonrigid registration algorithm [Finnis et al. 2003].

The Colin27 (also known as the CJH-27 dataset) brain was adopted as the reference MRI brain template (the registration target), as it has a high SNR, defines fine anatomical details within the deep brain, and has been popularly adopted in neuroscience community. Colin27 consists of a series of 27 T_1-weighted MR brain images (20×1 mm^3: TR/TE 18/10 ms, flip angle 30°, NEX 1; 7×0.78 mm^3: TR/TE 20/12 ms, flip angle 40°, NEX 1) of the same healthy individual obtained using a Philips 1.5T MR unit with a spoiled GRASS sequence. Twenty-six of the 27 images were rigidly registered to the 27th image and averaged into International Consortium for Brain Mapping (ICBM) brain space [Evans et al. 1994].

11.7   Image Registration

Two image registration steps are needed to successfully implement this system. The first is the rigid-body registration of the image with the patient (stereotactic frame), while the second performs the nonrigid mapping of the recorded electrophysiological data from each specific patient brain space to the coordinate system of the standard database, as well as inversely from the database to a patient.

1. *Patient-to-Image Registration*: This is achieved using an automatic procedure that fits a set of "N-bar" patterns similar to those on the frames, to their equivalents in the volumetric image, achieving a linear registration between the patient and the image. This fast frame extraction procedure establishes the transform between the coordinate system of the stereotactic frame and that of a patient preoperative brain image with 0.5 mm fiducial localization error.

2. *Data-to-Database and Database-to-Patient Registration*: Both require a nonrigid registration, and is usually accomplished in two steps. The first generates a global affine transformation that maximizes the normalized cross-correlation between the source and target image volumes. In addition, an arbitrary closed polygonal model enveloping different aspects of the image may be selected to act as a mask to constrain the search-space for the similarity measurement. Masking permits the user to bias the optimization of the affine transform so that specific regions, such as the diencephalon, may be brought into better registration at the expense of extra-cranial or cortical structures. The second step builds upon the affine registration by computing a deformation grid that maximizes the similarity metric on successively smaller subvolumes of the images. To achieve the nonrigid registration, we employed the same algorithm introduced above to accommodate the intersubject anatomical variability between each patient brain image and the Colin27 reference brain space. The registration algorithm incorporates a completely unsupervised, intensity-based, multiresolution registration approach built using

standard VTK classes. As reported by Finnis et al. [2003] this algorithm optimizes the registration in the deep brain region enclosed within a user-defined volume mask, and requires 8–12 min on a dual PIII 1 GHz machine to perform the deformation with an average registration error of 1.04 ± 0.64 mm [Guo et al. 2005]. The computational time can be further reduced by using a multiprocessor system (SGI Altix 8 processors: 5 min).

11.8   Surgical Targets

Surgical targets are chosen on the basis of the nature of the disease. The Ventralis intermedius (Vim) nucleus of the thalamus is targeted for tremor dominant diseases, the Ventralis caudalis (Vc) nucleus of the thalamus for chronic pain, the globus pallidus internus for Parkinson's disease (PD) or dystonia, and the subthalamic nucleus (STN) for PD. Typically, between two and nine trajectories are used for each thalamotomy or pallidotomy procedure and five trajectories for STN, thalamic, and pallidal DBS to refine the approximated target into a final location for lesioning or stimulator placement. Patients are awake and usually unmedicated during surgery. There are two types of targeting:

1. *Indirect Targeting*: Standard practice for identifying the best *initial-guess* targets involves MRI console-based planning on a single axial image thought to contain the target. The approximated target is identified on this image by AC-PC scaling of anatomical atlas-based coordinates to match the intercommissural distance of the patient. Stereotactic coordinates are assigned to the target relative to the frame center. It is important to note that this manual procedure for identifying the frame coordinates of the initial target from the MR console provides only an approximate estimate of the coordinates of the initial exploratory trajectory. As the coordinates of all electrophysiological measurements are read directly from the stereotactic frame, inaccuracies in this initial estimate have no effect on the overall accuracy of the process.

2. *Neurophysiological Target Verification*: Surgeons typically employ a combination of microelectrode recording (MER) and electrical stimulation to map the functional characteristics of the deep brain. A tungsten microelectrode (impedance at 1 KHz: 1 Mohm, maximum ground/reference impedance: 5 Kohm), capable of both recording neuronal activity and applying electrical current, is advanced to the estimated target region using a custom built, remote controlled motor microdrive. During MER, audio and visual representations displayed using the multichannel Medtronic Leadpoint neural activity monitoring system

(Medtronic Inc. Minneapolis, MN, USA) are used to visualize and listen to neuronal spike trains in real time. The electrode tip positions are noted for each event. Following MER exploration, microstimulation is typically applied using currents ranging from 5 to 120 μA (300 Hz, 0.2 ms pulse duration). Macrostimulation of 1–3 mA currents is usually administered using a monophasic square pulse with a pulse duration of 0.1 ms and a frequency of 200 Hz. Depending on the brain region being explored, suprathreshold stimulation commonly evokes visual phenomena, muscle contractions, or cutaneous sensory responses by the involvement of the optic tract, corticospinal tract, and somesthetic pathways, respectively.

Once the functional organization of the target anatomy is mapped and an ideal locus is determined, the target is either lesioned with a radio-frequency (rf) ablation tool or (more commonly) implanted with a stimulator. As opposed to ablative surgery, DBS is nondestructive, reversible, adjustable, and suitable for bilateral implantation.

11.8.1 Standardizing Electrophysiological Data in Patient Native MRI-Space

Both the stimulation-induced responses and micro-electrode recording (MER) data are standardized using a six-parameter code before being entered into the database. This code contains a patient identification number, a trajectory identification number (to identify the precise location of the electrophysiological measurements obtained through that trajectory), the data

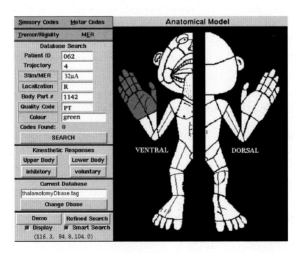

Fig. 11.2. Interactive GUI as used to retrieve from the database, data related to stimulation of the patient's right hand

acquisition method (including recording and stimulation parameters), the laterality of the response, a body part number assigned to a discrete region or a group of regions of the body, and a response code describing the characteristic of the response or changes in cell firing patterns.

The interactive GUI of this system is based on a homuncular graphic, loosely based on Tasker's version [Tasker et al. 1982] of the Woolsey figurine for physiological data recording (Fig. 11.2).

Each anatomical subdivision and groups of subdivisions on the homunculus model are assigned unique identification numbers that can be selected by the user for anatomically localizing each response. In addition, 80 response descriptors were created using a hierarchically organized user interface to permit rapid assignment of the appropriate standardized code to any given response. The user may also append free-form text to qualitatively describe the observed response.

Within this environment, coded functional data are plotted directly onto the patient's preoperative image along a virtual trajectory corresponding to the position and orientation of the actual surgical probe. Images are registered to the coordinate system defined by the stereotactic head frame. The image-to-frame transformation generated by this algorithm allows the display of the functional data codes on the appropriate anatomical area of the image in three-dimensional space.

Once annotated to their respective imaging volumes, the Cartesian coordinates of the patient-specific functional data, together with their corresponding codes, are saved in a text file for incorporation into the central database. A secondary code describing the sex, age, pathological condition, and the handedness of the patient, surgical procedure, and specifications of the probes used during the procedure are assigned to the header of each data file. When patient functional data are fully coded and annotated to their respective MRIs, the image and functional data are nonrigidly registered to the Colin27 common image space that defines the coordinate system of the central database.

11.8.2 Application to Deep-Brain Neurosurgery

This database currently contains over 15,000 individually coded data-points provided by 146 patients (199 procedures in total), and illustrates the effectiveness of this system in displaying the functional organization of basal ganglia structures.

11.8.3 Representative Database Searches

The intraoperatively obtained electrophysiological data, coded as described earlier, can be retrieved from the database and displayed either as clusters of spheres in 3D space or density maps on three intersecting orthogonal 2D image planes. Properties of the selected functional data, e.g., color, opacity, and shading, can be adjusted to facilitate interpretation of the search results.

Sensory Thalamus: The somatotopically organized sensory Vc nucleus is located in the postero-ventral aspect of the thalamus. During thalamotomy (therapeutic lesioning of the thalamus) for Parkinson's disease, essential tremor, and chronic pain, the functional borders of the Vc nucleus are determined by extensive electrophysiological mapping. A typical selective search of the database (for sensory responses characteristic of those obtained during Vc microstimulation at less than 100 μA and 300 Hz) is shown in Fig. 11.3. Note the presence of somatotopic organization that occurs naturally within these population data.

Motor Thalamus: Figure 11.4 demonstrates a probabilistic functional border between the Vim motor nucleus and the Vc sensory nucleus of the left thalamus.

Individual purple spheres (diameter = 0.2 mm) show data encoded for kinesthetic neurons detected by MER, whose activity has been activated or inhibited by specific movements around a joint. Green spheres represent tactile neurons detected by MER of induced neuronal excitation during mild physical stimulation of specific regions of the patient's body. Note that although moderate overlap exists between the two regions (as one would expect), there is an obvious transition between the population-based motor and tactile regions.

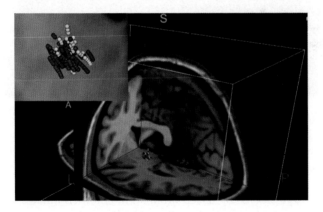

Fig. 11.3. Sensory responses manifesting on patient's right side retrieved from database during microstimulation

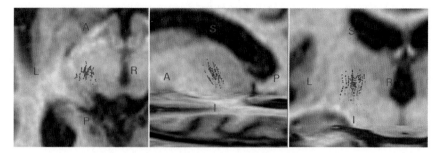

Fig. 11.4. Retrieval of microstimulation results from database and applied to the MRI of a new patient – shown in three different views. The purple and green clusters serve to identify the probabilistic functional border between the Vim motor and the Vc sensory nuclei, respectively

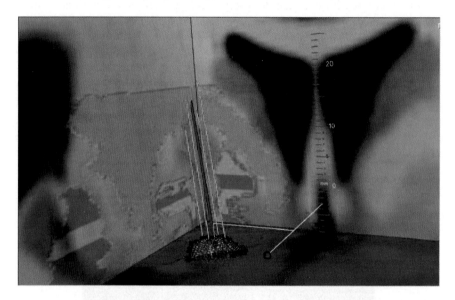

Fig. 11.5. DBS electrode combined with atlas data; *Mesh object*: segmented STN; *Color map*: digitized anatomical atlas of the deep brain region; *Purple line* (central): central electrode; *Cyan lines* (parallel to the central line): surgical trajectories; *Blue spheres*: tips of the five trajectories

Subthalamic Nucleus (STN): Deep brain stimulation eliminates excessive or abnormally patterned activity from the STN by implanting a multielectrode stimulator into a specific location of the nucleus, where, generated by a neuro-pacemaker, continuous high frequency electrical stimulation is delivered [Machado et al. 2006; Perlmutter and Mink 2006]. Decreasing STN hyperactivity through the use of chronic deep brain stimulation may slow or halt progression of Parkinson's disease by removing potentially excitotoxic effects [Rodriguez et al. 1998]. For this reason, the STN has recently received increased attention as a surgical target for treating Parkinson's disease and other movement disorders. The STN, although partially visible with T_2-weighted MRI sequences, must still be electrophysiologically defined to minimize stimulation effects on surrounding structures [Halpern et al. 2007; Sterio et al. 2002].

Figure 11.5 shows how the database may be employed to assist in the placement of DBS electrodes. The 3D model of a typical quadripolar DBS electrode faithfully displays the position and dimensions of the exposed contacts.

11.8.4 Target Prediction Using EP Atlases

Several groups have recently used anatomical and electrophysiological atlas-based approaches to automatically determine the optimal targeting for DBS implantation [D'Haese et al. 2005a; D'Haese et al. 2005b; Guo et al. 2006, 2007].

11.9   Integration of the Neurosurgical Visualization and Navigation System

Building on the fundamentals discussed earlier, we developed a 3D visualization and navigation system for stereotactic functional deep brain neurosurgery planning and guidance, and evaluated its effectiveness in predicting surgical targets for thalamotomy, pallidotomy, thalamic DBS, and STN DBS procedures. By the integration of the electrophysiological database, digitized three-dimensional brain atlases, segmented deep-brain nuclei, categorized surgical targets from previous procedures, plus representations of instruments, this system enables:

1. Interactive display of linked patient and standard brain images
2. Three-dimensional representation of the deep-brain nuclei
3. Accurate nonrigid accommodation of anatomical variability
4. Simultaneous and/or independent manipulation of multiple trajectories, and
5. Includes an intuitive graphical user interface

Standardized functional and anatomical data incorporated in this system are nonrigidly mapped to the patient brain, and play a crucial role in both preoperative surgical target planning and intraoperative surgical guidance.

11.9.1 Digitized Brain Atlas and Segmented Deep-Brain Nuclei

Because of its extensive use in the neuroscience community, the well-established stereotactic brain atlas of Schaltenbrand and Wahren [1977], in which different brain structures can easily be distinguished by unique color coding, was nonrigidly mapped to Colin27 brain-space to serve as one of our anatomical references. Each deep-brain nucleus is segmented, based on its anatomical representation in this atlas, and displayed either as a 3D object or as a triangulated mesh, allowing the visualization of trajectories inside the nucleus. This permits the probe trajectories to be placed at optimal functional subdivisions of certain nuclei, such as the dorsolateral STN, the posterolateral part of the GPi, and the Vim of the thalamus. The centroid of each segmented deep-brain nucleus can be calculated automatically and represented as a sphere.

11.9.2 Final Surgical Target Locations

During each surgical procedure, the location of the final target in patient brain space is saved and nonrigidly registered to Colin27. The registered final surgical target locations are collected into one of eight groups, categorized by the type of surgery. Surgical target initialization can be achieved by nonrigidly mapping the center of mass and the statistical map of a cluster of final surgical targets to the preoperative MR image of each individual patient.

11.9.3 Surgical Instrument Representation

Up to five multiple virtual probes, mimicking their physical counterparts, can be manipulated simultaneously or independently to simulate actual surgical procedures. Meanwhile, simultaneous display of the tip positions of these trajectories is available in both patient image space and stereotactic frame space.

11.9.4 Visualization and Navigation Platform

The user interface to this system comprises both an image display area and a function control panel. The 3D image volume and three orthogonal 2D slices of a patient, together with those of the standard brain template, can be interactively displayed in the adjustable viewing windows of the displaying area (Fig. 11.6). This platform is capable of registering and fusing the digitized brain atlases and T_2-weighted images with the preoperative patient and standard images. All three dimensional images may be reformatted along arbitrary axes. Additionally, coded functional data, along a virtual trajectory

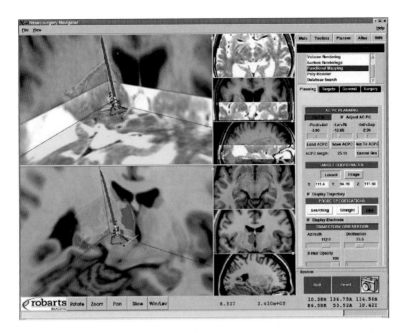

Fig. 11.6. The primary graphical user interface of the system displays the 3D image volume and 2D slices of a patient (top) and those of the standard brain template (bottom). The digitized atlas is registered and fused with each image. A T2-weighted image fused with the patient image is also shown. The control panel shows the tip location and the orientation of the central electrode trajectory

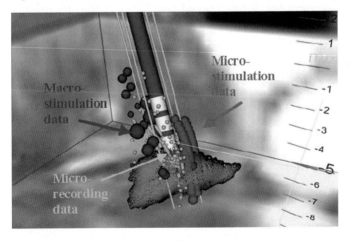

Fig. 11.7. The magnified version of Fig. 11.6. *Purple line* (central): central electrode; *Cyan lines* (parallel to the central line): surgical trajectories; *Green spheres* (small): microelectrode-recording data; *Magenta* spheres (medium): microstimulation data; *Blue spheres* (large): macrostimulation data; *Mesh object*: subthalamic nucleus (STN); the segmented STN and electro-physiological data are nonrigidly registered from the standard brain space to the patient brain image

that corresponds to the position and orientation of the physical probe, are registered to both the patient brain and the Colin27 brain template (Fig. 11.7). The intraoperatively acquired data are saved in a text file whose header contains the code describing the patient information and specifications of the probes used during the procedure. Meanwhile, these data, after mapping to Colin27, are stored in the functional database.

11.10 System Validation

11.10.1 Conventional Planning Approach

To evaluate this system, the neurosurgeon plans each patient's procedure using the standard planning technique immediately after the preoperative MRI acquisition. In this process, the benchmark anatomical structures such as the anterior commissure (AC) and posterior commissure (PC) in the MR image are first identified, and then the image is resampled to align axial slices with the AC-PC orientation. The initial target points for the procedure are determined on the basis of their locations relative to AC and PC (pallidotomy: 2–4 mm anterior to the mid AC-PC point, 19–22 mm lateral to the midline line, and 4–6 mm below the AC-PC plane; thalamotomy/thalamic DBS: 4–8 mm anterior to the PC, 12–15 mm lateral to the midline, and 0–2 mm superior to the AC-PC plane; STN DBS: 3 mm posterior to the mid AC-PC point, 11–12 mm lateral to the midline, and 4–6 mm below the AC-PC plane), and linear Tailarach mapping of the nearest atlas section from the Schaltenbrand and Wahren atlas [Schaltenbrand and Wahren 1977]. The final surgical targets are refined through multiple electrophysiological recording and stimulus/response measurements.

11.10.2 System-Based Planning Procedure

This system was employed by a nonexpert, who was familiar with deep-brain anatomy, to estimate the surgical target locations independently of the neurosurgeon. The preoperative MR image of each procedure was loaded into the neurosurgical system and nonrigidly registered to the Colin27 brain template. The inverse of both the resultant 3D transformation and the non-rigid displacement grid were then applied to map the data in the electro-physiological database, the collection of previous surgical targets, the digitized Schaltenbrand atlas, and the segmented deep-brain nuclei, from the standard coordinate system to the patient brain image. Three retrospect-tive studies and one prospective study were conducted to evaluate the effect-tiveness of this environment for surgical targeting by comparing the target locations estimated by the nonexpert with those identified by the neuro-surgeon. Twenty thalamotomy (10 left, 10 right), 20 pallidotomy (10 left, 10 right), 10 thalamic DBS (5 left, 5 right) procedures were included for the retrospective studies, and 20 STN DBS (10 left, 10 right) procedures for the prospective study.

An estimate of the target location for a particular patient can be achieved by nonrigidly registering the cluster of previous surgical targets determined from EP-guided searches and saved in the standard database to an individual patient image. To assess our registration algorithm in a clinical context, we nonrigidly mapped a cluster of 26 left STN DBS and a cluster of 21 right STN DBS surgical targets to the images of 10 patients who had received left STN DBS, and those of 10 patients undergoing right STN DBS, respectively. Similarly, 36 left and 16 right thalamotomy, 29 left and 27 right pallidotomy, and 10 left and 9 right thalamic DBS surgical targets were also transformed to the images of 10, 10, 10, 10, 5, and 5 patients who had the same sur-geries, respectively. The distances between centers of mass (or the most significant position on the probability map) of database-initialized target locations and the actual surgical targets are summarized in Table 11.1.

Table 11.1. Absolute distances between the database-initialized and the actual surgical targets

Difference (mm)	Pallidotomy	Thalamotomy	Thalamic DBS	STN DBS
Mean	2.33	2.18	2.29	2.21
Max	3.96	3.65	3.55	3.72
Min	1.52	1.21	1.26	1.48
Std	0.80	0.77	0.71	0.73

Figure 11.8 demonstrates the spatial correlation between a segmented left STN, the probability map of the registered cluster of previous surgical targets, as well as the actual surgical targets in a patient brain image.

Results show that this technique provides a reasonable initial estimate of the preoperative target location, which may be further refined with addi-tional functional and anatomical information available within the guidance platform.

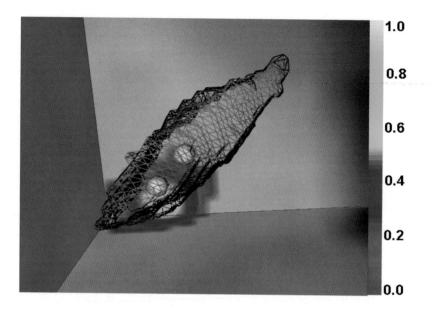

Fig. 11.8. *Mesh object*: STN; *Yellow sphere*: the centroid of STN; *Color-coded map*: the probability map of a collection of left STN DBS targets (1.0: the highest probability on the map; 0.0: the lowest on the map); *White sphere*: the actual surgical target

11.10.2.1 Application of the Segmented Deep-Brain Nuclei

Good nonrigid registration of intersubject brain images has been demonstrated previously [Guo et al. 2005]. When the deep brain nuclei, which have been segmented on the basis of the established anatomical brain atlas, are nonrigidly transformed to a specific patient brain image space using this method, they should overlap the patient's own homologous nuclei. We expected that the anatomical information provided by registering a segmented nucleus from the atlas coordinate system to a patient brain space would indicate an approximate location of the optimal surgical target within the nucleus. At our institution, the region of the Vim close to the border of the sensory thalamus (Vc) is considered to be the optimal target for tremor arrest with thalamotomy or thalamic DBS. The posterolateral part of the GPi is adopted as the ideal destination for pallidotomy, while the dorsolateral portion of STN is regarded as the most effective stimulation site for STN DBS. The distance between the centroid of the registered segmented Vim, GPi, or STN and the real target location of each patient who had been subject to thalamotomy, pallidotomy, or STN DBS procedure, respectively, was computed and evaluated (Table 11.2). The locations of more than 72% of the actual surgical targets are shown at the expected positions relative to the corresponding centroids.

Table 11.2. Absolute differences between the centroids of the segmented nuclei after nonrigid registration, and the real surgical targets.

Difference (mm)	Pallidotomy	Thalamotomy/thalamic DBS	STN DBS
Mean	2.53	2.24	2.80
Max	3.17	3.09	3.57
Min	0.97	1.05	1.21
Std	0.83	0.79	0.87

Clinical data are included from the thalamotomy, pallidotomy, thalamic DBS, and STN DBS procedures. System effectiveness in surgical targeting was assessed on 20 thalamotomy, 20 pallidotomy, 10 thalamic DBS procedures retrospectively, and 20 STN DBS procedures prospectively.

The results shown in Table 11.3 indicated that the average distance between the nonexpert-planned surgical targets and the expert-localized ones was on average less than 2 mm (thalamotomies: 1.95 ± 0.86 mm; pallidotomies: 1.83 ± 1.07 mm; thalamic DBS: 1.88 ± 0.89 mm; STN DBS: 1.61 ± 0.67 mm). Moreover, the final surgical targets chosen by the neurosurgeon were shown closer to the surgical sites determined with the combined information from both electrophysiological database and the anatomical resources than those defined either by standard image-based techniques, or by the mapping of a cluster of surgical targets onto the preoperative images. Hence, slight refinement of the target position initially estimated using this planning environment could enable the final surgical target to be reached with significantly less electrophysiological exploration. As a result, the duration required for the preoperative target/trajectory planning and intraoperative electrophysiological exploration can be greatly shortened without compromising surgical accuracy and precision, and the surgical procedure-elicited intracranial hemorrhage, brain tissue damage, and other related complications can be diminished by reducing the number of exploratory electrodes and the duration of the surgical process.

Table 11.3. Absolute distances between the real surgical targets and those estimated by a nonexpert on the basis of the database

Difference (mm)	Pallidotomy	Thalamotomy	Thalamic DBS	STN DBS
Mean	1.83	1.95	1.88	1.61
Max	2.79	2.69	2.41	2.82
Min	0.58	0.62	0.54	0.65
Std	1.07	0.86	0.89	0.67

11.11 Discussion

This chapter presents an overview of image-guided stereotactic neuro-surgical planning and guidance, including a demonstration of its specific application in the planning of therapy for Parkinson's disease and other movement disorders. This work emphasizes the value of moving beyond the structural image of the brain itself and incorporating functional information both from the individual patient and from a cohort of subjects who have already undergone similar procedures. By carefully collecting and labeling patient electrophysiological data and registering them, along with the preoperative images, to a standard reference image space, researchers made all of this information available to assist in the planning and guidance of procedures in new patients. Although this alone does not achieve the goal of "striking" the target on the first pass of a DBS probe, it does reduce the need for unnecessary additional exploratory trajectories that the surgeon would otherwise perform to refine the position of the ultimate target.

Although the studies for thalamotomy, pallidotomy, and thalamic DBS surgical targeting were carried out retrospectively, the surgical target estimation process for each case was performed according to those for STN DBS. The visualization capabilities, designed to present all the relevant functional and anatomical data with multiple virtual surgical instruments, make it possible to simulate actual surgical procedures. The relevant patient identification information, the physical parameters of the recording and stimulation probe used during the procedure, and the intraoperatively acquired electrophysiological data can be saved in a single file first, then nonrigidly mapped to the Colin27 template, and eventually stored in the functional database.

High quality anatomical and/or histological atlases [Chakravarty et al. 2006; Yelnick et al. 2007] containing more detailed deep brain information may enhance the accuracy of our system in surgical planning and targeting, and improve the reliability of the correlation between the anatomical structures and the electrophysiological organization. Although this system has reached a stage where prediction of surgical targets and trajectories has proved helpful, further clinical evaluation on the long-term surgical outcome is required for its thorough validation and application in stereotactic deep-brain neurosurgical procedures.

Acknowledgments

We thank Dr. David Gobbi, Dr. Yves Starreveld, and Kevin Wang for their assistance in the software development. The authors acknowledge financial support from the Canadian Institutes of Health Research (CIHR), the Ontario Research and Development Challenge Fund (ORDCF), the Canada Foundation for Innovation (CFI), and the Ontario Innovation Trust (OIT).

References

Alterman RL, Sterio D, Beric A, and Kelly PJ. (1999). "Microelectrode recording during posteroventral pallidotomy: Impact on target selection and complications." *Neurosurgery*, 44, 315–323.

Bertrand G, Oliver A, and Thompson CJ. (1973). "The computerized brain atlas: Its use in stereotaxic surgery." *Trans Am Neurol Assoc*, 98, 233–237.

Chakravarty MM, Sadikot AF, Mognia S, Bertrand G, and Collins DL. (2006). "Towards a multi-modal atlas for neurosurgical planning." *MICCAI Proceedings II,* Springer, Copenhagen, Denmark, 389–396.

Collins DL, Holmes CJ, Peters TM, and Evans AC. (1995). "Automatic 3-D model-based neuroanatomical segmentation." *Hum Brain Mapp*, 3, 190–208.

Cuny E, Guehl D, Burbaud P, Gross C, Dousset V, and Rougier A. (2002). "Lack of agreement between direct magnetic resonance imaging and statistical determination of a subthalamic target: The role of electrophysiological guidance." *J Neurosurg*, 97(3), 591–597.

D'Haese PF, Cetinkaya E, Konrad PE, Kao C, and Dawant BM. (2005a). "Computer-aided placement of deep brain stimulators: From planning to intraoperative guidance." *IEEE Trans Med Imag,* 24(11), 1469–1478.

D'Haese PF, Pallavaram S, Niermann K, Spooner J, Kao C, Konrad PE, and Dawant BM. (2005b). "Automatic selection of DBS target points using multiple electrophysiological atlases." *MICCAI*, 8 (Pt 2), 427–434.

Dawant BM, Hartmann SL, Pan S, and Gadamsetty S. (2002). "Brain atlas deformation in the presence of small and large space-occupying tumors." *Comput Aided Surg*, 7(1), 1–10.

Evans AC, Kamber M, Collins DL, MacDonald D, Shorvan SD, et al. (1994). "An MRI based probabilistic atlas of neuroanatomy." *Magnetic Resonance Scanning and Epilepsy*, Plenum Press, New York, 263–274.

Finnis KW, Starreveld YP, Parrent AG, Sadikot AF, and Peters TM. (2003). "Three-dimensional database of subcortical electrophysiology for image-guided stereotactic functional neurosurgery." *IEEE Trans Med Imag*, 22(1), 93–104.

Ganser KA, Dickhaus H, Metzner R, and Wirtz CR. (2004). "A deformable digital brain atlas system according to Talairach and Tournoux." *Med Image Anal*, 8(1), 3–22.

Giorgi C, Cerchiari U, Broggi G, Birk P, and Struppeler A. (1985). "Digital image processing to handle neuroanatomical information and neurophysiological data." *Appl Neurophysiol*, 48, 30–33.

Guo T, Finnis KW, Parrent AG, and Peters TM. (2005). "Development and application of functional databases for planning deep-brain neurosurgical procedures." *MICCAI*, 8(Pt 1), 835–842.

Guo T, Finnis KW, Parrent AG, and Peters TM. (2006). "Visualization and navigation system development and application for stereotactic deep-brain neurosurgeries." *Comput Aided Surg*, 11(5), 231–239.

Guo T, Parrent AG, Peters TM. (2007). "Surgical targeting accuracy analysis of six methods for subthalamic nucleus deep brain stimulation". *Comput Assist Surg*, 12(6): 325–334.

Guridi J, Gorospe A, Ramos E, Linazasoro G, Rodriguez MC, and Obeso JA. (1999). "Stereotactic targeting of the globus pallidus internus in Parkinson's disease: Imaging versus electrophysiological mapping." *Neurosurgery*, 45(2), 278–287; discussion 287–279.

Halpern C, Hurtig H, Jaggi J, Grossman M, Won M, and Baltuch G. (2007). "Deep brain stimulation in neurologic disorders." *Parkinsonism Relat Disord*, 13(1), 1–16.

Hamani C, Richter E, Schwalb JM, and Lozano AM. (2005). "Bilateral subthalamic nucleus stimulation for Parkinson's disease: A systematic review the clinical literature." *Neurosurgery*, 56(6), 1313–1321.

Holmes CJ, Hoge R, Collins L, Woods R, Toga AW, and Evans AC. (1998). "Enhancement of MR images using registration for signal averaging." *J Comput Assist Tomo*, 22(2), 324–333.

Kall BA, Kelly PJ, Goerss SJ, and Frieder G. (1985). "Methodology and clinical experience with computed tomography and a computer-resident stereotactic atlas." *Neurosurgery*, 17(3), 400–407.

Lehman RM, Zheng J, Hamilton JL, and Micheli-Tzanakou E. (2000). "Comparison of 3-D stereoscopic MR imaging with pre and post lesion recording in pallidotomy." *Acta Neurochirurgica*, 142, 319–328.

Machado A, Rezai AR, Kopell BH, Gross RE, Sharan AD, and Benabid AL. (2006). "Deep brain stimulation for Parkinson's disease: Surgical technique and perioperative management." *Mov Disord*, 21(14 Suppl), S247–S258.

Mark VH and Yakovlev PI. (1995). "A note on problems and methods in the preparation of a human stereotactic atlas." *Anat Rec*, 121, 745–752.

Nowinski W, Yeo T, and Yang GL. (1997). "Atlas-based system for functional neurosurgery." *SPIE Medical Imaging – The International Society for Optical Engineering*, Bellingham, WA, 92–103.

Nowinski WL, Belov D, and Benabid AL. (2003). "An algorithm for rapid calculation of a probabilistic functional atlas of subcortical structures from electrophysiological data collected during functional neurosurgery procedures." *NeuroImage*, 18(1), 143–155.

Nowinski WL, Belov D, Pollak P, and Benabid AL. (2005a). "Statistical analysis of 168 bilateral subthalamic nucleus implantations by means of the probabilistic functional atlas." *Neurosurgery*, 57(4 Suppl.), 319–330; discussion 319–330.

Nowinski WL, Belov D, Thirunavuukarasuu A, and Benabid AL. (2005b). "A probabilistic functional atlas of the VIM nucleus constructed from pre-, intra- and postoperative electrophysiological and neuroimaging data acquired during the surgical treatment of Parkinson's disease patients." *Stereotact Funct Neurosurg*, 83(5–6), 190–196.

Nowinski WL, Fang A, Nguyen BT, Raphel JK, Jagannathan L, Raghavan R, Bryan RN, and Miller GA. (1998). "Multiple brain atlas database and atlas-based neuroimaging system." *Comput Aided Surg*, 2, 42–66.

Perlmutter JS and Mink JW. (2006). "Deep brain stimulation." *Annu Rev Neurosci*, 29, 229–257.

Rodriguez MC, Obeso JA, and Olanow CW. (1998). "Subthalamic nucleus- mediated excitotoxicity in Parkinson's disease: A target for neuroprotection." *Ann Neurol*, 44(3 Suppl. 1), 175–188.

Schaltenbrand G and Wahren W. (1977). *Atlas for Stereotaxy of the Human Brain*, Thieme, Stuttgart.

St-Jean P, Sadikot AF, Collins DL, Clonda D, Kasrai R, Evans AC, and Peters TM. (1998). "Automated atlas integration and interactive 3-dimensional visuali- zation tools for planning and guidance in functional neurosurgery." *IEEE Trans Med Imag*, 17(5), 672–680.

Starr PA, Vitek JL, DeLong M, and Bakay RA. (1999). "Magnetic resonance imaging-based stereotactic localization of the globus pallidus and subthalamic nucleus." *Neurosurgery*, 44(2), 303–313.

Sterio D, Zonenshayn M, Mogilner A, Rezai AR, Kiprovski K, Kelly PJ, and Beric A. (2002). "Neurophysiological refinement of subthalamic nucleus targeting." *Neurosurgery*, 50, 58–69.

Talairach J and Tourneau P. (1988). *Co-planar Stereotaxic Atlas of the Human Brain*, Georg Thieme Verlag, Stuttgart.

Tasker RR, Organ LW, and Hawrylyshyn PA. (1982). *The Thalamus and Midbrain of Man*, Charles C. Thomas, Springfield.

Thompson CJ, Hardy TL, and Bertrand G. (1977). "A system for anatomical and functional mapping of the human thalamus." *Comput Biomed Res*, 10(1), 9–24.

Thompson PM, Toga AW, Brody W, and Zerhouni E. (2000). "Warping strategies for intersubject registration." In: *Handbook of Medical Imaging*, Bronzino J, ed., Academic Press, San Diego, 659–601.

Toga AW, Thompson PM, Mori S, Amunts K, and Zilles K. (2006). "Towards multimodal atlases of the human brain." *Nat Rev Neurosci*, 7(12), 952–966.

van Buren J and Borke R. (1972). *Variations and Connections of the Human Thalamus*, Springer, Berlin Heidelburg New York.

Yelnick J, Bardinet E, Dormont D, Malandain G, Ourselin S, Tande D, Karachi C, Ayache N, Cornu P, and Agid Y. (2007). "A three-dimensional, histological and deformable atlas of the human basal ganglia. I. Atlas construction based on immunohistochemical and MRI data." *NeuroImage*, 34(2), 618–638.

Yoshida M. (1987). "Creation of a three-dimensional atlas by interpolation from Schaltenbrand-Bailey's atlas." *Appl Neurophysiol*, 50(45), 48.

Yoshida M, Okada K, Nagase A, Kuga S, Shirahama M, Watanabe M, and Kuramoto S. (1982). "Neurophysiological atlas of the human thalamus and adjacent structures." *Appl Neurophysiol*, 45, 406–409.

Zonenshayn M, Rezai AR, Mogilner AY, Beric A, Sterio D, and Kelly PJ. (2000). "Comparison of anatomic and neurophysiological methods for subthalamic nucleus targeting." *Neurosurgery*, 47(2), 282–294.

Chapter 12

Computer-Assisted Orthopedic Surgery

Antony Hodgson

Abstract

Orthopedic surgeons treat musculoskeletal disorders such as arthritis, scoliosis, and trauma, which collectively affect hundreds of millions of people and are the leading cause of pain and disability. In this chapter, the main technical developments related to computer-assisted surgery (CAS) in several key areas of orthopedic surgery are reviewed: hip and knee replacements, spine surgery, and fracture repair. We also assess the evaluations of these systems performed to date, with a particular focus on the value proposition that CAS needs to deliver in order for it to become widely accepted. This means it must demonstrate better performance, less operating room time, and reduced costs.

We describe several systems for both hip and knee replacement that are based on computed tomographic (CT) images, intraoperative fluoroscopy, or image-free kinematic techniques, and in each domain consider both manual and robotic systems. Future work in computer-assisted orthopedic surgery will include efforts to develop newer technologies such as 3D ultrasound and ever less invasive procedures, but it must also concentrate on improving operative workflow, to transfer the benefits of improved accuracy to nonspecialist orthopedic surgeons working in community hospitals, where the case volumes are lower than in specialized centers. Linkages between improved accuracy during surgery and improved functional outcomes for the patients must be demonstrated for these technologies to be widely accepted.

12.1 Introduction

Orthopedics is the surgical discipline that treats musculoskeletal injuries and diseases, most notably fractures and various forms of arthritis. Although orthopedic problems do not have the same degree of public awareness as cancer and heart disease, because they are seldom life-threatening, their impact on public health is immense. Hundreds of millions of patients around the world suffer from musculoskeletal disorders, which are a leading cause of pain and disability and account for almost half of all chronic conditions

T. Peters and K. Cleary (eds.), *Image-Guided Interventions.*
© Springer Science + Business Media, LLC 2008

amongst people who are aged 50 and above in developed countries [CDC 2003]. Because of the *baby boomer* phenomenon, the number of patients with such conditions is expected to increase dramatically in the coming years.

The resulting costs to health care systems will be enormous. According to the Arthritis Foundation (http://www.arthritis.org/bone-joint-decade.php), musculoskeletal disorders account for 20% of all visits to outpatient facilities around the world and, in the USA in 1995, generated more visits to physicians (130 million per year) than any other category of illness, at a cost of $215B. There is, therefore, significant pressure on public health systems to prevent the disease processes, and on health care systems to provide effective, durable treatments when disease occurs. The focus of this chapter will be on this latter issue, in the use of computer-assisted technologies to improve treatment.

In general, orthopedics is a mature surgical discipline. Practitioners have developed effective techniques for treating both acute injuries and long-term degenerative diseases, and many orthopedic interventions offer immediate and long-lasting relief to their patients. Hip and knee joint replacement surgeries are prime examples of effective interventions, with success rates over 90% (as measured by percentage of implants surviving 10 or more years after implantation). However, because of the sheer number of these procedures performed (over 700,000 hip and knee replacement procedures performed annually in the USA alone) [Kozak et al. 2006], a 5–10% annual revision rate represents a substantial number of patients. Given that revision surgery for a failed joint implant costs upwards of $11,000 [Slover et al. 2006], annual direct surgical costs associated with these failures will soon approach $1 billion, providing considerable incentive to improve the effectiveness of these procedures.

In addition to the potential for improving the longevity of surgical interventions, other challenges faced by orthopedic surgeons relate to improving postoperative function, optimizing fracture repairs to avoid later development of osteoarthritis, minimizing hospital stays following surgery, minimizing the period of recovery and return to work, avoiding infection, and minimizing blood loss during surgery. As all these challenges are affected either by how accurately bone fragments or artificial components are aligned with respect to one another or by the degree of disruption to soft tissues, there is significant potential for computer-assisted surgical techniques to contribute to the refinement of orthopedic interventions by quantifying key aspects of these surgical procedures and enabling surgeons to more precisely control their surgical actions.

In many ways, orthopedic surgery is the most obvious and natural application domain for CAS techniques because so many procedures are performed on bones, which are essentially rigid. It is considerably easier to track bones or fragments across time than to monitor changes in deformable tissues, as occurs in neurosurgery (for more information, please see Chap. 11) and abdominal surgery (Chap. 13). Because of this, many of the early applications of CAS techniques were in fact in orthopedic surgery. However, despite well over a decade of development, CAS systems still have not been widely adopted by orthopedic surgeons, and there is continuing controversy over their value.

For example, a recent review of the factors influencing acceptance of computer-assisted orthopedic surgical (CAOS) technologies, conducted in 2005 by the University of Nottingham's Multidisciplinary Assessment of Technology Centre for Healthcare (MATCH) group [Craven et al. 2005], concluded that there was "poor validation of accuracy, lack of standardization, inappropriate outcomes measures for assessing and comparing technologies, unresolved debate about the effectiveness of minimally invasive surgery, and issues of medical device regulations, cost, autonomy of surgeons to choose equipment, ergonomics, and training." The authors went on to state that more dialogue is needed "between surgeons and manufacturers....to develop standardized measurements and outcomes scoring systems," and that increased attention should be paid to user requirements.

The opinion that the current state of CAOS technology is too premature for widespread market deployment has been echoed by numerous other bodies over the past few years. The US NIH Consensus Development Report on Total Knee Replacement [2003] concluded that although there was evidence that accuracy was enhanced, costs were higher, operating room time was generally increased, and the benefits were unclear. The Ontario Health Technology Advisory Committee [2004] noted that navigation and robotic technologies were still in an investigational phase. In September 2006, the California Blue Cross assessed whether or not navigated orthopedic surgical procedures should be eligible for reimbursement, and concluded that such procedures were considered investigational and not medically necessary. This Blue Cross study noted the relative lack of randomized control trials for femoral nail or pelvic fracture repairs, and with regard to total hip arthroplasty (THA), recognized the link between malignment of the components and a tendency toward subsequent dislocation, but again, there were no controlled trials for THA available. For total knee arthroplasty (TKA), only two randomized trials were identified [Saragaglia et al. 2001; Decking et al. 2005]. Saragaglia showed a tendency toward improvement in alignment (84% of 25 patients within 3° of target for CAS vs. 75% in the conventional group), but this result did not achieve statistical significance. Decking confirmed this result, showing a statistically significantly greater proportion of well-aligned limbs in the CAS group, although there was no significant difference between the groups in the clinical scores (Knee Society Score or Western Ontario and McMaster Universities Osteoarthritis Index), and no follow up beyond three months.

This chapter briefly presents the major areas of orthopedic surgery and the challenges faced by surgeons to identify the clinical opportunities for which computer-assisted techniques can provide a potential solution. The main technical developments in these various application areas over the past 20 years are reviewed, with a particular focus on the evaluations carried out to date. Finally, some promising directions for future development are highlighted.

12.2   Orthopedic Practice

12.2.1 Clinical Practice of Orthopedics

The term *orthopedics* was introduced in 1741 by a French physician, Nicolas Andre, and literally means *straight child*, reflecting the early orthopedists' concern with bracing of children suffering from limb and spine deformities. In the twentieth century, orthopedic practice became a surgical specialty as its practioners began treating war injuries, poliomyelitis, and other musculoskeletal diseases affecting the structural tissues of bone, ligament, tendon, muscle, and cartilage, as well as the associated nerves, arteries, and veins.

Broadly speaking, orthopedic practice can be divided according to the joints and bones of the body: upper limb (shoulder, elbow, and wrist), spine (neck and back), pelvis and hip, knee, and foot and ankle. The hand can be the domain of orthopedic surgeons as well, although many procedures are now normally handled by plastic surgeons. Clinical conditions addressed by orthopedic surgeons include congenital disorders (e.g., scoliosis), the various forms of arthritis, bone and soft tissue cancers, and trauma.

Another way of classifying orthopedic practice is according to the types of procedures commonly performed. A recent report from the Med-TechInsight consulting group (February 2007) summarizes the 33 million surgical procedures performed in all surgical specialties in the US in 2006. Their categorization of the subset of orthopedic procedures identifies the following five main groups:

1. Fracture repair (generally due to trauma)
2. Total joint arthroplasty (knee and hip)
3. Spine surgery
4. Disc replacement (discectomy, laminectomy and laminotomy, spinal fusion, and vertebroplasty)
5. Arthroscopy (knee, shoulder, and wrist)

Some key landmarks in the development of orthopedic practice have included the introduction of hip and knee joint replacements in the 1960s, arthroscopic repair of cartilage and ligament injuries in the 1970s and 1980s, rigid bone fixation techniques in the 1980s, and biologic agents in the 1990s.

12.2.2 CAOS Procedures

Within the five surgical areas identified earlier, the developers of CAS technologies have identified several situations where precise positioning or implant orientation could play a strong role in the clinical outcome. Other reasons for developing computer-assisted techniques include the promotion of minimally invasive surgical techniques, reducing radiation exposure, bringing younger surgeons more rapidly up the learning curve, reducing time and cost in the operating room, and documenting operating room actions for medicolegal reasons.

In a recent review volume, Stiehl et al. [2006a] classify CAOS systems as relating to the following five domains: total knee arthroplasty, anterior cruciate ligament reconstruction, total hip arthroplasty, reconstruction and trauma surgery, and spinal surgery. In an earlier volume, Nolte and Ganz [1999] identified the key applications for CAS as the spine (pedicle screw placement), the hip (acetabular osteotomies, total hip replacement, pelvic osteotomies, iliosacral screw placement), and the knee (arthroplasty, anterior cruciate ligament reconstruction). In addition to procedure-specific techniques, certain technologies such as virtual fluoroscopy (obtaining an initial set of X-rays and subsequently continuously monitoring the position of surgical tools on these images during the procedure as if fluoroscopic imaging were continuing) can be applied to multiple surgical tasks.

This chapter focuses on a set of orthopedic surgical applications that have received considerable attention from the developers of computer-assisted technologies, which are as follows:

1. Hip arthroplasty – total joint and resurfacing
2. Knee arthroplasty – total and unicompartmental
3. Pedicle screw insertions
4. Fracture fragment alignment and distal intramedullary nail locking.

Two other areas for which CAS systems have been developed, but which are not discussed in detail here, are:

1. Anterior cruciate ligament reconstruction
2. Pelvic and tibial osteotomies.

For each application, we discuss the clinical challenges associated with the traditional techniques, review the history of CAOS technology as applied to the application, assess the evaluations of the various CAOS systems that have been performed, and identify key directions for future research. Before discussing each application in detail, however, the existing technologies available to orthopedic surgeons are briefly reviewed.

12.2.3 Review of Quantitative Technologies Used in Orthopedics

In conventional orthopedic surgery practice, surgeons have access to a variety of imaging technologies, all of which are also used in CAS systems.

12.2.3.1 X-Rays, CT, and MRI

Orthopedic surgeons rely heavily on X-rays in their practice. Plain, two-dimensional X-rays are routinely acquired for virtually all orthopedic problems: trauma, varus (bowlegged) or valgus (knock-kneed) knees, arthritic hips, and spinal deformities, among others. Three-dimensional computed tomographic (CT) scans are more expensive than plain X-rays and involve higher radiation doses, so they are less commonly acquired, although they are used for more complex fracture cases, spinal deformation (e.g., scoliosis) and selected arthritic cases. Magnetic resonance imaging (MRI), another 3D imaging technology is occasionally used, but as it tends to be better suited for soft tissue imaging, it is most commonly employed when the problem is primarily related to soft tissues such as muscle or cartilage.

12.2.3.2 C-Arm Fluoroscopy

None of the technologies described earlier are commonly available in the operating room. However, a portable X-ray device known as a C-arm is widely used for intraoperative imaging. C-arms have an X-ray source at one end of a C-shaped arm and a detector at the other, which enables surgeons to obtain intraoperative images of any portion of the anatomy that can be placed within the cone-shaped radiation beam of the machine. These images are relatively small (up to about 15 cm in diameter), but can typically be acquired in under a minute. In addition, images can be acquired continuously at up to 30 frames per second, so continuous monitoring of a surgical intervention such as a fracture reduction is possible.

In the past 10 years, techniques have been developed for combining multiple images from different angular orientations over a period of several dozen seconds into a low-resolution 3D image similar to that produced by a CT scanner. New surgical techniques based on these capabilities are still in the early stages of development, and some of them are discussed later in conjunction with some recent computer-assisted techniques.

12.2.3.3 Ultrasound

Ultrasound is another imaging technology that is widely used in other areas of medicine, but is relatively uncommon in orthopedics. Its images have generally been considered too noisy for diagnostic purposes, but it has many desirable features as an intraoperative imaging modality; it is radiation-free, comparatively inexpensive, and can produce 3D images in real time. Several research groups, including our own, are currently experimenting with using ultrasound in conjunction with CAS systems to locate anatomical structures intraoperatively.

12.2.3.4 Statistical Shape Modeling

A significantly different way to obtain a 3D model of a bone for use in the operating room is to use a technique known as statistical shape modeling (or anatomical atlases). With this technique, the 3D shapes of a variety of sample bones are measured, and the resulting representations are stored in a database. The stored shapes are analyzed and decomposed into a relatively small number of *modes* describing the main ways in which different bones vary relative to one another. For example, the first mode might represent the average bone scaled for size, the second mode might represent thickness changes for a given size, and the third mode may represent some asymmetry. This is similar in concept to the various signal decomposition techniques used in various engineering domains (e.g., Fourier or wavelet decomposition). Intraoperatively, the patient's anatomy is measured by any of a variety of methods (fluoroscopy, direct digitization with a tracked pointer, ultrasound, or laser scanner) and the parameters of the most significant modes are adjusted to optimize the match between the adjusted model and the intraoperative measurements. In many situations, this technique can produce a well-described 3D model that is accurate to within 2–3 mm over its entire surface.

12.3   Evaluation

We noted earlier that health care funders generally regard computer-assisted orthopedic surgery as still being in a relatively early stage of development with insufficient evidence of value yet being available to justify reimbursement as procedures distinct from their conventional counterparts. The onus is therefore on developers of CAOS systems to demonstrate some combination of improved outcomes, reduced operative and recovery times, shorter learning curves for surgeons, and reduced costs (this set of considerations is sometimes summarized as *Better, Faster, Cheaper*), which can make acquisition of a CAOS system attractive to a hospital, an insurer, or a health maintenance organization, depending on how health care services are funded in a particular jurisdiction. In this section, we consider in more detail how system developers can establish these benefits for their systems.

12.3.1 Improved Technical and Functional Outcomes

To date, most evaluations of computer-assisted technologies or techniques have focused on short-term technical outcomes of the procedures. For example, in total knee replacement surgery, the most commonly reported outcome is the mechanical axis alignment (hip–knee–ankle (HKA) angle) in the frontal plane as evaluated on postoperative X-ray images. This outcome measure is based largely on a study of 115 total knee replacement surgery patients by Jeffery et al. [1991] in which they showed that the risk of early failure of knee implants was significantly increased when the HKA angle was more than 3° off neutral (24% failure rate at 8 years postsurgery in the one-third of patients in this group compared with a 3% failure rate in the two-thirds of patients with a mechanical alignment within this 3° window).

In total hip replacement surgery, the most commonly reported technical outcome is the alignment of the acetabular cup. For example, Haaker et al. [2007] reported that the standard deviation in cup placement was significantly lower using CAOS techniques (1.0° in inclination and 1.7° in version vs. 2.6° and 3.8° for the manual technique), although in both cases the range was large (28° in inclination and 33° in version for CAOS vs. 38° and 44° for the manual technique).

On the femoral side of total hip arthroplasty, an important issue has been the regularity of the hole that is formed to accept the femoral component. Conventionally, this hole is broached by hand, which produces an irregular hole with significant gaps (up to several millimeter) between the implant and the bone. With cemented implants, this is not a particularly significant problem, but there has been a long-standing debate in the surgical community as to the relative effectiveness of cemented vs. cementless implants. Bone can only effectively integrate into cementless implants if the gap between the implant and bone is in the order of 1 mm or less [Dalton et al. 1995], which cannot be achieved over more than a small portion of the implant surface with hand-broaching techniques. This limitation led to one of the earliest uses of robotics in surgery; Paul, Mittelstadt, and their colleagues adapted an industrial robot to mill the femoral cavity during total hip arthroplasty surgery [Paul et al. 1992]; this system eventually became a commercial product known as RoboDoc. In several papers, the RoboDoc developers and clinical users demonstrated improved accuracy of the femoral cavity [Schneider and Kalender 2003] and showed that the mean error produced by robotic milling was within 0.5 mm.

One final example of a short-term technical outcome is in the field of spinal fusion surgery. In such surgeries, the goal is to prevent relative motion of adjacent spinal segments by attaching mechanical hardware to two or more vertebrae, using screws inserted into the lateral channels of the vertebrae that link the posterior spinal processes to the vertebral body. These lateral channels are known as the pedicles, and the surgeon's task is to insert screws down these channels. If the screws are misdirected so that they pierce the medial side of the channel, they can impinge on the spinal cord and cause nerve injuries. This task is increasingly difficult as one moves up the spinal column because the vertebrae become smaller. Studies comparing computer-assisted to conventional techniques typically report the number of pedicular breaches, for example Lee et al. [2007].

Although these technical measures can serve as evidence that the computer-assisted techniques are generally capable of matching or exceeding the mechanical alignment accuracies achieved by well-trained surgeons using conventional manual techniques, by themselves, they have not been sufficient to allow funders to conclude that there are corresponding functional improvements for the patients that would justify either purchase or reimbursement. The challenge for researchers is to link improvements in these technical measures to demonstrable improvements in outcome measures. To date, there have been few such studies. One main reason for this in the case of arthroplasty procedures is that the success rates are already very good; often exceeding 90% survival at 10 years or longer, which makes it difficult to enroll a sufficient number of patients in a study and track them over a long enough period to show a significant difference in outcome. Furthermore, once an institution begins using CAS techniques, it becomes difficult to enroll patients in the control group; the patients naturally believe that the computer-assisted technique represents the state-of-the-art and are reluctant to be randomized to the control group. This implies that future comparative studies will increasingly become limited either to institutions that are introducing computer-assisted procedures, in which case the results are likely to be confounded with learning curve issues, or to interinstitutional studies in which differences between sites will likely confound the results.

The outcomes used in such studies are themselves an important matter for discussion. In arthroplasty studies, for example, the most common outcome measure used is the revision rate, but this measure does not adequately capture the broad range of ways in which a patient's life might be affected or improved by surgery. Other important considerations are how quickly the patient can return to their normal activities, how much their activities are affected by any deficits in function, and how much pain they continue to suffer. This latter issue has been surprisingly understudied. In a retrospective study performed at our institution [Anglin et al. 2004], we found that a significant fraction of patients reported an increase in the amount of pain they experienced following surgery, despite correction of their varus/valgus malalignment. Fortunately, increasing attention has been paid over the past decade to the need to acquire good measures of surgical outcomes, following some of the earlier studies that demonstrated that scores such as the Short Form 36 could be acquired in a cost-effective manner, which could show demonstrable improvements in several different aspects of a patient's subjective postoperative experience [Patt and Mauerhan 2005; Arslanian and Bond 1999].

A number of studies of computer-assisted orthopedic procedures have now reported a variety of functional outcome measurements ranging from more technical measures such as joint range of motion, to more task-related measures such as ability to walk specified distances or climb stairs. A number of procedure or joint-specific evaluation scores exist that have been shown to be reliable and repeatable measures both of functional results and impact on patients' lives, but many of these measures are relatively coarse and may not accurately reflect the specific aspects that are of most concern to patients. For example, in a study of the functional outcomes of acetabular fracture surgery, Moed et al. [2003] reported that despite achieving good to excellent results according to the modified Merle d'Aubigné clinical hip score, which "is the most generally accepted clinical grading system for evaluating the results of acetabular fracture treatment," the results of a functional assessment using the Musculoskeletal Function Assessment score showed that the patients still had not returned to their preinjury functional levels. The authors concluded that the clinical hip score has limited usefulness in assessing the results of acetabular fracture surgery.

12.3.2 Reduced Operative Times

Although proponents of CAOS systems often have envisioned that such techniques will be able to reduce the time needed to perform surgical procedures, to date most computer-assisted procedures in fact require additional time, both pre and interoperatively, due to the need to set up the equipment before the procedure and to perform various marker attachment and Registration steps during the surgery. The overall impact on operative time has occasionally been reported (for arthroplasty procedures, the increase in operative time is often reported as being in the range of 10–20 min), but few detailed studies yet exist to help researchers understand exactly where these increases in operative time arise, and the potential for decreasing the time impact.

In some selected procedures, time savings have been reported. For example, in spinal fusion procedures, considerable time is spent using fluoroscopy to target the pedicles, and CAS systems have succeeded in reducing both surgical time and fluoroscopy time [Sasso and Garrido 2007]. Time savings are important because of impacts on overall patient throughput, because operating room costs are high – on the order of $20 per minute [Weinbroum et al. 2003], and because extended anesthesia time can increase the risk to the patient.

12.3.3 Reduced Costs

Even if CAS procedures can be shown to improve patients' functional outcomes or to reduce time in the operating room, they are not cost-free. Early CAOS systems were very expensive, costing upwards of $300,000, which is comparable to a high-end fluoroscopy machine, and often involved per-procedure supply costs of several hundred dollars. Such costs have made it even more difficult for such procedures to be accepted. There have been some significant reductions in price of these systems in recent years, with simpler systems now selling in the $50–100,000 range (or available on a per-procedure basis for several hundred dollars, including supplies), but these expenses must nevertheless be more than compensated for by cost reductions elsewhere in the patient care process. Such reductions could potentially be realized in the form of decreased operating room time, decreased length of stay in hospital, decreased recovery times, decreased revision rates, or increased postoperative function. Accounting for some of these costs is often difficult, and there is often little connection between the entity incurring greater costs at the time of the operation (generally the hospital) and the entity receiving the long-term benefits (potentially the patient). It is, therefore, difficult to make the argument that the hospital incurs the additional costs if they are not going to benefit financially from the resulting benefits. Nonetheless, a full evaluation of CAOS technologies should include a careful assessment of any potential cost savings for any element of the health care system or for the patient [Beringer et al. 2007; Bozic and Beringer 2007].

12.3.4 Other Issues Affecting Adoption

In the end, issues other than direct cost-benefit considerations may drive adoption of computer-assisted technologies. Issues related to how the technologies affect surgical practice may be important, as may be legal considerations and marketing pressures. Although the comments below focus specifically on CAOS systems, they apply in general to the other computer-assisted interventional procedures discussed elsewhere in this book.

12.3.4.1 Surgical Practice Implications

Surgeons have a direct interest in CAOS systems because they affect how surgeons practice. Hüfner et al. [2004] point out that a navigation system must fit in with the set of equipment and case mix that a surgeon normally uses. An additional important reason for surgeons to consider adopting CAOS systems is the potential for reducing radiation exposure to themselves and the surgical team. As an increasing number of procedures are done under fluoroscopic or CT guidance, especially with the emergence of newer 3D fluoroscopy systems, surgeons and their teams are exposed to an increasing cumulative radiation dose over their working lifetimes, particularly if they perform particular surgeries or use particular techniques [Rampersaud et al. 2000].

12.3.4.2 Legal Considerations

On the legal side, there is considerable evidence now that computer-assisted procedures, particularly in knee arthroplasty and pedicle screw insertions, can reduce the number of outliers. Patients who have undergone a conventional procedure that produces an outlying result and who subsequently experience a poorer than expected outcome may increasingly decide to pursue a legal remedy on the basis of the argument that technology exists that could have prevented their poor outcome, and that the hospital is liable for not offering state-of-the-art care. This argument is unlikely to prevail in the short term, given the numerous assessments that deem CAOS technology to be premature, but it will likely become increasingly powerful over time given the number of cases brought against surgeons employing current practices [AAOS 1999]. At the same time, legal issues can potentially limit the introduction of new surgical technologies. In Germany, for example, there have been legal cases brought against the manufacturer of the RoboDoc system related to a purported increased rate of complications when using the device [Schräder 2005].

12.3.4.3 Marketing Pressures

In some jurisdictions, most notably the United States, many hospitals must compete for patients, and a key element in their marketing arsenal is the offer of state-of-the-art health technology. Such hospitals not only face enquiries from educated patients seeking particular types of procedures, but they actively advertise their technological capabilities to patients as an enticement to be treated at their facility. For example, a 2005 article in the Boston Globe described the aggressive marketing program conducted by a Massachusetts hospital, which had acquired a surgical robot. This hospital used billboard ads and sent information kits to potential patients who had enquired about prostate surgery, despite an absence of demonstrated long-term benefits of the robotic procedure, promising as it may be [Kowalczyk 2005]. A similar concern about such marketing efforts for surgical robots was expressed more recently in an editorial in the Medical Journal of Australia [Maddern 2007]: "[the purchase of robots by private hospitals] has caused some concern within segments of the surgical community, as the motives for installing these robotic machines appear to be more commercial and marketing-oriented than based on well-established science and surgical benefit. However, as more than half of the surgical procedures in our health system are performed in the private sector, it is hardly surprising that aggressive marketing and commercial interests should be factors in the availability of robotic surgery."

12.3.5 Prospective Randomized Clinical Trials

The standard for evaluating clinical evidence is often said to be the prospective randomized clinical trial (PRCT). In a PRCT trial, researchers compare a proposed technique against its conventional counterpart by controlling for as many variables as possible. In general, a well-defined patient population is randomly divided into a control and an intervention group: the control group receives the conventional treatment, while the intervention group receives the treatment that is hypothesized to be superior. The criteria for evaluation are specified in advance and are monitored prospectively, that is, after a suitable period of follow up, ideally by assessors who are blinded to the intervention a particular patient received. PRCTs avoid problems with selection or treatment bias and so are regarded as the most reliable type of evaluation study.

In the field of CAOS, however, relatively few such studies have been performed. A Medline search for "randomized computer-assisted orthopedic surgery" produced only three articles that described actual PRCTs, while searching for "prospective computer-assisted orthopedic surgery" added only one more. These studies are briefly outlined below; more detailed discussions of the issues raised can be found in the following sections describing particular procedures.

Three of these four studies relate to pedicle screw placement. Richards et al. [2007] reported that a CAOS system enabled junior surgeons to achieve a significantly higher successful placement rate for pedicle screws in a cadaveric porcine model. Seller et al. [2005] performed a prospective intraindividual comparison of pedicle screw placement in 16 patients undergoing spine surgery and also found a significantly increased successful placement rate. Laine et al. [1997] performed a prospective study of pedicle screw insertion, but did not randomize patients; only patients who could not be treated by the CAOS technique were treated conventionally, so the decreased malplacement rate in the CAOS-treated group may have been due to this group being easier to treat than the conventionally treated group.

In the fourth study, Parratte and Argenson [2007] recently reported a reduction in the variance of acetabular cup placement using an image-free CAOS system with no significant difference in the average position relative to the preplanned target orientation. The CAOS procedure took an average of 12 min longer than the conventional freehand procedure.

In summary, there is currently a paucity of evidence for the benefits of CAOS that meets the standard of the prospective, randomized clinical trial, and even the studies of decreased malplacement rates of pedicle screws do not show any significant difference in functional outcomes for patients. Although somewhat discouraging for those advocating adoption of CAOS systems, some researchers believe that PRCTs may themselves not be justified from a cost-effectiveness point of view. For example, Meikle [2005] argues that in the field of dentofacial interventions, PRCTs have not contributed significant new knowledge, but have served mainly to confirm what was already widely believed based on years of clinical experience.

12.4   Practice Areas

This section discusses in more detail four key practice areas in the field of orthopedic surgery where computer-assisted techniques have been developed. These four are:

1. Hip arthroplasty   – total joint and resurfacing
2. Knee arthroplasty – total and unicompartmental
3. Screw insertions   – pedicle, iliosacral, and femoral neck
4. Fracture fragment alignment and distal intramedullary nail locking

In each of these four areas, we discuss the clinical motivation for using computer guidance, describe examples of the major approaches used to address the clinical problem, and provide an overview of the evaluations of the computer-assisted approaches that have been carried out.

12.4.1 Hip Replacement

12.4.1.1 Clinical Motivation

A large number of people suffer from deterioration of the hip joint because of diseases such as osteoarthritis, rheumatoid arthritis, avascular necrosis, ankylosing spondilytis, tumors and trauma. These diseases cause significant pain and loss of mobility, so the impact on patients' quality of life is large. When these conditions have progressed to the point where more conservative treatments such as nonsteroidal antiinflammatory agents are no longer providing sufficient relief, joint replacement is often considered. The original low friction hip replacement was invented almost 50 years ago by Sir John Charnley, an orthopedic surgeon at the Centre for Hip Surgery in Wrightington, England, and has proven enormously successful with implant survival rates sometimes exceeding 90% at 15–20 years [Skutek et al. 2007]. It is also one of the most commonly performed orthopedic procedures with over 230,000 surgeries performed annually in the United States in 2004 [Kozak et al. 2006]. Nonetheless, for reasons such as increasing obesity at younger ages coupled with a general extension in lifespan, an increasing number of patients become candidates for joint replacement at a point where they can still expect to live another 30–50 years. As revision surgery to replace an implant is more difficult than the original procedure, and surgery places older patients at greater risk than younger ones, there is a strong incentive to take every step possible to maximize the lifespan of the implants.

Hip implants have been shown to fail prematurely for three main reasons: infection, instability, and wear. Infection is the most devastating complication of joint replacement, but infection rates are comparatively low.

Brander, for example, cites a rate of under 1% at her institution [Brander and Stulberg 2006] and points out that aseptic techniques, prophylactic antibiotics, including antibiotic-loaded bone cement, [Block and Stubbs 2005] and laminar airflow operating rooms are the most effective ways to prevent infection. Computer-assisted techniques likely will not play a significant role in further reducing these complications, though if they extend the operative time, they may actually increase infection risk.

Instability refers to the tendency of a hip to dislocate following joint replacement and early series resulted in dislocation rates as high as 10% or more [Etienne et al. 1978]. However, a review performed by Masonis and Bourne [2002] of 14 clinical studies conducted over the previous 30 years and involving over 13,000 primary total hip replacement procedures showed lower dislocation rates ranging from 0.55% to 3.95%, depending on the surgical approach (with the highest rates for the posterior approach) showed that rates of postoperative limp were comparable (up to 20%) for the different surgical approaches. A more recent review [Kwon et al. 2006] noted that performing soft tissue repair when a posterior approach was used had a significant impact on dislocation rates, decreasing them from 4.46% to 0.49% (lower than the 2.0% rate reported in Masonis and Bourne), which is comparable to the rates found for two other surgical approaches (0.43–0.7%) when soft tissue repair was performed. It is, therefore, fair to say that dislocation rates are now in the order of 1–2% when performed using optimal modern surgical techniques.

One important factor affecting dislocation rate is the orientation of the acetabular cup [Morrey 1997]. A number of authors have argued for the existence of a so-called *safe zone*; that is, they suggest that there is a range of angular orientations of the acetabular cup associated with a lower risk of dislocations [Lewinnek et al. 1978]. The conventional manual surgical technique produces such highly variable results that surgeons cannot guarantee that the cup orientation is within the desired bounds; for example, Parratte et al. [2007] found that these manual techniques produced a range of 27° in abduction and 37° in anteversion. Jaramaz et al. [1998] have argued that this large range of achieved orientations increases the occurrence of femoroacetabular impingement, reduces the safe range of motion, and increases the risk of dislocation and wear, and conclude that computer-assisted techniques may reduce the rate of occurrence of such problems. However, the low dislocation rate suggests that CAOS techniques may in fact be more beneficial in addressing suboptimal functional outcomes, which have not been so extensively investigated.

Harris [2001] identifies wear as the key long-term problem in total hip arthroplasty. Wear produces small particles, which can induce osteolysis around the implant, with subsequent loosening and failure. Although patient size and activity level can clearly affect wear, obesity by itself does not necessarily increase the risk of early implant failure, possibly because obese patients also tend to have lower activity levels than less heavy patients [Stukenborg-Colsman et al. 2005]. Impingement and extreme acetabular cup orientations have also been correlated with increased wear rates [Kennedy et al. 1998; Yamaguchi et al. 2000]. It is, therefore, clear that acetabular cup orientation plays an important role in preventing both dislocation and excessive wear. As cup orientation is not well-controlled using conventional manual techniques, there is a motivation for developing computer-assisted techniques.

In recent years, femoral head resurfacing has emerged as an alternative to total hip arthroplasty for younger, more active patients. The larger head enables greater loads to be carried, and by resecting less bone stock, the ability to perform a primary hip arthroplasty at a later date is preserved. Early failures of resurfaced hips have been correlated with varus placement of the implant, and this advice is supported by the results of recent laboratory experiments by our group [Anglin et al. 2007], where we found increased static failure loads when the implant was placed 10° in valgus relative to a neutral position, and by finite element analyses by others [Radcliffe and Taylor 2007]. However, surgeons find it difficult to reliably place the implant in the desired orientation and even harder to place it in an intentionally valgus orientation (personal communication with Dr. Bas Masri, Vancouver Hospital); a recent study found that experienced arthroplasty surgeons take upward of 60 cases to become proficient enough to place the implant within 5° of the targeted orientation [Back et al. 2007], so computer-assisted techniques may find a role in largely eliminating this learning curve.

Minimally invasive procedures for total hip arthroplasty have been developed in recent years to try to decrease soft tissue trauma, reduce postoperative pain, shorten in-patient stays and return to function, and to improve cosmesis. Although these benefits are still arguable, with some studies showing benefits in short-term outcomes such as reduced blood loss and shorter hospital stays [Vavken et al. 2007; Orozco et al. 2007], while other studies suggest that reliable evidence is still wanting [Woolson 2006], there is little debate that these procedures are technically more demanding and offer the surgeon less visibility and access than traditional techniques. The improved visualization offered by computer-assisted techniques may therefore find an important role in minimally invasive procedures if they prove superior to conventional approaches. At least one major trial is currently being planned to address the hypothesis that computer-navigated MIS will lead to a quicker recovery during the early postoperative period (3 months), and to an outcome at least as good 6 months postoperatively [Reininga et al. 2007].

A final motivation for developing CAS techniques for hip arthroplasty is related to medicolegal concerns. For example, the most common cause of lawsuits following hip surgery is leg-length discrepancy [Attarian and Vail

2005]. Edeen et al. [1995] found that almost a third of patients in a series of 68 patients were aware of the discrepancy, and half of these were disturbed by it. Visuri et al. [1993] showed that leg length discrepancy was linked to an increased risk of a need for revision because of aseptic loosening. As CAOS techniques are able to assess changes in the position of the limb intraoperatively, they can be used to prevent leg-length discrepancy, so potential reductions in legal costs should be weighed in any calculation of the costs and benefits of these technologies.

12.4.1.2 Computer-Assisted Hip Replacement Techniques

Computer-assisted hip procedures can be categorized in two main ways:

1. Operative site: does the system address the placement of the acetabular cup (pelvic side) or the preparation of the femoral canal and the positioning of the femoral component (femoral side)?
2. Anatomical reference: is the intervention based on preoperative CT images, intraoperative fluoroscopy, or image-free kinematic measures?

In this section, we will consider examples of each type of system.

RoboDoc

The first application of CAS techniques to hip replacements was on the femoral side. In the 1980s, cemented implants were commonly used, but these posed problems such as adverse cardiovascular responses, difficulties positioning the implant prior to the cement setting, and difficulty extracting cement during revision. Cementless implants were developed to address these problems, but bony ingrowth could only occur if the match between the bone cavity and the implant was accurate to submillimetric precision; this was not possible with manual broaching techniques, and fractures commonly occurred if the implant was forced into too small an opening. Paul and colleagues [1992] therefore proposed and developed a robot-based system in which the cavity was milled under computer control by a robot carrying a milling tool. The original system consisted of a CT-based planner (Orthodoc) and a modified industrial robot (Fig. 12.1).

Prior to the surgery, the surgeon could work with the planning station to select an implant and determine the optimal position relative to the femur. Views of the implant could be obtained from any orientation. During surgery, the femur was placed in a bone clamp and a registration procedure performed to be able to map the preoperative plan to the live operating situation. The original registration process used small titanium fiducial markers that were implanted under local or regional anesthetic in a brief procedure prior to the CT scan. During the procedure, the robot is equipped with a special end-effector that mates to the head of these pins so it can be brought into contact with them to identify their spatial position. From these data, the position of the femur in the robot's frame of reference can be calculated, as can the desired position of the femoral cavity. In later years, a pinless registration process was developed (Digimatch) in which points on the surface of the femur were acquired intraoperatively (a process that took approximately 5 min), but even recently this process has been described as "rather cumbersome" and in need of automation [Bauer 2004]. Following registration, the surgeon attaches a milling cutter to the robot, attaches air and irrigation lines, and moves the cutter into position. During autonomous cutting, the surgeon monitors the progress of the cutting and can shut down the process at any time.

For more information on this system and others, the reader is referred to Kazanzides [2007], who presents an excellent overview of a wide variety of robotic devices, which have been used in joint reconstruction.

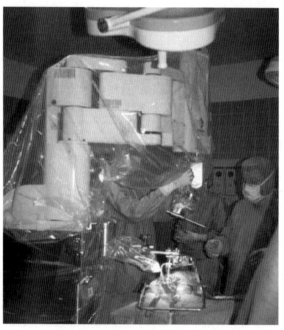

Fig. 12.1. RoboDoc in use in Oldenburg, Germany in 1996. Photo courtesy of Peter Kanzanzides, Johns Hopkins University, Baltimore, USA

HipNav

The potential for using CT images to control acetabular cup orientation was recognized at roughly the same time as the beginnings of RoboDoc [Mian et al. 1992], and navigation systems based on CT imaging emerged in the mid to late 1990s. The HipNav system from DiGioia and his colleagues in Pittsburgh was one of the first examples of this kind of system [Jaramaz et al. 1998]. In the HipNav system (Fig. 12.2), both the acetabular and femoral component positions were planned using a 3D planning workstation loaded with a patient's preoperatively acquired CT scan. Effects on leg length and hip offset were computed and presented to the surgeon so that the preoperative plan could be optimized. A new feature was a simulation of the range of motion of the hip. This allowed the surgeon to check for predicted impingement of the joint during a range of physiologically realistic situations such as sitting, stair-climbing, and walking.

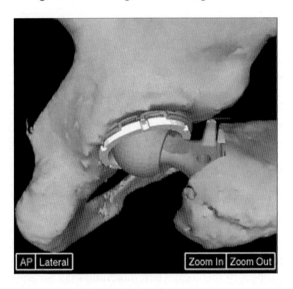

Fig. 12.2. Screenshot from HipNav planner showing predicted impingement of the prosthesis on the pelvis. Image courtesy of Branislav Jaramaz, Robotics Institute, Carnegie Mellon University, Pittsburgh, PA

Intraoperatively, an optical tracker is attached to the pelvis near the iliac crest to monitor movement of the bone during surgery. The pelvis is registered to the preoperative plan using a 3–5 min long surface point acquisition procedure in which points around the acetabulum, the sciatic notch, and the iliac crest are acquired with an optically tracked pointer probe (the latter percutaneously). The insertion tool for the acetabular cup is also tracked, which permits its position to be displayed on the screen as the surgeon aligns it prior to pressfitting the cup into place. In early versions of the system, the femoral reamer was not tracked, although the capability to do so was built into the system from the beginning.

Fluoroscopy-Based Procedures

The research group at the Müller Institute in Bern developed a CT-free navigation system for acetabular cup placement [Zheng et al. 2002] that was based on a hybrid combination of direct landmark digitization and use of virtual fluoroscopy. Virtual fluoroscopy is a technique in which two or more calibrated fluoroscopic images are taken at an angle to one another, which allows optically tracked tools to be located relative to the original images and projected into these images in real time, producing the effect of taking a continuous X-ray image. Using this technique, the pelvic landmarks are identified to define the anatomical reference planes, and the acetabular cup insertion tool is monitored in real-time on the virtual fluoroscopic images.

Image-Free Procedures

Although not much discussed in the research literature, various CAOS companies have introduced image-free hip arthroplasty techniques, as have a small number of independent developers (see Dorr et al. [2005] for one example). A commercial example is the Stryker Hip Navigation System (Stryker Leibinger, Freiburg, Germany) that offers a landmark digitization technique in which the key landmarks (anterosuperior iliac spines (ASIS) and both pubic tubercles) are digitized percutaneously [Nogler et al. 2004].

Hip Resurfacing

Two main CAOS techniques have been described for hip resurfacing.

1. OrthoSOFT and Brainlab have both introduced an image-free point-based surface digitization approach, in which points are acquired on all aspects of the femoral neck, with a particular emphasis on the superior aspect of the neck where notching may potentially occur.
2. Our group has developed an approach on the basis of the surgeon using preoperative plain film X-rays to determine the desired valgus/varus angle, and then rapidly transferring this plan to the patient intra-operatively using an optically tracked registration plate [Hodgson et al. 2005, 2007].

Ante/retroversion is determined intraoperatively in both systems; with the commercial systems, the proposed axis position is shown relative to the acquired points, and the surgeon adjusts the targeted axis until satisfied. With our system, the version is determined by acquiring estimated vertical center lines along the femoral neck using a tracked caliper and fitting a line to where these center lines pierce an anteroposterior plane lying at the desired valgus/varus orientation (Fig. 12.3).

Once the desired orientation has been found, the surgeon places an optically tracked drill guide against the head of the femur, orients it using a computer-based targeting display, and drills a guide pin along the indicated axis. The rest of the procedure proceeds conventionally.

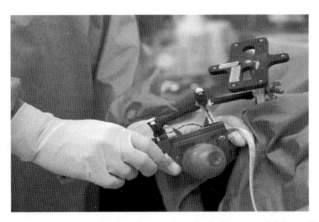

Fig. 12.3. Tracked caliper applied to femoral neck during acquisition of center lines along the neck in the author's femoral head resurfacing system

Evaluation

For the most part, the various hip arthroplasty systems have been relatively well evaluated from a technical point of view. Quantities such as accuracy and repeatability have been reported for a variety of systems. Perhaps one of the most detailed and comprehensive technical evaluations performed to date is that of the fluoroscopy-based Medtronic StealthStation Treon Plus system, which was assessed by an independent research group [Stiehl et al. 2005]. In their assessment, they used a National Institute of Standards and Technology (NIST) traceable coordinate measuring machine (CMM) to determine the location of an acetabular cup implanted in a nominal position of 45° inclination and 17.5° anteversion. They found that the CMM method had a repeatability of 1.1° in inclination and 0.4° in anteversion. The intra-surgeon repeatability was 1.5° in inclination and 3.0° in anteversion, which was similar to the intersurgeon reproducibility of 0.9° in inclination and 2.5° in anteversion, which indicates that the technique is relatively insensitive to who is using the system. The increased variability in the anteversion direction was suggested to be due to difficulties in predictably identifying the relevant anatomical points from the fluoroscopic image. This same investigator was involved in a later study [Stiehl et al. 2007] that used a similar evaluation protocol to compare both fluoroscopic and image-free navigation methods against CT and CMM-based reference methods. The CT technique produced excellent repeatability (better than the CMM-based method). The results for the fluoroscopic-based system were comparable to the earlier study, but the image-free technique was significantly better with an intra-surgeon repeatability of 0.5° in inclination and 0.8° in anteversion and an inter-surgeon reproducibility of 0.8° in inclination and 1.1° in anteversion. Based on the Six Sigma Cp and Cpk capability indices, they concluded that the image-free system was "process capable," but that fluoroscopic referencing posed problems for controlling anteversion.

In comparison with conventional manual acetabular cup placement techniques, navigated techniques do appear to reduce the variability in cup orientation. Nogler et al. [2004], for example, shows a significant reduction in variability of cup placement when using the commercial image-free navigation system described earlier (Fig. 12.4); the 90th percentile limits spanned a much larger range for the conventional procedure (16° inclination; 19° anteversion) than the navigated procedure (4° inclination; 7° anteversion).

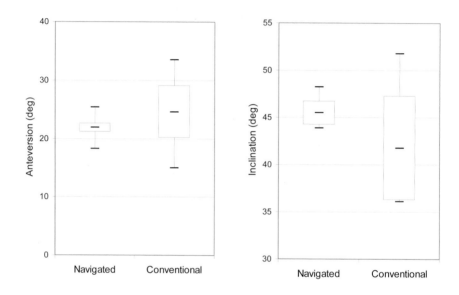

Fig. 12.4. Comparison of variability of cup placement when using the image-free Stryker Hip Navigation System. *Cross-bars* indicate the 90th percentile limits. Data derived from Nogler [2004]

Similarly, [Kalteis et al. 2006] showed reductions in the ranges of acetabular cup orientation when using two navigated techniques: one CT-based and one image-free (both available as part of the Brainlab VectorVision hip 3.0 system (BrainLAB, Heimstetten, Germany). With the manual technique, the standard deviation was 7° in inclination and 14° in anteversion, whereas the comparable figures were 4.0° in inclination and 5.3–5.5° in anteversion for the two navigated techniques. Figure 12.5 shows that 53% of the cups positioned manually lie outside the *safe zone* defined by Lewinnek, whereas only 7% and 17% of those positioned by the image-free and CT-based techniques, respectively, lay outside this zone. Kalteis also reported that the image-free and CT-based systems took slightly longer than the manual technique at 7 and 17 min, respectively.

These orientation results are consistent with several other studies quoted by Kalteis: both Saxler et al. [2004] and DiGioia et al. [2002] found that three quarters of manually implanted cups were malpositioned, and numerous other authors have found reductions in variability with CT-based techniques [DiGioia et al. 1998; Leenders et al. 2002; Jaramaz et al. 1998; Widmer and Grutzner 2004].

Von Recum et al. [2003] (see also Wentzensen et al. [2003] for an earlier report of the first portion of this patient series) evaluated a hybrid fluoroscopy/digitization technique (part of the SurgiGATE application by Medivision) and showed in a series of 256 patients that the variability in cup placement as evaluated by a postoperative CT analysis was relatively low: 3.0° in inclination and 3.9° in anteversion. The authors concluded that this technique was equivalent in performance to the established CT-based systems.

On the basis of the studies summarized earlier, we can conclude that there is evidence that both fluoroscopy-based and image-free navigation techniques can produce acetabular cup alignment results that are comparable

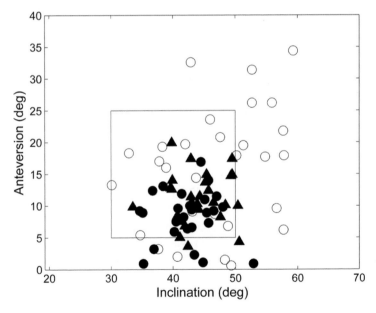

Fig. 12.5. Positions of acetabular cup relative to the "safe zone" defined by Lewinnek when using the conventional freehand (*open circle*) and two navigated techniques: CT-based (*filled circle*) and an image-free technique (*filled triangle*). Derived from Kalteis et al. [2006]

to those produced by CT-based systems. Hube et al. [2003] also compared a fluoroscopy-based system with a CT-based system and concluded that there was no difference in final alignment variability (although there was a slight increase in operating time relative to manual techniques; 9 and 13 min for the CT and fluoroscopy-based systems, respectively). Given the lack of difference in performance and the need for a separate preoperative scan and planning process with the CT-based system, these authors recommended reserving CT-based interventions for cases with significant congenital or posttraumatic abnormalities.

To date, there have been no studies attempting to show improved functional outcomes from using navigated acetabular cup placement techniques, so it is unclear whether the improvements in repeatability achieved to date will be sufficient to justify widespread acceptance of computer-assisted approaches. A small number of studies have identified factors contributing to the final implant orientation error, and such models will be useful in future if further refinements to the techniques become necessary [Wolf et al. 2005a; Tannast et al. 2005].

While the potential for computer assistance with femoral side of a total hip arthroplasty has been recognized for some years [Noble et al. 2003], there has to date been comparatively little evaluation of the outcomes following computer-assisted interventions on the femoral side. Lazovic and Zigan [2006] report that the commercially available Orthopilot system proved useful in inserting short stem prostheses with modular necks by helping to control leg length and femoral head offset.

The RoboDoc system has undergone more scrutiny. Several authors (e.g., Nishihara et al. 2004; Schneider and Kalender 2003] have demonstrated that the robot has indeed been able to improve the shaping of the femoral cavity, with accuracies of better than 1 mm. Bauer [2004] reports that the operating room time requirement has stabilized at about 90 min (20–30 min longer than the manual technique), that there is some evidence of earlier weight bearing and faster rehabilitation, and that intraoperative fractures could largely be avoided. Honl et al. [2003] reported on a prospective randomized study involving 154 patients that found that the RoboDoc system did improve the accuracy of the implantation, but that its use was associated with higher early revision rates, higher dislocation rates, longer surgery, an increased amount of muscle damage, and an increase in operating room cost of approximately $700. They concluded that the system required further development before it could be widely recommended. The results of 10-year follow ups will be available shortly as 3,800 cases were performed in Germany between 1994 and 1998.

With regard to computer-assisted femoral head resurfacing, very few results are yet available as the technique has been in use for only about 2 years. In our first cadaver study [Hodgson et al. 2005], we found that our CAOS technique had a standard deviation of only 2.2° in the varus/valgus direction in the hands of residents, compared with 5.5° for the conventional manual procedure performed by expert surgeons; the time needed to align the drill guide was comparable in the two cases, despite the difference in experience level, which suggests that a CAOS approach could enable surgeons to avoid the 60-case learning curve described by Back (2007). As a change in orientation of 10° can cause a 28% change in static failure load [Anglin et al. 2007], surgeons would like to be able to control placement to an accuracy substantially better than this. Beaulé et al. [2004] found that the difference in the mean implant alignment relative to the femoral shaft between a group of successful and problematic resurfacing patients was on the order of 6°, which suggests that it may be beneficial to control the implant's accuracy of placement to even less than this value.

Davis et al. [2007] showed that a CAOS technique reduced the range of implant placement from 12° with the manual technique to 8° with the CAOS technique. However, to date there have been no reports of functional outcome data. Kruger et al. [2007] compared 9 patients treated with a CAOS technique to 9 with a manual approach and found no statistically significant difference in femoral component orientation.

12.4.2 Knee Replacement

12.4.2.1 Clinical Motivation

The knee is subject to the same kinds of degenerative processes as described earlier for the hip, and in fact has become the most commonly replaced major joint. According to a projection presented at the 2006 American Academy of Orthopedic Surgeons Annual Meeting that was based on combining National Inpatient Sample data from 1990 to 2002 with census data to estimate demographic trends, primary total hip replacements in the United States are likely to increase from a little over 200,000 in 2005 to 450,000 by 2030 [Kurtz et al. 2006]. More dramatically, primary total knee replacements are expected to grow from 430,000 in 2005 to what the authors describe as a *staggering* 2.2 million procedures by 2030. Revision hip procedures will rise from 41,000 in 2005 to almost 100,000 in 2030 (roughly 20%), while revision knee procedures will increase even more dramatically from 37,000 in 2005 to almost 200,000 in 2030 (under 10%). Hernandez et al. [2006] estimates the average cost of these total knee revision surgeries at $56,000 each, so hospital costs for revisions could exceed $10 billion per year by 2030. To accommodate this massive increase in demand, significant improvements in both operative efficiency and implant longevity will be required.

Total knee replacement, like total hip arthroplasty, is considered to be an excellent surgical procedure. Sorrells and Capps [2006] reviewed the outcome date for primary, cementless, low-contact stress, total knee arthroplasty and found that fewer than 1% had patellar difficulties or significant radiological evidence of joint failure, and that over 99% of patients had good to excellent knee scores at follow up. Buechel et al. [2002] evaluated 233 cemented and cementless rotating platform knee replacement implants with a minimum 10-year follow up period and found a survivorship of 98% at 10 and 20 years, with 47% having excellent results in the cemented group and 68% in the cementless group. Different implants have been developed to better approximate the natural kinematics of the knee, but the clinical results are similar (Hospital for Special Surgery knee scores of 89.4 vs. 88.6) [Kim et al. 2004]. Other studies report similarly excellent results (e.g. Papachristou et al. [2006]), although these studies are likely drawn from centers with extensive experience in performing TKAs; the overall revision rate of roughly 10% reported by Kurtz et al. [2006] suggests that not all surgeons are capable of obtaining such results; this figure is in line with the results at 10 years of follow-up from the Swedish Knee Arthroplasty Registry [Robertsson 2001]. Indeed, there is evidence that revision rates are strongly linked to the volume of surgeries a surgeon performs (NIH Consensus Statement 2003). Callahan et al. [1994] presented a meta-analysis of 130 studies with a total of 9,879 patients. The mean complication rate was 18%, and the overall rate of revision at an average of 4.1 years was 3.8%. In a different international multicenter study of 4,743 primary total knee arthroplasty with mobile bearing design, the overall survivorship at 16 years' follow up was 79%, and revisions were performed in 5.4% of the knees [Stiehl et al. 2006b]. Approximately half the revisions (2.3%) were due to bearing-related issues such as instability, wear or dislocation. Similar problems occurred in significant proportions of revision cases treated in Canada in 2004 [CJRR 2004]: aseptic loosening (39%), poly wear (36%), instability (26%), and osteolysis (20%).

Despite these successful survival results in well-established surgical centers, we cannot conclude that there is no potential for improvement. When patients are asked about their postoperative experience, not all are satisfied. Hawker [2006] reported that up to 30% experience a suboptimal outcome or are otherwise dissatisfied with the results. Callaghan et al. [2000] reported 100% implant survival at 9–12 years, but found that 10% of the patients in that study experienced anterior knee pain. In another study, Brander and Stulberg [2003] found that 44% of their patients report moderate to severe pain one month after surgery, declining to 13% at one year. Resurfacing the patella plays an important role in avoiding anterior knee pain – several recent metaanalyses have shown that anterior knee pain occurs in over 20% of patients whose patellas are not resurfaced (range: 21–24%), but in less than 10% of patients whose patellas are resurfaced (range: 6–12%) [Nizard et al. 2005; Parvizi et al. 2005; Pakos et al. 2005] – but has not entirely eliminated the problem.

Postoperative range of motion (ROM) of the knee is important for function, particularly for being able to rise from sitting, but according to Jones et al. [2007], the link between ROM and measures of well-being or patient satisfaction are not well-established, even though various other quality of life measures related to social function, mental health, and vitality do increase postoperatively.

Even though knee replacement does reduce pain and increase mobility, patients rarely recover to the level of health exhibited by age and sex-adjusted control groups who have not required surgery [Jones et al. 2007], and TKR patients do not experience as much of an improvement as THR patients. There is also considerable evidence that surgeons express more satisfaction with patients' result than the patients themselves. Overall, as many as 15–30% of patients report "little or no improvement after surgery or are unsatisfied with the results after a few months" [Jones et al. 2007].

In summary, then, modern total knee replacement procedures produce extremely high success rates, which poses a challenge to developers of computer-assisted techniques to demonstrate impact. However, it is widely accepted by surgeons that implant loosening is more common when the alignment of the implant is off neutral. This finding was first reported by Rand and Coventry [1988], who found that the 10-year survival rate of a geometric total knee implant was 73% if the knee was in varus, 90% if in up to 4° of valgus, and 73% if between 5° and 9° of valgus. Jeffery et al. [1991] found that the incidence of loosening at up to 12 years' follow up was 3% if the line connecting the hip and ankle centers passed through the middle third of the prosthesis (approximately ±3° from neutral), but 24% if outside this zone. Other research found that 5/35 patients with varus alignment required revision, 3/234 patients with 0–4° of valgus, and 0/82 patients with more than 4° of valgus [Ritter et al. 1994].

In addition to the issue of varus/valgus alignment, surgeons must ensure stability of the reconstructed knee joint complex to provide satisfactory function for the patient. Otherwise, patients experience their knees giving way during loading. Stability is primarily governed by the collateral ligaments and the posterior cruciate ligament (or equivalent with PCL-sacrificing implant designs). The primary task for the surgeon is to ensure that the gaps between the prepared femoral and tibial bone surfaces are rectangular and equal in both flexion and extension. Griffin et al. [2000] showed that careful attention on the part of the surgeon can generally ensure that the gaps are rectangular in both flexion and extension (84–89%), but that it is considerably more difficult to ensure that they are equal (roughly half were within 1 mm); any resulting differences can lead to either laxity or tightness at different points in the flexion cycle.

A third important consideration that has not received much attention among CAOS system developers until recently has been patellofemoral instability, which can occur when the line of action of the quadriceps tendon pulls the patella too far laterally, particularly close to extension; this can result in subluxation of the patella and knee pain [Kelly 2001]. Parker et al. [2003] and Eisenhuth et al. [2006] both state that patellofemoral complications are the most common cause of postoperative pain and of revision. Avoiding these problems requires careful attention to implant alignment and soft tissue balance.

12.4.2.2 Computer-Assisted Knee Replacement Technique

In knee replacement surgery procedures, the surgeon typically makes a transverse planar cut across the superior aspect of the tibia, followed by a set of five cuts at the distal end of the femur: a distal cut, which determines the varus/valgus orientation of the implant, an anterior and a posterior cut, which determine the rotational orientation of the implant, and two chamfer cuts to accommodate the implant. In addition, a box cut is typically made to accommodate stabilizing lobes designed to augment or replace the function of the cruciate ligaments. In the conventional manual procedure, these cuts are made by using mechanical instruments to position a cutting block (or cutting guide) against the bone, pinning it in place with so-called Kirchner (K) wires, and then inserting an oscillating saw through a slot in the cutting guide to actually make the cut.

Historically, the first goal of CAOS systems for the knee was to control the varus/valgus (or coronal plane) alignment. In subsequent years, it has been increasingly important to control the rotation as well, as that determines the soft tissue balance. As with the hip, several different types of CAOS systems have been developed for total knee replacement surgery. There are two major types of TKA systems: CT-based systems in which a preoperative scan is acquired for planning, and image-free systems in which the key anatomical landmarks are identified intraoperatively (although, as with hip surgery, fluoroscopy-based systems have also been developed). We briefly present examples of each type of system.

Image-Free

One of the most popular types of CAOS system for TKA is an image-free system. This type of system was originally developed over 12 years ago at the Université Joseph Fourier in Grenoble and has since evolved into a variety of different commercial systems. Stulberg et al. [2004] describes a surgical technique on the basis of the Aesculap Orthopilot system. With image-free systems, no preoperative planning is necessary as all anatomical landmarks are determined during the surgery. After conventional draping and exposure, optically tracked marker arrays are attached to the femur and tibia, and optionally to the pelvis. To position the prosthetic implant, the surgeon must identify key anatomical landmarks, particularly the hip center, the ankle center, and landmarks around the knee such as the medial and lateral epicondyles; these allow the system to determine the appropriate rotational orientation for the implant.

The first step in the procedure is to identify the center of rotation of the femoral head. This is accomplished by rotating the femur relative to the acetabulum such that each marker will trace out a path on a surface of a sphere centered on the femoral head. By applying an optimization algorithm to the collected data, the computer is able to calculate an offset vector relative to the femoral marker array that moves least in the pelvic reference frame. This approach is known as a kinematic registration technique.

A similar approach is used to identify the ankle center. A marker array is strapped to the foot and the foot taken through a series of flexion and abduction motions. Alternatively, the ankle center may be found by directly digitizing the medial and lateral malleoli and using the geometric center as an estimate for the ankle center. The knee joint is also flexed, which allows the system to estimate the preoperative axis of rotation of the joint; this is later used as a rotational reference for the femoral component. Several points on the surface of the joint are also acquired for use in setting the joint line and the anteroposterior placement of the implants. On the tibial side, the deepest point on the least damaged side of the plateau is digitized as a reference for the tibial resection depth. The intercondylar eminence is also digitized as a reference for mediolateral placement of the tibial component.

On the femoral side, the posterior aspects of the two condyles are digitized, along with the anterior surface of the femur. This latter point is used to prevent anterior notching. Finally, the origins of the medial and lateral epicondyles are digitized to aid in determining the rotation of the femoral component.

Once these measurements are made, the computer has enough information to construct reference frames and define the desired locations of the bone cuts. The tibial cut is made after placing a slotted cutting block against the anterior surface of the tibia, positioning it under computer guidance, and pinning it in place. The femoral cuts are made in two stages: first, a distal cutting block is positioned under computer guidance and the distal cut made; then a second cutting block is mounted to the resected bone, positioned to ensure that the implant's rotational alignment will be correct, and the anterior, posterior, and chamfer cuts made. Following a trial reduction, the balance of the procedure proceeds as with the conventional manual procedure.

Numerous variants on this basic approach are used in other systems. The methods of identifying the hip and ankle centers may vary, and there is considerable debate as to the most appropriate reference for controlling the femoral component's rotation; the transepicondylar axis, the perpendicular to the so-called Whiteside's line (an anteroposterior line drawn through the femoral notch), and an offset from the posterior condylar line have all been proposed [Siston et al. 2006]. Many surgeons advocate using a direct evaluation of the flexion and extension gaps instead of an explicit geometric reference, because this will relate more directly to function (some systems incorporate some measure of soft tissue balance into their workflows, either manually or with a special tensing device) [Marmignon et al. 2005]. Other systems use the bone-morphing technology described earlier to create a full 3D model of the distal femur, and the surgical plan is defined in relation to this morphed model instead of on the basis of digitized points (Fig. 12.6).

An interesting variant on this image-free system is a technique known as Navigated Freehand Cutting in which the cutting blocks are dispensed with altogether and the surgeon simply places the saw against the bone and relies only on the computer screen to position it correctly [Haider et al. 2007]. The developers of this technique have demonstrated in a cast-foam model that the cutting time is decreased by 15% and the overall alignment of the implant is significantly improved, albeit at the cost of increased surface roughness of the sawn bone models.

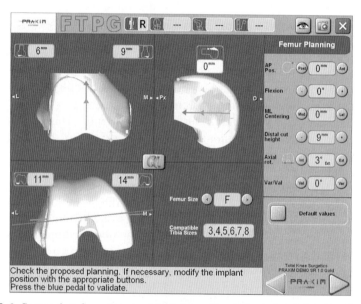

Fig. 12.6. Screenshot from Praxim-Medivision Total Knee Surgetics (TKS) image-free navigation application, based on bone-morphing algorithm. Used with permission.

CT-Based

A number of authors, including our group, have identified significant errors related to the bone sawing process [Plaskos et al. 2002] and have recommended using milling techniques instead. A group of researchers at Imperial College in London has designed a robot that carries a milling tool to perform both unicompartmental and total knee arthroplasty procedures and has coupled their robot with a CT-based surgical planning system [Davies et al. 2007]. Their philosophy is that a preoperative CT scan is justified because of the opportunity it presents to create a full 3D preoperative plan. The primary justification for such a system is to enhance unicompartmental knee replacements, where it is more difficult to gain access to the bone and to properly visualize its orientation underneath the overlying tissue.

The distinguishing feature of their robot, which is known as ACROBOT (Active Constraint ROBOT), is that it does not operate under autonomous control, but in a servo-enhanced cooperative mode in which the surgeon operates a handle located close to the milling tool and the robot interprets forces applied to the handle as instructions to move in the indicated direction. Because the motors are backdrivable, the surgeon can sense when the tool encounters changes in the environment, such as a sudden change in bone density. In addition, there is a supervisory level built in, which prevents the robot from moving outside of zones that have been predefined as safe. This feature can be used, for example, to avoid cutting the collateral ligaments. In use, the robot is wheeled into the operating theatre and the base put into position using a four degree of freedom gross positioning unit. The tibia and femur are immobilized using clamps that penetrate through 5 mm incisions and engage with the bone. Registration is performed by attaching a small ball-ended probe to the robot's end effector and touching several dozen points on the bone surface; these are matched to the preoperative CT model.

The ACROBOT is not the only robot that has been developed for use in TKA surgery. Siebert et al. [2002] describes the modification of a commercially available robot (CASPAR) for use in TKA procedures. Both

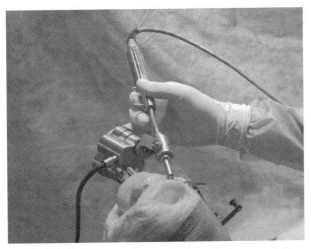

Fig. 12.7. Praxiteles miniature bone-mounted robot mounted to a cadaveric knee during a cutting trial in 2006. Photo courtesy of Dr. Jacques Rit of Center Hospitalier Princesse Grace, Monaco.

our group [Plaskos et al. 2005] and a group in Pittsburgh [Wolf et al. 2005b] have recently developed miniature bone-mounted robots to facilitate both the standard TKA surgical exposure and less invasive approaches (Fig. 12.7).

Evaluation

As with total hip arthroplasty, the impact of computer assistance in total knee arthroplasty has largely been demonstrated on the basis of technical measures such as the accuracy of varus/valgus (coronal) alignment. Lüring et al. [2006], for example, identified six prospective and randomized clinical studies with more than 30 patients per group that met the requirements for being a level 1 or level 2 study. They consolidated all these data from these six studies and found that 95% of the 375 implants placed using navigation had a mechanical axis alignment that was within the 3° window commonly used to define optimal placement, compared with 82% of the same number of implants placed conventionally. In the sagittal plane, only two of the six studies demonstrated improved alignment of the femoral component. On average, the CAS technique took 20 min longer than the conventional procedure (range: 15–40 min). The authors point out that the alignment results should be judged somewhat critically because the standard method used to evaluate alignment is the weight-bearing, long-leg X-ray, which can introduce errors of up to 4° in the estimated varus/valgus angle.

A slightly more recent study by this same group [Bäthis et al. 2006] involving 1,784 implants reached similar conclusions. Of the 919 CAS implants from 13 studies, 94% were within the optimal 3° window, compared with only 76% of the 865 conventional implants. No remarkable differences in any other clinical indicators were found.

The most comprehensive meta-analysis to date involved 3,423 patients from 33 studies, including 11 randomized trials [Bauwens et al. 2007]. The principle finding of this study was that the relative risk of the mechanical alignment being outside a 3° window from the desired neutral value when a computer-assisted technique was used was less than 80% of the risk for the manual technique. Assuming that the risk of being outside this window using the manual technique is similar to the studies reported above (i.e., 18–24%), we would expect that CAOS procedures would reduce this by approximately 5%, which appears to be a lower benefit than was found by Lüring or Bäthis. Bauwens also reports that the mean duration of surgery was increased from 73 to 90 min when using CAOS techniques. Only four of the studies investigated functional assessment and no consequential differences were found, with the possible exception of some evidence of improved stiffness scores with CAOS.

From these assessments, we can conclude that CAOS systems have generally proven to produce better coronal alignment outcomes, although little evidence of impact on other functional measures, such as pain or ability to perform various activities of daily living has been produced. This general picture was recently echoed by Ulrich et al. [2007] in an overview of the scientific evidence supporting computer-assisted surgery for TKA. Ulrich concluded that there was sufficient evidence to justify some expectation of increased success in future, and that this has proven to be enough to motivate manufacturers to develop appropriate surgical tools and updated designs to take advantage of CAOS capabilities. Holt et al. [2006] concurred, and argued that from an ethical point of view, there is sufficient merit to CAOS systems to justify their use on the grounds that they produce at least technically equivalent results. In contrast, Holt regarded the evidence for minimally invasive techniques as insufficient to support widespread use, because of a higher likelihood that long term outcomes would not be as good as those of the current technique.

Davies et al. [2007] notes that concerns about the cost-effectiveness have only recently been recognized. Dong and Buxton [2006] recently applied one of the first economic benefit analyses of computer-assisted surgery to total knee arthroplasty, albeit with a number of assumed values for key estimates of probabilities of different outcomes. Using reasonable point estimates, they showed the potential for CAOS techniques to save over $1,000 per operation when potential reductions in revision procedures were taken into account, although they admitted that this reduction needed to be verified in longer term studies. To strengthen the case for adopting CAOS systems for TKA, more attention must be paid to measuring the impact of more consistent and accurate implant placement and soft tissue balancing on the patient's quality of life. To whatever extent is possible, these impacts should also be assessed in economic terms so that their value may be evaluated against any increased costs because of the use of the CAOS system. Time savings should also be sought whenever possible. Darmanis et al. [2007] showed that paying attention to simple details such as providing feedback via a laser pointer as to where the optical tracker is pointed can save significant amounts of time; in this case, they saved 11 min using this simple innovation alone.

Finally, given the discrepancy between revision rates in the most successful case sets reported (in the order of 0–2% at 10–20 years) and the actual number of revisions performed in the United States each year (~8%; Kurtz et al. [2005]), we hypothesize that many of the cases ultimately resulting in revision are performed by surgeons with lower case volumes [Kreder et al. 2003]. If this is the case, then CAOS systems face a significant economic obstacle, because in order for them to be adopted in the surgical settings where they will likely do the most good, that is, in community hospitals where surgeons do a relatively low number of TKAs annually, the system costs must be proportionately lower to induce the surgeons and hospitals to purchase the equipment.

12.4.3 Pedicle Screw Insertion

12.4.3.1 Clinical Motivation

A variety of spinal injuries, as well as disorders resulting from congenital deformities such as scoliosis, or progressive conditions such as osteoporotic vertebral collapse, arthritis, spondylolisthesis, and tumors, can potentially benefit from a treatment known as spinal fusion. In spinal fusion, two or more adjacent vertebrae are fixed relative to one another and bony connections are allowed to form between them so as to prevent further relative motion, thereby reducing or eliminating pain and reducing the risk of future compromise of neural function or paralysis.

Historically, a variety of different kinds of hardware (known as instrumentation) was used to secure one vertebra to another. These included hooks, sublaminar wires, and anterior screws. In recent years, however, pedicle screws have come into widespread use, particularly for the lumbar and thoracic spine, and are commonly regarded as offering mechanical fixation superior to these other instruments [Van Brussel et al. 1996]. The screws, however, must be inserted into the vertebra's pedicles, the channels of bone connecting the anterior vertebral body to the posterior spinal processes and which pass around and enclose the spinal cord. When inserting the screws with conventional freehand or fluoroscopically guided techniques, there is a significant risk of perforating the pedicle and damaging either the nerves passing out of the spinal cord above and below the pedicle or the spinal cord itself if the screw perforates the medial wall of the pedicle. The misplacement rate can vary significantly from institution to institution, and rates as high as 40% have been reported [Castro et al 1996]. However, the significance of this is uncertain. Kim et al. [2004] reported on the safety of over 3,200 freehand pedicle screw placements in the thoracic spine using a palpation technique, and found that, although the cortical perforation rate was 6.2%, they experienced no neurological, vascular, or visceral complications at up to 10 years follow up, and so concluded that this technique was safe and reliable. Similar safety records have been obtained by others [Faraj and Webb 1997]. Overall, outcomes are generally good; Rivet et al. [2004], for example, reported that 73% of a group of 42 consecutive patients experienced a good or excellent outcome as measured by the modified Prolo scale and that 90% of patients would choose to undergo the procedure again.

Perhaps the most detailed look at the outcomes associated with spine surgery on a broader scale was that carried out by the Japan Spine Research Society in 2004 [Nohara et al. 2004]. They surveyed the outcomes of over 16,000 spine patients from nearly 200 institutes during the year 2001. Spinal instrumentation was used on just over one third of this patient group, and pedicle screws were used in 55% of these cases. The most common clinical indications for instrumentation surgery were spinal deformity, trauma, rheumatoid arthritis, osteoporotic vertebral collapse, spondylolisthesis, and spinal tumors. Instrumentation was employed roughly twice as frequently in the lower thoracic region (~75% of the time) as in the upper thoracic and cervical regions (35–38% of the time).

Overall, the complication rate for instrumentation surgery was 12.1%, with lower rates of about 6% for decompression procedures and higher rates of 12% for fusion, or fusion with decompression, and 17% if fusion was combined with correction or reduction. Complication rates were not specifically coupled to the choice of instrumentation in this report, but the four most common complications across the entire cohort of 16,000 patients (representing approximately 55% of all complications) were neurological complications (1.7% of the cases), dural tear and fluid leakage (1.4%), infection (0.9%), and instrumentation failure (0.5%). Neurological complications produced a residual disorder in 40% of patients, whereas 90–93% of those suffering dural tears or infection experienced significant or complete recovery. On the basis of this study, we can conclude that it is highly likely that there were a significant number of patients who suffered persistent neurological complication from misplaced pedicle screws.

An additional consideration in pedicle screw surgery is the radiation exposure experienced by the patient and the surgical team, but particularly the latter as they are subject to radiation on an ongoing basis whereas the patient is exposed on a single occasion. As imaging techniques have been more commonly used in orthopedic surgery, there has been increased concern about the radiation exposure surgeons face [Dewey and Incoll 1998; Hynes et al. 1992], with the hands of the orthopedic surgeon being particularly at risk [Gwynne Jones and Stoddart 1998; Smith et al. 1992].

12.4.3.2 Computer-Assisted Screw Insertion Techniques

As with the arthroplasty procedures, computer-assisted screw insertion techniques can be based on intraoperative fluoroscopy or preoperative CT scans, or can be performed image-free. In this section, we present examples of two image-based techniques.

One of the earliest CAOS pedicle screw insertion techniques was a CT-based approach described by Amiot et al. [1995], who reported promising results on a set of three sheep vertebrae and successfully drilled five of the six targeted holes. The estimated accuracy of the system was reported to be 4.5 mm and 1.6° RMS. A more recent description of a CT-based system is found in Gebhard et al. [2004]. In the system described there, the patient undergoes a preoperative CT scan, which is used initially in a preoperative planning process, and is then transferred to the operating room for the surgery. Intraoperatively, the surgeon attaches a dynamic reference frame to each vertebra that is to have a pedicle screw inserted, uses a tracked pointing tool to digitize a set of 4–5 index points that have been previously identified on the CT image, along with another dozen or so points distributed across the visible surface of the vertebra, and a combination paired-point/surface matching registration algorithm is executed. The T-handle used to orient and drive the pedicle is then either positioned according to the preoperative plan or tracked in real-time to allow the surgeon to choose the final trajectory on the fly.

Gebhard also describes a C-arm-based technique on the basis of the concept of *virtual fluoroscopy*, originally introduced by Foley et al. [2001]. Virtual fluoroscopy is a clever way to provide the surgeon with the effect of having continuously updated fluoroscopic images from multiple simultaneous perspectives, even though the fluoroscopy machine is not active. This effect is achieved by taking two or more calibrated fluoroscopic images from multiple viewing directions, computing their spatial locations, tracking one or more surgical tools using an optical tracking system, computing the location of the tracked tool(s) relative to the known positions of the fluoroscopic images, and overlaying a representation of the surgical tool onto these images in real-time. In the context of pedicle screw insertion, the surgeon can manipulate a tracked insertion tool and view an instantly updated representation from multiple perspectives of where the screw is relative to the vertebra. In most systems, the axis of the screw can be projected forward from its current location, which assists in targeting the screw.

Related CAOS systems have also been applied to similar screw insertion procedures at the pelvis (iliosacral screw insertions) [Kahler and Zura 1997; Kahler and Mallick 1999; Schep et al. 2004] and the hip [Hamelinck et al. 2007].

As with total knee arthroplasty, some researchers believe that there is an advantage to be gained by using small bone-mounted robots to assist with the surgical intervention. Barzilay et al. [2006] described the design and use of a miniature robot that can be attached to the posterior processes of the spine to position a drill guide. This system was used in nine surgical cases and several relatively minor implementation issues were identified, which the authors expect to address in future cases.

12.4.3.3 Evaluation

The major technical outcome described for pedicle screw insertion techniques is the rate of cortical perforation. In the most comprehensive meta-analysis presented to date, Kosmopoulos and Schizas [2007] reported on 130 studies over the past 40 years involving over 37,000 pedicle screw insertions in both live patients, and cadavers implanted using both conventional and navigated techniques. Overall, 90% of the screws were considered accurately placed amongst 12,299 screws placed in patients using a conventional technique (32 studies), while over 95% of 3,059 screws placed under navigation were accurately placed (21 studies) (Fig. 12.8), so the general claim that navigation systems improve pedicle screw placement appears to be substantiated.

Similar advantages for CAOS systems have been found in detailed laboratory studies. For example, Arand et al. [2006] showed that CT and fluoroscopy-based systems were generally superior to the conventional procedure, although they caution that neither type of CAOS system can offer submillimetric accuracy and conclude that it is unrealistic to expect these systems to completely prevent perforation of the pedicle's cortex.

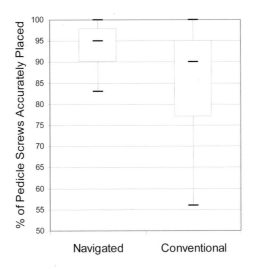

Fig. 12.8. Percentage of pedicle screws accurately placed using either a navigated (21 studies) or a conventional (32 studies) technique. *Cross bars* indicate maximum, median, and minimum results (excluding the single worst study in each group) and the *boxes* indicate the interquartile ranges (25th to 75th percentile results). Data derived from Kosmopoulos and Schizas [2007]

Although no studies to date have demonstrated a decrease in neurological complication rates, there are studies that have shown reduction both in the amount of radiation used during surgery, and in the time taken. Sasso and Garrido [2007] found that in a retrospective review of 105 patients undergoing posterior L5-S1 spine fusion, either with or without virtual fluoroscopic guidance, the virtual fluoroscopic technique reduced the operative time by an average of 40 min ($p < 0.001$; Fig. 12.9).

When only the last 20 cases in each group were considered (in case there were learning effects), the average times in both groups had decreased and the average difference had narrowed to only 22 min in favor of virtual fluoroscopy, although because of the smaller group size, this difference was only on the margins of being statistically significant (p just over 0.05).

Rajasekaran et al. [2007] also recently demonstrated in a study of 478 screw placements that a CAOS technique based on the Iso-C technology was able to reduce operative time (from 4.6 min per screw in the conventional group to 2.4 min in the navigated group), and radiation exposure (1.5 movements of the C-arm into the field were required per screw in the conventional group vs. 0.09 movements per screw in the navigated group, indicating that multiple screws could be placed with a single exposure when using navigation).

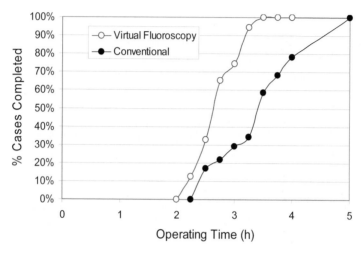

Fig. 12.9. Time needed to complete spinal fusion surgery using either conventional or virtual fluoroscopic procedures. Data derived from Sasso and Garrido [2007]

Given these demonstrated advantages, some surgeons have raised the question of whether or not spinal navigation should now be considered the standard of care. Schröder and Wassmann [2006] reported the results of a survey of German neurosurgery departments. With 107 responses (84% response rate), they found that almost two-thirds of the responding departments (64%) were using spinal navigation systems, and that 58% of the departments not currently having access would like access. Currently, just under half (49%) of the responders believe that spinal navigation enhances safety, and 94% reject the suggestion that it should now be considered mandatory. For now, conventional pedicle screw insertion is still considered acceptable practice.

12.4.4 Fracture Repair

12.4.4.1 Clinical Motivation

When bones are fractured, the surgeon is faced with the problem of placing the fragments back in nominal alignment with one another (reduction) and securing the fragments in place (fixation), so that the bone can heal.

Fractures are extremely common. As a group, they represent one of the most common reasons for presenting at emergency rooms, and long bone fractures of the humerus, radius, ulna, femur, and tibia are among the most frequently occurring fractures. Van Staa et al. [2001] report that in England and Wales, these long bone fractures occur at a rate of 0.55% per year, and in the United States, closed reduction of fractures is the most frequently performed orthopedic trauma procedure, with over 400,000 performed annually [Joskowicz et al. 1998].

The standard treatment for femoral shaft fractures is now the intramedullary nail [Bong et al. 2007], a hollow metal tube inserted down the intramedullary canal of the bone and secured in place at both ends with pairs of transverse bicortical screws. Union rates are normally close to 100% [Winquist et al. 1984] and there is a low incidence of infection. Despite this, femur fractures represent the single most prevalent and the third most expensive type of malpractice suit brought against orthopedic surgeons [AAOS 1999]. The main reason for patient dissatisfaction is most likely related to difficulties achieving proper alignment of the two fragments; according to Westphal et al. [2006], malalignment in the sagittal and frontal planes occurs in up to 18% of cases and rotations of the bone beyond 10° occur in upwards of 40% of cases. Braten et al. [1995] similarly found rotations of more than 15° in 19% of cases.

From a surgical point of view, it is difficult to be confident that the rotation is correct. In addition, the distal locking process is particularly time consuming and radiation intensive. The reason distal locking is so difficult is that the process of inserting the nail through the femur produces significant deformations in the nail [Krettek et al. 1998a] both laterally and in torsion, which prevent the surgeon from being able to locate the holes relative to the proximal portion of the nail that is accessible. The standard operative technique therefore uses fluoroscopy. The patient's leg is immobilized and a C-arm fluoroscope is repositioned repeatedly until a view is obtained in which the distal locking holes appear circular, which means that the fluoroscope is aimed directly down the holes. A radiolucent drill guide is then pressed against the bone, and when an X-ray image confirms that it is aligned, the surgeon taps it against the bone and drills a screw through the guide.

This fluoroscopic method has two major disadvantages: it is not time efficient, and it exposes the surgical team to a significant amount of radiation. In an in vitro study, Krettek et al. [1998b] found that distal locking of the implant took 22 min out of a total of 31 min for the simulated surgical time. In live surgeries, Suhm et al. [2004] reported that distal locking of two screws was accomplished in a mean time of 27.4 min. Okcu and Aktuglu [2003] reported a total surgical time of 141.6 ± 20.2 min for intramedullary nailing of the femur. Distal locking therefore accounts for approximately 20% of total surgical time. As operating room time costs roughly $20 per minute, a significantly more rapid distal locking procedure could save hundreds of dollars per case.

In the *in vitro* study mentioned earlier [Krettek et al. 1999], the distal locking process required 88 s of fluoroscopic screening time out of a total of 93 s for the whole procedure. Total fluoroscopic screening times as low as 0.52 min have been reported for senior orthopedic surgeons performing live surgeries [Madan and Blakeway 2002] but are more commonly reported to be in the range of 4–7 min [Blattert et al. 2004; Muller et al. 1998]. The wide range of reported screening times is likely due to the complexity of reducing comminuted fractures and the variations in experience of orthopedic surgeons [Blattert et al. 2004; Madan and Blakeway 2002; Hafez et al. 2005]. Radiation exposure during distal locking is particularly important because the surgeon's hands are typically either in the beam or very close to it during this process, whereas during guide wire insertion, their hands are further away. Numerous studies in recent years have called attention to the possibility that orthopedic surgeons' cumulative exposure is underestimated [Mehlman and DiPasquale 1997; Herscovici and Sanders 2000; Madan and Blakeway 2002; Hafez et al. 2005; Singer 2005]. Hafez argues that previous studies have significantly underestimated the actual radiation exposure received at a surgeon's fingertips, and found that doses there were as much as 75 times higher than at the base of the fingers. This suggests that techniques that can reduce radiation exposure would be welcomed by surgeons.

The primary motivations for using navigation techniques in fracture repair are therefore to more accurately control the rotational alignment of the bone fragments, to shorten the operative time, and to decrease the radiation exposure of the surgeon.

12.4.4.2 Computer-Assisted Fracture Reduction and Distal Locking

There are currently two major navigated approaches to dealing with long bone fractures: virtual fluoroscopy-based systems for targeting the distal locking screws and CT-based systems for controlling rotational alignment of the bone fragments.

Two early virtual-fluoroscopy-based systems were developed by Phillips et al. [1995] (see also Viant et al. [1997]; and Hofstetter et al. [1999]). The Phillips/Viant system used a mechanical arm with optical encoders to make the intraoperative measurements, while Hofstetter used optical trackers. In use, a pair of calibrated fluoroscopic images were obtained and the 3D locations of the distal locking holes found. A calibrated screw insertion guide was then positioned under computer guidance using guidance displays similar to those described earlier in the section on pedicle screw insertions.

To control the rotational alignment of the bone fragments, a 3D representation of the fragments must be created. Joskowicz et al. [1998]

proposed using a preoperative CT scan to identify the fragments, and intra-operative fluoroscopy to register the preoperative 3D model to the patient. In this technique, known as FRACAS (fracture computer-assisted surgery), a preoperative CT is acquired of both the injured and the normal leg, the mirror image of which serves as a reference for setting the relative rotation of the bone fragments. Intraoperatively, a rigid body with optical markers attached is screwed onto each major bone fragment. Two fluoroscopic images are then acquired, and a 2D/3D registration procedure is performed. In effect, the computer generates simulated X-ray images on the basis of an assumed position and orientation of the 3D CT model and compares the simulated outlines with those of the actual images (Fig. 12.10). The estimated spatial position of the CT model is then manipulated to optimize the match between the real and simulated X-ray bone contours. Once registered, the relative position of the fragments can be displayed on a computer monitor in real time, and the fragments are manipulated by the surgeon until an optimal relative alignment is achieved. At this point, a guide wire is inserted, followed by the intramedullary nail itself.

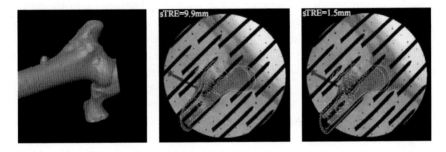

Fig. 12.10. FRACAS system: Anatomic model derived from CT on *left*, fluoroscopic images with projected X-ray contours shown in *white* at initial (*center*) and final pose (*right*). Reproduced with permission from Joskowicz et al. [2004]

In addition to these two major approaches to fracture reduction and nail locking, in recent years, several researchers have developed robotic systems to address various aspects of this type of surgery. For example, Fuchtmeier et al. [2004] adapted a Staubli industrial robot to apply the relatively large distraction forces necessary for reduction, while Westphal and his colleagues [2006] also used a Staubli robot to assist in reduction, although to date no reduction in radiation or time has been achieved. Wang et al. [2006a] presented the design of a robot, which assisted in the distal locking process; all screws were correctly positioned and the fluoroscopy time was reduced to under 2 s per screw. Grützner et al. [2005] describe a novel application of virtual reality techniques to assist the surgeon in visualizing the 3D relationships between bone fragments during reduction.

Most recently, our group introduced a radiation-free technique for intramedullary nail locking on the basis of electromagnetic tracking of a small 6 DOF position sensor less than 3 mm in diameter, which is inserted down the central channel of the intramedullary nail [Beadon et al. 2007]. In this technique, the sensor is contained in a plastic carrier designed to engage in the distal locking holes, thereby placing the sensor in a precalibrated position relative to the holes. The surgeon then uses computer guidance to position a tracked drill guide in the correct location to make the holes for the bicortical screws. The accuracy of this technique has been validated in the laboratory and plans are underway for a clinical evaluation. Because the C-arm is not needed for the locking process, the operative time required is expected to be less than for the conventional procedure.

12.4.4.3 Evaluation

Joskowicz's group reported results of the FRACAS system in Ron et al. [2002]. In a study performed using five dry femurs, they found that their system was able to recreate the torsion of the healthy side with a mean absolute difference of 1.8° (range: −4.4° to 1.7°). The repeatability on the given specimens was characterized by standard deviations ranging from 0.4° to 0.9°. They concluded that their technique was sufficiently accurate in the laboratory setting to move to clinical trials. To date, we are not aware of any clinical studies reported in the peer-reviewed literature.

Virtual fluoroscopy-based (VF) systems have proven effective in the distal locking process in several studies. The system described by Hofstetter has been evaluated in two studies [Hofstetter et al. 2000; Slomczykowski et al. 2001]. In the first of these studies, the torsion angle produced by the VF system on average was found to be 1.5° off the torsion produced by a full 3D CT-based system. The second study explored the ability of the system to lock the distal holes in a variety of bone models, cadaveric specimens, and one clinical case. All 76 holes attempted were successfully locked, with contact between the drill bit and the nail in 11% of the cases. The fluoroscopy time per pair of screws was 1.67 s (compared with 0.5–7 min with the conventional procedure). This is consistent with the 2.23 s per screw pair reported by Wang et al. [2006b]. Malek et al. [2005] reported more specifically on the accuracy of the virtual fluoroscopy approach described by Phillips and Viant. In this lab-based study, they found excellent accuracy results; the positional accuracy was within 0.3 mm and the angular accuracy within 0.2°. This is consistent with the accuracy reported by Zheng et al. [2007].

Suhm et al. [2004] found similar results to Hofstetter, also for a VF-based system used with a set of 42 patients divided into conventional fluoroscopic and navigated groups. The fluoroscopic time for the conventional procedure was 108 s vs. 7.3 s for the navigated group. The navigated procedure took slightly longer, at 17.9 min per screw compared with 13.7 min per screw in the conventional group. In a different study performed a little earlier with 50 patients, in which a mechanical guide was compared with navigation, Suhm et al. [2003] found that the manual technique failed on one screw, while navigation failed on two screws. The time per screw was 6.9 min for the manual technique and 37.6 min for the navigated process, considerably longer than in the 2004 study. The navigation system required an additional 44 min of setup time in the operating theater before and after the patient was present.

In summary, CT-based systems exist that can align femoral fracture fragments in rotation with good accuracy, and virtual fluoroscopy-based systems have been shown to produce successful targeting rates comparable to the conventional fluoroscopic procedure, but with markedly reduced radiation exposure and comparable, although generally slightly increased, operative times.

12.5   Summary and Future Trends

In this chapter, we have explored a variety of clinical situations in orthopedic surgery in which there is a need for increased accuracy when performing the surgery. Very significant progress has been made in the past decade on the technical side, and in every area there have been demonstrations of improved performance as measured by such outcomes as implant alignment or percentage of implantations within specified bounds. However, demonstrations of long-term benefits relative to the conventional approaches are few in number and significant progress is still required to make computer-assisted approaches less disruptive to the surgical process, require less time, and cost less. A recent opinion was expressed by a group of surgeons in an editorial in the Journal of Arthroplasty that computer-assisted surgery was "a wine before its time" [Callaghan et al. 2006], and a number of organizations responsible for approving widespread use of computer-assisted procedures in broader health care systems have reached similar conclusions in the past year or two.

The challenge is therefore before us. Although more advances in technology are clearly possible, ranging from new imaging techniques such as 3D ultrasound to implants combining mechanical and biological functions, widespread adoption of computer-assisted orthopedic surgical techniques will be greatly encouraged by concerted research efforts directed toward workflow improvements, cost reductions, and time savings. Finally, given that the majority of orthopedic procedures are currently performed by general orthopedic surgeons who practice in the community and perform a wide variety of procedures, special attention must be paid to their needs.

References

AAOS Committee on Professional Liability. (1999). "Managing Orthopaedic Malpractice Risk" (2nd Edn.). AAOS, Rosemont, IL.

Amiot LP, Labelle H, DeGuise JA, Sati M, Brodeur P, Rivard CH. (1995). "Computer-assisted pedicle screw fixation. A feasibility study." *Spine* 20(10):1208–1212.

Anglin C, Hodgson AJ, Masri BA, Greidanus NV, Garbuz DS. (2004). "Quality of life before and after total knee arthroplasty." *Canadian Orthopaedic Association*, June 3–6, Montreal, Canada.

Anglin C, Masri BA, Tonetti J, Hodgson AJ, Greidanus NV. (2007). "Hip resurfacing femoral neck fracture influenced by valgus placement." *Clin. Orthop Relat Res.* 465:71–79.

Arand M, Schempf M, Fleiter T, Kinzl L, Gebhard F. (2006). "Qualitative and quantitative accuracy of CAOS in a standardized *in vitro* spine model." *Clin. Orthop. Relat. Res.* 450:118–128.

Arslanian C, Bond M. (1999). "Computer assisted outcomes research in orthopedics: Total joint replacement." *J. Med. Syst.* 23(3):239–247.

Attarian DE, Vail TP. (2005). "Medicolegal aspects of hip and knee arthroplasty." *Clin. Orthop. Relat. Res.* 433:72–76.

Back DL, Smith JD, Dalziel RE, et al. (2007). "Establishing a learning curve for hip resurfacing." *74th Annual Meeting of American Academy of Orthopaedic Surgeons.* February 14–18, San Diego, USA.

Barzilay Y, Liebergall M, Fridlander A, Knoller N. (2006). "Miniature robotic guidance for spine surgery–introduction of a novel system and analysis of challenges encountered during the clinical development phase at two spine centres. " *Int. J. Med. Robot.* (2):146–153.

Bäthis H, Shafizadeh S, Paffrath T, Simanski C, Grifka J, Lüring C. (2006). "[Are computer assisted total knee replacements more accurately placed? A meta-analysis of comparative studies]. " *Orthopade.* 35(10):1056–1065.

Bauer A. (2004). "Total hip replacement–robotic-assisted technique." In *Computer and Robotic Assisted Hip and Knee Surgery*, DiGioia AM (Ed.). Oxford University Press, Oxford, New York, pp. 83–96.

Bauwens K, Matthes G, Wich M, Gebhard F, Hanson B, Ekkernkamp A, Stengel D. (2007). "Navigated total knee replacement. A meta-analysis." *J. Bone Joint Surg. Am.* 89(2):261–269.

Beadon K, Stanley J, O'Brien PJ, Guy P, Hodgson AJ. (2007). "Electromagnetic tracking for navigation in computer-assisted distal locking for intramedullary nailing of the femur: A feasibility study." *7th Annual Meeting of the International Society for Computer Assisted Orthopaedic Surgery Conference*, June 20–23, Heidelberg, Germany.

Beaulé PE, Lee JL, Le Duff MJ, Amstutz HC, Ebramzadeh EJ. (2004). "Orientation of the femoral component in surface arthroplasty of the hip. A biomechanical and clinical analysis." *Bone Joint Surg Am.* Sep. 86-A(9):2015–21.

Beringer DC, Patel JJ, Bozic KJ. (2007). " An overview of economic issues in computer-assisted total joint arthroplasty." *Clin Orthop Relat Res.* Oct. 463:26–30.

Blattert TR, Fill UA, Kunz E, Panzer W, Weckbach A, Regulla DF. (2004). "Skill dependence of radiation exposure for the orthopaedic surgeon during interlocking nailing of long-bone shaft fractures: A clinical study." *Arch. Orthop. Trauma Surg.* 124(10):659–664.

Block JE, Stubbs HA. (2005). "Reducing the risk of deep wound infection in primary joint arthroplasty with antibiotic bone cement." *Orthopedics*. 28(11):1334–1345.

Bong MR, Kummer FJ, Koval KJ, Egol KA. (2007). "Intramedullary nailing of the lower extremity: Biomechanics and biology." *J. Am. Acad. Orthop. Surg.* 15(2):97–106.

Bozic KJ and Beringer D. (2007). "Economic considerations in minimally invasive total joint arthroplasty." *Clin Orthop Relat Res*. Oct. 463:20–25.

Brander V, Stulberg SD. (2006). "Rehabilitation after hip- and knee-joint replacement: An experience- and evidence-based approach to care." *Am. J. Phys. Med. Rehabil*. 85(Suppl): S98–S118.

Brander VA, Stulberg SD, Adams AD, Harden RN, Bruehl S, Stanos SP, Houle T. (2003). "Predicting total knee replacement pain: A prospective, observational study." *Clin. Orthop. Relat. Res*. 416:27–36.

Braten M, Terjesen T, Rossvoll I. (1995). "Femoral shaft fractures treated by intramedullary nailing. A follow-up study focusing on problems related to the method." *Injury* 26(6):379–383.

Buechel FF Sr, Buechel FF Jr, Pappas MJ, Dalessio J. (2002). "Twenty-year evaluation of the New Jersey LCS rotating platform knee replacement." *J. Knee. Surg*. 15(2):84–89.

Callaghan JJ, Liu SS, Warth LC. (2006). "Computer-assisted surgery: A wine before its time: In the affirmative." *J. Arthroplasty* 21(4 Suppl 1):27–28.

Callaghan JJ, Squire MW, Goetz DD, Sullivan PM, Johnston RC. (2000). "Cemented rotating-platform total knee replacement: A nine to twelve-year follow-up study." *J. Bone Joint Surg. Am*. 82(5):705–711.

Callahan CM, Drake B, Heck D, Dittus RS. (1994). "Patient outcomes following tricompartmental total knee replacement. A meta-analysis." *JAMA* 271(17): 1349–1357.

Canadian Joint Replacement Registry (CJRR). (2004). "Report on Total Hip and Knee Replacements in Canada." Canadian Institute for Health Information.

Castro WH, Halm H, Jerosch J, Malms J, Steinbeck J, Blasius S. (1996). "Accuracy of pedicle screw placement in lumbar vertebrae." *Spine* 21(11):1320–1324.

Centers for Disease Control and Prevention (CDC). (2003). "Targeting Arthritis: The Leading Cause of Disability", Report from the Centers for Disease Control and Prevention, Atlanta, USA.

Craven MP, Davey SM, Martin JL. (2005). "Factors influencing wider acceptance of Computer Assisted Orthopaedic Surgery (CAOS) technologies for total joint arthroplasty", MATCH CAOS Review, December 2005.

Dalton JE, Cook SD, Thomas KA, Kay JF. (1995). "The effect of operative fit and hydroxyapatite coating on the mechanical and biological response to porous implants." *J. Bone Joint Surg. Am*. 77(1):97–110.

Darmanis S, Toms A, Durman R, Moore D, Eyres K. (2007). "A technical innovation for improving identification of the trackers by the LED cameras in navigation-assisted total knee arthroplasty." *Comput. Aided Surg*. 12(4):247–251.

Davies BL, Rodriguez y Baena FM, Barrett AR, Gomes MP, Harris SJ, Jakopec M, Cobb JP. (2007). "Robotic control in knee joint replacement surgery." *Proc. Inst. Mech. Eng. [H]*. 221(1):71–80.

Davis ET, Gallie P, Macgroarty K, Waddell JP, Schemitsch E. (2007). "The accuracy of image-free computer navigation in the placement of the femoral component of the Birmingham hip resurfacing: A cadaver study." *J. Bone Joint Surg. Br.* 89-B(4):557–560.

Decking R, Markmann Y, Fuchs J, Puhl W, Scharf HP. (2005). "Leg axis after computer-navigated total knee arthroplasty: A prospective randomized trial comparing computer-navigated and manual implantation." *J. Arthroplasty* 20(3):282–288.

Dewey P, Incoll I. (1998). "Evaluation of thyroid shields for reduction of radiation exposure to orthopaedic surgeons." *Aust. NZ J. Surg.* 68:635–636.

DiGioia AM, Jaramaz B, Blackwell M, et al. (1998). "The Otto Aufranc Award: Image-guided navigation system to measure intraoperatively acetabular implant alignment." *Clin. Orthop.* 355:8–22.

DiGioia AM, Jaramaz B, Plakseychuk AY, et al. (2002). "Comparison of a mechanical acetabular alignment guide with computer placement of the socket." *J. Arthroplasty* 17:359–364.

Dong H, Buxton M. (2006). "Early assessment of the likely cost-effectiveness of a new technology: A Markov model with probabilistic sensitivity analysis of computer-assisted total knee replacement." *Int. J. Technol. Assess Health Care.* 22(2):191–202.

Dorr LD, Hishiki Y, Wan Z, Newton D, Yun A. (2005). "Development of imageless computer navigation for acetabular component position in total hip replacement." *Iowa Orthop. J.* 25:1–9.

Edeen J, Sharkey PF, Alexander AH. (1995). "Clinical significance of leg-length inequality after total hip arthroplasty." *Am. J. Orthop.* 24(4):347–351.

Eisenhuth SA, Saleh KJ, Cui Q, Clark CR, Brown TE. (2006). "Patellofemoral instability after total knee arthroplasty." *Clin. Orthop. Relat. Res.* 446:149–160.

Etienne A, Cupic Z, Charnley J. (1978). "Postoperative dislocation afterCharnley low-friction arthroplasty." *Clin. Orthop.* 132:19–23

Faraj AA, Webb JK. (1997). "Early complications of spinal pedicle screw." *Eur. Spine J.* 6(5):324–326.

Foley KT, Simon DA, Rampersaud YR. (2001). "Virtual fluoroscopy: Computer-assisted fluoroscopic navigation." *Spine* 26(4):347–351.

Fuchtmeier B, Egersdoerfer S, Mai R, Hente R, Dragoi D, Monkman G, Nerlich M. (2004). "Reduction of femoral shaft fractures in vitro by a new developed reduction robot system 'RepoRobo'." *Injury* 35(1):113–119.

Gebhard F, Weidner A, Liener UC, Stockle U, Arand M. (2004). "Navigation at the spine." *Injury* 35(1):35–45.

Griffin FM, Insall JN, Scuderi GR. (2000). "Accuracy of soft tissue balancing in total knee arthroplasty." *J. Arthroplasty* 15(8):970–973.

Grützner PA, Langlotz F, Zheng G, von Recum J, Keil C, Nolte LP, Wentzensen A, Wendl K. (2005). "Computer-assisted LISS plate osteosynthesis of proximal tibia fractures: Feasibility study and first clinical results." *Comput. Aided Surg.* 10(3):141–149.

Gwynne Jones DP, Stoddart J. (1998). "Radiation use in the orthopaedic theatre a prospective audit". *Aust. NZ J. Surg.* 68:782–784.

Haaker RG, Tiedjen K, Ottersbach A, Rubenthaler F, Stockheim M, Stiehl JB. (2007). "Comparison of conventional versus computer-navigated acetabular component insertion." *J. Arthroplasty* 22(2):151–159.

Hafez MA, Smith RM, Matthews SJ, Kalap G, Sherman KP. (2005). "Radiation exposure to the hands of orthopaedic surgeons: Are we underestimating the risk?" *Arch. Orthop. Trauma Surg.* 125(5):330–335.

Haider H, Barrera OA, Garvin KL. (2007). "Minimally invasive total knee arthroplasty surgery through navigated freehand bone cutting." *J. Arthroplasty* 22(4):535–542.

Hamelinck HK, Haagmans M, Snoeren MM, Biert J, van Vugt AB, Frolke JP. (2007). "Safety of computer-assisted surgery for cannulated hip screws." *Clin. Orthop. Relat. Res.* 455:241–245.

Harris WH. (2001). "Wear and periprosthetic osteolysis: The problem." *Clin. Orthop. Relat. Res.* 393:66–70.

Hawker GA. (2006). "Who, when, and why total joint replacement surgery? The patient's perspective." *Curr. Opin. Rheumatol.* 18(5):526–530.

Hernandez VH, D'Apuzzo MR, Lee D, Lavernia CJ. (2006). "Projections of total knee revision. A cost analysis." AAOS Annual Meeting, March 22–24, Chicago, USA.

Herscovici D Jr, Sanders RW. (2000). "The effects, risks, and guidelines for radiation use in orthopaedic surgery." *Clin. Orthop. Relat. Res.* 375:126–132.

Hodgson AJ, Inkpen KB, Shekhman M, Anglin C, Tonetti J, Masri BA, Duncan CP, Garbuz DS, Greidanus NV. (2005). "Computer-assisted femoral head resurfacing." *Comput. Aided Surg.* 10(5–6):337–343.

Hodgson AJ, Helmy N, Masri BA, Greidanus NV, Inkpen KB, Duncan CP, Garbuz DS, Anglin C. (2007). "Comparative repeatability of guide-pin axis positioning in computer-assisted and manual femoral head resurfacing arthroplasty." *Proc. Inst. Mech. Eng. (H) J. Eng. Med.* 221(7):713–724.

Hofstetter R, Slomczykowski M, Krettek C, Koppen G, Sati M, Nolte LP. (2000). "Computer-assisted fluoroscopy-based reduction of femoral fractures and antetorsion correction." *Comput. Aided Surg.* 5(5):311–325.

Hofstetter R, Slomczykowski M, Sati M, Nolte LP. (1999). "Fluoroscopy as an imaging means for computer-assisted surgical navigation." *Comput. Aided Surg.* 4(2):65–76.

Holt G, Wheelan K, Gregori A. (2006). "The ethical implications of recent innovations in knee arthroplasty. "*J. Bone Joint Surg. Am.* 88:226–229.

Honl M, Dierk O, Gauck C, Carrero V, Lampe F, Dries S, Quante M, Schwieger K, Hille E, Morlock MM. (2003). "Comparison of robotic-assisted and manual implantation of a primary total hip replacement. A prospective study." *J. Bone Joint Surg. Am.* 85-A(8):1470–1478.

Hube R, Birke A, Hein W, Klima S. (2003). "CT-based and fluoroscopy-based navigation for cup implantation in total hip arthroplasty (THA)." *Surg. Technol. Int.* 11:275–280.

Hüfner T, Gebhard F, Grützner PA, Messmer P, Stöckle U, Krettek C. (2004). "Which navigation when?" *Injury* 35(1):30–34.

Hynes DE, Conere T, Mee MB, Cashman WF. (1992). "Ionising radiation and the orthopaedic surgeon." *J. Bone Joint Surg. Br.* 74:332–334.

Jaramaz B, DiGioia AM III, Blackwell M, Nikou C. (1998). "Computer assisted measurement of cup placement in total hip replacement." *Clin. Orthop. Relat. Res.* 354:70–81.

Jeffery RS, Morris RW, Denham RA. (1991). "Coronal alignment after total knee replacement." *J. Bone Joint Surg. Br.* 73(5):709–714.

Jones CA, Beaupre LA, Johnston DW, Suarez-Almazor ME. (2007). "Total joint arthroplasties: Current concepts of patient outcomes after surgery." *Rheum. Dis. Clin. N. Am.* 33(1):71–86.

Joskowicz L, Knaan D. (2004). "How to achieve fast, accurate and robust rigid registration between fluoroscopic X-ray and CT images". *CARS* 2004, June 23–26, Chicago, USA.

Joskowicz L, Milgrom C, Simkin A, Tockus L, Yaniv Z. (1998). "FRACAS: A system for computer-aided image-guided long bone fracture surgery." *Comput. Aided Surg.* 3(6):271–288.

Kahler DM, Mallik K. (1999). "Computer assisted iliosacral screw placement compared to stafndard fluoroscopic technique." *Comput. Aided Surg.* 4:348.

Kahler DM, Zura R. (1997). "Evaluation of a computer-assisted surgical technique for percutaneous internal fixation in a transverse acetabular fracture model." *Lecture Notes in Computer Science.* Springer, Berlin, pp. 565–572.

Kalteis T, Handel M, Bathis H, Perlick L, Tingart M, Grifka J. (2006). "Imageless navigation for insertion of the acetabular component in total hip arthroplasty: Is it as accurate as CT-based navigation?" *J. Bone Joint Surg. Br.* 88(2):163–167.

Kazanzides P. (2007). "Robots for orthopaedic joint reconstruction." In: *Robotics in Surgery: History, Current and Future Applications* (Ed. Faust RA), Nova Science, New York, pp. 61–94.

Kelly MA. (2001). "Patellofemoral complications following total knee arthroplasty." *Instr Course Lect.* 50:403–407.

Kennedy JG, Rogers WB, Soffe KE, Sullivan RJ, Griffen DG, Sheehan LJ. (1998). "Effect of acetabular component orientation on recurrent dislocation, pelvic osteolysis, polyethylene wear, and component migration." *J. Arthroplasty* 13(5):530–534.

Kim YJ, Lenke LG, Bridwell KH, Cho YS, Riew KD. (2004). "Free hand pedicle screw placement in the thoracic spine: Is it safe?" *Spine* 29(3):333–342.

Kosmopoulos V, Schizas C. (2007). "Pedicle screw placement accuracy: A meta-analysis." *Spine* 32(3):111–120.

Kowalczyk L. (2005). "Robotic surgery gets new push: Long-term prostate benefits unclear." Boston Globe, October 1, 2005.

Kozak LJ, DeFrances CJ, Hall MJ. (2006). "National hospital discharge survey: 2004 annual summary with detailed diagnosis and procedure data." *Vital Health Statistics* 13. Oct. (162):1–209.

Kreder HJ, Grosso P, Williams JI, Jaglal S, Axcell T, Wal EK, Stephen DJ. (2003). "Provider volume and other predictors of outcome after total knee arthroplasty: A population study in Ontario." *Can. J. Surg.* 46(1):15–22.

Krettek C, Mannss J, Miclau T, Schandelmaier P, Linnemann I, Tscherne H. (1998a). "Deformation of femoral nails with intramedullary insertion." *J. Orthop. Res.* 16(5):572–575.

Krettek C, Konemann B, Farouk O, Miclau T, Kromm A, Tscherne H. (1998b). "Experimental study of distal interlocking of a solid tibial nail: Radiation-independent Distal Aiming Device (DAD) versus Free Hand Technique (FHT)." *J. Orthop. Trauma.* 12(6):373–378.

Krettek C, Konemann B, Miclau T, Kolbli R, Machreich T, Tscherne H. (1999). "A mechanical distal aiming device for distal locking in femoral nails." *Clin Orthop Relat Res.* (364):267–275.

Kruger S, Zambelli PY, Leyvraz PF, Jolles BM. (2007). "Computer-assisted placement technique in hip resurfacing arthroplasty: Improvement in accuracy?" *Int Orthop.* (Published online on Aug 24)

Kurtz S, Mowat F, Ong K, Chan N, Lau E, Halpern M. (2005). "Prevalence of primary and revision total hip and knee arthroplasty in the United States from 1990 through 2002." *J. Bone Joint Surg. Am.* 87(7):1487–1497.

Kurtz SM, Lau E, Zhao K, Mowat F, Ong K, Halpern MT. (2006). "The future burden of hip and knee revisions: U.S. projections from 2005 to 2030", *AAOS Annual Meeting*, March 22–24, Chicago, IL, USA.

Kwon MS, Kuskowski M, Mulhall KJ, Macaulay W, Brown TE, Saleh KJ. (2006). "Does surgical approach affect total hip arthroplasty dislocation rates?" *Clin. Orthop. Relat. Res.* 447:34–38.

Laine T, Schlenzka D, Mäkitalo K, Tallroth K, Nolte LP, Visarius H. (1997). "Improved accuracy of pedicle screw insertion with computer-assisted surgery. A prospective clinical trial of 30 patients." *Spine* 22(11):1254–1258.

Lazovic D, Zigan R. (2006). "Navigation of short-stem implants." *Orthopedics.* 29(10 Suppl):S125–S129.

Lee GY, Massicotte EM, Rampersaud YR (2007). "Clinical accuracy of cervicothoracic pedicle screw placement: A comparison of the 'open' lamino-foraminotomy and computer-assisted techniques." *J. Spinal Disord. Tech.* 20(1):25–32.

Leenders T, Vandevelde D, Mahieu G, Nuyts R. (2002). "Reduction in variability of acetabular cup abduction using computer-assisted surgery: A prospective and randomized study." *Comput. Aided Surg.* 7:99–106.

Lewinnek GE, Lewis JL, Tarr R, Compere CL, Zimmerman JR. (1978). "Dislocations after total hip-replacement arthroplasties." *J. Bone Joint Surg. Am.* 60(2):217–220.

Lüring C, Bäthis H, Tingart M, Perlick L, Grifka J. (2006). "Computer assistance in total knee replacement – a critical assessment of current health care technology." *Comput. Aided Surg.* 11(2):77–80.

Madan S, Blakeway C. (2002). "Radiation exposure to surgeon and patient in intramedullary nailing of the lower limb." *Injury* 33(8):723–727.

Maddern GJ. (2007). "Robotic surgery: Will it be evidence-based or just "toys for boys"?" *MJA* 186(5):221–222.

Malek S, Phillips R, Mohsen A, Viant W, Bielby M, Sherman K. (2005). "Computer assisted orthopaedic surgical system for insertion of distal locking screws in intra-medullary nails: A valid and reliable navigation system." *Int. J. Med. Robot.* 1(4):34–44.

Marmignon C, Leimnei A, Lavallée S, Cinquin P. (2005). "Automated hydraulic tensor for total knee arthroplasty." *Int. J. Med. Robot.* 1(4):51–57.

Masonis JL, Bourne RB. (2002). "Surgical approach, abductor function, and total hip arthroplasty dislocation." *Clin. Orthop. Relat. Res.* (405):46–53.

Mehlman CT, DiPasquale TG. (1997). "Radiation exposure to the orthopaedic surgical team during fluoroscopy: How far away is far enough?" *J. Orthop. Trauma.* 11(6):392–398.

Meikle MC. (2005). "Guest editorial: What do prospective randomized clinical trials tell us about the treatment of class II malocclusions? A personal viewpoint." *Eur. J. Orthod.* 27(2):105–114.

Mian SW, Truchly G, Pflum FA. (1992). "Computed tomography measurement of acetabular cup anteversion and retroversion in total hip arthroplasty." *Clin. Orthop. Relat. Res.* 276:206–209.

Moed BR, Yu PH, Gruson KI. (2003). "Functional Outcomes of Acetabular Fractures." *J. Bone Joint Surg. Am.* 85:1879–1883.

Morrey BF. (1997). "Difficult complications after hip joint replacement: Dislocation." *Clin. Orthop. Relat. Res.* 344:179–187.

Muller LP, Suffner J, Wenda K, Mohr W, Rommens PM. (1998). "Radiation exposure to the hands and the thyroid of the surgeon during intramedullary nailing." *Injury* 29(6):461–468.

National Institutes of Health (NIH) Consensus Statement on Total Knee Replacement. (2003). *NIH Consensus and State-of-the-Science Statements.* December 8–10, 20(1):1–34.

Nishihara S, Sugano N, Nishii T, Tanaka H, Nakamura N, Yoshikawa H, Ochi T. (2004). "Clinical accuracy evaluation of femoral canal preparation using the ROBODOC system." *J. Orthop. Sci.* 9(5):452–461.

Nizard RS, Biau D, Porcher R, Ravaud P, Bizot P, Hannouche D, Sedel L. (2005). "A meta-analysis of patellar replacement in total knee arthroplasty." *Clin. Orthop. Relat. Res.* Mar. (432):196–203.

Noble PC, Sugano N, Johnston JD, Thompson MT, Conditt MA, Engh CA, Mathis KB. (2003). "Computer simulation: How can it help the surgeon optimize implant position?" *Clin. Orthop. Relat. Res.* 417:242–252.

Nogler M, Kessler O, Prassl A, Donnelly B, Streicher R, Sledge JB, Krismer M. (2004). "Reduced variability of acetabular cup positioning with use of an imageless navigation system." *Clin. Orthop.* 426:159–163.

Nohara Y, Taneichi H, Ueyama K, Kawahara N, Shiba K, Tokuhashi Y, Tani T, Nakahara S, Iida T. (2004). "Nationwide survey on complications of spine surgery in Japan." *J. Orthop. Sci.* 9(5):424–433.

Nolte LP, Ganz R (Eds.). (1999). "Computer-Assisted Orthopedic Surgery (CAOS)", Hogrefe and Huber, Seattle, WA, USA.

Okcu G, Aktuglu K. (2003) "Antegrade nailing of femoral shaft fractures combined with neck or distal femur fractures. A retrospective review of 25 cases, with a follow-up of 36-150 months." *Arch. Orthop. Trauma Surg.* 123(10):544–550.

Ontario Health Technology Advisory Committee. (2004). *"Review of Computer-Assisted Hip and Knee Arthroplasty: Navigation and Robotic Systems".* Medical Advisory Secretariat, Ontario Ministry of Health and Long-term Care. February/March 2004.

Orozco FR, Ong A, Rothman RH. (2007). "The role of minimally invasive hip surgery in reducing pain." *Instr. Course Lect.* 56:121–124.

Pakos EE, Ntzani EE, Trikalinos TA. (2005). "Patellar resurfacing in total knee arthroplasty. A meta-analysis." *J Bone Joint Surg Am.* Jul. 87(7):1438–1445.

Papachristou G, Plessas S, Sourlas J, Chronopoulos E, Levidiotis C, Pnevmaticos S. (2006). "Cementless LCS rotating-platform knee arthroplasty in patients over 60 years without patella replacement: A mid-term clinical-outcome study." *Med. Sci. Monit.* 12(6):CR264–268.

Parker DA, Dunbar MJ, Rorabeck CH. (2003). "Extensor mechanism failure associated with total knee arthroplasty: Prevention and management." *J. Am. Acad. Orthop. Surg.* 11(4):238–247.

Parratte S, Argenson JN, Flecher X, Aubaniac JM. (2007). "[Computer-assisted surgery for acetabular cup positioning in total hip arthroplasty: Comparative prospective randomized study]." *Rev. Chir. Orthop. Reparatrice Appar. Mot.* 93(3):238–246.

Parratte S, Argenson JN. (2007). "Validation and usefulness of a computer-assisted cup-positioning system in total hip arthroplasty. A prospective, randomized, controlled study." *J. Bone Joint Surg. Am.* 89(3):494–499.

Parvizi J, Rapuri VR, Saleh KJ, Kuskowski MA, Sharkey PF, Mont MA. (2005). "Failure to resurface the patellar during total knee arthroplasty may result in more knee pain and secondary surgery." *Clin. Orthop. Rel. Res.* Sep. 438:191–196.

Patt JC, Mauerhan DR. (2005). "Outcomes research in total joint replacement: A critical review and commentary." *Am. J. Orthop.* 34(4):167–172.

Paul HA, Bargar WL, Mittlestadt B, Musits B, Taylor RH, Kazanzides P, Zuhars J, Williamson B, Hanson W. (1992). "Development of a surgical robot for cementless total hip arthroplasty." *Clin. Orthop. Relat. Res.* 285:57–66.

Phillips R, Viant WJ, Moshen AMMA, Griffiths JG, Bell MA, Cain TJ, Sherman KP, Karpinski MRK. (1995). "Image-guided orthopaedic surgery: Design and analysis." *Trans. Inst. Measure Control* 17:251–265

Plaskos C, Cinquin P, Lavallee S, Hodgson AJ. (2005). "Praxiteles: A miniature bone-mounted robot for minimal access total knee arthroplasty." *Int. J. Med. Robot.* 1(4):67–79.

Plaskos C, Hodgson AJ, Inkpen K, McGraw RW. (2002). "Bone cutting errors in total knee arthroplasty." *J. Arthroplasty* 17(6):698–705.

Radcliffe IA, Taylor M. (2007). "Investigation into the effect of varus-valgus orientation on load transfer in the resurfaced femoral head: A multi-femur finite element analysis." *Clin. Biomech. (Bristol, Avon).* 22(7):780–786.

Rajasekaran S, Vidyadhara S, Ramesh P, Shetty AP. (2007). "Randomized clinical study to compare the accuracy of navigated and non-navigated thoracic pedicle screws in deformity correction surgeries." *Spine* 32(2):E56–64.

Rampersaud YR, Foley KT, Shen AC, Williams S, Solomito M. (2000). "Radiation exposure to the spine surgeon during fluoroscopically assisted pedicle screw insertion." *Spine* 25(20):2637–2645.

Rand JA, Coventry MB. (1988). "Ten-year evaluation of geometric total knee arthroplasty." *Clin. Orthop. Relat. Res.* 232:168–173.

Reininga IH, Wagenmakers R, van den Akker-Scheek I, Stant AD, Groothoff JW, Bulstra SK, Zijlstra W, Stevens M. (2007). "Effectiveness of computer-navigated minimally invasive total hip surgery compared to conventional total hip arthroplasty: Design of a randomized controlled trial." *BMC Musculoskelet. Disord.* 8(1):4.

Richards PJ, Kurta IC, Jasani V, Jones CH, Rahmatalla A, Mackenzie G, Dove J. (2007). "Assessment of CAOS as a training model in spinal surgery: A randomised study." *Eur. Spine J.* 16(2):239–244.

Ritter MA, Faris PM, Keating EM, Meding JB. (1994). "Postoperative alignment of total knee replacement. Its effect on survival." *Clin. Orthop. Relat. Res.* 299:153–156.

Rivet DJ, Jeck D, Brennan J, Epstein A, Lauryssen C. (2004). "Clinical outcomes and complications associated with pedicle screw fixation-augmented lumbar interbody fusion." *J. Neurosurg. Spine.* 1(3):261–266.

Robertsson O, Knutson K, Lewold S, Lidgren L. (2001). "The Swedish Knee Arthroplasty Register 1975–1997: An update with special emphasis on 41,223 knees operated on in 1988–1997." *Acta. Orthop. Scand.* 72(5):503–513.

Ron O, Joskowicz L, Milgrom C, Simkin A. (2002). "Computer-based periaxial rotation measurement for aligning fractured femur fragments from CT: A feasibility study." *Comput. Aided Surg.* 7(6):332–341.

Saragaglia D, Picard F, Chaussard C, Montbarbon E, Leitner F, Cinquin P. (2001). "[Computer-assisted knee arthroplasty: Comparison with a conventional procedure. Results of 50 cases in a prospective randomized study]." *Rev. Chir. Orthop. Reparatrice Appar. Mot.* 87(1):18–28.

Sasso RC, Garrido BJ. (2007). "Computer-assisted spinal navigation versus serial radiography and operative time for posterior spinal fusion at L5-S1." *J. Spinal Disord. Tech.* 20(2):118–122.

Saxler G, Marx A, Vandevelde D, Langlotz U, Tannast M, Wiese M, Michaelis U, Kemper G, Grützner PA, Steffen R, von Knoch M, Holland-Letz T, Bernsmann K. (2004). "The accuracy of free-hand cup positioning: A CT based measurement of cup placement in 105 total hip arthroplasties." *Int. Orthop.* 28(4):198–201.

Schep NW, Haverlag R, van Vugt AB. (2004). "Computer-assisted versus conventional surgery for insertion of 96 cannulated iliosacral screws in patients with postpartum pelvic pain." *J. Trauma.* 57(6):1299–1302.

Schneider J, Kalender W. (2003). "Geometric accuracy in robot-assisted total hip replacement surgery." *Comput. Aided. Surg.* 8(3):135–145.

Schräder P. (2005). "[Consequence of evidence-based medicine and individual case appraisal of the Robodoc method for the MDK, and the malpractice management of insurance funds and the principles of managing innovations]." *Gesundheitswesen.* 67(6):389–395.

Schröder J, Wassmann H. (2006). "Spinal navigation: An accepted standard of care?" *Zentralbl. Neurochir.* 67(3):123–128.

Seller K, Wild A, Urselmann L, Krauspe R. (2005). "[Prospective screw misplacement analysis after conventional and navigated pedicle screw implantation]." *Biomed Tech (Berl).* 50(9):287–292

Siebert W, Mai S, Kober R, Heeckt PF. (2002). "Technique and first clinical results of robot-assisted total knee replacement". *Knee.* 9(3):173–180.

Singer G. (2005). "Radiation exposure in hand surgery." *J. Hand Surg. Am.* 30(6):1317.

Siston RA, Goodman SB, Patel JJ, Delp SL, Giori NJ. (2006). "The high variability of tibial rotational alignment in total knee arthroplasty." *Clin. Orthop. Relat. Res.* 452:65–69.

Skutek M, Bourne RB, Rorabeck CH, Burns A, Kearns S, Krishna G. (2007). "The twenty to twenty-five-year outcomes of the Harris design-2 matte-finished cemented total hip replacement. A concise follow-up of a previous report." *J. Bone Joint Surg. Am.* 89(4):814–818.

Slomczykowski MA, Hofstetter R, Sati M, Krettek C, Nolte LP. (2001). "Novel computer-assisted fluoroscopy system for intraoperative guidance: Feasibility study for distal locking of femoral nails." *J. Orthop. Trauma.* 15(2):122–131.

Slover J, Espehaug B, Havelin LI, Engesaeter LB, Furnes O, Tomek I, Tosteson A. (2006). "Cost-effectiveness of unicompartmental and total knee arthroplasty in elderly low-demand patients. A Markov decision analysis." *J. Bone Joint Surg. Am.* 88(11):2348–2355.

Smith GL, Briggs TWR, Lavy CBD, Nordeen H. (1992). "Ionising radiation: Are orthopaedic surgeons at risk." *Ann. R Coll. Surg. Engl.* 74:326–328.

Sorrells RB, Capps SG. (2006). "Clinical results of primary low contact stress cementless total knee arthroplasty." *Orthopedics* 29(9 Suppl):S42–S44.

Stiehl JB, Konerman WH, Haaker RG, DiGioia III AM, (Eds.). (2006a). "*Navigation and MIS in Orthopedic Surgery*", Springer, Berlin Heidelberg New York.

Stiehl JB, Hamelynck KJ, Voorhorst PE. (2006b). "International multi-centre survivorship analysis of mobile bearing total knee arthroplasty." *Int. Orthop.* 30(3):190–199.

Stiehl JB, Heck DA, Jaramaz B, Amiot LP. (2007). "Comparison of fluoroscopic and imageless registration in surgical navigation of the acetabular component." *Comput. Aided Surg.* 12(2):116–124.

Stiehl JB, Heck DA, Lazzeri M. (2005). "Accuracy of acetabular component positioning with a fluoroscopically referenced CAOS system." *Comput. Aided Surg.* 10(5–6):321–327.

Stukenborg-Colsman C, Ostermeier S, Windhagen H. (2005). "[What effect does obesity have on the outcome of total hip and knee arthroplasty. Review of the literature]." *Orthopade* 34(7):664–667.

Stulberg SD, Saragaglia D, Miehlke R. (2004). "Total knee replacement: Navigation technique intraoperative model system." In *Computer and Robotic Assisted Knee and Hip Surgery*, Digioia III AM , Jaramaz B, Picard F, Nolte LP (Eds.). Oxford University Press, pp 157–178.

Suhm N, Jacob LA, Zuna I, Regazzoni P, Messmer P. (2003). "[Fluoroscopy based surgical navigation vs. mechanical guidance system for percutaneous interventions. A controlled prospective study exemplified by distal locking of intramedullary nails]." *Unfallchirurg.* 106(11):921–928.

Suhm N, Messmer P, Zuna I, Jacob LA, Regazzoni P. (2004). "Fluoroscopic guidance versus surgical navigation for distal locking of intramedullary implants. A prospective, controlled clinical study." *Injury* 35(6):567–574.

Tannast M, Langlotz F, Kubiak-Langer M, Langlotz U, Siebenrock KA. (2005). "Accuracy and potential pitfalls of fluoroscopy-guided acetabular cup placement." *Comput. Aided Surg.* 10(5–6):329–36.

Ulrich SD, Mont MA, Bonutti PM, Seyler TM, Marker DR, Jones LC. (2007). "Scientific evidence supporting computer-assisted surgery and minimally invasive surgery for total knee arthroplasty." *Expert Rev. Med. Devices* 4(4): 497–505.

Van Brussel K, Vander Sloten J, Van Audekercke R, Fabry G. (1996). "Internal fixation of the spine in traumatic and scoliotic cases. The potential of pedicle screws." *Technol. Health Care* 4(4):365–384.

van Staa TP, Dennison EM, Leufkens HG, Cooper C. (2001). "Epidemiology of fractures in England and Wales." *Bone* 29(6):517–522.

Vavken P, Kotz R, Dorotka R. (2007). "[Minimally invasive hip replacement--a meta-analysis]." *Z Orthop. Unfall.* 145(2):152–156.

Viant WJ, Phillips R, Griffiths JG, Ozanian TO, Mohsen AM, Cain TJ, Karpinski MR, Sherman KP. (1997). "A computer assisted orthopaedic surgical system for distal locking of intramedullary nails." *Proc. Inst Mech. Eng [H].* 211(4):293–300.

Visuri T, Lindholm TS, Antti-Poika I, Koskenvuo M. (1993). "The role of overlength of the leg in aseptic loosening after total hip arthroplasty." *Ital. J. Orthop. Traumatol.* 19(1):107–111.

Von Recum J, Wendl K, Korber J, Wentzensen A, Grützner PA. (2003). "[CT-free image guided acetabulum navigation in clinical routine]." *Unfallchirurg.* 106(11):929–934.

Wang JQ, Wang JF, Hu L, Su YG, Wang Y, Zhao CP, Zhou L, Wang TM, Wang MY. (2006a). "[Effects of medical robot-assisted surgical navigation system in distal locking of femoral intramedullary nails: An experimental study]." *Zhonghua Yi Xue Za Zhi* 86(9):614–618.

Wang JQ, Zhao CP, Wang MY, Su YG, Hu L, Sun L, Zhang LD, Liu WY, Zhang H, Gao YF, Wang TM. (2006b). "Computer-assisted auto-frame navigation system for distal locking of tibial intramedullary nails: A preliminary report on clinical application." *Chin. J. Traumatol.* 9(3):138–145.

Weinbroum AA, Ekstein P, Ezri T. (2003). "Efficiency of the operating room suite." *Am. J. Surg.* 185(3):244–250.

Wentzensen A, Zheng G, Vock B, Langlotz U, Korber J, Nolte LP, Grutzner PA. (2003). "Image-based hip navigation." *Int. Orthop.* 27(Suppl 1):S43–S46.

Westphal R, Winkelbach S, Gösling T, Hüfner T, Faulstich J, Martin P, Krettek C, Wahl FM. (2006). "A surgical telemanipulator for femur shaft fracture reduction." *Int. J. Med. Robot.* 2(3):238–250.

Widmer KH, Grutzner PA. (2004). "Joint replacement-total hip replacement with CT-based navigation." *Injury* 35(1 Suppl 1):84–89.

Winquist RA, Hansen ST Jr, Clawson DK. (1984). "Closed intramedullary nailing of femoral fractures. A report of five hundred and twenty cases." *J. Bone Joint Surg. Am.* 66(4):529–539.

Wolf A, Digioia AM, Mor AB, Jaramaz B. (2005a). "Cup alignment error model for total hip arthroplasty." *Clin. Orthop. Relat. Res.* 437:132–137.

Wolf A, Jaramaz B, Lisien B, DiGioia AM. (2005b). "MBARS: Mini bone-attached robotic system for joint arthroplasty." *Int. J. Med. Robot.* 1(2):101–121.

Woolson ST. (2006). "In the absence of evidence--why bother? A literature review of minimally invasive total hip replacement surgery." *Instr. Course Lect.* 55:189–193.

Yamaguchi M, Akisue T, Bauer TW, Hashimoto Y. (2000). "The spatial location of impingement in total hip arthroplasty." *J. Arthroplasty* 15(3):305–313.

Zheng G, Marx A, Langlotz U, Widmer KH, Buttaro M, Nolte LP.(2002). "A hybrid CT-free navigation system for total hip arthroplasty." *Comput. Aided Surg.* 7(3):129–145.

Zheng G, Zhang X, Haschtmann D, Gédet P, Langlotz F, Nolte LP. (2007). "Accurate and reliable pose recovery of distal locking holes in computer-assisted intra-medullary nailing of femoral shaft fractures: A preliminary study." *Comput. Aided Surg.* 12(3):138–151.

Chapter 13
Thoracoabdominal Interventions

Filip Banovac, Jill Bruno, Jason Wright, and Kevin Cleary

Abstract

This chapter introduces the application of image-guided intervention to the internal organs of the thorax and abdomen. In the strict sense, image-guided therapy is any therapy that uses fluoroscopy, ultrasound, computed tomography, or magnetic resonance imaging to assist the physician in placing an instrument to a desired target in the body. In this chapter, the concept of image-guided surgery and intervention applies to more recent concepts that rely on computer-assisted guidance. This new paradigm still uses the conventional imaging modalities listed above, but also adds a tracking system and probe position sensors to couple the images with the anatomic space of interest. Therefore, the concepts of visualization, three-dimensional (3D) image reconstruction, segmentation, and registration discussed in earlier chapters are intimately tied to the procedures performed with these systems. Some of the challenges with visualization and registration related to patient motion and respiration become particularly apparent when working in the thoracoabdominal regions of the body. This chapter surveys the work performed in animal tests and early human trials, but omits most of the benchtop testing in phantoms. It is therefore a brief review of clinical applications that have been investigated using these emerging guidance systems.

13.1   Introduction

This chapter reviews the state-of-the-art of image-guided systems for thoracoabdominal interventions. While most image-guided systems to date have been based on optical tracking, the line-of-sight limitation of this tracking technique makes it unsuitable for tracking inside the body (for more information, see Chap. 2: Tracking Devices). Therefore, the image-guided systems described in this chapter are based on electromagnetic tracking, which, while not as accurate as optical tracking, is capable of tracking inside the body. The successful development of most of the systems presented here has been enabled by the recent improvement and miniaturization of electromagnetic

T. Peters and K. Cleary (eds.), *Image-Guided Interventions.*
© Springer Science + Business Media, LLC 2008

tracking devices. It should be noted that many of these systems have been developed for research purposes to date, and there are only a few FDA approved systems for abdominal interventions at the time of this writing.

This chapter describes the efforts of various researchers by organ system and also includes work in tracked laparoscopy. We have attempted to include the major studies as listed in Table 13.1. Most of this work is relatively recent, beginning with the work of Solomon in the late 1990s. The table includes the following columns:

1. Organ/method: describes the organ of interest, or the method used as in laparoscopy
2. The specific procedure or type of procedure under investigation

Table 13.1. Major Studies Incorporating Tracking for Thoracoabdominal Interventions

Organ/ Method	Procedure	Tracking System	Trial	Modality	Reference
Lung	Bronchoscopic biopsy	Biosense	8 Swine, 15 Humans	CT	[Solomon et al. 1998, 2000]
		Super Dimension	4 Swine, 13 Humans, 30 Humans	CT	[Becker et al. 2005; Schwarz et al. 2003, 2006]
		Aurora	16 Humans	CT	[Hautmann et al. 2005]
Liver/ Abdomen	TIPS	Biosense	5 Swine	CT	[Solomon et al. 1999]
		Aurora	Swine	CT	[Levy et al. 2007]
	Biopsy	Aurora	Phantoms, 3 Swine	CT	[Banovac et al. 2005, 2006]
		UltraGuide	43 Humans	US	[Howard et al. 2001]
		UltraGuide	39 Humans	US	[Birth et al. 2003]
	Liver surgery	Optotrak, laser range scanner	Phantoms, Cow livers, Humans	CT or MRI	[Bao et al. 2007; Rauth et al. 2007]
Kidney	Nephrostomy	Ultraguide	7 Swine	US	[Krombach et al. 2001]
	Biopsy	Ultraguide	18 Humans	US	[Wallace et al. 2006]
Laparoscopy	Interventional procedures	Aurora	Phantom	US, CT	[Krucker et al. 2005]
	Surgery	miniBird	Phantom, swine	US, CT	[Ellsmere 2004]

3. The tracking system used
4. The type of trial (phantoms/animals/humans)
5. The primary imaging modality used for guidance.

13.2   Lung: Bronchoscopic Biopsy

Bronchoscopy is the examination of the airways with an optical camera mounted on a rigid or flexible guide. It is used to evaluate the endobronchial structures and mucosa and can be used as both a diagnostic and a therapeutic tool. Bronchoscopy is frequently performed using a flexible bronchoscope with a mounted fiberoptic camera. The bronchoscope also has a working channel through which instruments may be used to take tissue samples or provide therapy. An illustration of bronchoscopy is shown in Fig. 13.1. Several researchers have investigated the use of image-guided systems for bronchoscopy, and one commercial system is available as described in the following text.

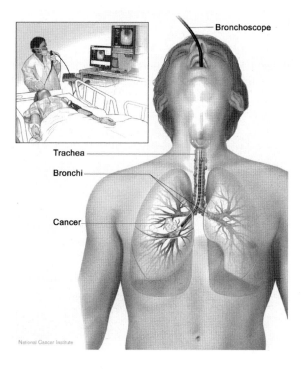

Fig. 13.1. Bronchoscopy (public domain image from U.S. National Cancer Institute: http://visualsonline.cancer.gov/details.cfm?imageid=4161)

13.2.1 *Beginnings of Guided Bronchoscopy: Biosense*

The integration of electromagnetic tracking with preprocedure CT for navigation in bronchoscopy was first reported by Solomon et al. [1998].

This work was based on the Biosense system and used a 1.5 mm diameter six degree-of-freedom (DOF) position sensor (Fig. 13.2), which was placed at the tip of a flexible bronchoscope (Fig. 13.3). The Biosense system uses three external electromagnetic emitters that can track within an approximately $20 \times 20 \times 20$ cm^3 region.

Two studies were completed by Solomon: the first study [Solomon et al. 1998] was in eight swine and the second study [Solomon et al. 2000]

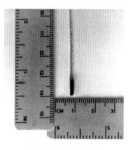

Fig. 13.2. Biosense 1.5 mm long position sensor with attached electrical wire. Reprinted with permission of the American College of Chest Physicians from Solomon et al. [1998]

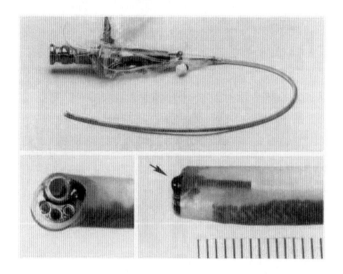

Fig. 13.3. *Top*: Fiberoptic bronchoscope (Vision Sciences, Natick, MA). *Bottom left*: End view of bronchoscope tip. *Bottom right*: Arrow indicates position sensor within the disposable bronchoscopic sheath. Reprinted with permission of the American College of Chest Physicians from Solomon et al. [1998]

was in 15 humans. The swine study used 35 kg animals. Synthetic para-tracheal lesions ~2 cm in diameter were created to serve as targets, using a mixture of radiographic contrast and tissue adhesive. Next, 10–20 metallic nipple markers of 1 cm diameter were secured on the anterior chest wall for use in registration. The images of the swine thorax were acquired on a CT scanner after administration of intravenous contrast and the images were reconstructed with 2 mm spacing. End-expiration breath hold was achieved during scanning by turning off the ventilator during the scan while the swine were paralyzed with pancuronium.

For the bronchoscopy, the swine were intubated with an 8–9 mm inside diameter tube. The CT data set was transferred to the Biosense system. The Biosense position sensor was touched to four of the nipple markers to register the animal's chest with the CT images. An additional position sensor was placed on the chest wall to gate respiratory motion. The position of the bronchoscope was updated on the image monitor when the swine was within a 1 mm threshold of end expiration and this time was indicated by an audible tone. The accompanying display is shown in Fig. 13.4.

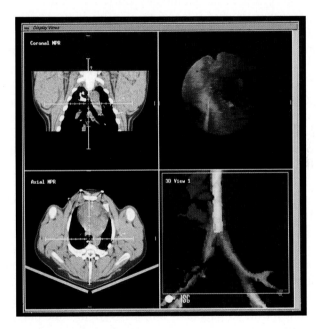

Fig. 13.4. Monitor display during bronchoscopy showing the fiberoptic view (*top right*), coronal (*top left*), axial (*bottom left*), and 3D view (*bottom right*). The yellow crosshairs in the coronal and axial views indicate the tip of the bronchoscope. The yellow bar in the 3D image indicates the orientation of the bronchoscope tip. Reprinted with permission of the American College of Chest Physicians from [Solomon et al. 1998]

Solomon and colleagues then extended their work in this area by conducting a clinical trial in 15 patients [Solomon et al. 2000]. They compared two registration techniques to assess if there were any differences between skin fiducial-based registration and endotracheal anatomy-based registration.

They achieved a registration error of 5.6 ± 2.7 mm using the skin fiducial method. They were unable to measure the registration error of the second method, but subjectively judged it to be more accurate, based on the fiberoptic view of the endobronchial tree. The disadvantage of the second method was that it took more bronchoscopy time as the registration was performed during the bronchoscopy session.

13.2.2 *Clinical Evolution: SuperDimension*

Bronchoscopy is the one abdominal procedure where an FDA approved system exists, which is the Bronchus from superDimension Ltd (Hertzliya, Israel). The system was FDA approved in November 2005 for guiding endoscopic instruments in the pulmonary tract. The system is a traditional image-guided system in that it consists of a tracking device, tracked instruments, and computer-based display.

The tracking system is proprietary and based on a 1 cm thick and 47×56 cm^2 wide localization board that is placed underneath the patient [Schwarz et al. 2006]. The board emits low-frequency electromagnetic waves that are detected by a sensor probe of 1 mm diameter by 8 mm in length. This probe is incorporated into the tip of a flexible catheter 130 cm in length and 1.9 mm in diameter, which can be inserted into the working channel of the bronchoscope. The registration technique is based on anatomic landmarks and the system does not use artificially placed fiducials.

In their initial animal studies, Schwarz and his colleagues achieved a 4.5 ± 2.5 mm fiducial target registration error in four animals with a total of 10 artificially created lesions [Schwarz et al. 2003]. This same group then completed a clinical trial in 30 patients with peripheral lung lesions (mean distance to pleura 1.9 mm) and reported a 69% diagnostic biopsy yield [Becker et al. 2005]. They used a registration technique based on touching anatomic landmarks such as the main carina or the left, right, or middle lobe carina. An average target registration error of 6.12 ± 1.7 mm was achieved. In a related study with 15 patients using this system, nine diagnostic transbronchial biopsies were achieved [Schwarz et al. 2006]. The authors also reported a false negative biopsy in four patients in this cohort. A diagnostic biopsy for these patients was then achieved by conventional CT-guided fine needle aspiration or surgery.

These initial trials illustrated both the usefulness and the limitations of this system. It is unclear whether the failures were due to misregistration, technique, or a combination of these factors. Conventional, albeit more invasive methods were needed in the cases where the system was not successful.

13.2.3 *Aurora-Based System*

Another image-guided bronchoscopy system was developed at the Medical Center of the Technical University of Munich [Hautmann et al. 2005]. This system was based on the Aurora electromagnetic tracking device from Northern Digital Inc. (Waterloo, Ontario, Canada). Sixteen patients were studied for the diagnosis of peripheral infiltrates or solid pulmonary nodules.

The Aurora system was described in Chap. 2: Tracking Devices, and consists of a field generator, control unit, and small sensors (diameter 0.8 mm, length 10mm), which were encapsulated in the tip of a flexible catheter (diameter 1.5mm). The navigation software (Syngo, Siemens Medical Solutions, Erlangen, Germany) runs on a standard personal computer. The field generator was located on the left side of the examination table with its height adjusted to the level of the patient's thorax.

Anatomic landmark registration was performed using four discernible points on the human anatomy. The same points were then manually selected in CT space and paired-point registration was performed. The authors showed the utility of using electromagnetic navigation to guide the bronchoscope into three out of five solitary pulmonary nodules, and all pulmonary infiltrates in a group of 16 patients. The addition of electromagnetic navigation added 3.9 ± 1.3 min to the entire procedure. One clear advantage was that the bronchoscope could be guided to otherwise fluoroscopically invisible infiltrates and lesions [Hautmann et al. 2005]. Diagnostic material could therefore be obtained and electromagnetic navigation was therefore an enabling technology in these cases.

In summary, electromagnetic navigation for bronchoscopic guidance has become commercially available and early clinical trials are promising, although the overall impact of this technology remains to be seen. The systems are still largely investigational and require additional steps, including preprocedural imaging, registration, software and hardware support, and modification of the clinical workflow.

13.3 Liver

The liver, much like the lung, is subject to considerable respiratory motion. The predominant motion is cranio-caudal and subject to respiratory excursion of the diaphragm [Clifford et al. 2002]. Therefore, the targeting of the internal structures of the liver such as the vasculature and the bile ducts might be made easier using image guidance. Specifically, the creation of a transjugular intrahepatic portosystemic shunt (TIPS), as is frequently carried out in the setting of acute gastric variceal hemorrhage, was attempted with electromagnetic guidance. The biopsy of intrahepatic targets was also investigated, and these topics are described in the following section.

13.3.1 *Transjugular Intrahepatic Shunt Placement (TIPS)*

TIPS is a fluoroscopically guided procedure performed by interventional radiologists. The procedure is carried out in patients with acute gastric or esophageal bleeding, which can be life threatening. The goal of the procedure is to create an intrahepatic connection (shunt) between the portal venous system and the hepatic venous system. This connection shunts the blood through the metallic stent placed in the liver and reduces the portal venous pressure, which in turn decreases or stops the bleeding from the gastric and esophageal varices. The procedure is considered technically challenging and is even more difficult in emergency settings. Providing navigational guidance with electromagnetically tracked instruments potentially could overcome some of the technical challenges associated with this procedure.

The first paper in this area was by Solomon et al. [1999] and investigated the use of the Biosense electromagnetic navigation system for this procedure. A 16-gauge, 50 cm curved needle was used to create a connection between the hepatic vein and the portal vein. Prior to CT scanning, five domestic swine had 10–20 one millimeter metallic nipple markers placed on the abdominal wall to allow for later image registration. The swine were scanned with spiral CT using intravenous contrast and the images were reconstructed with 2 mm spacing. End-expiration breath hold was achieved during scanning by turning off the ventilator during the scan while the swine were paralyzed with pancuronium.

As described earlier in this chapter, the Biosense system uses a locator pad situated beneath the procedure table. The position sensor was passed through the long curved needle to provide the position and orientation of the needle tip. An additional position sensor was placed on the swine's abdomen and used to monitor respiratory motion. The position of the needle tip was updated on the monitor only when the swine was within a 1 mm threshold of end expiration. During the procedure, image registration was performed by touching eight nipple markers with the position sensor. The accuracy of the system was then estimated by touching the other 12 nipple markers and comparing their perceived location on the CT scan with the actual location. The average difference found was 3 mm. Multiplanar reconstructed images were then used, together with tracking of the needle tip, to access the portal vein.

Successful TIPS formation was performed in four out of five animals and the one failure was attributed to a dull needle. The system was found to be useful for providing a better visualization of the anatomy and needle tip localization during the procedure.

Graphical User Interface

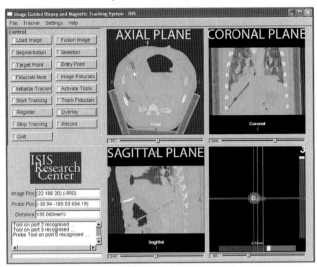

Needle Trajectory Monitoring Windows

a.

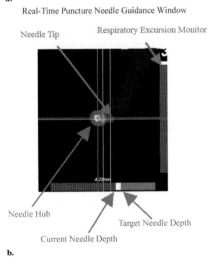

b.

Fig. 13.5. (a) GUI target planning and monitoring windows (axial, coronal, sagittal) with puncture needle in terminal position. Puncture needle position is superimposed upon planned trajectory in the trajectory monitoring windows. **(b)** GUI needle-guidance window. Color-coded crosshairs represent target, needle tip, and needle hub, which must be overlapped for successful puncture. Reprinted with permission from Levy et al. [2007]

More recently, Levy and colleagues used an Aurora-based navigation system to create a modified version of the TIPS procedure in swine [Levy et al. 2007]. Using four skin fiducials and four active needle based fiducials, this group created a successful transhepatic puncture using electromagnetic guidance. This was done by puncturing the portal vein, hepatic vein, and inferior vena cava in a single percutaneous transabdominal puncture, followed by placement of an intrahepatic stent.

The graphical user interface and needle targeting window is shown in Fig. 13.5. Needle advancement was performed only when the GUI indicated that respiratory-related organ motion had ceased during the typically observed ~1.4 s regular end-expiratory phase pause. The system tracks the motion of an electromagnetically tracked internal fiducial to determine the timing of the pause in respiratory-related organ motion and indirectly the optimal target position. The GUI displays (a) the depth of the needle tip relative to the target depth in graphical fashion and (b) the position of the needle tip registered with the preoperative CT data set. The needle procedure can therefore be terminated by the operator based on the real-time information and guidance provided by the GUI.

13.3.2 *Biopsy and Thermoablation*

Our research group at Georgetown has been focusing on electromagnetic tracking for delivery of instruments into small liver targets to enable more precise biopsies, and we have developed a new image-guided system based on the Aurora electromagnetic tracking device. Initially, image-guided biopsy of synthetic liver lesions and small nodules in phantoms and anesthetized swine was performed in an angiography suite [Banovac et al. 2005].

The mean RMS error of needle placement was 6.4 mm in the phantom and 8.3 mm in the swine. More importantly, the system enabled less experienced operators to perform just as well as fellowship trained interventional radiologists in terms of procedure time and accuracy of needle probe delivery (Fig. 13.6).

Some system improvements were then made and biopsy needle insertion was carried out in the CT-fluoroscopy suite [Banovac et al. 2006]. We demonstrated in swine that by using electromagnetic tracking and image guidance alone, one can achieve at least equivalent accuracy as with CT-fluoroscopy guided needle insertion (Fig. 13.7). There was a trend towards improved accuracy with electromagnetic tracking and image guidance, but the results were not statistically significant. In addition, radiation dose and total time of needle manipulation were significantly reduced using our system.

In parallel with our efforts, Wood et al. also used the Aurora system to show the feasibility of in vivo tracking on a catheter and needle based systems using coregistration with multiple modalities such as CT, MRI, and

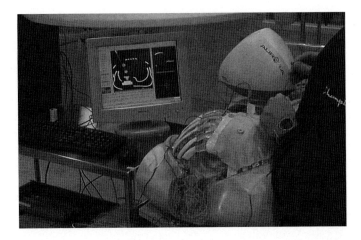

Fig. 13.6. Electromagnetic navigation system and GUI in phantom tests at George-town. Reprinted with permission from Banovac et al. [2005]

PET [Wood et al. 2007; Wood et al. 2005]. These studies demonstrated the versatility of electromagnetic tracking as an adjunctive guidance modality across the spectrum of imaging methods used for imaging and intervention.

An early clinical system incorporating electromagnetic tracking was the Ultraguide 1000 (Fig. 13.8, UltraGuide Ltd., Tirat Hacarmel, Israel). The Ultraguide system consists of a computer, a monitor, and a proprietary electromagnetic tracking system. All components are mounted on a movable trolley, including the magnetic field generating coils of the tracking system. A magnetic field sensor is then attached to the transducer and a second field sensor is attached to the hub of the needle. The navigation volume is a 50 cm cube. The system allows for in-plane or out-of-plane navigation of the needle.

Howard et al. [2001] showed the clinical utility of this system in a 43-patient study that included a biopsy of solid organs in 24 patients, including 14 livers. They formulated a subjective scoring system of physicians' impressions while using the device, and concluded that the system would be beneficial as an adjunctive technology in approximately half the ultrasound-guided procedures in their practice.

In related work, Birth et al. [2003] performed 39 interventional procedures under OR conditions using an improved system called the Ultraguide 2000 (Tirat Hacarmel, Israel). Twenty-three of these procedures were thermal ablations of the liver malignancies, and 16 were diagnostic biopsies. The authors reported technical success with out-of-plane probe insertion in all cases and reported no complications. They concluded that the system increases the safety of the procedures, particularly when lesions are difficult to reach or next to critical structures.

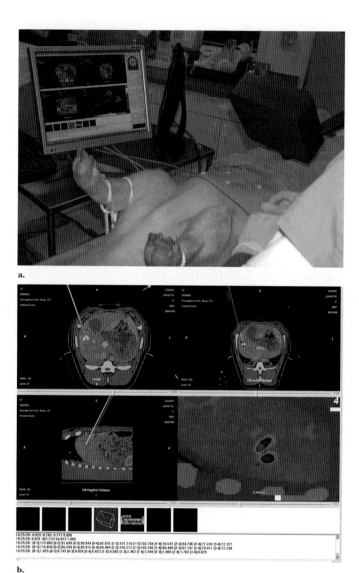

Fig. 13.7. (a) Experimental setup in the CT suite. The operator performs the puncture without real-time imaging, with only electromagnetic navigation and software guidance. **(b)** Image-guided biopsy user interface for navigation-guided trials. Sagittal image in the graphic interface (*bottom left*) shows a representative needle planning pass in which the craniocaudal angle of planned approach is greater than the possible mechanical tilt of the CT gantry. Reprinted with permission from Banovac et al. [2006]

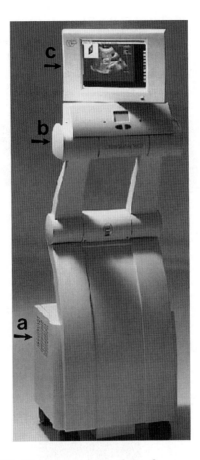

Fig. 13.8. UltraGuide 1000. The base unit consists of a computer (**a**), a magnetic field generator (**b**), and a display screen (**c**). The field generator can be raised and lowered according to the height of the table, and the screen can be swiveled in all directions to match the viewing angle. Reprinted with permission of the Radiological Society of North America from [Howard et al. 2001]

In summary, the use of electromagnetic tracking and image-guidance in liver applications is still evolving, and preclinical studies in swine and early clinical studies with humans have shown promise. The inherent error introduced by liver motion and deformation is still a major roadblock in accurate registration and will continue to be a topic of research.

13.3.3 *Image-Guided Liver Surgery*

Another approach toward image-guided liver surgery is being developed by Galloway and colleagues at Vanderbilt University (Nashville, TN). A spin-off company called Pathfinder Therapeutics is developing the platform shown in Fig. 13.9. The software is based on the Orion platform, which has been developed by the Vanderbilt group for over 10 years. A typical view as presented to the surgeon is shown in Fig. 13.10.

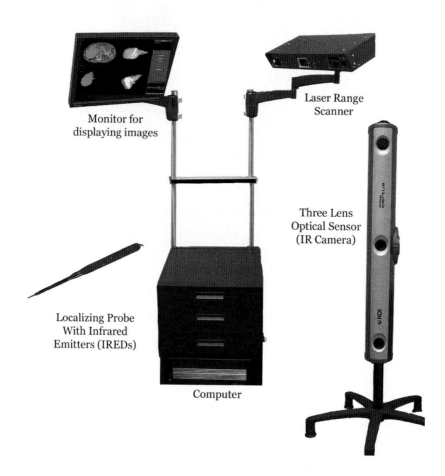

Fig. 13.9. Image-guided liver surgery technology platform under development by Pathfinder Therapeutics Inc. (Nashville, TN). All the components of the system are connected to one central computer located in the bottom of the mobile cart. The three lens optical sensor detects the infrared light and determines the physical position of the probe. The monitor then displays the appropriate images of the organ using data acquired by the laser range scanner and the current probe location. Figure courtesy of Pathfinder Therapeutics Inc.

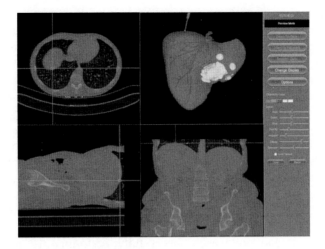

Fig. 13.10. System GUI showing four-quadrant view and 3D view of the liver, vasculature, and tumor in the upper right. Figure courtesy of Pathfinder Therapeutics Inc.

In related research, this team has investigated the use of this system for laparoscopic radiofrequency ablation of the liver in phantom studies [Bao et al. 2007]. A tracked needle was directed to a phantom target and a targeting accuracy of 5–10 mm was achieved. The use of an endoscopic laser range scanner for registration was also studied [Rauth et al. 2007]. Six radio-opaque targets were placed in an ex vivo bovine liver and a CT data set was obtained. The liver surface was then scanned with the laser range scanner and surface-based registration performed. The target registration error (TRE) obtained was 2.4 ± 1.0 mm.

13.4   Kidney: Ultrasound-Guided Nephrostomy

A nephrostomy is an artificial connection created between the kidney and the skin to allow drainage of urine directly from the kidney into an external collection bag. A nephrostomy is performed whenever an obstruction of the urinary system, most commonly in the ureters, keeps urine from passing from the kidneys to the ureter and into the bladder. The procedure is usually performed by interventional radiologists using a combination of ultrasound guidance and fluoroscopic guidance. In situations where the obstruction is significant or chronic, the renal pelvis tends to dilate substantially and the task of guiding the needle into a markedly dilated collecting system is relatively easy. However, there are many situations where the renal pelvis does not dilate significantly and consequently placement of the needle can be more difficult.

Some investigators have explored adjunct guidance modalities to facilitate the needle puncture of the renal pelvis. A swine study was conducted to evaluate the utility of the UltraGuide 1000 navigation system described earlier as a guidance tool for nephrostomy [Krombach et al. 2001]. Twelve percutaneous nephrostomy procedures were performed in seven pigs. For in-plane intervention in this system, the needle and the target are both kept in the imaging plane. The transducer is placed above the target and the insertion point for the needle is chosen. The navigation device displays the schematic display of the needle in relation to the ultrasound transducer in real-time. For out-of-plane intervention, the needle and the transducer are not in the same imaging plane. The system allows for needle insertion from any angle, and the puncture path is determined and displayed by the system to eventually insert the needle into a target. The needle tip is visualized by real-time ultrasound only when it reaches the target.

Krombach and colleagues successfully performed 12 nephrostomy placements using this system. Nine were carried out using in-plane guidance and three using out-of-plane guidance. The total time taken for nephrostomy placement was approximately 30–40 min and the diameter of the target renal calyces was 5–10 mm. The authors noted that they had to perform the first few guidance attempts 2–3 times before eventually switching to a stiffer needle, and they also experienced needle bending during insertion. This bending illustrates one of the problems with electromagnetic guidance systems that do not place the sensor in the tip of the instrument, but rather on the hub or the back end. In these situations, needle bending introduces error and needle tip position cannot be accurately accounted for by the image guidance systems. Placing the sensor in the needle or catheter requires developing special instruments, and this has been achieved by several vendors.

Wallace and colleagues used an updated version of the UltraGuide system made specifically for assisted guidance in the CT scanner to successfully biopsy seven adrenal lesions, using an out-of-plane approach as shown in Fig. 13.11 [Wallace et al. 2006]. Their study examined the use of this device in multiple organ systems, including the adrenal gland, liver, lung, and pancreas. This group did not report the overall error of needle placement, but did note that their mean insertion point at the skin was 40 mm (with a range of 18–90 mm) away in the axial plane from their final target. This, in essence, demonstrated the potential benefit of using navigation assistance to enable out-of-plane CT-guided biopsies.

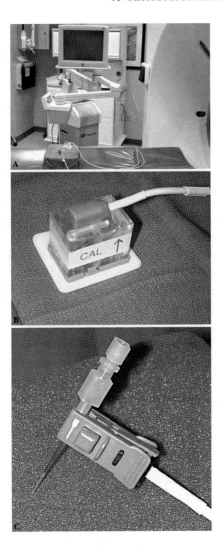

Fig. 13.11. Components of the magnetic-field-based navigation system include the base unit (**a**), the skin-based sensor (**b**), and the needle-based sensor (**c**). Reprinted with permission of Springer Science and Business Media from [Wallace et al. 2006]

13.5   Laparoscopic Guidance

Laparoscopic surgery is a popular minimally invasive technique in which physicians operate through small incisions. A video camera is usually one of the laparoscopic instruments through which the physician can view the anatomy. However, the field of view of the video camera is limited to the local anatomy. Therefore, several researchers have investigated integrating laparoscopy with electromagnetic tracking and preprocedure images to provide additional guidance information. Two such efforts are described in the following section.

13.5.1 *Phantom Investigations*

The use of electromagnetic tracking with laparoscopic ultrasound and Registration with preprocedure CT was investigated by Krucker et al. [2005]. A six DOF sensor was placed at the tip of the ultrasound probe and tracked with the Aurora system. Proof of concept experiments were completed using an interventional abdominal phantom (Model 57, CIRS, Norfolk, Virginia). The phantom was customized to include ~10 hypo-echoic lesions with diameters of 10–20 mm in the liver region.

For registration with a preprocedure CT, landmarks in physical space were identified using three methods: (1) pointing with an electromagnetic tracker; (2) pointing with the laparoscope tip; and (3) manual identification using laparoscopic ultrasound. The RMS registration error using these three methods was 1.5, 1.4, and 1.1 mm, respectively. The system was then used to guide a 19-gauge electromagnetically tracked stylet to a user-defined target location as identified in the CT scan. The resulting accuracy for all the needle placement tests was less than 2 mm.

13.5.2 *Swine Studies*

A navigation system for augmenting laparoscopic ultrasound was developed by Ellsmere et al. [2004]. The system provides a virtual reality visualization of the region of interest as shown in Fig. 13.12. The navigation system consists of four major components: (1) a laparoscopic ultrasound transducer; (2) a surgical pointer; (3) an electromagnetic tracking device (miniBird, Ascension Technology, Burlington, VT); and (4) a laptop computer.

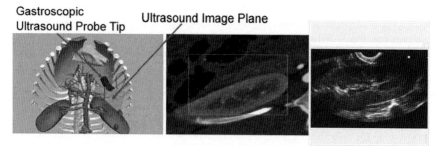

Fig. 13.12. Gastroscopic ultrasound navigation system showing a virtual reality 3D orientation display (*left*), a matched oblique slice from the preprocedure CT volume (*center*), and the gastroscopic ultrasound image (*right*). Figure courtesy of Kirby Vosburgh, PhD and Raul San Jose Estepar, PhD

The initial feasibility studies were carried out using the Model 57 phantom from CIRS mentioned earlier. This was followed by an animal study using a 25 kg swine. The tips of several ribs were used in the registration process. The average registration error was 5 mm, but was reduced to 3 mm when vasculature features were used to update the registration. Overall, the system was found to be helpful in teaching surgeons how to use laparoscopic ultrasound.

13.6   Summary and Research Issues

As can be seen from the systems presented in this chapter, image guidance in the abdomen has been tried for many different organs and many different procedures. However, it is fair to say that image guidance in the abdomen is still in its infancy. All the systems proposed still rely on rigid body assumptions for navigation, and none of them is capable of handling deformation of the anatomy or respiratory motion in any robust manner.

The following are some of the key issues that need to be considered when designing a new image-guided system for any abdominal procedure:

1. Which tracking system is most appropriate? While the current state of the art is electromagnetic tracking, which is limited to a few vendors, issues of robustness, tracking volume, and sensor size must be considered.
2. What imaging modality or combination of modalities will be most useful to the physician, taking into account issues such as resolution, radiation exposure, and real-time requirements?
3. How can the GUI be designed to present the essential information to the physician without developing a complicated display that is more suited for engineers?

One specification that should be briefly discussed is the necessary degree of accuracy for these procedures. For abdominal procedures, it is not feasible to develop image-guided systems that have the millimetric accuracy, which might be possible with systems designed for bony landmarks. However, as a rule of thumb, it is suggested that an accuracy requirement of 3–5 mm is sufficient for abdominal interventions.

In terms of the major research issues, improved tracking systems and improved accuracy and tracking volume are certainly desirable, but an even more important need is for partnerships of scientists and clinicians to continue to build prototype systems that are tested in the clinical environment. Although advances in deformable modeling and respiratory compensation are important, a crucial point is how these advances are validated. It is highly unlikely that a clinician would trust a display built on a predictive deformable model, unless that model had been extensively validated in the clinical environment.

References

Banovac F., Tang J., Xu S., Lindisch D., Chung H. Y., Levy E. B., Chang T., McCullough M. F., Yaniv Z., Wood B. J., and Cleary K. (2005). Precision targeting of liver lesions using a novel electromagnetic navigation device in physiologic phantom and swine. *Med. Phys.*, 32(8), 2698–2705

Banovac F., Wilson E., Zhang H., and Cleary K. (2006). Needle biopsy of anatomically unfavorable liver lesions with an electromagnetic navigation assist device in a computed tomography environment. *J. Vasc. Interv. Radiol.*, 17(10), 1671–1675

Bao P., Sinha T. K., Chen C. C., Warmath J. R., Galloway R. L., and Herline A. J. (2007). A prototype ultrasound-guided laparoscopic radiofrequency ablation system. *Surg. Endosc.*, 21(1), 74–79

Becker H., Herth F., Ernst A., and Schwarz Y. (2005). Bronchoscopic biopsy of peripheral lung lesions under electromagnetic guidance: A pilot study. *J. Bronchol.*, 12(1), 9–13

Birth M., Iblher P., Hildebrand P., Nolde J., and Bruch H. P. (2003). Ultrasound-guided interventions using magnetic field navigation: First experiences with Ultra-Guide 2000 under operative conditions. *Ultraschall. Med.*, (2), 90–95

Clifford M. A., Banovac F., Levy E., and Cleary K. (2002). Assessment of hepatic motion secondary to respiration for computer assisted interventions. *Comput. Aided Surg.*, 7(5), 291–299

Ellsmere J., Stoll J., Wells W., Kikinis R., Vosburgh K., Kane R., Brooks D., and Rattner D. (2004). A new visualization technique for laparoscopic ultrasonography. *Surgery*, 136(1), 84–92

Hautmann H., Schneider A., Pinkau T., Peltz F., and Feussner H. (2005). Electromagnetic catheter navigation during bronchoscopy: validation of a novel method by conventional fluoroscopy. *Chest*, 128(1), 382–387

Howard M. H., Nelson R. C., Paulson E. K., Kliewer M. A., and Sheafor D. H. (2001). An electronic device for needle placement during sonographically guided percutaneous intervention. *Radiology*, 218(3), 905–911

Krombach G. A., Mahnken A., Tacke J., Staatz G., Haller S., Nolte-Ernsting C. C. A., Meyer J., Haage P., and Gunther R. W. (2001). US-guided nephrostomy with the aid of a magnetic field-based navigation device in the porcine pelvicaliceal system. *J. Vasc. Interv. Radiol.*, 12(5), 623–628

Krucker J., Viswanathan A., Borgert J., Glossop N., Yang Y., and Wood B. J. (2005). An electro-magnetically tracked laparoscopic ultrasound for multi-modality minimally invasive surgery. *Int. Congr. Ser.*, 1281, 746–751

Levy E. B., Zhang H., Lindisch D., Wood B. J., and Cleary K. (2007). Electromagnetic tracking-guided percutaneous intrahepatic portosystemic shunt creation in a swine model. *J. Vasc. Interv. Radiol.*, 18(2), 303–307

Rauth T. P., Bao P. Q., Galloway R. L., Bieszczad J., Friets E. M., Knaus D. A., Kynor D. B., and Herline A. J. (2007). Laparoscopic surface scanning and subsurface targeting: implications for image-guided laparoscopic liver surgery. *Surgery*, 142(2), 207–214

Schwarz Y., Greif J., Becker H. D., Ernst A., and Mehta A. (2006). Real-time electromagnetic navigation bronchoscopy to peripheral lung lesions using overlaid CT images: the first human study. *Chest*, 129(4), 988–994

Schwarz Y., Mehta A. C., Ernst A., Herth F., Engel A., Besser D., and Becker H. D. (2003). Electromagnetic navigation during flexible bronchoscopy. *Respiration*, 70(5), 516–522

Solomon S. B., Magee C., Acker D. E., and Venbrux A. C. (1999). TIPS placement in swine, guided by electromagnetic real-time needle tip localization displayed on previously acquired 3D CT. *Cardiovasc. Intervent. Radiol.*, 22(5), 411–414

Solomon S. B., White P., Jr., Acker D. E., Strandberg J., and Venbrux A. C. (1998). Real-time bronchoscope tip localization enables three-dimensional CT image guidance for transbronchial needle aspiration in swine. *Chest*, 114(5), 1405–1410

Solomon S. B., White P., Jr., Wiener C. M., Orens J. B., and Wang K. P. (2000). Three-dimensional CT-guided bronchoscopy with a real-time electromagnetic position sensor: a comparison of two image registration methods. *Chest*, 118(6), 1783–1787

Wallace M. J., Gupta S., and Hicks M. E. (2006). Out-of-plane computed-tomography-guided biopsy using a magnetic-field-based navigation system. *Cardiovasc. Intervent. Radiol.*, 29(1), 108–113

Wood B. J., Locklin J. K., Viswanathan A., Kruecker J., Haemmerich D., Cebral J., Sofer A., Cheng R., McCreedy E., Cleary K., McAuliffe M. J., Glossop N., and Yanof J. (2007). Technologies for guidance of radiofrequency ablation in the multimodality interventional suite of the future. *J. Vasc. Interv. Radiol.*, 18(1, Part 1), 9–24

Wood B. J., Zhang H., Durrani A., Glossop N., Ranjan S., Lindisch D., Levy E., Banovac F., Borgert J., Krueger S., Kruecker J., Viswanathan A., and Cleary K. (2005). Navigation with electromagnetic tracking for interventional radiology procedures: a feasibility study. *J. Vasc. Interv. Radiol.*, 16(4), 493–505

Chapter 14

Real-Time Interactive MRI for Guiding Cardiovascular Surgical Interventions

Michael Guttman, Keith Horvath, Robert Lederman,

and Elliot McVeigh

Abstract

Real-time magnetic resonance imaging (rtMRI) is a compelling modality for guidance of surgical interventions. An effective toolkit for planning and guidance of surgery using rtMRI includes continuously updated images with excellent soft tissue contrast, devices that are visible in the images, interactively adjustable imaging parameters, simultaneous imaging and display of multiple intersecting oblique planes, and the ability to measure blood flow and perfusion. MRI has the benefit of not exposing the patient, physician, or staff to ionizing radiation from X-rays. This chapter describes the initial experience in the development of minimally invasive surgical implantation of an aortic valve in the beating heart, using continuously updated rtMRI. The potential benefits of this approach include reduction of patient trauma from open heart surgery using cardiopulmonary bypass, and the ability to implant a more robust device than can be delivered by catheter-based methods. Since the heart is a moving target, the surgeon is guided by continuously updated images, rather than those previously acquired as in stereotactic procedures.

14.1 Introduction

Minimally invasive approaches to cardiac surgical therapies are under active investigation to reduce trauma and recovery time [Doty et al. 2000; Vassiliades et al. 2005; Lutter et al. 2004]. Therapies traditionally requiring open-chest access are now being carried out through small incisions. Without direct access to the target, approaches under development deploy robotic tools under the surgeon's control to administer therapy with fiber optics, providing visual guidance. However, these approaches still require emptying the heart of blood to allow unobstructed visualization, and the heart is arrested to operate on a stationary target.

Real-time magnetic resonance imaging (rtMRI) provides views of anatomy and invasive devices in a beating heart with circulating blood.

Excellent anatomical detail is available due to inherent soft tissue contrast and oblique thin-slice imaging. Complementary functional information such as flow, ventricular ejection fraction, and perfusion are readily obtained. The effect of interventional therapies such as radiofrequency ablation, cryo-ablation, and direct injections can be observed quickly in rtMRI.

Advantages of MR arise not only from the superior soft tissue contrast, but from the many different ways in which MR signal may be produced and processed, offering a variety of contrast mechanisms and flexible slice positioning. For example, pulse sequence parameters can be changed dynamically during real-time imaging [Hardy et al. 1993; Holsinger et al. 1990; Kerr et al. 1997] to alter the imaging slice position or contrast as needed for different stages of an examination or invasive procedure [Lederman et al. 2002]. These capabilities have been used for delivery and immediate visualization of intra-myocardial injections of stem cells mixed with a contrast agent [Dick et al. 2003; Kraitchman et al. 2003], and for renal artery stenting [Elgort et al. 2006], among others [Henk et al. 2005; Lederman 2005]. Multiple parallel or oblique slices may be imaged in rapid succession to provide more complete views of a tortuous blood vessel or other anatomical structures such as heart valves, and these slices can be displayed together in a three-dimensional (3D) rendering [Guttman et al. 2002; Lorenz et al. 2005; Quick et al. 2003]. Receiver coils embedded in interventional and surgical devices can be used for device tracking [Feng et al. 2005; McVeigh et al. 2006; Zuehlsdorff et al. 2004], near-field imaging [Atalar et al. 1998; Hillenbrand et al. 2004], or the coil locations may be visualized by colorizing images reconstructed from device coil signals and blending them with gray-scale images produced from surface coil signals [Aksit et al. 2002; Guttman et al. 2002; Quick et al. 2003; Serfaty et al. 2000]. The color-highlighted images indicate the positions of invasive devices with anatomical context.

Many of the techniques used for intravascular interventions can be applied directly to the guidance of minimally invasive surgical procedures. For some surgical procedures such as heart valve replacement and repair, percutaneous intravascular methods [Babaliaros et al. 2006; Kuehne et al. 2004] as well as minimally invasive surgical approaches [Horvath et al. 2007] are under active investigation. These techniques present different balances between risk and benefit. The open-chest surgical approach is associated with higher morbidity, but direct access allows superior visualization of anatomy anatomy and manipulation of devices for a more durable therapy. The percutaneous methods reduce trauma, but therapeutic devices must be designed for catheter delivery through blood vessels, a constraint which may compromise the performance and durability of the device and therapy. In addition, some patients with stenotic cardiovascular disease may not be candidates for the percutaneous intervention. With a minimally invasive surgical approach, it may be possible to achieve the best of both surgical and percutaneous techniques reducing trauma while providing durable therapy. This goal is feasible using rtMRI to guide the procedure and monitor the progress of therapy.

14.2   Interventional MR Imaging System

14.2.1 Magnet Configuration

Older generations of MR imaging systems used magnets either of the so-called, closed "doughnut" configuration, with a bore too deep and narrow to allow adequate access to the surgical site, or the open "double pancake" configuration, which allowed superior access but at reduced gradient performance and image quality/speed. These systems have been used in MR-guided therapeutic interventions with success [Blanco et al. 2005; Schulz et al. 2004], but with imaging performance below that which is obtainable on a scanner designed for cardiac applications.

Newer technologies have yielded an effective compromise. Closed bore designs with shorter depth and wider opening, such as the 1.5 T Magnetom Espree (Siemens Medical Solutions Diagnostics, Tarrytown, N.Y. and Los Angeles, CA) with a bore opening 120 cm long by 70 cm wide, are providing greater accessibility with imaging performance rivaling that of many cardiac scanners. Imaging field-of-view (FOV) is reduced to 30 cm, but this has been demonstrated to be adequate for many cardiac interventions. This magnet bore is sufficiently short for a surgeon to reach the center of the magnet, and wide enough to allow placement and manipulation of instruments over the patient's body. With the heart positioned at the center of the magnet, the short bore also allows better access to the head by anesthesiologists and nurses.

14.2.2 Interventional Imaging Platform

The platform that we have developed at the National Heart, Lung, and Blood Institute (NHLBI) at the National Institutes of Health (NIH) for interventional rtMRI utilizes clinical MR 1.5 T scanners (Sonata with eight receiver channels, Espree with 12 channels, and Avanto with 32 channels, Siemens Medical Solutions Diagnostics), with additional software for sockets communication over Gigabit Ethernet with a Linux workstation (8-CPU, 64-bit, AMD Opteron, HPC Systems, San Jose, CA) running custom software for rapid image reconstruction, display, and 3D rendering [Guttman et al. 2002, 2003a]. The workstation is connected directly to the image reconstruction computer of the MR scanner for quick access to the raw echo data. The reconstruction and display software takes advantage of parallel processing by farming out tasks to different computing threads, which can run concurrently on different CPUs. Threads are created for individual processing of data from each receiver channel, combination of the data, graphical display, communications, and other tasks that can be executed in parallel. Open source packages and standards are used wherever possible: Fast Fourier transforms are performed using the FFTW library (fftw.org), graphics and user interface are implemented using OpenGL and GLUT (opengl.org).

At the beginning of a scan, imaging parameters are sent from the scanner to the workstation for initialization of the reconstruction program. At the end of each image acquisition, a packet of data containing dynamic imaging parameters and the raw MR data is sent to the workstation. Commands are sent to the scanner in response to user input via the same network interface.

14.2.3 Pulse Sequences and Image Reconstruction

MR data is acquired in the frequency domain (k-space) and reconstructed into an image by Fourier transformation. Real-time MR imaging requires an efficient pulse sequence, i.e., one that covers k-space in a short time. This is often accomplished by acquiring many data points in each repetition, such as in echo-planar or spiral, or by using sequences with inherently short repetition times (TR), such as gradient-recalled echo or steady-state free precession (SSFP, a.k.a. True FISP, b-FFE, FIESTA) [Oppelt et al. 1986]. The NHLBI implementation uses SSFP for rapid, high signal-to-noise ratio (SNR) consecutive imaging of multiple slices. Imaging parameters are tailored to the procedure: although high frame rates are available, spatial resolution and image quality are given priority over imaging speed, thus reported frame rates are well below the maximum attainable. The imaging frame rate is then increased using variable rate view sharing or TSENSE [Guttman et al. 2003a; Kellman et al. 2001]. Both of these methods accelerate image acquisition by skipping phase encoding lines. For example, at acceleration rate 2, odd and even lines are acquired in alternating acquisitions. For acceleration rate N, every Nth line is acquired, incrementing the starting line for each image acquisition. This causes ghosting artifacts of moving objects, which are suppressed by TSENSE using dynamic estimates of the coil sensitivities.

TSENSE is one of the several parallel imaging techniques such as SMASH [Sodickson and Manning 1997], SENSE [Pruessmann et al. 1999], and GRAPPA [Griswold et al. 2002], which accelerate imaging by undersampling k-space, and use the local sensitivity map of each coil element to either fill in the gaps in k-space or remove undersampling artifacts in image space. Modern scanners feature up to 32 channels, which provide enough independent information for parallel imaging methods to achieve an acceleration factor of four with good image quality. Other acceleration methods do not require multiple coils and use the fact that the samples in a typical time series of image data are correlated in time (UNFOLD [Madore et al. 1999], or both *k*-space and time (*k-t* BLAST [Tsao et al. 2003]).

Since SSFP is a steady-state imaging sequence, care must be taken when disrupting the steady state for multiple slice imaging or image preparation such as fat suppression. In the NHLBI implementation for these cases, the magnetization is stored longitudinally (along the *z*-axis) after each image acquisition, using a "closing" sequence ($-\alpha/2$; gradient spoil) [Scheffler et al. 2001], followed by the preparation and an "opening" sequence (gradient spoil; $\alpha/2$; $-\alpha$; dummy pulses) on the new slice. Fat-selective saturation is achieved by either a typical fat selective RF pulse or one of the quicker off-resonance saturation schemes as described elsewhere [Derbyshire et al. 2005; Santos et al. 2003].

14.2.4 Interactive Imaging Features

Graphical user interfaces for rtMRI guidance of interventional procedures have been under active development. The first systems allowed basic real-time imaging with a single adjustable imaging plane [Holsinger et al. 1990; Morton et al. 1997]. Subsequent systems added many of the features described above [Aksit et al. 2002; Guttman et al. 2002; Nayak et al. 2001; Quick et al. 2003]. Automatic image parameter adjustment in response to motion of a device being tracked has also been investigated [Elgort et al. 2003; Zuehlsdorff et al. 2004].

Recent work has shown the utility of device-only projection imaging, an interactive imaging mode where slice-selection is turned off and images are produced using signal from only the invasive devices [Peters et al. 2003], for views that resemble X-ray fluoroscopy. The entire active portion of the device is displayed against a dark background. This mode can be switched on and off during scanning for any slice to give a quick glance at an active device that may have escaped the thin-slice imaging plane.

Derived from this technique is adaptively oriented projection navigation (PRONAV), which is designed to facilitate steering of an active device towards target tissue. A device-only projection image and at least one standard thin-slice image are displayed together in a 3D rendering, all updated using real-time imaging. As the user interactively rotates the 3D rendering, the scanner automatically changes the projection direction, analogous to changing X-ray gantry position during fluoroscopy. This provides a real-time 3D view of the catheter position and trajectory with respect to the thin-slice image plane. For anatomical context, the thin-slice image is positioned to contain target tissue, and the combination of projection and thin-slice views can be used to navigate the device towards the target.

The NHLBI rtMRI implementation contains the projection imaging features and many other interactive features, which can be controlled by simple keyboard or mouse operation without stopping the scanner. Below is an abbreviated list of interactive features available [Guttman et al. 2002, 2003a; Raman et al. 2005]:

1. Display each slice in separate windows, as well as a 3D rendering where they are shown at their respective locations in space (see Fig. 14.1 and Fig. 14.2). This provided simultaneous views of all slices and devices in one window from any angle.

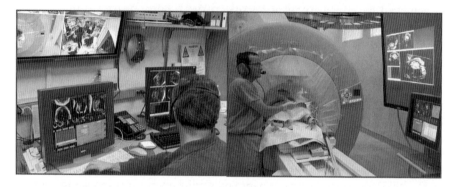

Fig. 14.1. The console room (*left*) and inside magnet room (*right*) during a swine experiment. Output from the custom reconstruction engine is rear projected onto the magnet room screen. The MRI scanner console is displayed on a remote monitor (*right*). MRI scanner console. Headsets are used for communication during scans

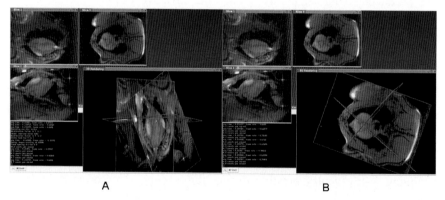

A   B

Fig. 14.2. Real-time multislice imaging before placement of a bioprosthetic aortic valve in swine. Three 2D slices are shown both individually and in a 3D rendering at their respective positions. On the live display, colored dots mark the positions of LAD and RCA ostia and the level of the aortic valve annulus. Two viewing angles of the 3D rendering are displayed A and B, showing long and short axis views of the multiple slice scan, respectively. A Video (Movie 14.1) demonstrating the dynamic interaction depicted by this figure is included with the DVD accompanying this book

Device channel   Device channel
intensities not squared   intensities squared

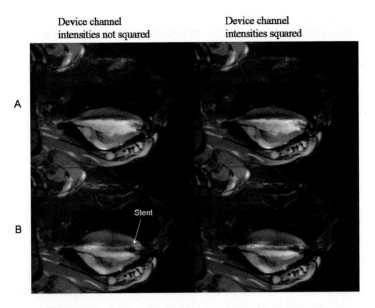

Fig. 14.3. (**A**) The central guide wire (*green*) is advanced through the LV and aortic valve. (**B**) The catheter with the stent/valve (*dark region* on the catheter) and second guide wire attached to the side of the stent (*red*) is advanced along the central lumen guide wire. The right column shows how squaring the intensity of the device images sharpens the appearance of the devices in the images and reduces the background noise from the device channels

2. Change the slice position/orientation using the standard scanner slice prescription interface.
3. Enable/disable acquisition of selected slices. This was often used when slices were initially prescribed for all stages of the procedure, and then only those needed at the time were enabled.
4. Highlight device channels in different colors, blended with grayscale images from surface coils (see Fig. 14.2). The device signal magnitude can be squared to sharpen the device profile.
5. Marking of reference points. Reference points are displayed in the 3D rendering and persist until deleted. This was used to mark anatomical features for device positioning (see Fig. 14.2).
6. Enable/disable squaring of device channel intensity. Squaring sharpens the device profile for more accurate localization.
7. Enable/disable device-only projection view on selected slices to show entire device if it exited from the thin slice.
8. Enable/disable adaptive projection navigation (PRONAV) mode for 3D projection views of the device.
9. Use non-selective saturation to darken background and isolate T1-shortening contrast agent (see Fig. 14.3).

10. Change acceleration factor.
11. Enable subtraction imaging for enhancing contrast injections.
12. Enable saving of raw data to files. The same program can be used at a later time to review the images with the same or different options for reconstruction or display. Several display and rendering parameters (such as 3D rendering orientation, highlight colors, window positions) are also saved. Post-procedure review therefore can mimic how the images were displayed during the actual procedure.

14.2.5 Invasive Devices and Experiments

Several custom-made active interventional devices, such as guide wires and catheters incorporating an active solenoid coil at the distal tip or loopless antenna [Ocali and Atalar 1997], were employed for in vivo experiments to develop the features described above.

One such device is a dual-channel injection catheter designed by S. Smith and G. Scott [Dick et al. 2003], based on the X-ray compatible Stiletto catheter (Boston Scientific, Inc.), which had an antenna along its shaft and a small coil near the tip. Experiments were performed on swine with previously induced infarcts, as described by Dick et al. [2003]. Two imaging planes were prescribed for real-time imaging: (1) Long-axis "candy cane" view showing ascending and descending aorta, aortic valve, and left ventricle (LV); (2) LV short-axis plane containing infarcted tissue, seen by delayed hyper-enhancement after contrast injection. The catheter was steered into the LV using the candy cane view. Then the short-axis view was turned on and PRONAV enabled on the candy cane view to guide navigation of the catheter towards the border regions of the infarcts.

Another device is an active loopless antenna guide-wire with a flexible tip [Raval et al. 2006b]. Two of these devices were used to guide minimally invasive surgical implantation of bioprosthetic aortic valves. One active guide-wire was used to cross the native aortic valve antegrade via a left ventricular transapical approach. The valve was affixed to a platinum stent and compressed onto the outer balloon of a BiB catheter. The second guide-wire was loosely sutured to the outside of the stent, along one of the commissures of the valve. Three oblique slices were prescribed: (1) axial view of the aortic valve; (2) long axis image containing the LAD ostium, aortic valve, and trocar; and (3) long axis image containing the RCA ostium, aortic valve, and trocar. The axial image was interactively translated above the valve to show the ostia of the LAD and RCA, which were then marked for reference. The aortic valve annulus position was similarly marked on one of the long-axis images. Multiple-slice imaging with color-highlighted active guide-wires and anatomical reference markers were then used to guide the delivery trajectory and positioning of the stent/valve.

Typical imaging parameters for cardiac interventional experiments were as follows: matrix size of 108×192; TR/TE = 3.84/1.92 ms; bandwidth,

1,000 Hz/pixel or higher; excitation RF pulse $\alpha = 45°$; ¾ partial phase-encode acquisition with homodyne detection for *k*-space filling [Noll et al. 1991]; and acceleration rate of 2. For higher quality imaging of more stationary tissues such as peripheral vessels, the parameters were typically changed to 168 × 224 matrix, 800 Hz/pixel bandwidth, full phase-encode acquisition, and acceleration rate of 2 or 3. Frame rate ranged from 3 to 8 per second, depending on the choice of imaging parameters.

The Siemens torso phased-array coil or a custom design surface coil (Nova Medical, Wilmington, MA) was placed on the ventral surface. Spine coils were turned on only when necessary, e.g., for imaging the aorta or some peripheral vessels, otherwise they were turned off to allow smaller FOV and increased spatial resolution. One or two receiver channels were used for device-mounted coils. The scanner was set up to function normally while MR echo data were simultaneously transferred to the workstation for custom reconstruction and display. Image reconstruction on the scanner can be turned off in case a high data rate (e.g., from using many receiver channels) causes it to lag behind data acquisition.

14.2.6 Room Setup

Figure 14.1 shows the console room (left) and magnet room (right), representative of our typical configuration during interventional experiments on animal models. Several displays are used in both rooms to monitor

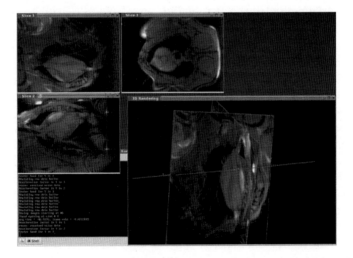

Movie 14.1. (This movie can be found on the DVD accompanying this book). Real-time multislice imaging before placement of a bioprosthetic aortic valve in swine. Three 2D slices are shown individually and in a 3D rendering at their respective positions. *Cyan dots* mark the positions of LAD and RCA ostia; the *yellow dot* marks the level of the aortic valve annulus. The 3D rendering is rotated to view the slices from different angles, for better understanding of the slice positions in anatomical context.

the function of the scanner, external workstation, and physiology [Guttman et al. 2003b]. Team members wear custom-designed communication headsets (Magnacoustics, Atlantic Beach, NY) with noise-canceling optical microphones (Phone-Or, Or-Yehuda, Israel) to talk to each other during scanning for imaging parameter changes, timing during injections, or saving data. Slice position and orientation changes were performed interactively in the graphical prescription interface on the scanner console. Complex scanner controls dictate that someone other than the surgeon will adjust imaging parameters, and thus good voice communication between the physician and operator is essential.

14.3   Initial Preclinical Procedures

Some of the important features of the system are illustrated in Fig. 14.2. This figure shows a screen capture on the external workstation before place-ment of a bioprosthetic aortic valve in swine. Multiple oblique slices were acquired in succession and displayed at their respective locations on the 3D rendering. Heart function can be monitored in either long-axis view if a single slice is enabled. The trocar is seen in the long-axis images, having been inserted through the LV apex. The coronary ostia and aortic valve annulus were visible in the real-time images. For anatomical reference, their positions were marked in the 2D images and were displayed in the 3D rendering (ostia and annulus in cyan and yellow dots, respectively). Two viewing angles of the 3D rendering are displayed (Fig. 14.2a,b), showing long and short axis views of the multiple slice scan, respectively. There is a movie (Movie 14.1) on the CD included with this book, which shows this with interactive rotations of the 3D rendering are shown in Movie 14.1, which is on the DVD included with this book.

Figure 14.3 shows images where signal from the active guide-wires was reconstructed separately from that of the surface coils, color highlighted, and blended. The central active guide-wire was clearly seen (green) as it was steered through the aortic valve (Fig. 14.3a). The second active guide-wire affixed to the side of the stent (red) as well as the stent itself (darkened region from RF shielding) were easily seen as the device was advanced through the LV (Fig. 14.3b). Note that the red and green colors blend to yellow in regions where both active guide wires are visible. The right column shows how squaring the intensity of the device images sharpens the appearance of the devices in the images and reduces the background noise from the device channels.

The axial image in Fig. 14.4 provided feedback when rotating the valve to position a commissure between the coronary ostia (cyan dots) before deployment. The active guide wire affixed to the side of the stent (green) indicated the commissure position. In Fig. 14.5, the proximal edge of the stent/valve was lined up with the annulus marker (yellow dot, c). This integrated information facilitated placement of the stent/valve at the correct location using real-time MRI guidance.

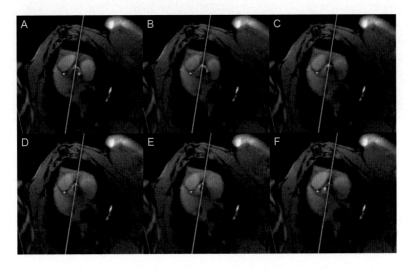

Fig. 14.4. The stent/valve is rotated using rtMRI feedback. The guide wire affixed to the side of the stent (*green*) indicates the position of a commissure. The practitioner rotates the catheter to position the commissure between the coronary ostia

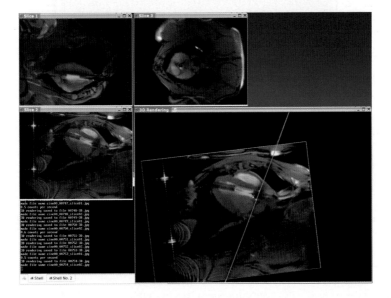

Fig. 14.5. The practitioner advances the stent until the proximal edge lines up with the marker, indicating the aortic valve annulus level (*yellow dot*)

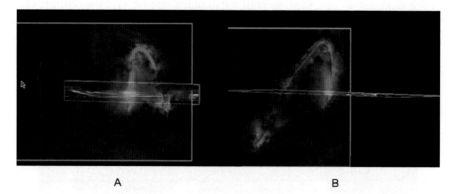

A   B

Fig. 14.6. Adaptive projection navigation (PRONAV) is illustrated in this basic example. The projection image is displayed along with a thin slice image **A**. When the 3D rendering is interactively rotated **B**, the projection direction is automatically updated, providing a different view of the device. The device is an injection catheter containing two receivers: a small coil at the tip (*red*) and a loopless antenna along the shaft (*green*)

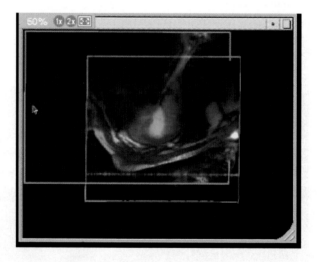

Movie 14.2. (This movie can be found on the DVD accompanying this book). Adaptive projection navigation (PRONAV) is illustrated in this basic example. At first, an LV short axis image is seen. The full extent of the device is seen when device-only projection imaging is turned on. The 3D rendering is then rotated down then horizontally, revealing the trajectory of the injection catheter. The projection image is displayed along with a thin slice image. When the 3D rendering is interactively rotated, the projection direction is automatically updated, providing a different view of the device. The device is an injection catheter containing two receivers: a small coil at the tip (*red*) and a loopless antenna along the shaft (*green*).

Figure 14.6 and Movie 14.2 (on the included CD) demonstrate the basic function of adaptive projection navigation (PRONAV) in a percutaneous targeting experiment, using an active injection catheter containing two

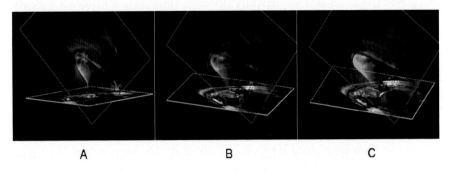

A   B   C

Fig. 14.7. PRONAV is used for real-time 3D visualization of an active catheter and navigation towards infarct border tissue in a 2D image plane. A *yellow dot* marks the target tissue. The device is the same as that in Fig. 14.6. The rendering is manually rotated during the scan to see the device trajectory from different angles, giving a 3D effect. Knowledge of the device trajectory is used to advance the tip of the device toward the target tissue

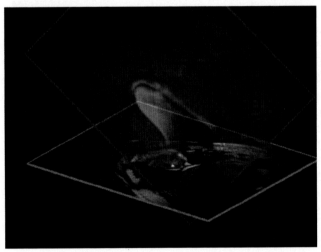

Movie 14.3. (This movie can be found on the DVD accompanying this book). PRONAV imaging is used in an intra-myocardial injection experiment. This 3D rendering shows a thin-slice image, a device-only projection image, and a yellow marker indicating a target on the endocardium. As the user rotates the rendering, the projection direction is continually oriented normal to the viewing screen. This allows appreciation of the full trajectory of the device from any angle, imparting a 3D viewing effect. Updating of the thin-slice image stops while rotating the rendering for better interactivity with the projection image. Knowledge of the device trajectory is used to advance the tip of the device toward the target tissue.

receivers: a small coil at the tip (red) and a loopless antenna along the shaft (green). The projection image of the device only is displayed together with a thin slice image (a). When the 3D rendering is interactively rotated (b), the projection direction is automatically updated, providing a different view of the device. The interactive technique gives a 3D perception of device trajectory, better appreciated in moving rather than static pictures. In Fig. 14.7 and Movie 14.3 (on the included CD), PRONAV is used for navigation towards infarct border tissue in a 2D image plane [Dick et al. 2003].

Projection imaging allowed continuous visualization of the device in 3D when the rendering was rotated. Targeting of infarct borders was enhanced, since regions of reduced cardiac function and delayed hyper-enhancement (post-contrast) were observable in the thin-slice image. This interactive technique gave 3D feedback about device trajectory with respect to the imaging slice and simplified catheter steering toward target tissue in the imaging plane.

14.4   Discussion

An interactive real-time MR imaging environment initially developed for use in intravascular procedures [Guttman et al. 2003b] has been adapted to guide minimally invasive cardiovascular surgical procedures such as aortic valve placement. Many features were implemented that exploit the advantages of MRI: enhancing visualization of separate antennae or coils mounted on invasive devices, providing multiple oblique slices that are easily adjusted, rendering all slices and landmarks in 3D, accelerated imaging and projection imaging modes to see the entire trajectory of a device receiving signal along its shaft.

The system has been used by our group in a number of preclinical studies in swine, including intra-myocardial injection of stem cells [Dick et al. 2003], endovascular repair of abdominal aortic aneurysms [Raman et al. 2005], stenting of aortic coarctation [Raval et al. 2005], recanalization of chronic total occlusions [Raval et al. 2006b], atrial–septal puncture and balloon septostomy [Raval et al. 2006a], and catheterization in humans [Dick et al. 2005]. In this chapter, we have shown results from feasibility experiments in which the system was used to guide minimally invasive aortic valve replacement. Separate experiments were previously performed to improve catheter navigation for intra-myocardial injection, all using rtMRI for visual feedback while manipulating invasive devices. The particular needs of these applications have driven the development of the system over the last several years.

Real-time imaging of multiple oblique slices offers many potential advantages. Different views of complicated anatomy may be simultaneously displayed and individual slices can be interactively turned on or off during a scan as needed. Another important use would be to provide continuous monitoring of function (e.g., heart motion) in one view during an intervention requiring a different view. Also of benefit would be to allow a different sequence or parameters to be run for different slices. This would increase the range of information provided by the real-time imaging.

High performance hardware was used to minimize image reconstruction latency. As reported, typical frame rates ranged from 3 to 8 per second, depending on choice of parameters. Much higher frame rates, in excess of 30 per second, were sustainable by the system when using small k-space matrix (such as 64×128), view sharing, and eight receiver channels. This small matrix does not result in adequate image quality, but was useful to gauge the limits of the reconstruction and display pipeline. As of this writing, better raw data throughput and a faster reconstruction computer are required to handle real-time processing of 32-channel data with high acceleration rates and larger matrix.

The minimally invasive valve replacement experiment was performed on a Siemens 1.5 T Espree scanner. This magnet features a bore with wider diameter (70 cm) and shorter length (120 cm) than has been common until now, which provided easier access to the worksite than the typical 1.5 T magnet bore. One compromise is a smaller imaging volume, which is especially evident using a refocused sequence such as SSFP. However, our experience is that the imaging volume is adequate to perform this intervention without moving the patient table.

Further advancements will incorporate more advanced real-time volume rendering modes, other interactive control modes such as PRONAV, and closed-loop techniques for automatically changing image parameters [Elgort et al. 2006]. An imaging suite such as this can be of benefit to a variety of interventional procedures using real-time MRI guidance.

MRI offers the advantage that the surgeon can see "through" the blood, and morphological landmarks for positioning the device are visible. New short magnet design makes it possible to have high performance real-time MRI available while manipulating the prosthetic valve under image guidance. These advantages render real-time MRI an attractive method to guide interventional procedures. In additional to the aortic valve procedure discussed here, additional target applications are mitral, pulmonary, and tricuspid valve replacements or repairs [Boudjemline et al. 2004, 2005; Buchbinder and Cosgrove 1998; Mihaljevic et al. 2004].

Acknowledgment

The authors thank Joni Taylor, Kathy Lucas, Shawn Kozlov, and Timothy Hunt for animal care and support. Much of the development of rtMRI interventional procedures was a collaboration with the following investigators: Cenghizhan Ozturk, MD, PhD; Parag V. Karmarkar, MS; Amish N. Raval, MD; Venkatesh K. Raman, MD; Alexander J. Dick, MD; Ranil DeSilva, MBBS, PhD; Ming Li, PhD. This work was supported through the Intramural Research Program of the National Heart Lung and Blood Institute, NIH, DHHS.

References

Aksit P, Derbyshire JA, Serfaty JM, and Atalar E. (2002). Multiple field of view MR fluoroscopy. *Magn Reson Med*, 47(1), 53–60

Atalar E, Kraitchman DL, Carkhuff B, Lesho J, Ocali O, Solaiyappan M, Guttman MA, and Charles HK, Jr. (1998). Catheter-tracking FOV MR fluoroscopy. *Magn Reson Med*, 40(6), 865–872

Babaliaros V, Cribier A, and Agatiello C. (2006). Surgery insight: Current advances in percutaneous heart valve replacement and repair. *Nat Clin Pract Cardiovasc Med*, 3(5), 256–264

Blanco RT, Ojala R, Kariniemi J, Perala J, Niinimaki J, and Tervonen O. (2005). Interventional and intraoperative MRI at low field scanner – A review. *Eur J Radiol*, 56(2), 130–142

Boudjemline Y, Agnoletti G, Bonnet D, Sidi D, and Bonhoeffer P. (2004). Percutaneous pulmonary valve replacement in a large right ventricular outflow tract: An experimental study. *J Am Coll Cardiol*, 43(6), 1082–1087

Boudjemline Y, Pineau E, Borenstein N, Behr L, and Bonhoeffer P. (2005). New insights in minimally invasive valve replacement: Description of a cooperative approach for the off-pump replacement of mitral valves. *Eur Heart J*, 26(19), 2013–2017

Buchbinder BR and Cosgrove GR. (1998). Cortical activation MR studies in brain disorders. *Magn Reson Imaging Clin N Am*, 6(1), 67–93

Derbyshire JA, Herzka DA, and McVeigh ER. (2005). S5FP: Spectrally selective suppression with steady state free precession. *Magn Reson Med*, 54(4), 918–928

Dick AJ, Guttman MA, Raman VK, Peters DC, Pessanha BS, Hill JM, Smith S, Scott G, McVeigh ER, and Lederman RJ. (2003). Magnetic resonance fluoroscopy allows targeted delivery of mesenchymal stem cells to infarct borders in Swine. *Circulation*, 108(23), 2899–2904

Dick AJ, Raman VK, Raval AN, Guttman MA, Thompson RB, Ozturk C, Peters DC, Stine AM, Wright VJ, Schenke WH, and Lederman RJ. (2005). Invasive human magnetic resonance imaging: Feasibility during revascularization in a combined XMR suite. *Catheter Cardiovasc Interv*, 64(3), 265–274

Doty DB, Flores JH, and Doty JR. (2000). Cardiac valve operations using a partial sternotomy (lower half) technique. *J Card Surg*, 15(1), 35–42

Elgort DR, Hillenbrand CM, Zhang S, Wong EY, Rafie S, Lewin JS, and Duerk JL. (2006). Image-guided and -monitored renal artery stenting using only MRI. *J Magn Reson Imaging*, 23(5), 619–627

Elgort DR, Wong EY, Hillenbrand CM, Wacker FK, Lewin JS, and Duerk JL. (2003). Real-time catheter tracking and adaptive imaging. *J Magn Reson Imaging*, 18(5), 621–626

Feng L, Dumoulin CL, Dashnaw S, Darrow RD, Guhde R, Delapaz RL, Bishop PL, and Pile-Spellman J. (2005). Transfemoral catheterization of carotid arteries with real-time MR imaging guidance in pigs. *Radiology*, 234(2), 551–557

Griswold MA, Jakob PM, Heidemann RM, Nittka M, Jellus V, Wang J, Kiefer B, and Haase A. (2002). Generalized autocalibrating partially parallel acquisi-tions (GRAPPA). *Magn Reson Med*, 47(6), 1202–1210

Guttman MA, Kellman P, Dick AJ, Lederman RJ, and McVeigh ER. (2003a). Real-time accelerated interactive MRI with adaptive TSENSE and UNFOLD. *Magn Reson Med*, 50(2), 315–321

Guttman MA, Lederman RJ, and McVeigh ER. (2003b). The cardiovascular interventional MRI suite: Design considerations. in *Cardiovascular Magnetic Resonance: Established and Emerging Applications*, ed. by Lardo A, Fayad ZA, Fuster V, and Chronos N, (Martin Dunitz, London)

Guttman MA, Lederman RJ, Sorger JM, and McVeigh ER. (2002). Real-time volume rendered MRI for interventional guidance. *J Cardiovasc Magn Reson*, 4(4), 431–442

Hardy CJ, Darrow RD, Nieters EJ, Roemer PB, Watkins RD, Adams WJ, Hattes NR, and Maier JK. (1993). Real-time acquisition, display, and interactive graphic control of NMR cardiac profiles and images. *Magn Reson Med*, 29(5), 667–673

Henk CB, Higgins CB, and Saeed M. (2005). Endovascular interventional MRI. *J Magn Reson Imaging*, 22(4), 451–460

Hillenbrand CM, Elgort DR, Wong EY, Reykowski A, Wacker FK, Lewin JS, and Duerk JL. (2004). Active device tracking and high-resolution intravascular MRI using a novel catheter-based, opposed-solenoid phased array coil. *Magn Reson Med*, 51(4), 668–675

Holsinger AE, Wright RC, Riederer SJ, Farzaneh F, Grimm RC, and Maier JK. (1990). Real-time interactive magnetic resonance imaging. *Magn Reson Med*, 14(3), 547–553

Horvath KA, Guttman M, Li M, Lederman RJ, Mazilu D, Kocaturk O, Karmarkar PV, Parag V, Hunt T, Kozlov S, and McVeigh ER. (2007). Beating heart aortic valve replacement using real-time MRI guidance. Innovations: Technology and Techniques in Cardiothoracic and Vascular Surgery. 2(2): 51–55

Kellman P, Epstein FH, and McVeigh ER. (2001). Adaptive sensitivity encoding incorporating temporal filtering (TSENSE). *Magn Reson Med*, 45(5), 846–852

Kerr AB, Pauly JM, Hu BS, Li KC, Hardy CJ, Meyer CH, Macovski A, and Nishimura DG. (1997). Real-time interactive MRI on a conventional scanner. *Magn Reson Med*, 38(3), 355–367

Kraitchman DL, Heldman AW, Atalar E, Amado LC, Martin BJ, Pittenger MF, Hare JM, and Bulte JW. (2003). *In vivo* magnetic resonance imaging of mesenchymal stem cells in myocardial infarction. *Circulation*, 107(18), 2290–2293

Kuehne T, Yilmaz S, Meinus C, Moore P, Saeed M, Weber O, Higgins CB, Blank T, Elsaesser E, Schnackenburg B, Ewert P, Lange PE, and Nagel E. (2004). Magnetic resonance imaging-guided transcatheter implantation of a prosthetic valve in aortic valve position: Feasibility study in swine. *J Am Coll Cardiol*, 44(11), 2247–2249

Lederman RJ. (2005). Cardiovascular interventional magnetic resonance imaging. *Circulation*, 112(19), 3009–3017

Lederman RJ, Guttman MA, Peters DC, Thompson RB, Sorger JM, Dick AJ, Raman VK, and McVeigh ER. (2002). Catheter-based endomyocardial injection with real-time magnetic resonance imaging. *Circulation*, 105(11), 1282–1284

Lorenz CH, Kirchberg KJ, Zuehlsdorff S, Speier P, Caylus M, Borys W, Moeller T, and Guttman MA. (2005). Interactive Frontend (IFE): A Platform for Graphical MR Scanner Control and Scan Automation. *ISMRM*, Miami, 7–13 May

Lutter G, Ardehali R, Cremer J, and Bonhoeffer P. (2004). Percutaneous valve replacement: Current state and future prospects. *Ann Thorac Surg*, 78(6), 2199–2206

Madore B, Glover GH, and Pelc NJ. (1999). Unaliasing by fourier-encoding the overlaps using the temporal dimension (UNFOLD), applied to cardiac imaging and fMRI. *Magn Reson Med*, 42(5), 813–828

McVeigh ER, Guttman MA, Lederman RJ, Li M, Kocaturk O, Hunt T, Kozlov S, and Horvath KA. (2006). Real-time interactive MRI guided cardiac surgery: aortic valve replacement using a direct apical approach. *Magn Reson Med*, 56(5), 958–964

Mihaljevic T, Cohn LH, Unic D, Aranki SF, Couper GS, and Byrne JG. (2004). One thousand minimally invasive valve operations: Early and late results. *Ann Surg*, 240(3), 529–534

Morton RE, Bonas R, Minford J, Kerr A, and Ellis RE. (1997). Feeding ability in Rett syndrome. *Dev Med Child Neurol*. 39(5), 331–335

Nayak KS, Pauly JM, Nishimura DG, and Hu BS. (2001). Rapid ventricular assessment using real-time interactive multislice MRI. *Magn Reson Med*, 45(3), 371–375

Noll DC, Nishimura DG, and Macovski A. (1991). Homodyne detection in magnetic resonance imaging. *IEEE Trans Med Imag*, 10(2), 154–163

Ocali O and Atalar E. (1997). Intravascular magnetic resonance imaging using a loopless catheter antenna. *Magn Reson Med*, 37(1), 112–118

Oppelt A, Graumann R, Barfuß H, Fischer H, Hartl W, and Scajor W. (1986). FISP – A new fast MRI sequence. *Electromedica*, 54(1), 15–18

Peters DC, Lederman RJ, Dick AJ, Raman VK, Guttman MA, Derbyshire JA, and McVeigh ER. (2003). Undersampled projection reconstruction for active catheter imaging with adaptable temporal resolution and catheter-only views. *Magn Reson Med*, 49(2), 216–222

Pruessmann KP, Weiger M, Scheidegger MB, and Boesiger P. (1999). SENSE: sensitivity encoding for fast MRI. *Magn Reson Med*, 42(5), 952–962

Quick HH, Kuehl H, Kaiser G, Hornscheidt D, Mikolajczyk KP, Aker S, Debatin JF, and Ladd ME. (2003). Interventional MRA using actively visualized catheters, TrueFISP, and real-time image fusion. *Magn Reson Med*, 49(1), 129–137

Raman VK, Karmarkar PV, Guttman MA, Dick AJ, Peters DC, Ozturk C, Pessanha BS, Thompson RB, Raval AN, DeSilva R, Aviles RJ, Atalar E, McVeigh ER, and Lederman RJ. (2005). Real-time magnetic resonance-guided endovascular repair of experimental abdominal aortic aneurysm in swine. *J Am Coll Cardiol*, 45(12), 2069–2077

Raval AN, Karmarkar PV, Guttman MA, Ozturk C, Desilva R, Aviles RJ, Wright VJ, Schenke WH, Atalar E, McVeigh ER, and Lederman RJ. (2006a). Real-time MRI guided atrial septal puncture and balloon septostomy in swine. *Catheter Cardiovasc Interv*, 67(4), 637–643

Raval AN, Karmarkar PV, Guttman MA, Ozturk C, Sampath S, DeSilva R, Aviles RJ, Xu M, Wright VJ, Schenke WH, Kocaturk O, Dick AJ, Raman VK, Atalar E, McVeigh ER, and Lederman RJ. (2006b). Real-time magnetic resonance imaging-guided endovascular recanalization of chronic total arterial occlusion in a swine model. *Circulation*, 113(8), 1101–1107

Raval AN, Telep JD, Guttman MA, Ozturk C, Jones M, Thompson RB, Wright VJ, Schenke WH, DeSilva R, Aviles RJ, Raman VK, Slack MC, and Lederman RJ. (2005). Real-time magnetic resonance imaging-guided stenting of aortic coarctation with commercially available catheter devices in Swine. *Circulation*, 112(5), 699–706

Santos JM, Hargreaves BA, Nayak KS, and Pauly JM. (2003). Real-Time Fat Supressed SSFP *Proc 11th ISMRM*, Toronto, p. 982

Scheffler K, Heid O, and Hennig J. (2001). Magnetization preparation during the steady state: Fat-saturated 3D TrueFISP. *Magn Reson Med*, 45(6), 1075–1080

Schulz T, Puccini S, Schneider JP, and Kahn T. (2004). Interventional and intraoperative MR: Review and update of techniques and clinical experience. *Eur Radiol*, 14(12), 2212–2227

Serfaty JM, Yang X, Aksit P, Quick HH, Solaiyappan M, and Atalar E. (2000). Toward MRI-guided coronary catheterization: visualization of guiding catheters, guidewires, and anatomy in real time. *J Magn Reson Imaging*, 12(4), 590–594

Sodickson DK and Manning WJ. (1997). Simultaneous acquisition of spatial harmonics (SMASH): Fast imaging with radiofrequency coil arrays. *Magn Reson Med*, 38(4), 591–603

Tsao J, Boesiger P, and Pruessmann KP. (2003). *k-t* BLAST and *k-t* SENSE: Dynamic MRI with high frame rate exploiting spatiotemporal correlations. *Magn Reson Med*, 50(5), 1031–1042

Vassiliades TA, Jr., Block PC, Cohn LH, Adams DH, Borer JS, Feldman T, Holmes DR, Laskey WK, Lytle BW, Mack MJ, and Williams DO. (2005). The clinical development of percutaneous heart valve technology. *J Thorac Cardiovasc Surg*, 129(5), 970–976

Zuehlsdorff S, Umathum R, Volz S, Hallscheidt P, Fink C, Semmler W, and Bock M. (2004). MR coil design for simultaneous tip tracking and curvature delineation of a catheter. *Magn Reson Med*, 52(1), 214–218

Chapter 15

Three-Dimensional Ultrasound Guidance and Robot Assistance for Prostate Brachytherapy

Zhouping Wei, Lori Gardi, Chandima Edirisinghe, Dónal Downey, and Aaron Fenster

Abstract

Current transperineal prostate brachytherapy uses transrectal ultrasound (TRUS) guidance and a template at a fixed position to guide needles along parallel trajectories. However, pubic arch interference (PAI) with the implant path obstructs part of the prostate from being targeted by the brachytherapy needles along parallel trajectories. To solve the PAI problem, some investigators have explored other insertion trajectories, such as oblique, but the parallel trajectory constraints in current brachytherapy procedure also do not allow oblique insertion. This chapter describes a robot-assisted, three-dimensional (3D) TRUS guided approach to solve this problem. Our prototype consists of a commercial robot, plus a 3D TRUS imaging system comprising an ultrasound machine, image acquisition apparatus using 3D TRUS image reconstruction, and display software. The robot positions the needle before insertion, but the physician inserts the needle into the patient's prostate. By unifying the robot, ultrasound transducer, and the 3D TRUS image coordinate systems, the position of the template hole can be accurately related to the 3D TRUS image coordinate system, allowing accurate and consistent insertion of the needle via the template hole into the targeted position in the prostate.

15.1 Introduction

The prostate is a variably sized gland, approximately the size of a walnut, located in the male pelvis. The urethra is surrounded by the prostate, traveling through the center of the prostate, carrying urine from the bladder to the penis. Three problems can occur within a prostate:

T. Peters and K. Cleary (eds.), *Image-Guided Interventions.*
© Springer Science + Business Media, LLC 2008

1. Benign prostatic hyperplasia (BPH) (nonmalignant enlargement of the prostate gland)
2. Prostatitis (inflammation of the prostate due to a bacterial infection)
3. Prostate cancer (an abnormal growth of malignant cells that usually starts in the peripheral zone of the prostate)

Autopsies have revealed small prostatic carcinomas in up to 29% of men aged 30–40 years of age, and in up to 64% of men aged 60–70 years of age [Sakr et al. 1994]. In 2006, Canadian Cancer Statistics report that 20,700 Canadians will be diagnosed with prostate cancer and 4,200 will die from the disease [McLaughlin et al. 2006]. In the United States, it is estimated that 234,460 new cases of prostate cancer will be diagnosed and 27,350 men will due from prostate cancer in 2006 [Jemal et al. 2006].

Initially, cancer cells are confined within the prostate ducts and glands; but over time, the cancer develops the ability to exit the ducts and migrates into the blood and lymphatic system. Prostate cancer can spread not only through lymphatic channels, producing metastases in pelvic lymph nodes, but also through the blood, producing metastases elsewhere in the body, particularly in the bones.

Currently, there are four standard treatments used for clinically localized prostate cancer, i.e., cancer that is still confined within the prostate: watchful waiting, radical prostatectomy (RP), external beam radiation therapy (EBRT), and brachytherapy [Bangma et al. 2001].

1. *Watchful waiting.* During this period, the physician closely observes the cancer without initiating treatment. Watchful waiting represents a practical approach to those patients who are not at significant risk of dying from prostate cancer. Patients considered for this approach are typically men over the age of 70, or men at a lower risk of dying from prostate cancer.
2. *Radical prostatectomy (RP).* This approach involves the surgical removal of the prostate gland, seminal vesicles, and a varying number of pelvic lymph nodes. RP offers the complete removal of prostate cancer within the patient. Patients who are considered candidates for RP are those who are in good health and those with a life expectancy of 10 years or more.
3. *External beam radiation therapy (EBRT).* In EBRT, radiation is emitted from a linear accelerator. EBRT can potentially kill prostate cancer cells using a series of radiation treatments administered for a length of time. This approach has been recommended as a potential treatment option for patients who have localized cancer, who have a life expectancy of more than 10 years, and who are unable or unwilling to undergo RP.

4. *Brachytherapy*. Brachytherapy is a form of radiation therapy in which radioactive sources are implanted into the prostate permanently or temporarily. Candidates for the implantation of permanent radioactive sources are men with prostate volumes less than 60 cm^3, Gleason histologic scores < 6, and PSA < 10 ng ml^{-1}. However, candidates for the temporary implantation of radioactive sources are less limited. Patients with variably sized prostates, PSA levels, and Gleason scores are eligible to receive temporary implantations of radioactive sources.

15.1.1 Prostate Brachytherapy

While watchful waiting is an option for some low risk patients, most North American patients expect, and may require, active treatment. However, although it has an excellent cure rate, RP may cause serious complications, such as incontinence, impotence, and contracture of the bladder neck. Compared with RP, EBRT has a lower risk for impotence and incontinence. Because the radiation beam passes through normal tissues on its way to the prostate, some healthy cells are killed. In addition, EBRT needs daily dose treatment, each of which requires realignment of the beams. A study has shown that for over half of the patients treated with EBRT, realignment errors of 5 mm or greater had occurred within EBRT treatments [Lattanzi et al. 2000]. Therefore, EBRT can miss cancer cells, while seriously damaging nearby normal cells.

Compared with RP, brachytherapy is minimally invasive. It involves no incisions or sutures and it essentially produces no blood loss. With accurate placement, brachytherapy can confine high doses of radiation to the prostate, dramatically limiting treatment-related complications by minimizing the radiation to nearby organs [Ash et al. 1998]. The results of treatment from the limited number of available comparative studies did not show any significant difference in the clinical effectiveness of RP, EBRT, or brachytherapy [Norderhaug et al. 2003]. In addition, brachytherapy has the potential to achieve sharp demarcation between irradiated volume and healthy structures, achieving superior tumor control with significantly reduced morbidity and side effects in comparison to other treatment modalities and techniques [Blasko et al. 2002].

Currently, two different approaches to prostate brachytherapy are possible: temporary afterloading high dose rate (HDR) radioactive source (e.g., iridium-192) and permanent implantation of low dose rate (LDR) isotopes with low energy and short half-lives (e.g., iodine-125 and palladium-103) [Butler et al. 1997]. An HDR procedure involves the placement of a hollowed catheter array into the prostate followed by the insertion of iridium-192. After the treatment is completed, iridium-192 and the catheters are removed and no radiation is left in the patient. In an LDR procedure, the radioactive seeds (iodine-125 or palladium-103) are permanently implanted into the prostate, and over the course of their radioactive lives the seeds continuously emit low levels of radiation. Permanent seed implantation is technically easier to implement and perform, and so it tends to receive the most clinical interest. Since Holm et al. [1983] first described the use of transrectal ultrasound (TRUS) to guide transperineal insertion of needles into the prostate to permanently deposit iodine-125 sources into the gland, two-dimensional (2D) TRUS guided LDR prostate brachytherapy has become the standard approach to prostate therapy. This chapter discusses the method of applying three-dimensional (3D) TRUS guidance with robot assistance to improve current LDR prostate brachytherapy procedures. For the remainder of this chapter, LDR brachytherapy is referred to simply as brachytherapy.

In an effort to achieve an optimal geometry of the implanted sources, a template is currently used in prostate brachytherapy. With the patient in the lithotomic position, the template, which acts as a guide for each needle placement, is held rigidly in place over the perineum. This placement allows the physician to control the entire prostate target volume and to specify the placement of each radioactive source at any point within the gland. If the prostate is imaged in 3D, then any point within the prostate can be given a unique set of coordinates using the grid on the template to determine the X and Y coordinates, and then using the distance from the plane of the template at the perineum to define the Z coordinate. For every increment of 5 mm from the "zero plane" at the base of the prostate to the apex, TRUS can be used to map the area of the gland onto this grid. This mapping creates a series of 2D images that can be used to create a 3D target volume. An integrated computer performs the treatment planning using this target volume to develop a pattern for radioactive source placement that will deliver the desired dose. This treatment pattern is called the preimplant plan (or preplan). The position of each source is defined by the grid coordinate system of the chosen template together with its depth or distance from the template.

Implantation is performed during a subsequent visit. The patient is positioned in a similar orientation to the preplanning position. Each of the needles is placed in the pattern determined by the preplan. The number of seeds to be placed in each needle and the spacing between seeds is determined by the preplan; however, it may be modified intraoperatively using real-time adjustments in the 2D TRUS image planes to improve the accuracy of the final distribution. These adjustments are made to compensate for the errors caused by the displacement of the prostate.

Amongst physicians, it is generally agreed that postoperative dosimetry must be performed to assess the adequacy of implantation and to determine the actual dose received by the prostate and normal tissues [Prete et al. 1998]. This process usually requires a post implantation CT scan so that the position of the seeds in the prostate capsule (as well as critical tissues) can be outlined, and a full reconstruction of dose and volume can be made [Roy et al. 1993].

15.1.2 Limitations of Current Brachytherapy

Although current prostate brachytherapy is widely accepted, it still suffers from limitations and variability due to the following four factors that have limited the full potential of prostate brachytherapy: pubic arch interference (PAI), geometric changes in the prostate, prostate trauma due to seed implantation, and prostate variations.

PAI with the implant path occurs in many patients with large prostates (>60 cm^3) and in some patients with a small pelvis. When using parallel needle trajectories guided by a fixed template, the anterior and/or the antero-lateral parts of their prostate are blocked by the pubic bone. The patients in whom PAI occurs cannot be treated with current brachytherapy until their prostates have been reduced in size using hormonal therapy, a separate process that typically takes between 3–9 months [Pathak et al. 1998; Strang et al. 2001]

Geometric changes occurring in the prostate between the preplan scan and the implantation scan lead to incorrect seed placement. It has been shown that the prostate volume can change by as much as 50% in the time between the preplan and implantation [Messing et al. 1999].

Seed implant procedures induce trauma and cause the prostate to swell due to edema [Badiozamani et al. 1999]. Clearly, variations of prostate shape and volume during the procedure may result in "misplaced" seeds and lack of proper dose coverage. The AAPM TASK Group 64 has identified this as an issue to be resolved [Yu et al. 1999]. Prostate variations and changes between seed implantation, postoperative dosimetry (and other factors such as TRUS imaging artifacts), migration of the seeds in the needle tracks, and needle deflection also lead to potential inaccuracies [Wan et al. 2005]. Discrepancies have also been reported between CT- and TRUS-based prostate volume measurements [Bangma et al. 1995]. These factors can result in incorrect determination of dose coverage.

15.1.3 Potential Solutions

To solve several of the aforementioned problems associated with current prostate brachytherapy, some researchers have proposed a dynamic intra-operative procedure, encompassing all the processes in one session, including planning, monitoring of prostate changes, dynamic replanning, and optimal needle implantation (including oblique trajectories) [Cheng et al. 2001].

TRUS-guided prostate planning and seed implantation are being used extensively in current prostate brachytherapy procedures, as 2D TRUS imaging with 3D reconstruction provides an excellent visualization of the

3D space. In recent years, many advances have been made in 3D ultrasound (US) imaging of the prostate [Fenster et al. 2001; Tong et al. 1996], US image processing for prostate boundary segmentation [Ding et al. 2003b; Hu et al. 2003; Ladak et al. 2000; Shen et al. 2003; Wang et al. 2003], pubic arch detection [Pathak et al. 1998], needle segmentation [Ding et al. 2003a; Ding and Fenster 2003], and seed segmentation [Wei et al. 2006]. These advances have greatly enhanced the role of US in clinical diagnosis and image-guided interventions.

Because a robot can position, orient, and manipulate surgical tools along various trajectories accurately and consistently in three-dimensional space, medical robotic systems have been playing an increasing role in various image-guided interventions. The mobility of the robot is important because it helps to free the insertion of the needle from the constraints of the parallel trajectory, allowing an oblique insertion of the needle to occur. Robotic systems also can be dynamically programmed, controlled, and effectively integrated with 3D imaging systems, and so the robot can be instructed to target any point identified in the 3D image. Although they introduce more complex instrumentation and increased hardware costs, robotic approaches provide significant advantages and cost saving techniques. As a result, medical robotic approaches are being extensively explored. Several research teams have already investigated the possibilities of using robots during prostate therapy [Fichtinger et al. 2006; Wei et al. 2004; Yu et al. 2006].

15.2   System Description

Before the approach for robotic assistance is described, some consideration will be given to the tasks required for robot-assisted brachytherapy with 3D TRUS guidance. These tasks can be divided into two sections: preimplantation planning (preplanning) and seed implantation. For the preplanning stage, the physician's tasks include positioning the patient, obtaining the 3D TRUS images of the prostate, and sending the 3D TRUS images to a medical physicist, who determines the placement of the seeds. During seed implantation, the needles that implant seeds at various preplanned locations are inserted into the prostate so that the total amount of preplanned radioactive dose is delivered. Therefore, before the implantation of seeds can begin, a method of registering the patient to the implantation system (i.e., the robot system) is required. This registration method differs amongst varying system designs.

15.2.1 Hardware Components

Figures 15.1 and 15.2 show the prototype of the robotic-assisted system using 3D TRUS guidance for prostate brachytherapy. The prototype consists of a 3D TRUS imaging system, developed in our laboratory [Fenster et al. 2001; Tong et al. 1996], and a robot with 6 degrees-of-freedom (DOF).

To evaluate the feasibility of the proposed approach, we used a CRS *A465* commercial robot system (Thermo-CRS, Burlington, Ontario, Canada), but we have developed software to allow for the integration of the 3D TRUS imaging system with any robot with 6 DOF.

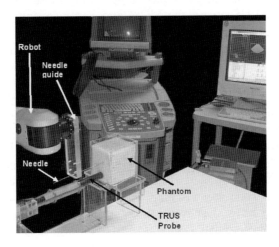

Fig. 15.1. The prototype of the robot-assisted and 3D TRUS-guided prostate brachytherapy system

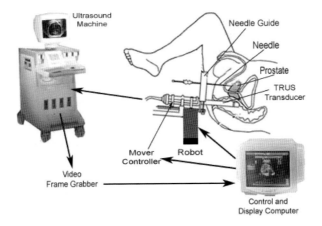

Fig. 15.2. Diagram of the robot-assisted and 3D TRUS-guided prostate brachy-therapy system. The rotation of the TRUS transducer is controlled by the mover controller. A video frame grabber is used for image acquisition. The acquired images are reconstructed into a 3D image and displayed in the computer. The robot is controlled to move to a position, so that the needle can be guided via the needle-guide to a target identified in the 3D TRUS image

The 3D TRUS imaging system consists of a Pentium III personal computer (PC) with a 1.2 GHz processor (for 3D image acquisition, reconstruction, and display), a Matrox Meteor II video frame grabber (for 30 Hz video image acquisition), a mover controller module (MCM) that controls the rotation of the transducer–mover assembly via the serial port of the computer, and a B-K Medical 2102 Hawk ultrasound machine (B-K, Denmark) with an 8558/S 7.5 MHz side-firing linear array transducer. To produce a 3D US image, the MCM and motor assembly rotate the transducer over an angle of approximately 120° about its long axis while a series of 2D US images are digitized at 0.7° intervals by a frame grabber. These acquired images are reconstructed into a 3D volume, which is available for viewing as the 2D images are being acquired.

The 3D US image can be viewed using 3D visualization software, which includes measurement and multiplanar reformatting tools for viewing any plane in the image in 3D.

The robot includes a robotic arm assembly with 6 DOF (three translational, three rotational), a PC-based kinematics positioning software system, and a robot controller. The positioning software of the robot system can control the robotic arm assembly via the controller in terms of world/tool coordinate systems. The world coordinate system is fixed to the ground, while the tool coordinate system is fixed to the arm of the robot. As the arms of the robot move, the position and orientation of the tool coordinate system change as well. The robot control software has been integrated together with the 3D visualization software, so that precise image-based planning of the robot path can be performed. Multiple potential trajectories can also be viewed by using a graphical user interface. The needle guide for manually inserting the needle is attached to the arm of the robot, which has a hole for needle guidance. Because the needle guide is attached to the arm of the robot, the position and orientation of the needle guide hole (in the robot tool coordinate system) is known. A transformation is performed by a software module, calibrating the robot tool coordinate system to the world coordinate system so that the guidance hole can be described in the robot world coordinate system.

15.2.2 System Calibration

Integration of the 3D TRUS image-based coordinate system with the robotic coordinate system is required to allow for accurate needle target planning and insertion under 3D TRUS guidance. This approach involves two calibration steps: (1) calibration of the 3D US image to the coordinate system of the transducer (image calibration), and (2) calibration of the transducer to the coordinate system of the robot (robot calibration).

The transformation between any two different coordinate systems is found by solving the orthogonal Procrustes problem as follows [Gower and Dijksterhuis 2004]:

Given two 3D sets of points, $K = \{k_j\}$, $L = \{l_j\}$ for $j = 1, 2, K, N$, we determine a rigid-body transformation such that $\mathcal{F} : l_j = \mathcal{F}\{k_j\} = \mathbf{R}k_j + \mathbf{T}$, where $\mathbf{R}$ is a 3×3 rotation matrix, and $\mathbf{T}$ is a 3×1 translation vector obtained by minimizing the cost function:

$$C = \frac{1}{N}\sum_{j=1}^{N}\left\| l_j - \left(\mathbf{R}k_j + \mathbf{T}\right)\right\|^2 . \tag{15.1}$$

A unique solution to (15.1) exists if and only if the sets of points, K and L, contain at least four noncoplanar points [Arun et al. 1987].

As shown in Fig. 15.3, the phantom used for the calibration of the image is comprised of seven 1 mm diameter nylon strings positioned in a $14 \times 14 \times 14$ cm^3 Plexiglas box.

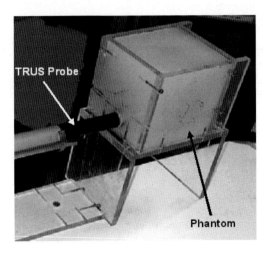

Fig. 15.3. Photograph of the image calibration phantom with the transducer inserted into the simulated rectum

The side of the Plexiglas box has a hole to simulate the rectum and to accommodate the TRUS transducer. The nylon strings are immersed in agar and placed in three layers 1 cm apart. The strings are arranged with known separations, forming noncoplanar intersections. In the coordinate system of the transducer, the coordinates of these intersections are known from the phantom design; in the 3D TRUS coordinate system, the coordinates of the intersections were determined by scanning the intersections. Using the coordinates of the string intersections in both coordinate systems, we solved (15.1) to determine the transformation linking the two coordinate systems.

For the calibration of the robot, two orthogonal plates mounted on the transducer holder were used and drilled with 10 hemispherical divots. Figure 15.4 shows these calibration plates along with the divots on each of the plates. Homologous points in the coordinate systems of the transducer and the robot are provided by the centers of the hemispherical divots on the two plates. The coordinates of these divot centers in the robot coordinate system were determined by moving the robot, sequentially touching the divots with a stylus tip attached to the arm of the robot. Using the co-ordinates of the divots in the two coordinate systems, we solved (15.1) to determine the transformation linking the two coordinate systems.

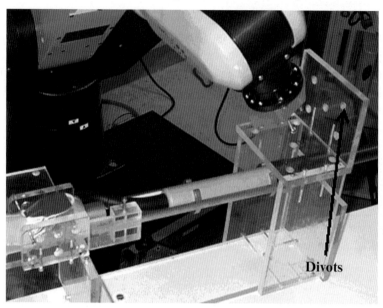

Fig. 15.4. The plates for robot calibration. The positions of the divots in the transducer coordinate system are all known through the phantom design. The positions of the divots in the robot coordinate system are determined by moving the robot to touch these divots as shown in this figure

15.2.3   Software Tools

Software tools are indispensable components in a 3D TRUS-guided, robot-assisted system for prostate brachytherapy, and should include the following items: prostate segmentation, needle segmentation, seed segmentation, and dosimetry.

15.2.3.1 Prostate Segmentation

Outlining the margins of the prostate manually is time consuming and te-dious, so an accurate, reproducible, and fast semi- or fully-automated prostate segmentation technique would greatly improve the process. Because 3D US images suffer from shadowing, speckle, and poor contrast, fully auto-mated segmentation procedures sometimes result in unacceptable errors. Our approach has been to develop a semi-automated prostate segmentation technique that allows the user to correct errors [Hu et al. 2003].

The prostate is segmented as a series of cross-sectional 2D images obtained from the 3D TRUS image. The resulting set of boundaries is assembled into a single 3D prostate boundary. This segmentation algorithm has been described in detail in previous publications [Hu et al. 2003].

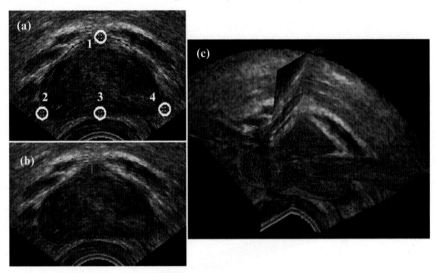

Fig. 15.5. Images showing the steps of the 3D prostate segmentation algorithm; (**a**) the 3D TRUS image is first resliced into 2D slices; (**b**) the user initializes the algorithm by placing four or more points on the boundary as shown. A model-based interpolation approach is used to generate an initial contour; (**c**) A deformable dynamic contour (DDC) approach is used to refine the initial contour until it matches the prostate boundary. The contour is propagated to adjacent 2D slices of the 3D TRUS image and refined using the DDC. The process is repeated until the complete prostate is segmented as shown

As shown in Fig. 15.5, this algorithm consists of the following three steps:

1. The operator manually initializes the algorithm by selecting four or more points on the prostate boundary (in one central prostate 2D slice). A curve passing through these points is then calculated and is used as the initial estimate of the prostate boundary (Fig. 15.5a).
2. The curve is converted to a polygon with equally spaced points, which are then deformed using a Discrete Dynamic Contour algorithm until reaching equilibrium (Fig. 15.5b). If required, the polygon can be edited by manually repositioning selected vertices.
3. The boundary of the 2D segmented prostate in one slice is extended to 3D by propagating the contour to an adjacent slice and repeating the

deformation process (Fig. 15.5c). This process is accomplished by slicing the prostate in radial slices separated by a constant angle (e.g., 3°) intersecting along an axis approximately in the center of the prostate.

15.2.3.2 Needle Segmentation

As described in Sect. 15.2.1 and 15.2.2, 3D TRUS-guided, robot-assisted prostate brachytherapy allows oblique needle insertion during seed implant-ation. So the needle may be inserted in an oblique trajectory, which results in the image of the needle passing out of the real-time 2D US image (Fig. 15.6).

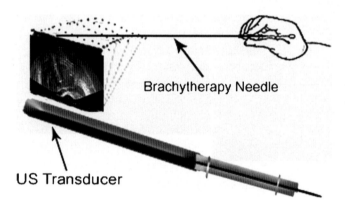

Fig. 15.6. The brachytherapy needle leaves the real-time 2D TRUS image for an oblique insertion, and the needle will only appear as a dot in the 2D US image, leading to sub-optimal guidance

Although the robot possesses high positioning and angulation accuracies and the robot and 3D US systems can be accurately related to each other through a careful calibration, due to needle deflection, the needle co-ordinates reported by the robot do not describe the actual needle trajectories [Wan et al. 2005]. While the needle is inserted into the prostate, visual tracking of the needle tip in an US image is necessary to ensure proper placement, and to avoid implanting seeds outside the prostate. Automated segmentation of the needle during an oblique (as well as parallel) needle insertion would allow the position and orientation of the needle to be determined. As a result, rapid dynamic replanning could be performed based on the actual needle trajectory and seed locations to obtain an optimum 3D dose distribution within a prostate. Thus, we developed a technique to track the needle as it is being inserted obliquely [Wei et al. 2005].

A grey-level change detection technique is used (i.e., values derived by comparing the grey-level values of the images before and after the needle has been inserted and processed). As the needle may be angled maximally 20° from the orientation of the 2D US plane, and 2D images may be acquired at 30 images per second, a new 3D image can be formed in less than 1 s. From these 3D images, the needle may be segmented automatically, and the three planes needed to visualize the needle insertion displayed. The needle segmentation algorithm is composed of the following five steps:

1. A 3D difference image of the grey-level change between the prescan and the live-scan is generated. The needle contrast in the difference image can be enhanced by suppressing the background noise caused by the implanted seeds and needle tracks.
2. The needle candidate voxels from the background are segmented through a thresholding operation.
3. Spurious needle candidate voxels are removed.
4. Linear regression of the needle candidate voxels is performed to determine the orientation of the needle in 3D space.
5. The position of the needle top in 3D space is determined.

Figure 15.7 shows the result of the needle segmentation algorithm using a chicken phantom, which simulates the clinical environment. Figure 15.7a,b displays the needle in the reconstructed oblique sagittal and coronal planes.

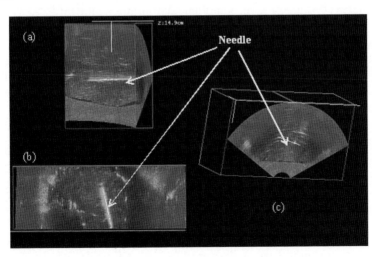

Fig. 15.7. A result of needle segmentation during insertion of a needle into a chicken phantom simulating clinical environment. (**a**) Oblique sagittal view; (**b**) oblique coronal plane; (**c**) transverse view with needle projected

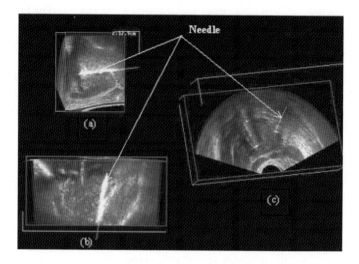

Fig. 15.8. A result of oblique needle segmentation during insertion of a needle into a patient's prostate. (**a**) Oblique sagittal view; (**b**) oblique coronal plane; (**c**) transverse view with needle projected

Figure 15.8 shows the result of the needle segmentation algorithm in a patient image that was obtained during a prostate cryotherapy procedure.

15.2.3.3 Seed Segmentation

Post-implant dosimetry is an important step in the treatment process. Thus, the American Brachytherapy Society (ABS) has recommended that post-implant dosimetry should be performed on all patients undergoing permanent prostate brachytherapy [Nag et al. 2000]. However, segmentation of the implanted radioactive seeds in US images of the prostate is made difficult by image speckle, low contrast, signal loss due to shadowing, and refraction and reverberation artifacts. To solve these problems, we proposed an algorithm [Wei et al. 2006] that uses 3D TRUS imaging and *prior* knowledge of the needle position described in Sect. 15.2.3.2. The following six steps describe the algorithm:

1. A 3D difference image of the grey-level change is generated by subtracting the image before the needle has been inserted, from the image after the seeds have been implanted and the needle has been withdrawn from the prostate.
2. The algorithm narrows the searching space from the whole 3D TRUS image to contain a smaller cylinder around the needle.
3. The seed candidate voxels are segmented from the background in the search cylinder using a thresholding operation.
4. The seed candidate voxels are grouped to find the candidate seeds.

5. The center location, orientation, and size of a seed are determined using 3D principal component analysis (PCA).
6. Spurious seeds are removed from the candidate seeds.

Steps 1–6 are repeated until all the seeds have been implanted and localized. Figure 15.9 shows the flowchart of the seed segmentation algorithm. Figure 15.10 shows an image of the segmented seeds in 3D TRUS images of chicken phantoms using the seed segmentation algorithm.

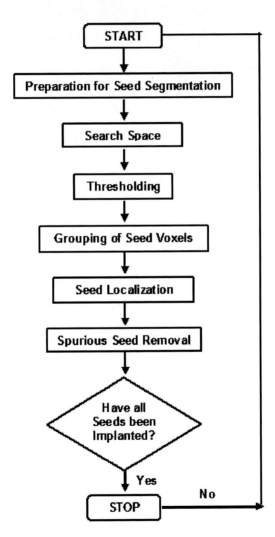

Fig. 15.9. Flowchart of the intraoperative seed segmentation algorithm

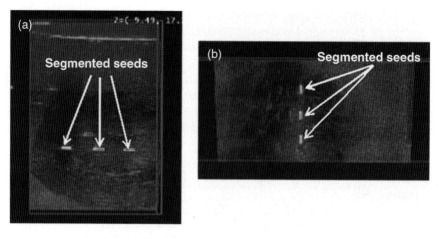

Fig. 15.10. An example image of the segmented seeds in a 3D TRUS image of the chicken phantom. (**a**) Sagittal view; (**b**) coronal view

15.2.3.4 Dosimetry

We use the AAPM TG-43 formalism, which uses predetermined dosimetry data from dose rate evaluation [Nath et al. 1995]. The dose can be calculated either by considering the sources oriented in a line in any trajectory or as point sources where source orientation is ignored. After delineating the organs, the user selects the type of source to be used and enters its calibration data. Considering the effects of pubic arch interference, the area of possible needle insertions is outlined and the preplan is produced. The preplan uses about 20 needles, which can be oriented in oblique trajectories to avoid pubic arch interference. The isodose curves are displayed on the 3D TRUS image in real-time, as well as on a surface-rendered view with the needles and the seeds. Each needle can also be activated and deactivated individually and the modified isodose curves can be observed instantly. The user can evaluate the plan using dose volume histograms for each organ and make necessary modifications. Figure 15.11 shows an example of the use of the preplan software for oblique trajectory needle planning.

During a live planning procedure in the operating room (OR), after each needle is inserted, its location is determined and the isodose curves are modified and displayed in real-time. This procedure helps the user to decide whether the needle position is satisfactory. After retracting the needle, the actual seed locations are determined (currently we use assumed positions) and the new isodose curves are displayed. At this time, the user has the option of modifying the rest of the plan according to the "real" seed locations after the needle retraction.

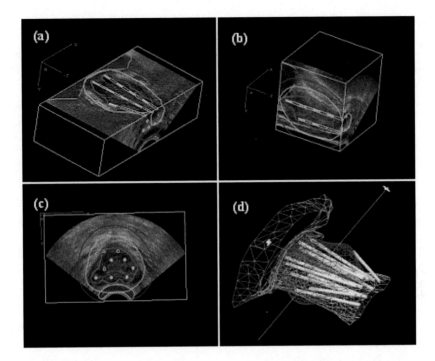

Fig. 15.11. Display of a typical dose plan with oblique needle trajectories for use with 3D TRUS guidance and robotic aids. Our 3D visualization approach allows display of a texture-mapped 3D view of the prostate, extracted planes, and graphical overlays of surfaces and contours. (**a**) Coronal view with delineated organs, needles, seeds, and isodose curves; (**b**) sagittal view; (**c**) transverse view; (**d**) surface rendered view showing the organs and needles with seeds

15.3   System Evaluation

The following experiments were performed to evaluate our 3D TRUS-guided, robot-assisted prostate brachytherapy system, as described in Sect. 15.2.

15.3.1 Evaluation of Calibration

15.3.1.1 Method

Accuracy analysis of the image and robot calibrations was performed using the method for analyzing accuracy of point-based, rigid-body registration [Maurer et al. 1998]. This method involves the analysis of three errors: fiducial localization error (FLE), fiducial registration error (FRE), and target registration error (TRE). These error parameters are discussed in detail in Chap. 6, Sect. 6.4. The following discussion illustrates their relevance to the assessment of a clinical system.

FLE: The FLE is defined as the error in locating fiducial points used in the registration procedure [Fitzpatrick et al. 1998]. We assumed that the mean value of the error in locating the fiducial points is zero, and we calculated the root-mean-square (rms) distance between the exact and calculated fiducial positions [Maurer et al. 1993]:

$$\begin{cases} \text{FLE}_i^2 = \sigma_{ix}^2 + \sigma_{iy}^2 + \sigma_{iz}^2, \\ \text{FLE}^2 = \dfrac{1}{N} \sum_{i=1}^{N} \text{FLE}_i^2. \end{cases} \tag{15.2}$$

The variances of the error in locating the fiducials points along the three orthogonal axes are σ_x^2, σ_y^2, and σ_z^2. Each of the terms in (15.2) is calculated as follows:

$$\sigma_{ij}^2 = \frac{1}{n-1} \sum_{k=1}^{n} \left(x_{ijk} - \overline{x}_{ijk} \right)^2. \tag{15.3}$$

The components (i.e., x, y, or z) are represented by $j = 1, 2, 3$; x_{ijk} is the kth measurement for ith fiducial point (for image calibration, $i = 1, 2, 3, 4$, and for robot calibration, $i = 1, 2, \ldots, 6$); and k is the number of measurements for each fiducial point. For both calibrations of image and robot, $n = 10$, and, $\overline{x}_{ij} = \dfrac{1}{10} \sum_{k=1}^{10} x_{ijk}$ is the mean measurement for the jth component of the ith fiducial point.

FRE: The exact positions of N fiducials in the transducer coordinate system, $P = \{\mathbf{p}_j; j = 1, \ldots, N\}$, are known for either the image calibration phantom (Fig. 15.3) or the robot calibration plates (Fig. 15.4). For image calibration, we measured the positions of N fiducials (from the intersection of the nylon strings) in 3D TRUS image coordinate systems, $Q = \{\mathbf{q}_j; j = 1, \ldots, N\}$. For robot calibration, we measured the positions of N fiducials (small divots), $Q = \{\mathbf{q}_j; j = 1, \ldots, N\}$, in robot coordinate system by moving the robot to touch the small divots. The FRE is calculated as the rms distance between the corresponding fiducial positions, before and after registration:

$$\text{FRE} = \sqrt{\frac{\sum_{j=1}^{N} \left\| q_j - F\left(p_j \right) \right\|^2}{N}}. \tag{15.4}$$

The rigid body transformation, F, registers the exact fiducial positions, P, with the measured fiducial positions, Q.

TRE: TRE is defined as the distance between the corresponding points (other than the fiducial points) before and after registration. The TRE is calculated by (15.4). We used four targets in the image calibration phantom to determine the TRE for image calibration; four other markers on the plates were used to determine the TRE for robot calibration [Wei et al. 2004].

15.3.1.2 Results

Our ability to localize the intersections of the nylon strings in the 3D TRUS image for the calibration of the image was analyzed along the *X*-, *Y*-, and *Z*-directions; Table 15.1 shows the average fiducial localization error (FLE). From Table 15.1, it can be seen that the FLE for localizing the intersection of the strings is similar in the *X*- or *Y*-directions and larger in the *Z*-direction. This is attributed to the fact that the resolution in the *X*- and *Y*-directions (i.e., lateral and axial direction in the original acquired images) is best. The larger FLE in the *Z*-direction, which corresponded to the elevation (i.e., out-of-plane) direction of the acquired 2D images, is due to the poorer out-of-plane resolution in the 3D TRUS image [Fenster et al. 2001].

Table 15.1. The standard deviation (SD) used to describe the FLE (in mm) for the localization of the nylon intersections (fiducial points) for image calibration

Intersection No. (i)	σ_{ij} (mm)			FLE_i
	σ_{ix}	σ_{iy}	σ_{iz}	
1	0.04	0.05	0.12	0.12
2	0.06	0.05	0.10	0.13
3	0.05	0.08	0.12	0.15
4	0.06	0.06	0.10	0.13
Total				*0.13*

Each σ_{ij}, determined by (15.3), describes the FLE of one nylon intersection in one direction. The total FLE in this table, i.e., FLE as described in (15.2), is the vector composition of SD components in various directions

Table 15.2 shows the FLE for localizing the divots on the two orthogonal plates used for robot calibration. From Table 15.2, it can be seen that the FLE for the divot localization was approximately the same in the three directions. The measured error of the divots in the robot coordinate system is caused by such factors as the flexibility of the robot arm and the calibration plates, and the backlash in the robot arm joint. Comparing Table 15.2 with Table 15.1, it can be seen that the FLE for the divot localization (i.e., robot calibration) is greater than that for the string intersection localization (i.e., image calibration). Therefore, the FLE for robot calibration will dominate the overall calibration errors affecting the accuracy of the whole system.

Table 15.2. The SD used to describe the FLE (in mm) for the localization of divots (fiducial points) in the phantom used for robot calibration

Divot No. (i)	σ_{ix}	σ_{ij} σ_{iy}	σ_{iz}	FLE$_i$
1	0.17	0.10	0.26	0.33
2	0.11	0.13	0.30	0.35
3	0.12	0.28	0.10	0.32
4	0.21	0.31	0.14	0.40
5	0.29	0.09	0.33	0.45
6	0.10	0.32	0.11	0.35
Total				*0.37*

The meanings of σ_{ij} and total FLE are the same as those used in Table 1

The FRE and TRE values for robot calibration are shown in Table 15.3. The mean FRE for the calibration of the robot was 0.52 ± 0.18 mm, and the mean TRE was 0.68 ± 0.29 mm; these means being greater than those for image calibration. As discussed above, this results from the greater FLE for robot calibration. Because system errors will result from both the image and robot calibrations, the errors in robot calibration dominate the accuracy of integration of the two coordinate systems.

Table 15.3. FRE and TRE (in mm) for image and robot calibrations

	Image Calibration		Robot Calibration	
	FRE	TRE	FRE	TRE
Mean	0.12	0.23	0.52	0.68
SD	0.07	0.11	0.18	0.29
Max	0.25	0.39	0.78	1.02
Min	0.03	0.08	0.3	0.33

The FRE and TRE for each point in either image calibration or robot calibration are described by (15.5)

15.3.2 Needle Positioning and Orientation Accuracy by Robot

The accuracies of the needle position and orientation by the robot on the skin of the "patient" (i.e., before the needle has been inserted into the prostate) are described by the accuracy of the needle placement and the accuracy of the needle angulation.

15.3.2.1 Needle Placement Accuracy

We determined the needle placement accuracy by using the robot to move the needle tip to nine locations on a 5×5 cm^2 grid that represented the skin of the patient (i.e., 3×3 grid of targeting points) [Wei et al. 2004]. A three-axis stage (Parker Hannifin Co., Irwin, PA) with a measuring accuracy of 2 µm was then used to locate the tip of the needle. The displacement, ε_d, between the measured and targeted positions of the needle tip was found as follows:

$$\varepsilon_d = \sqrt{\left(x - x_i\right)^2 + \left(y - y_i\right)^2 + \left(z - z_i\right)^2} \qquad (15.5)$$

The coordinates for the targeted point are (x, y, z), where (x_i, y_i, z_i) are the coordinates for the ith measured point. The mean needle placement error, $\overline{\varepsilon}_d$, and the standard deviation (STD) from 10 measurements at each position were found to be 0.15 ± 0.06 mm.

15.3.2.2 Needle Angulation Accuracy

To measure the accuracy of needle angulation using the robot, we attached a small plate to the needle holder and used the robot to tilt the plate in four angles vertically and laterally ($0°$, $5°$, $10°$, $15°$). After each tilt, we measured the orientation of the plate using the three-axis stage and determined the angulation error by comparing the measured and planned plate angle.

Table 15.4 shows the mean angle differences between the measured and planned angulation by the robot and its STDs.

As seen in Table 15.4, all mean angle differences were less than $0.12°$ with a mean of $0.07°$. Because the angulation error will cause an increasing displacement error with increasing needle insertion distances, we estimated the displacement error after an insertion of 10 cm from the needle guide. Using the mean and maximum angulation errors, we determined the mean and maximum displacement errors for a 10 cm insertion to be ±0.13 and ±0.50 mm, respectively [Wei et al. 2004].

Table 15.4. Accuracy analysis of the needle angulation by the robot for vertical and lateral tilts

	Vertical angulation			Lateral angulation		
Targeted angles (i)	1(5°)	2(10°)	3(15°)	1(5°)	2(10°)	3(15°)
Mean angle difference $(\bar{\varepsilon}_a)_i$	0.02°	0.04°	0.06°	0.07°	0.10°	0.12°
Standard deviation (SD_{ai})	0.02°	0.06°	0.05°	0.05°	0.03°	0.08°
Max($\Delta\theta_{ik}$)	0.08°	0.22°	0.18°	0.15°	0.15°	0.28°

15.3.3 Needle Targeting Accuracy

The accuracy of the needle targeting reflects the accuracy of the needle tip after the needle has been inserted into the prostate under the guidance of 3D TRUS image with robotic assistance, as described in Sect. 15.2.

15.3.3.1 Method

We used tissue-mimicking phantoms made from agar [Rickey et al. 1995], which were contained in a Plexiglas box, to determine the accuracy of needle insertion [Wei et al. 2004]. One side of the box was removable, allowing the insertion of the needle. As shown in Fig. 15.12, each of two phantoms contained two rows of 0.8 mm diameter stainless beads [Smith et al. 2001]. This approach provided four different bead-targeting configurations: two different needle insertion depths and two different distances from the ultrasound transducer. These bead configurations formed a $4 \times 4 \times 4 \text{ cm}^3$ cube to simulate the approximate size of a prostate.

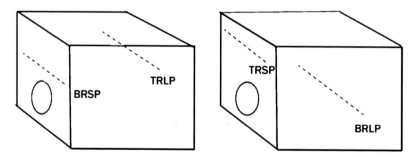

Fig. 15.12. Diagram of the prostate phantom used for evaluation of needle targeting accuracy. The four rows of circles represent the four different bead configurations. The needle entered the phantom from the front, parallel to the *x*-axis. *TRLP* top row, long penetration, *TRSP* top row, short penetration, *BRLP* bottom row, long penetration, *BRSP* bottom row, short penetration

15.3.3.2 Results

Figure 15.13 shows a 3D ellipsoid representing the 95% confidence intervals for displacement errors of the needle insertion at one of the four targeting configurations, each of which is shown in Fig. 15.12. We plotted these ellipsoids using the axis that accounted for the least variation in needle targeting. Projections through the needle positions and 95% confidence intervals on the X-Y, X-Z, and Y-Z planes are also shown.

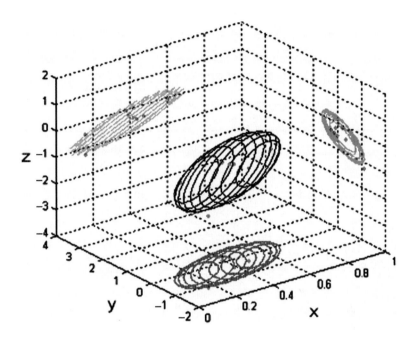

Fig. 15.13. Needle targeting accuracy is displayed as a 95% confidence intervals ellipsoid. The origin of the coordinate system represents the target, and the needle tip positions after insertion (relative to the targets) are represented by the squares. The projections of the needle tip positions and the ellipsoid (on the three orthogonal planes) are also shown. These results are for the targets near the transducer and for a short penetration as shown in Fig. 15.12

Table 15.5 lists the widths of the 95% confidence intervals along the primary, secondary, and tertiary axes plotted in Fig. 15.13. The 95% confidence interval is widest (i.e., the primary axis is greatest) for the predefined points on the top row, i.e., long penetration, and smallest for the bottom row, i.e., short penetration. The ellipsoid volumes (i.e., the volume encompassed by the 95% confidence intervals) were greater for the points further from the ultrasound transducer than for those closer to the ultrasound transducer. As shown in Table 15.4 (and Fig. 15.13), the confidence widths were not centered at the origin of the coordinate system, (i.e., the positions of the predefined points), but, rather, at the average needle targeting position for each of the four targeting configurations as shown in Fig. 15.12. The error of the needle targeting, obtained by averaging all 32 needle targeting errors, was 0.79 ± 0.32 mm. The greatest targeting error was found to be in Z-direction of the TRLP, and the smallest targeting error was found to be in the X-direction of the TRSP [Wei et al. 2004].

Table 15.5. A description of the 95% uncertainty intervals for brachytherapy needle insertion

Targeting configuration	Width of the 95% uncertainty interval (mm)			Center of confidence interval (mm)	Ellipsoid volume (mm³)
	Primary axis	Secondary axis	Tertiary axis		
Top row, long penetration (TRLP)	1.95	1.02	0.23	(−0.46, 0.57, −0.98)	1.92
Bottom row, short penetration (BRSP)	1.06	0.55	0.22	(0.38, −0.22, −0.44)	0.54
Top row, short penetration (TRSP)	1.77	0.94	0.24	(0.03, 0.49, −0.04)	1.68
Bottom row, long penetration (BRLP)	1.38	0.60	0.19	(0.17, 0.39, 0.68)	0.66

15.3.4 Evaluation of the Prostate Segmentation Algorithm

15.3.4.1 Method

To evaluate the performance of the prostate segmentation algorithm, the surfaces segmented using the algorithm were compared with the surfaces manually outlined by a trained technician. The technician was representative of users working in a radiological oncology department. Manual segmentation was performed using a multiplane reformatting image display tool

[Fenster and Downey 1996]. The 3D prostate images were resliced into sets of transverse parallel 2D slices along the length of the prostate. Intervals of 2 mm were used at mid-gland, and at 1 mm near the ends of the prostate where the prostate shape changes more rapidly from one slice to the next. The prostate boundary was outlined in each slice, resulting in a stack of 2D contours. The contours were then tessellated into a 3D meshed surface. Manual outlining of each prostate from the 2D slices required approximately 30 min.

15.3.4.2 Results

Figure 15.14 shows not only the quality of the fit of the algorithm, but also the manually segmented meshes to the actual boundary of the prostate.

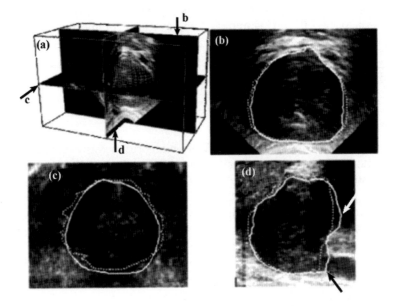

Fig. 15.14. Cross sections of a prostate showing the algorithm segmentation (*solid line*) and manual segmentation (*dotted line*). (**a**) 3D ultrasound image of the prostate with transverse, coronal, and sagittal cutting planes indicated by b, c, and d, respectively, to show 2D cross-sectional images. (**b**) Transverse cross section of the image and the boundaries corresponding to the plane shown in (**a**). (**c**) Coronal cross section of the image and the boundaries. (**d**) Sagittal cross section of the image and the boundaries

Figure 15.14a shows the algorithm mesh in the 3D ultrasound image with (b) transverse, (c) coronal, and (d) sagittal cutting planes of the 2D cross-sectional images. Figure 15.14b shows a 2D transverse mid-gland slice of the 3D image with corresponding cross sections through the algorithm and manually segmented meshes superimposed. Figure 15.14c shows a coronal section with the corresponding cross section of the meshes, and Fig. 15.14d shows a sagittal section with the corresponding cross section of the meshes. The manual and algorithm contours in Fig. 15.14 are similar to each other. Each of the contours follows the prostate boundary well in regions where the contrast is high and the prostate is clearly separated from other tissues. In regions where the signal is low, the actual boundary is difficult to discern: the outlines generated by a manual segmentation differ from the outlines generated by the algorithm. As shown in Fig. 15.14d, these regions include images near the bladder (indicated by the white arrow) and the seminal vesicle (indicated by the black arrow).

Error analysis showed that the average difference between the boundaries generated by a manual segmentation compared to boundaries generated by the algorithm boundaries was 0.20 ± 0.28 mm; the average absolute difference was shown to be 1.19 ± 0.14 mm, the average maximum difference was shown to be 7.01 ± 1.04 mm, and the average volume difference was shown to be $7.16\% \pm 3.45\%$ [Hu et al. 2003].

15.3.5 Evaluation of the Needle Segmentation Algorithm

15.3.5.1 Method

The performance of the needle segmentation algorithm was evaluated using agar phantoms. To test the accuracy of the needle segmentation algorithm, a rigid rod with a 1.2 mm diameter was used, which is the same size as a typical 18-gauge prostate brachytherapy needle. The rigid rod was used to avoid the effect of needle deflection, allowing us to test the accuracy of the algorithm under ideal conditions. The position of the needle tip and the orientation of the needle were determined by the needle segmentation algorithm. Because the robot possesses high angulation accuracy, the position of the needle tip and the orientation of the needle were compared with the measurements of the robot (see Sect. 15.3.2).

15.3.5.2 Results

The accuracy of the needle segmentation algorithm depends on the distance of needle insertion into the 3D TRUS images, angulations of the needle with respect to the TRUS transducer, and the distance of the needle from the TRUS transducer. Generally, the segmentation error and its standard deviation are larger at smaller insertion distances. Because more information about the needle can be obtained for segmentation (as the needle is inserted deeper into an image, resulting in a more accurate determination of the needle trajectory), the segmentation error and its standard deviation tend to decrease with increasing insertion distances. In addition, the errors appear to be larger at larger insertion angulations when the needle is angulated in both the horizontal and the vertical planes. In general, the segmentation error and its standard deviation tend to decrease with decreasing insertion angulations. The mean errors (and their corresponding standard deviations) also increase slightly with the increase in the distance of the needle from the transducer. This increase is due to the lower image resolution at larger distances away from the TRUS transducer [Wei et al. 2005]. Figure 15.15 shows the needle segmentation errors in respect to the different needle angulations.

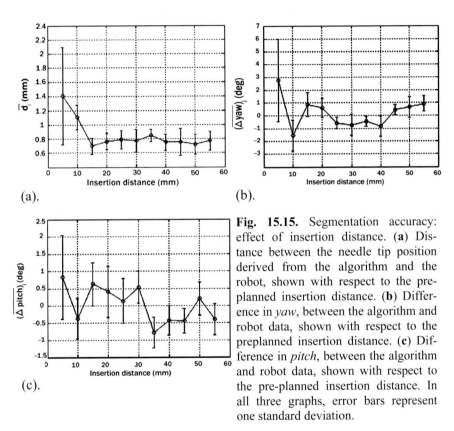

(a).

(b).

(c).

Fig. 15.15. Segmentation accuracy: effect of insertion distance. (**a**) Distance between the needle tip position derived from the algorithm and the robot, shown with respect to the pre-planned insertion distance. (**b**) Difference in *yaw*, between the algorithm and robot data, shown with respect to the preplanned insertion distance. (**c**) Difference in *pitch*, between the algorithm and robot data, shown with respect to the pre-planned insertion distance. In all three graphs, error bars represent one standard deviation.

15.3.6 Evaluation of the Seed Segmentation Algorithm

15.3.6.1 Method

The seed segmentation algorithm was evaluated by implanting 22 dummy iodine-125 seeds into a chicken phantom in three layers. The locations of those seeds were determined by the seed segmentation algorithm in the 3D TRUS image first. This phantom was scanned using the eXplore Locus Ultra Pre-clinical cone-beam CT scanner (GE Healthcare Canada, London, Ontario, Canada), which possesses an isotropic voxel size of 154 μm. The seed positions were determined manually in the CT image. These seed positions were registered to the 3D TRUS image and compared with the algorithm-determined seed positions [Wei et al. 2006].

15.3.6.2 Results

We evaluated the accuracy of registration by using the fiducial localization error (FLE), fiducial registration error (FRE), and target registration error (TRE). The FLE in the 3D TRUS image was 0.22 mm, and in the CT image, the FLE was 0.15 mm. The FRE was 0.21 mm and the TRE was 0.35 mm. In our test, all 22 seeds were successfully segmented [Wei et al. 2006].

Table 15.6 lists the widths of the 95% confidence intervals along the primary, secondary, and tertiary axes. The 95% confidence interval is widest (i.e., the primary axis is greatest for the seeds on the top layer and smallest for the seeds on the bottom layer). The ellipsoid volume for the seeds in the bottom layer was determined to be the smallest (0.68 mm^3), followed by the ellipsoid volume for the seeds in the middle layer (0.92 mm^3). The ellipsoid volume for the seeds in the top layer was the largest at 1.15 mm^3. The ellipsoid volume for the seeds in the bottom layer was the smallest (1.07 mm^3), followed by the ellipsoid volume for the seeds in the middle layer (1.30 mm^3.). The ellipsoid volume for the seeds in the top layer was the largest (1.40 mm^3). The ellipsoid volume for all of the seeds was 2.07 mm^3. The confidence widths also were not centered at the origin of the 3D TRUS coordinate system. A mean distance of 0.30 mm was determined [Wei et al. 2006].

Table 15.6. A description of the 95% uncertainty intervals for seed segmentation in an agar phantom

	Width of the 95% uncertainty interval (mm)			Center of confidence interval (mm)	Ellipsoid volume (mm^3)	Rms Distance (mm)
	Primary axis	Secondary axis	Tertiary axis			
Top layer	1.92	0.42	0.34	(0.07, −0.01, −0.07)	1.15	1.02
Middle layer	1.36	0.49	0.33	(−0.05, −0.02, −0.65)	0.92	0.95
Bottom layer	1.68	0.42	0.23	(0.18, 0.06, −0.40)	0.68	0.95
Overall	1.60	0.64	0.31	(0.07, 0.01, −0.37)	1.33	0.98

15.4 Discussion

Our prototype 3D TRUS-guided system with robotic assistance was developed for prostate brachytherapy. The fundamental motivation to apply robotic assistance in prostate brachytherapy originated from the motion features of a robot system. The motion features of a robot system include accuracy, consistency, and flexibility, i.e., the robot system can be controlled to move to any position in any orientation along any trajectory at sufficiently high accuracies and consistencies within its 3D workspace. In addition, the 3D US image can provide a direct delineation of the volume of interest, providing radiologists a direct impression of the 3D anatomy and pathology of the prostate.

It also has been reported that measurements of prostate volume in 3D are more accurate than those in 2D US images [Tong et al. 1998]. Therefore, by including 3D TRUS guidance and robotic assistance into the prostate brachytherapy system, we can remove the parallel trajectory constraints. As a result, needles can be guided to target a point identified in 3D US images along any trajectory (including oblique trajectories) to avoid pubic arch interference.

The procedures detailed in this chapter form a valuable precursor to the development of an intraoperative prostate brachytherapy system. The test results are promising, giving clinically relevant results in needle targeting accuracy. The prototype 3D TRUS-guided and robotic-assisted prostate brachytherapy system has the ability to target a location accurately and consistently. We believe that these results imply that the 3D TRUS-guided and robotic-assisted transperineal prostate brachytherapy, together with the progress in developing special software tools for prostate segmentation, dynamic replanning, needle, and seed segmentation, will soon provide a suitable intraoperative alternative, in which all the steps of a prostate brachytherapy procedure may be carried out in a single session.

Acknowledgments

The authors gratefully acknowledge the financial support provided by the Canadian Institute of Health Research and the Ontario R & D Challenge Fund. Dr. Fenster holds a Canada Research Chair in Biomedical Engineering, and acknowledges the support of the Canada Research Chair Program. The authors also thank Kerry Knight for editing the manuscript.

References

Arun KS, Huang TS, Blostein SD. (1987). Least-square fitting of two 3D point sets. *IEEE Trans Pattern Anal Mach Intell*, 9, 698–799

Ash D, Bottomley DM, Carey BM. (1998). Prostate brachytherapy. *Prostate Cancer Prostatic Dis*, 1(4), 185–188

Badiozamani KR, Wallner K, Sutlief S, Ellis W, Blasko J, Russell K. (1999). Anticipating prostatic volume changes due to prostate brachytherapy. *Radiat Oncol Investig*, 7(6), 360–364

Bangma CH, Hengeveld EJ, Niemer AQ, Schroder FH. (1995). Errors in transrectal ultrasonic planimetry of the prostate: Computer simulation of volumetric errors applied to a screening population. *Ultrasound Med Biol*, 21(1), 11–16

Bangma CH, Huland H, Schroder FH, van Cangh PJ. (2001). Early diagnosis and treatment of localized prostate cancer. *Eur Urol*, 40(3), 361–370

Blasko JC, Mate T, Sylvester JE, Grimm PD, Cavanagh W. (2002). Brachytherapy for carcinoma of the prostate: Techniques, patient selection, and clinical outcomes. *Semin Radiat Oncol*, 12(1), 81–94

Butler EB, Scardino PT, Teh BS, Uhl BM, Guerriero WG, Carlton CE, Berner BM, Dennis WS, Carpenter LS, Lu HH, Chiu JK, Kent TS, Woo SY. (1997). The Baylor College of Medicine experience with gold seed implantation. *Semin Surg Oncol*, 13(6), 406–418

Cheng G, Liu H, Liao L, Yu Y. (2001). Dynamic brachytherapy of the prostate under active image guidance. *Proc MICCAI 2001*, 2208 (LNCS), 351–359

Ding M, Cardinal HN, Fenster A. (2003a). Automatic needle segmentation in three-dimensional ultrasound images using two orthogonal two-dimensional image projections. *Med Phys*, 30(2), 222–234

Ding M, Chen C, Wang Y, Gyacskov I, Fenster A. (2003b). Prostate segmentation in 3D US images using the cardinal-spline-based discrete dynamic contour. *Proc SPIE*, 5029, 69–76

Ding M, Fenster A. (2003). A real-time biopsy needle segmentation technique using Hough transform. *Med Phys*, 30(8), 2222–2233

Fenster A, Downey D. (1996). Three-dimensional ultrasound imaging: A review. *IEEE Eng Med Biol*, 15, 41–51

Fenster A, Downey DB, Cardinal HN. (2001). Three-dimensional ultrasound imaging. *Phys Med Biol*, 46(5), R67–99

Fichtinger G, Burdette EC, Tanacs A, Patriciu A, Mazilu D, Whitcomb LL, Stoianovici D. (2006). Robotically assisted prostate brachytherapy with transrectal ultrasound guidance-Phantom experiments. *Brachytherapy*, 5(1), 14–26

Fitzpatrick JM, West JB, Maurer CR, Jr. (1998). Predicting error in rigid-body point-based registration. *IEEE Trans Med Imaging*, 17(5), 694–702

Gower JC, Dijksterhuis GB. (2004). *Procrustes Problems*, Oxford University Press, New York

Holm HH, Juul N, Pedersen JF, Hansen H, Stroyer I. (1983). Transperineal 125iodine seed implantation in prostatic cancer guided by transrectal ultra-sonography. *J Urol*, 130(2), 283–286

Hu N, Downey DB, Fenster A, Ladak HM. (2003). Prostate boundary segmentation from 3D ultrasound images. *Med Phys*, 30(7), 1648–1659

Jemal A, Siegel R, Ward E, Murray T, Xu J, Smigal C, Thun MJ. (2006). Cancer statistics. *CA Cancer J Clin*, 56(2), 106–130

Ladak HM, Mao F, Wang Y, Downey DB, Steinman DA, Fenster A. (2000). Prostate boundary segmentation from 2D ultrasound images. *Med Phys*, 27(8), 1777–1788

Lattanzi J, McNeeley S, Donnelly S, Palacio E, Hanlon A, Schultheiss TE, Hanks GE. (2000). Ultrasound-based stereotactic guidance in prostate cancer – Quantification of organ motion and set-up errors in external beam radiation therapy. *Comput Aided Surg*, 5(4), 289–295

Maurer CR, Jr., Maciunas RJ, Fitzpatrick JM. (1998). Registration of head CT images to physical space using a weighted combination of points and surfaces. *IEEE Trans Med Imaging*, 17(5), 753–761

Maurer CR, Jr., McCrory JJ, Fitzpatrick JM. (1993). Estimation of accuracy in localizing externally attached markers in multimodal volume head images. *Proc SPIE*, 1898, 43–54

McLaughlin J, Dryer D, Mao Y, Marrett L, Morrison H, Schacter B, Villeneuve G. (2006). *Canadian Cancer Statistics*, National Cancer Institute of Canada, Toronto, Ontario, Canada

Messing EM, Zhang JB, Rubens DJ, Brasacchio RA, Strang JG, Soni A, Schell MC, Okunieff PG, Yu Y. (1999). Intraoperative optimized inverse planning for prostate brachytherapy: Early experience. *Int J Radiat Oncol Biol Phys*, 44(4), 801–808

Nag S, Bice W, DeWyngaert K, Prestidge B, Stock R, Yu Y. (2000). The American Brachytherapy Society recommendations for permanent prostate brachytherapy post-implant dosimetric analysis. *Int J Radiat Oncol Biol Phys*, 46(1), 221–230

Nath R, Anderson LL, Luxton G, Weaver KA, Williamson JF, Meigooni AS. (1995). Dosimetry of interstitial brachytherapy sources: Recommendations of the AAPM Radiation Therapy Committee Task Group No. 43. American Association of Physicists in Medicine. *Med Phys*, 22(2), 209–234

Norderhaug I, Dahl O, Hoisaeter PA, Heikkila R, Klepp O, Olsen DR, Kristiansen IS, Waehre H, Bjerklund Johansen TE. (2003). Brachytherapy for prostate cancer: A systematic review of clinical and cost effectiveness. *Eur Urol*, 44(1), 40–46

Pathak SD, Grimm PD, Chalana V, Kim Y. (1998). Pubic arch detection in trans-rectal ultrasound guided prostate cancer therapy. *IEEE Trans Med Imaging*, 17(5), 762–771

Prete JJ, Prestidge BR, Bice WS, Friedland JL, Stock RG, Grimm PD. (1998). A survey of physics and dosimetry practice of permanent prostate brachytherapy in the United States. *Int J Radiat Oncol Biol Phys*, 40(4), 1001–1005

Rickey DW, Picot PA, Christopher DA, Fenster A. (1995). A wall-less vessel phantom for Doppler ultrasound studies. *Ultrasound Med Biol*, 21(9), 1163–1176

Roy JN, Wallner KE, Harrington PJ, Ling CC, Anderson LL. (1993). A CT-based evaluation method for permanent implants: Application to prostate. *Int J Radiat Oncol Biol Phys*, 26(1), 163–169

Sakr WA, Grignon DJ, Crissman JD, Heilbrun LK, Cassin BJ, Pontes JJ, Haas GP. (1994). High grade prostatic intraepithelial neoplasia (HGPIN) prostatic adenocarcinoma between the ages of 20–69: An autopsy study of 249 cases. *In Vivo*, 8(3), 439–443

Shen D, Zhan Y, Davatzikos C. (2003). Segmentation of prostate boundaries from ultrasound images using statistical shape model. *IEEE Trans Med Imaging*, 22(4), 539–551

Smith WL, Surry KJ, Mills GR, Downey DB, Fenster A. (2001). Three-dimensional ultrasound-guided core needle breast biopsy. *Ultrasound Med Biol*, 27(8), 1025–1034

Strang JG, Rubens DJ, Brasacchio RA, Yu Y, Messing EM. (2001). Real-time US versus CT determination of pubic arch interference for brachytherapy. *Radiology*, 219(2), 387–393

Tong S, Cardinal HN, McLoughlin RF, Downey DB, Fenster A. (1998). Intra- and inter-observer variability and reliability of prostate volume measurement via two-dimensional and three-dimensional ultrasound imaging. *Ultrasound Med Biol*, 24(5), 673–681

Tong S, Downey DB, Cardinal HN, Fenster A. (1996). A three-dimensional ultrasound prostate imaging system. *Ultrasound Med Biol*, 22(6), 735–746

Wan G, Wei Z, Gardi L, Downey DB, Fenster A. (2005). Brachytherapy needle deflection evaluation and correction. *Med Phys*, 32(4), 902–909

Wang Y, Cardinal HN, Downey DB, Fenster A. (2003). Semiautomatic three-dimensional segmentation of the prostate using two-dimensional ultrasound images. *Med Phys*, 30(5), 887–897

Wei Z, Gardi L, Downey DB, Fenster A. (2005). Oblique needle segmentation and tracking for 3D TRUS guided prostate brachytherapy. *Med Phys*, 32(9), 2928–2941

Wei Z, Gardi L, Downey DB, Fenster A. (2006). Automated localization of implanted seeds in 3D TRUS images used for prostate brachytherapy. *Med Phys*, 33(7), 2404–2417

Wei Z, Wan G, Gardi L, Mills G, Downey D, Fenster A. (2004). Robot-assisted 3D-TRUS guided prostate brachytherapy: System integration and validation. *Med Phys*, 31(3), 539–548

Yu Y, Anderson LL, Li Z, Mellenberg DE, Nath R, Schell MC, Waterman FM, Wu A, Blasko JC. (1999). Permanent prostate seed implant brachytherapy: Report of the American Association of Physicists in Medicine Task Group No. 64. *Med Phys*, 26(10), 2054–2076

Yu Y, Podder T, Zhang YD, Ng WS, Misic V, Sherman J, Fu L, Fuller, D, Messing E, Rubens D, Strang J, Brasacchio R. (2006). Robot-assisted prostate brachytherapy. *Proc MICCAI*, 4191 (LNCS), 41–49

Chapter 16

Radiosurgery

Sonja Dieterich, James Rodgers, and Rosanna Chan

Abstract

Radiosurgery involves the use of radiation to treat tumors and is often an alternative to surgery. Many of the same advances in technology that have enabled the development of image-guided interventions have been applied in radiosurgery as well. In particular, the development of high resolution tomographic imaging for identification of the target treatment volume, as well as new methods for precisely delivering the radiation beam, have enabled more exact treatments. This chapter begins with a definition of radiosurgery and a brief historical review, followed by a description of the Gamma Knife® system for noninvasive treatment of intracranial brain disorders. The chapter describes conventional LINAC-based radiosurgery systems, and the CyberKnife® system robotic radiosurgery system, which can account for respiratory motion in the thorax and abdomen. The chapter concludes with a look at future tracking technologies.

16.1 Introduction

16.1.1 Definition of Radiosurgery

The concept of radiosurgery was developed by neurosurgeon Lars Leksell in 1951 [Leksell 1951]. Leksell translated the concept of destroying deep-seated tumors in the brain by electrocoagulation into the use of small radiation beams to achieve the same goal. The sources of these small radiation beams changed over the decades from orthovoltage X-rays (100 – 350 kVp) to higher X-ray energies delivered by proton beams, cobalt-60 sources, or high-voltage linear accelerators. One technique that tied the use of these different radiation sources together was a stereotactic localization frame to immobilize the patient. The later implementation of frameless radiosurgery systems meant that treatments could be fractionated (spread out over time), which led to a new definition of what is, or is not, included in the term stereotactic radiosurgery (SRS) [Adler et al. 2004].

T. Peters and K. Cleary (eds.), *Image-Guided Interventions.*
© Springer Science + Business Media, LLC 2008

16.1.2 Review of Body Sites Treated with Radiosurgery

The strict immobilization requirements to achieve accuracy in SRS limited its application in intracranial tumors. Depending on the shape and size of the patient's skull, lesions located in the skull base or peripherally in the brain could not be treated.

Development of body frames enabled the expansion of SRS, first to extra-cranial central nervous system (CNS) applications, and later to other body sites. For extracranial use, SRS is commonly labeled stereotactic body radiosurgery (SBRS). The spine is relatively easily immobilized and hardly moves, if at all, with respiration. When image-guided SRS techniques became available, the range of body sites was rapidly expanded to any location in the human body that was not moving with respiration.

Organs that move during respiration such as lung, liver, and pancreas were the last in which SRS techniques were applied, as immobilization proved to be the main obstacle. Early techniques, such as breath-hold and abdominal compression, were aimed at temporarily interrupting or minimizing respiration. Gating techniques still allowed for some amount of residual motion, but were much easier for patients to tolerate.

Recent research efforts have focused on developing SRS delivery technology to adapt in real-time to respiratory motion. Currently, there are four approaches:

1. Moving the patient in a chair or couch [D'Souza et al. 2005]
2. Dynamically moving multileaf collimators [Keall et al. 2006]
3. Sliding apertures [Neicu et al. 2003]
4. Dynamic robot [Adler et al. 1997; Kuo et al. 2003; Quinn 2002]

Of these technologies, only the dynamic robot has been in clinical use since receiving FDA approval in 2004.

Of the body sites now being treated using dynamic SBRS, the lung and pancreas stand out, although for very different reasons. Pancreatic cancer is relatively rare, but has a very poor prognosis and causes significant levels of abdominal pain. The pancreas is surrounded by the radiation-sensitive small bowel, and due to the structure of the organ, surgery is challenging and often limited to partial tumor resection. Dynamic SBRS can minimize the dose to the small bowel, thereby lowering the complication rates, while at the same time delivering very high doses of radiation to the pancreatic tumor.

Lung cancer is much more prevalent than pancreatic cancer, but with almost equally poor prognostics. Typical lung cancer patients who are good candidates for dynamic SBRT have either multiple comorbidities that disqualify them for surgery, or too little remaining healthy lung tissue for surgery or conventional radiation treatments. In addition, nonsmall cell lung cancers (NSCLC) are radiation resistant and do not respond well to conventional fractionation schemes.

Another category of lung cancer treated with dynamic SBRS is stage I cancers. The standard of care for those patients is still surgery (lobectomy), but with the approach of early lung cancer screening trials, a larger proportion of lung cancers are diagnosed in early stage. This means that the number of patients diagnosed with Stage I lung cancers who are not surgical candidates is increasing.

16.1.3   What is Image-Guided Radiosurgery (IGRT)?

The use of the term image guidance is, surprisingly, not very well defined in the Radiation Therapy Community. In this section, we will discuss some of the past and current usage of the term image guidance and define the context in which it is used in this chapter.

Image guidance was implemented into radiation treatments when it was realized that tattoos on the skin were not a reliable navigation device for correctly aiming at a hidden target inside the human body. As a response, the simulation process was developed, where kV X-ray films were taken of the anatomy within the treatment field. These X-ray films were then compared to MV X-ray films (port films) taken after the external landmark setup (based on the tattoos) was complete, but before the radiation treatment started. Setup errors could be corrected before starting the treatment. This early method could be considered an image-guided setup procedure for radiation treatments.

The imaging technology to guide the accuracy of setup has developed rapidly in recent years. Orthogonal kV imagers mounted in the room, rather than on the treatment machine, were developed [Willoughby et al. 2006], while some companies developed cone-beam CTs to provide volumetric imaging information [Groh et al. 2002; Jaffray et al. 2002].

There are two criteria to distinguish image-guided setup procedures from truly image-guided treatments. The first is that image guidance must be available during the treatment process without significantly interrupting the treatment. A significant interruption would be defined as an interaction that required the system to leave the treatment mode and return to setup mode, or the necessity for a therapist to enter the treatment room to adjust the patient setup. The second criterion for image-guided treatment is that the delivery system is able to act on the information provided by the image guidance, i.e., to make adjustments to the treatment based on the image guidance. Adjustments can be done either using the couch, gantry, multileaf collimator or, for the CyberKnife, a robot to change the beam position relative to the patient.

16.2   Gamma Knife®

The Gamma Knife®, manufactured by Elekta Instrument AB (Stockholm, Sweden), is a stereotactic radiosurgery unit for noninvasive treatment of intracranial brain disorders. A single fraction of high dose radiation is generated by focusing 201 cobalt-60 beams onto one fixed isocenter. Fig. 16.1 shows a schematic layout of the Leksell Gamma Knife® system. The unit consists of a hemispherical shield, a fixed primary collimator, four interchangeable helmets, and a couch with a head positioning system.

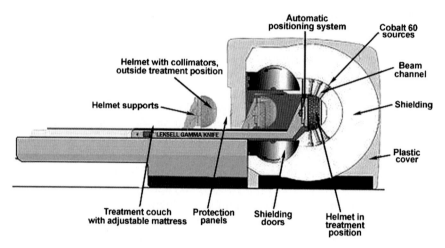

Fig. 16.1. Leksell Gamma Knife® Unit (Courtesy of Elekta Instrument Inc., Norcross, Georgia)

The shield serves as the protective housing for the 201 radioactive sources used to deliver the radiation, and a door to shield scatter radiation when not in use. Each of these sources is made up of 20 cobalt-60 pellets packed in a double encapsulated steel capsule 1 mm in diameter and 20 mm in height and loaded into a bushing assembly that locks into the shield unit (Fig. 16.2). The activity of each pellet is measured and matched with extreme care so that all sources will have a similar total activity of about 30 Ci at the time of loading. Each source assembly is labeled and loading is performed on site after the unit is installed. The primary collimator that is fixed to the shield has 201 channels, each machined to align with the sources. All channels are designed to focus each individual beam onto the center of the unit, the isocenter, which is 40 cm away (Fig. 16.3).

The four interchangeable helmets further collimate the beam to a fixed diameter of 4, 8, 14, or 18 mm at isocenter (Fig. 16.4).

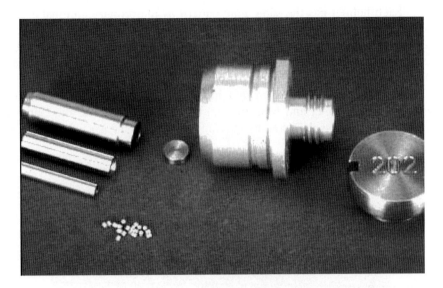

Fig. 16.2. Gamma sources – Cobalt-60 pallets, capsule, and the bushing assembly (Courtesy of Elekta Instrument, Inc., Norcross, Georgia)

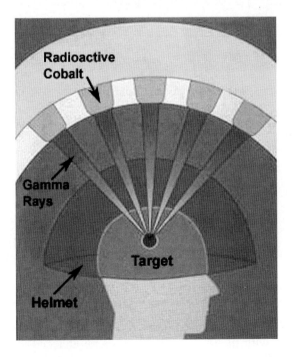

Fig. 16.3. Basic principle of the Leksell Gamma Knife® (Courtesy of Elekta Instrument Inc., Norcross, Georgia)

Each helmet has the same hole pattern as the primary collimator and docks onto the latter during treatment. Individual plugs with fixed aperture conform the beam to size. Minor shaping of the beam is made possible by replacing one or more of these individual plugs with an occlusive one (Fig. 16.5a,b).

To cover a larger area, or to achieve dose conformity, multiple shots with different helmet and head positions must be used. With the Gamma Knife®, treatment is delivered by moving the target to the isocenter, which is

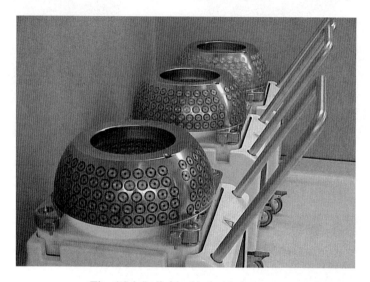

Fig. 16.4. Individual helmets on carts

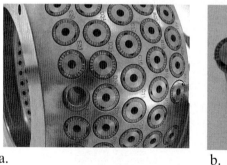
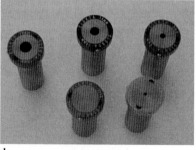

a.   b.

Fig. 16.5. (a) 18 mm diameter helmet with a plug removed. **(b)** The four different diameter plugs available for individual helmet plus occlusion plug used for shaping.

then exposed for a predetermined amount of time. The patient lies on the treatment couch with the stereotactic head frame attached to a positioning system. The patient's head position is set as planned, either with an automatic positioning system (APS) (Fig. 16.6), or manually via a set of trunnions (Fig. 16.7).

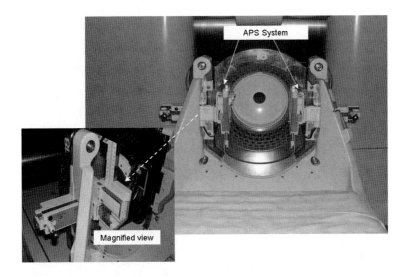

Fig. 16.6. Automatic positioning system (APS) with magnified scales

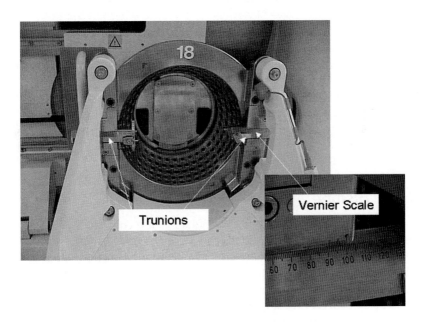

Fig. 16.7. Trunnions with magnified Vernier scale view

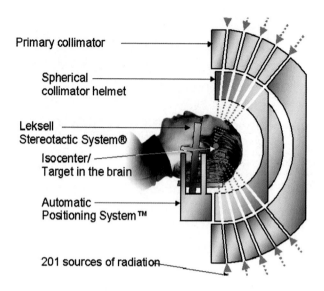

Primary collimator

Spherical collimator helmet

Leksell Stereotactic System®

Isocenter/ Target in the brain

Automatic Positioning System™

201 sources of radiation

Fig. 16.8. Schematic diagram showing patient at treatment position (Courtesy of Elekta Instrument Inc., Norcross, Georgia)

At the start of treatment, the shielding door in the head unit opens, allowing the couch to move inside. Microswitches at the end of the helmet ensure the precision of docking between the two collimators. Once docked to the primary collimator, all channels are in line and the timer begins. With the APS system, position change is done automatically at the end of a shot. A slight pull back of the couch forces the helmet out of alignment with the primary collimator, and blocks all primary beams to the patient. The APS system then moves the head to the next position for treatment (Fig. 16.8). With trunnions, the x, y, z coordinates for each shot must be done manually.

16.2.1 History

As mentioned at the beginning of this chapter, the concept of radiosurgery was first introduced by Professor Lars Leksell in 1951. While working on his stereotactic frame for image-guided intervention to the brain, Leksell realized that the target point always coincided with the center of the arc system (Fig. 16.9). This led him to the idea of using radiation for minimally invasive neurosurgery. Multiple radiation beams, which are harmless singly, traverse from various positions of the arc, and when directed towards the target deliver a destructive dose at the center, while sparing the normal tissues along the way. This revolutionary concept was first tested on a linear accelerator, but it lacked the precision and accuracy needed. Next, he attempted to

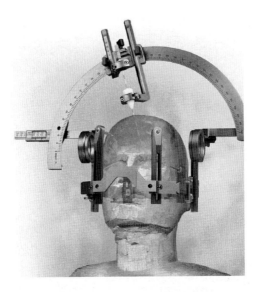

Fig. 16.9. Stereotactic neurosurgery – underlying principle for the development of stereotatic radiosurgery (Courtesy of Elekta Instrument Inc., Norcross, Georgia)

use a proton beam generated by a cyclotron, but the equipment was very costly. Since gamma radiation has similar radiobiological characteristics as a proton beam, the alternative was to use the gamma radiation produced by natural radioactive decay. This eventually led to the choice of cobalt-60 as the radioactive source.

Leksell, together with Larson, a radiobiologist, went on to design the first multiple cobalt source unit. The first patient was treated at the nuclear plant in Studsvik, Sweden in November 1967. The radiation field produced from the original design was small, therefore treatment was limited to small pathological volumes only. Since its first prototype, the design has been focused on noninvasive procedures for surgery of neurological diseases. The goal was to use high dose radiation to abrade the tumor in one treatment, without using open surgery and with minimal damage to the surrounding normal tissues. In 1987, the first commercially available Gamma Knife® Model U changed its design to house 201 sources arranged in an arc of 160° along the transverse axis of the table, with 96° along the long axis of the table (Fig. 16.10). As a result, the isodose line was more elongated in the superior inferior orientation. This model was discontinued in 1988 and replaced by the B series (Fig. 16.11). The central body unit was redesigned to simplify the source loading and reloading process. The source pattern arrangement was changed to a full 360° covering a spherical segment of 30°, thereby giving the isodose line a more left-right spread [Yamamoto 1999; Wu et al. 1990; Kondziolka et al. 2002].

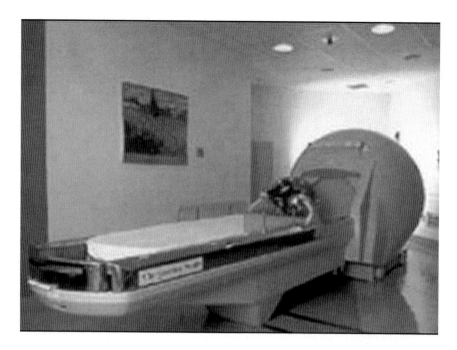

Fig. 16.10. Model U – First installation 1987 (Courtesy of Elekta Instrument, Inc., Norcross, Georgia)

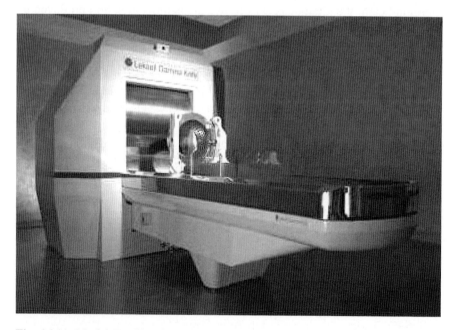

Fig. 16.11. Model B – First installation 1996 (Courtesy of Elekta Instrument Inc., Norcross, Georgia)

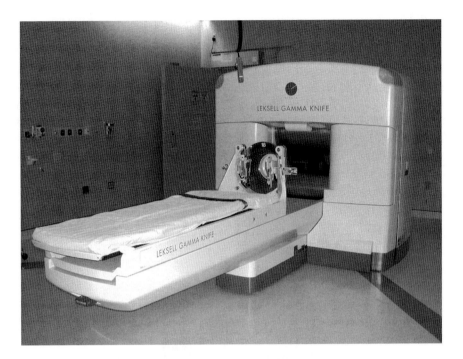

Fig. 16.12. Model C – First Installation 1999

The next major change came in 1999 with the Model C (Fig. 16.12), when a new automatic positioning system (APS) was added to the existing manual trunnion system. One drawback of the earlier model was the time for manually repositioning each shot with the attendant risks of human error. With a computer controlled module, the APS first defocuses the beam by moving the couch outwards by 28 cm. Precision motors then move the head slowly to the next position before moving the couch back into position for the next treatment. This procedure saves time as the staff does not have to enter and exit the room for each shot. However, the APS system does occupy more space, which limits the mechanical travel in all directions inside the helmet, thereby making frame placement more critical.

16.2.2 Current Status

The Gamma Knife® has always been a frame-based system. The stereotactic radiosurgery procedure using Gamma Knife® can be divided into four major steps: frame placement, target localization, treatment planning, and delivery.

16.2.2.1 Frame Placement

To begin, a Leksell Coordinate Frame Model G is attached to the patient's skull for target localization. The frame is made up of four bars with a fixation pole that is attached to each of the four corners. A set of fixation screws threaded through the hole at the top of each pole is used to secure the frame to the patient's head. Positioning of the frame is crucial, because treatment positions are limited by the physical size of the helmet and the head position within the frame. Ideally, the frame should be placed with the target center at the frame center. For spatial reference, a rectilinear coordinate system is used with the origin located at a point superior, lateral, and posterior to the frame on the right side of the patient. The coordinate scale is engraved on all sides of the frame in millimeter graduations and conforms with the X, Y, and Z directions used for imaging (Fig. 16.13).

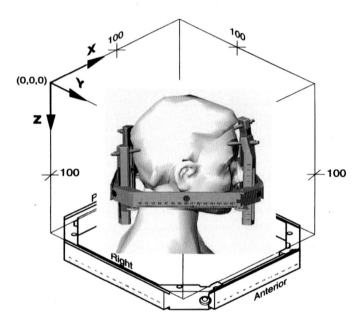

Fig. 16.13. Orientation of the Leksell Coordinate Frame – Model G (Courtesy of Elekta Instrument Inc., Norcross, Georgia)

16.2.2.2 Target Localization

Tumor location is determined either by MR or CT. Although MR is the preferred imaging modality for the brain, there are circumstances when only CT can be performed. A fiducial marker box especially designed for each of the imaging modalities is placed over the respective frame before scanning. For CT and MR, the fiducials used for determining the target coordinates are arranged in the shape of an N in each panel of the box (Fig. 16.14). During scanning, the fiducials are superimposed on the images of the patient. Each slice has four sets of fiducials, each with three separate markers

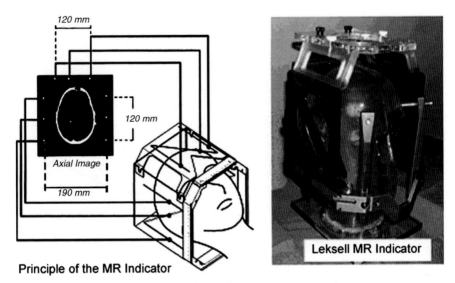

120 mm

120 mm

Axial Image

190 mm

Principle of the MR Indicator

Leksell MR Indicator

Fig. 16.14. MR indicator – N shaped fiducials as shown on axial scans (Courtesy of Elekta Instrument Inc., Norcross, Georgia)

superimposed upon it. By identifying these markers on each slice, the target localization software can determine the coordinates of the treatment area in stereotactic space.

16.2.2.3 Treatment Planning

Once the treatment area is located, a 3D conformal treatment plan on one or more target areas is designed with image reconstruction. Dose calculation requires that the distance between the center of the beam and the entrance point is known. To reduce the number of slices needed and thus speed up the calculation process, the planning system uses a skull scaling instrument to determine the skull size (Fig. 16.15). This partial sphere, designed to dock onto the Leksell frame, has a total of 33 holes arranged in eight longitudinal columns and four lateral rings, plus a top radius. By inserting a graduated pole through these holes, the distance is measured from the center of the Leksell stereotactic space to the outer surface of the patient's skull. From these measured data, the computer generates a three-dimensional skull model for dose calculation.

Using the Gamma Knife®, dose conformity is achieved by super-imposing shots of different helmet sizes and isocenters [Kondziolka et al. 2002; Bank and Timmerman 2002]. The total dose to a point within the patient's head is calculated by summing the dose contribution from all 201 non-coplanar beams, while taking account of the patient's head shape

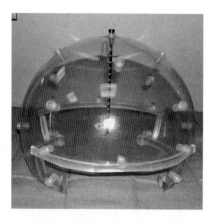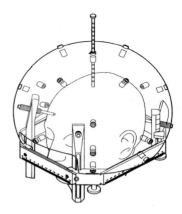

Fig. 16.15. Skull scaling instrument (Courtesy of Elekta Instrument Inc., Norcross, Georgia)

and size, the size of the collimators, the linear attenuation coefficient of cobalt-60, and the transverse beam profile. To simplify the dose calculation process, a single-beam dose profile is used for all individual beams [Wu et al. 1990; Cheung et al. 1998]. Since all the individual beams are small and circular, corrections for oblique beam incidence and heterogeneities can be ignored. The ideal objective for treatment planning is dose conformity to the target volume with high homogeneity inside. However, with a small target volume, dose conformity often takes priority. For Gamma Knife® radiosurgery, it is typical to prescribe to the 50% isodose line. Treatment time for each shot is determined based on the total dose desired, size of the collimator used, weighting of the beam, and source activity. After a plan is established, the location and time for each shot are sent to the console via a computer network. The coordinates for each shot are downloaded to the APS system for treatment delivery.

16.2.2.4 Treatment Delivery

The greatest advantage of the Gamma Knife® for SRS is its fixed isocenter. Treatment accuracy is limited only by the ability to set up the treatment position. There are two ways to secure the patient's head frame to the collimator helmet: the manually set trunnion or the computer controlled APS. The frame secures the patient's head onto the trunnion, which is a set of calipers capable of moving the frame in all three directions. Traditionally, treatment coordinates are set manually on the trunnion and the couch moves the patient into the head unit for treatment. The accuracy of the treatment depends solely on the equipment operator. With APS, treatment positions are set by the computer, which reduces the chances for human error. Multiple shots are grouped into different runs so as to minimize staff interventions, such as helmet changes. This results in more shots being delivered over a shorter period of time.

16.2.3 Developments

Gamma Knife® treatment has proven effective for thousands of patients with benign or malignant brain tumors. However, the treatment sites have been limited to areas within the head, with the exception of very peripheral lesions. With APS, the usable area within the helmet is further reduced making it difficult to treat laterally located lesions or lesions that are located too inferiorly.

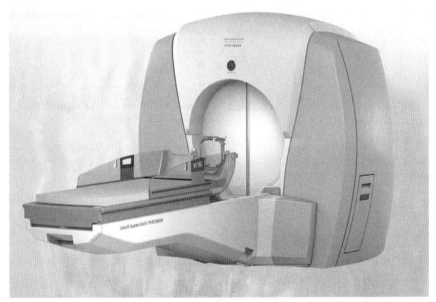

Fig. 16.16. Gamma Knife® PerfexionTM – First installation 2006 (Courtesy of Elekta Instrument Inc., Norcross, Georgia)

In July 2006, the Gamma Knife® Perfexion^{TM} (Fig. 16.16) was introduced. This next generation system was designed to accommodate head and neck radiosurgery with minimal operator intervention. This new design does not use interchangeable helmets, but instead has a robotic collimator that is permanently fixed with openings for collimations of three difference diameters, 4, 8, and 16 mm, plus a beam off control. The collimator is divided into eight segments, each with an independently moveable sector housing 24 cobalt-60 sources (Fig. 16.17a,b). By the use of a servo system, each sector can be moved individually or in unison to achieve dynamic shaping of dose pattern (Fig. 16.18). The treatment planning system provides a fast and easy way to compute all composite shots for treatment delivery and provide better dose conformity. In addition, the larger collimator opening significantly improves target accessibility (Fig. 16.19). Instead of repositioning the head after each shot as in previous models, the couch is part of the integrated system and is capable of movement in all directions. This enables the patient to be moved into treatment position and reduces stress on the neck. This design has revolutionized the Gamma Knife® technology, although it is too new to have made a major impact as yet.

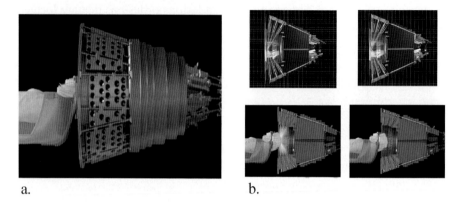

a.   b.

Fig. 16.17. (**a**) Robotic collimator of PerfexionTM. (**b**) Schematic diagram showing the sector position change (Courtesy of Elekta Instrument, Incorporated, Norcross, Georgia)

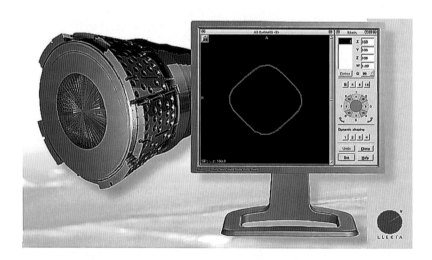

Fig. 16.18. Effect on dose pattern with composite sector diameter (Courtesy of Elekta Instrument Inc., Norcross, Georgia)

Side View

Leksell Gamma Knife® Perfexion™

Leksell Gamma Knife® C

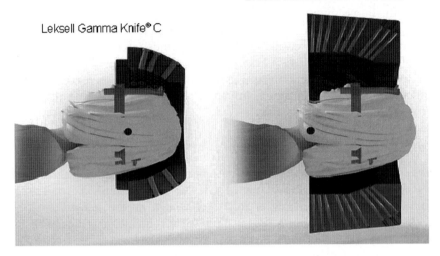

Front View

Leksell Gamma Knife® Perfexion™

Leksell Gamma Knife® C

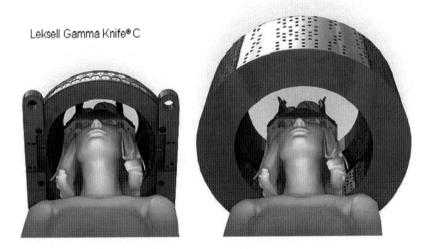

Fig. 16.19. Comparison of the old and new collimators (Courtesy of Elekta Instrument Inc., Norcross, Georgia)

16.3   Conventional Linac-Based Radiosurgery Systems

Following the standards established by the Gamma Knife®, the initial linear accelerator (linac) based cranial SRS procedure used a head frame attached to the patient's skull. More recent linac-based, cranial radiosurgery systems rely on image-guided treatment setup without using a head frame. The first generation of extracranial or body radiosurgery procedures also started out using a body frame to guide set-up prior to treatment. The shortcomings of the body frame approach gave way to image guidance (primarily X-ray orthogonal pairs or CT) to achieve precise set-up prior to treatment. Several systems have become available for image-guided (cranial and/or body) setup in the last few years. These systems use the treatment couch rotation (or translation for TomoTherapy as described later) to achieve the third dimension in beam orientations around the isocenter (or axis of rotation for TomoTherapy).

16.3.1 Frame-Based Systems

The frame-based cranial SRS was designed to achieve setup accuracy and precision on par with the Gamma Knife®. These systems had no image guidance for setup verification and so depended on the transfer of localization information from a diagnostic (kV) CT image set taken with the frame on the patient. The neurosurgeon attaches the head frame (using four screws) to the patient's skull under local anesthesia. After CT scanning, localization, and tumor contouring, treatment dose planning is performed. Once these tasks are completed, the head frame is then mounted to a rigid surgical floor stand and the treatment isocenter is subsequently positioned by verniers at the accelerator's isocenter. Alternatively, the head frame is secured to a linac couchtop adapter and the couchtop locked down once the frame is positioned, using room lasers focused on the machine isocenter. Both techniques depend on the precision of couch rotation (up to about 190°) about its axis during treatment. The Novalis system designed and marketed by BrainLab (Feldkirchen, Germany) is an example of such a system. For the couch-mounted frame in the TomoTherapy system (Madison, USA), the precision of couch translations during treatment delivery is vital.

Of the above frame-based localization systems, only the TomoTherapy system offers image guidance for cranial treatment setup. The TomoTherapy system delivers treatment using a 6 MV X-ray beam that is modulated by a pair of opposed multileaf collimator (MLC) leaves that cross the beam while the patient is translated along the super-inferior axis, and the X-ray source is rotated in the plane perpendicular to the translation axis. These motions produce a helical path for the X-ray source relative to the patient. Image-guided setup for TomoTherapy is performed by MV-CT obtained from the same 6 MV X-ray treatment beam just prior to treatment. The MV-CT images are compared to the planning kV-CT images to obtain corrections for setup positioning.

For all the cranial SRS treatment systems (frame-based or not), CT images are used to plan treatment and define the reference point for treatment setup. Frequently, MRI (and possibly PET) images are fused to the CT images to better define the tumor (target) volume. Since no images are used for set-up and treatment delivery (except for TomoTherapy), rigorous quality assurance is performed prior to treatment to assure localization accuracy.

Quality assurance primarily consists of verification that the radiation beam isocenter (including both gantry and couch rotations) is coincident with isocenter pointers (room lasers or mechanical pointer on the floor stand).

The treatment delivery options available vary with the equipment. A brief summary is given in Table 16.1.

Table 16.1. Head frame-based SRS treatment techniques

	Floor stand mounted	Novalis	TomoTherapy
Noncoplanar arcs with cones	Yes	Yes	No
Noncoplanar arcs with MLC	Possible	Yes	No
Helical path with milk	No	No	Yes
IMRT with MLC	Possible	Yes	Yes

Non-coplanar arc techniques typically use 3–6 gantry arcs in different coaxial planes through the patient's head, which are achieved by rotating the treatment couch (and couch base plate to which a floor stand may be secured). The sharpest radiation field falloff is achieved using circular cones attached to the linac head relatively close to the patient. Tumors having irregular shapes usually can be best conformed to by the MLC leaves being dynamically shaped to match the target volume outline as seen from the X-ray source as it travels along the arc. The helical path of the Tomo-Therapy treatment delivery offers dynamic shaping, but only in a continuous sequence of axial planes. TomoTherapy also provides one version of intensity modulated radiation therapy (IMRT) delivery, which is dynamic helical. The Novalis system from BrainLab, with its gantry mounted linac and micro MLC, offers the more traditional type of IMRT where the radiation beams are modulated by the MLC and which originate from 4–12 static orientations of the X-ray source around the target volume (determined by gantry and couch rotations).

One advantage of IMRT treatment delivery is that the planning process can be much more sophisticated since it permits inverse planning. Inverse planning allows the treatment goals (minimum dose to the target volume, maximum doses to the critical normal tissues and organs, and other constraints) to be predefined and an optimum solution can then be computed. Conventional (or forward) planning is an iterative process to achieve the same goals based on intuition and persistence.

Body or extracranial stereotactic setup can be performed with one of the several body frames composed of a radio-translucent three-sided box with built-in rods and other fiducial markers, plus a body conforming vacuum bag for patient positioning and comfort. When the patient in the body frame is sent through a CT scanner, a coordinate system is defined and the tumor volume can then be defined relative to this coordinate system at the time of the CT examination. The treatment setup is relative to the body frame coordinate system, which can be placed on the treatment couch to about 2 mm precision. Patients with tumors that move with respiratory motion may have a reduced range of motion imposed by body frame devices. In general, body frame setup is not image-guided although it is certainly possible to use imaging implanted fiducials (in or around the tumor) at the time of treatment. However, this procedure would reduce the role of the body frame to a fancy immobilizer. Patients with relatively immobile tumors in the body are much more likely to benefit from the body frame setup in the absence of daily image guidance during treatment.

16.3.2 *Image-Guided Setup Systems*

The concept of image-guided setup is that prior to each treatment session the patient's tumor is imaged, compared to a reference location, and adjusted so that the tumor is accurately centered before treatment commences. For stereotactic body radiosurgery, the imaging is performed either with an orthogonal pair of diagnostic X-ray beams or with a CT scanner. Bony anatomy or other fixed landmarks relative to the tumor may also be used for localization. Alternatively, implanted fiducial markers (e.g., gold seeds) placed in proximity to the tumor are used for tumor localization. The goal of image-guided setup is to correct for day-to-day variations of the tumor in the body and/or the patient on the couch. Such corrections can be made to a precision of about 1 mm. If the tumor is relatively fixed with respect to respiration, then treatment may commence, assuming no other causes of tumor motion during treatment delivery.

As described previously, the TomoTherapy system uses the MV therapy beam to acquire a CT scan, and information in the MV-CT image is compared with the planning kV-CT for tumor localization. Although the MV-CT images provide 3D anatomy, they have less soft tissue contrast than the planning kV-CT images. For applications where fiducials are used as surrogate markers, the soft tissue contrast is acceptable. The Novalis system uses a pair of X-ray imagers (source and receptor) fixed in the room (floor and ceiling) in a specified geometry that is roughly orthogonal. The Varian (Palo Alto, USA) image-guided radiotherapy (IGRT) systems use an imager mounted to the accelerator gantry at 90°, and in the rotational plane of the MV X-ray beam axis.

Both approaches (diagnostic imagers or MV-CT) work quickly and provide the information needed to improve stationary target localization at the time of treatment setup. These systems can be used to verify and reposition the patient at the beginning of the treatment. However, it is currently not common practice to interrupt treatment for additional imaging and repositioning.

16.3.3   Image-Guided Treatment with Respiratory Motion

Respiratory motion of a target volume in the thorax or abdomen can have a range of a few millimeters up to several centimeters in each of the three dimensions. Tumor rotations are not uncommon, nor are respiratory induced deformations. This situation is clearly a challenge even for the most advanced technologies of image guidance. There are two fundamental techniques employed to compensate for respiratory movement during treatment delivery. For the gated treatment delivery method, rapid beam on/off technology is used to start/stop the irradiation based on the phase of the respiratory cycle. One implementation employs a patient breath-hold at full inspiration to trigger the beam on and off. Another gating technique uses normal breathing, and the beam is turned on at the full expiration phase. The determination of respiratory phase can be based on external markers placed on the patient and then monitored continuously, as used by the Novalis system, for example. The advent of 4D CT scanning permits quantitative assessment of respiratory motion and aids the process of planning the gating. The Varian and Novalis systems have adopted the gated delivery approach.

The second technique to respiratory motion compensation is model-based. This means that a patient-specific correlation model is built to predict tumor position based on the continuous tracking of chest or abdominal surface markers, and on the tumor position tracking with time-stamped X-ray images. This approach is currently used by the CyberKnife. The Cyber-Knife also periodically verifies the accuracy of the motion correlation during treatment delivery and rebuilds the model as needed.

A continuing challenge for respiratory compensation is that respiration for a given patient may change significantly in frequency and amplitude during the course of treatment delivery, and the tumor location relative to phase also can change.

16.4   Image-Guided Robotic Radiosurgery

16.4.1   History and Description of the CyberKnife

The CyberKnife   is based on a concept developed by neurosurgeon John Adler of Stanford University. Adler, who was trained by Lars Leksell on the Gamma Knife®, was looking for a way to deliver SRS without inflicting head-frame placements on patients. The essential problem was how to determine the patient's position before treatment. The solution was image guidance using a pair of orthogonal X-ray cameras.

Instead of using a conventional linac with its geometric motion limitations, or an array of X-ray sources, Adler decided to use a 6 MV X-band miniature accelerator mounted on top of an industrial robot. The accuracy and reproducibility of the robot was capable of meeting radio-surgical standards with an accuracy of better than 0.5 mm.

The CyberKnife SRS system (Accuray Inc, Sunnyvale, California) currently consists of an X-band linear accelerator mounted on a robotic arm (KUKA, Augsburg, Germany). The patient is placed on a treatment couch and images from two orthogonal X-ray cameras mounted on the ceiling are compared with digitally reconstructed radiographs (DRRs) from the treat-ment planning CT. Internal gold fiducial markers or bony landmarks can be used for coregistration.

During the treatment, images are taken before every treatment beam. The robot corrects for patient motions up to 10 mm in each translational direction, for 1° of roll and pitch rotation and 3° of yaw. The relevant clinical accuracy is determined by the so-called end-to-end test and com-bines the robot pointing accuracy, camera image tracking system, and target localization accuracy. For fiducial tracking and CT slice thickness between 0.625 and 1.25 mm, the system accuracy has been shown to be 0.7 ± 0.3 mm [Yu et al. 2004].

For the simulation, the patient is immobilized. Cranial immobilization is done using a thermoplastic mask, while for extracranial cases, a vacuum-bag, such as the Acculoc bag or other similar devices may be used. The immobilization does not need to be rigid, but mainly serves as a reminder for the patient to abstain from sudden, large movements as well as stabi-lizing the patient position during treatment. It is very important that the patient can lie comfortably and be relaxed in the immobilization device during the treatment time, which takes approximately 1 h.

16.4.2   Frameless Tracking Technology for Cranial Surgery, Spine, and Body

The frameless image guidance system can be considered the center of the technology. The image guidance hardware, together with the tracking algorithm, provides the CyberKnife system with the information on the amount and direction of adjustment required to correct for patient motion. The adjustments are made using the automated couch or the robot couch during the setup phase of the treatment. During the treatment, the robot corrects for patient motion up to 10 mm in each translational direction, 1° rotation in roll and pitch, and 3° rotation in yaw rotation. The coordinate systems are defined in Fig. 16.20. Roll rotation is around the patient long

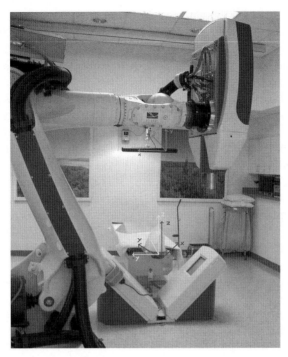

Fig. 16.20. Coordinate systems in the CyberKnife room. The robot, patient, and the Synchrony camera all have separate coordinate systems associated with them that are displayed in different colors.

axis in the *y-z* plane, pitch in the *x-z* plane, and yaw rotation in the *x-y* plane of the patient coordinate system.

There are currently four different tracking algorithms depending on the body site treated: cranial, spine, and lung tumor tracking, and fiducial-based tracking. The tracking workflow remains the same across all four tracking algorithms.

Tracking starts with the simulation CT scan of the patient. The slice thickness is typically chosen to be 1.25 mm or less, because a larger slice thickness would decrease the spatial accuracy of the tracking algorithm. After the CT images are imported into the treatment planning system, a CT center has to be defined. This CT center not only provides the landmark for the contouring and planning process, but also defines the patient origin during treatment. In an ideal treatment setup, this CT center would be perfectly aligned with the imaging coordinate system origin. The placement of the CT center also defines the section of the patient anatomy, which is in the field of view of the imaging system. After the CT center is selected, a set of digitally reconstructed radiographs (DRRs) is created from the CT image. The DRRs are used during treatment to match the X-ray images of the patient to a position change relative to the simulation position used as a baseline.

For the image guidance during treatment, an X-ray image is first taken by the two orthogonal cameras. The images captured by the two cameras are processed by the tracking algorithm to provide a 6 degrees-of-freedom localization of the patient in the patient coordinate system. The patient coordinates are then transformed into the robot coordinate system, which is rotated 45° relative to the patient coordinate system. This data is then provided as input into the software driving the robot. The robot then adjusts its position from the default beam position to the corrected position. The special case of real-time motion adaptive tracking will be discussed in Sect. 16.4.2.5. In the following paragraphs, each tracking mode is described in more detail.

16.4.2.1 Cranial Tracking

The cranial tracking mode was the first to be implemented, to transition from traditional frame-based SRS in the brain to frameless tracking. The brain is also the easiest site for which to develop tracking technology. The brain does not move relative to the bony anatomy of the cranium. The cranium itself does not vary much in shape and size between humans, with the exception of children and adolescents. However, the variations in shape of the cranial bones between humans are sufficiently different so as to be distinguished by the software, which provides an additional safeguard against delivering a treatment plan to the wrong patient.

The CT center for cranial tracking is typically selected to be on the patient midline between the sphenoid bones. This results in optimum coverage of the imagers, without cutting off the structurally rich area of the facial bones (Fig. 16.21). For pediatric and adolescent patients, the CT center placement has to be shifted more superiorly in the skull, or too much of the mandible would be visible in the DRRs. The mandible's position can move sufficiently even in immobilized patients, which can cause failure of the tracking algorithm.

In cranial tracking, the brightness and brightness gradient of the live X-ray images is compared to a library of DRRs. The image brightness and gradient is compared to the closest match in the library.

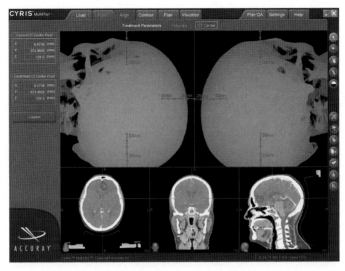

Fig. 16.21. CT center selection for cranial tracking. The lower screens, from left to right, show an axial, sagittal, and coronal cross section of a patient CT. The green lines intersect at the CT center. The upper screens show the DRRs for the perfectly aligned patient in the 45° view of the ceiling cameras. The view of the DRRs is from the amorphous silicon detector up towards the ceiling camera

16.4.2.2 Fiducial Tracking

Except for certain lung tumors, treatment sites located in soft tissue cannot be tracked using kV X-ray images because the contrast is not high enough. For those sites, multiple cylindrical gold markers of at least 3 mm in length and 1.5 mm in diameter are implanted in or around the tumor [Shirato et al. 2003]. Implantation techniques include trans-thoracic [Pishvaian et al. 2006], trans-bronchial [Reichner 2005], and trans-esophageal [Yousefi et al. 2007] techniques.

The location of the gold markers is registered in the treatment planning system (Fig. 16.22). The registration can be done either manually or by defining a seed point for automated registration. The CT center is defined automatically as the center of mass of all registered fiducials.

During the treatment, the tracking software analyzes both X-ray images for high-density objects that satisfy the criteria for a gold fiducial. The tracking algorithm is described in detail in Mu et al. [2006]. In each X-ray image, a number of potential fiducial candidates (blobs) are identified. To improve the signal-to-noise ratio for detecting fiducials in the live X-ray image, a band-pass filter is employed. The frequency range for the filter is determined by the specific fiducial being used; the properties of the fiducials recommended for use with the CyberKnife are predefined in the software.

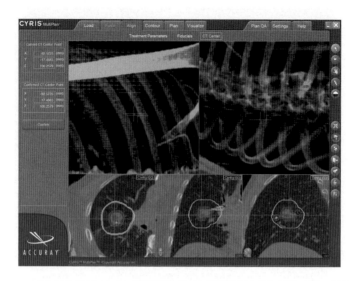

Fig. 16.22. Gold marker registration during planning. The lower left and right images show a clearly visible gold marker implanted into a lung lesion. The DRRs on top show the registered fiducials with the coordinates of the center of mass listed on the upper left in the CT coordinate system.

Once the fiducial candidates have been identified, the candidates are ranked using several criteria based on the known shapes of the screws and gold fiducials: blob size, contrast, position on both cameras, and fiducial-to-fiducial distance. A modified Hidden Markov Model (HMM) is employed to identify the fiducials. Because some of the information about the fiducial candidates is redundant, e.g., the x-coordinate is determined by both camera systems, the special case of this second order HMM was solved by using a modified Concurrent Viterbi Algorithm with Association. After the fiducial positions have been determined, a 6D transformation is calculated, transforming the fiducial coordinates identified in the live image into the configuration identified in the simulation scan.

The result of this approach is a robust fiducial tracking algorithm with a limited number of parameters (Fig. 16.23), which can be used to optimize tracking for specific patients. The user can change the criteria within a certain range to filter out objects that were incorrectly identified as fiducials. Typical examples of high-density shapes resembling fiducials are surgical clips or crossing ribs in the oblique views of the cameras.

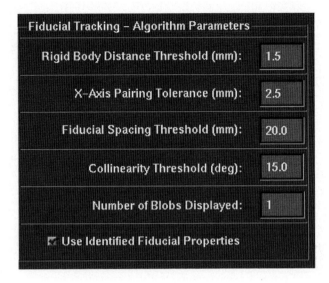

Fig. 16.23. Fiducial tracking algorithm parameters

16.4.2.3   Spine Tracking

The spine tracking algorithm was developed to avoid the invasive procedure of placing gold fiducials into the spine [Gerszten et al. 2003a,b; Ryu et al. 2001]. In addition, fiducial placement in many cancer patients proved to be a challenge, because dense scar tissue and eroded bone is often present close to tumor locations, due to previous surgeries. Muacevic et al. [2006] report on the clinical experience using the fiducial-free spine tracking algorithm described in Fu and Kuduvalli [2006] and Fu et al. [2006].

The algorithm uses a combination of digital image enhancement features to improve the visualization of the skeletal anatomy. The 2D–3D image registration is achieved by using similarity measures to match a region of interest, defined by a mesh that is centered on the user-defined CT center, to the live radiograph. The optimum CT center placement is in the midline of the vertebral body a few millimeters above the spinal canal (Fig. 16.24). To maximize the amount of information contained in the mesh grid, the initial user-defined CT center is refined automatically.

During the treatment, the 2D–3D image registration determines the patient position. Grid nodes for which the registration fails are marked in purple in the live image (Fig. 16.25 - please see color version of this figure on the DVD supplied with the book). The misalignment of the patient is corrected by the robot during the treatment.

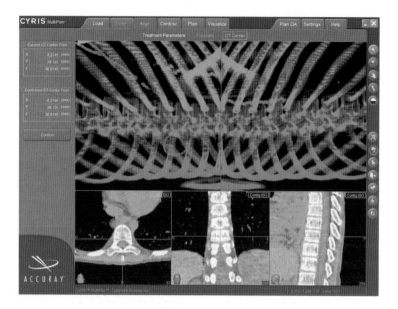

Fig. 16.24. CT center selection for spine tracking

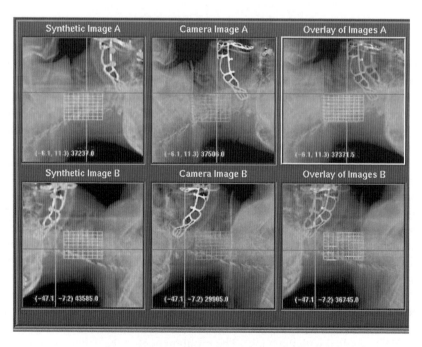

Fig. 16.25. Grid used for fiducial-free spinal tracking

16.4.2.4 Lung Tumor Tracking

Implanting fiducials in a lung tumor is an invasive procedure and includes the associated risks of pneumothorax [Kupelian et al. 2007]. Developing a method to use the relatively high contrast in a diagnostic X-ray between lung tumor tissue and lung is therefore highly desirable. To be visible, lung tumors typically have to be located in the peripheral lung to avoid obstructing the tumor by the mediastinum in the oblique camera angle view. A minimum tumor diameter of about 15 mm is also necessary to provide visibility (Fig. 16.26).

The first step in the lung tumor tracking method is to automatically segment the spine in the treatment planning CT (Fig. 16.27) and remove it visually from the DRRs (Fig. 16.28).

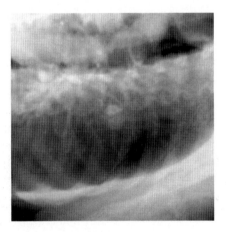

Fig. 16.26. DRR of a peripheral lung tumor with diameter >15 mm. The tumor is partially obstructed by the bony anatomy of the spine

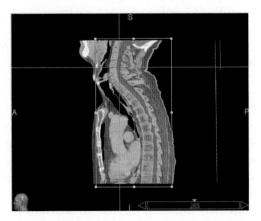

Fig. 16.27. Spine segmentation during the treatment planning stage

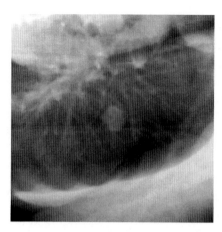

Fig. 16.28. DRR after the spine was segmented out. The tumor is now clearly visible

After the tumor is contoured by the physician, the 2D oblique projections of the contour are calculated in the DRR. A 2D window just bounding the tumor contour is created in each DRR. These windows contain the entire 2D tumor information with some background, and form the basic unit for the matching algorithm. During treatment, a number of matching windows are placed onto the live X-ray images within a search window and a similarity measure is calculated between the matching windows and the 2D bounding window created in the treatment planning system.

16.4.3 Treatment Planning

Once the tracking mode has been established and the appropriate CT center has been selected, the treatment planning process can begin. The first step in the treatment planning process is the selection of the treatment paths. Each treatment path has a fixed number of robot positions (nodes). The number, position, and order of the nodes do not change after initial installation to avoid potential collision between the robot and objects in the room. At each of the nodes, the robot can point in up to twelve beam directions. The product of node number and beam direction, depending on path set chosen, allows for a library of about 500–1,400 beam orientations from which the planning system can choose.

The user has two options for planning: the isocentric mode, which mimics a Gamma Knife® plan, and inverse planning. In isocentric planning, a set of one or more isocenters is defined. Beams can either have the same number of monitor units as in Gamma Knife® planning, or be weighted using an an isocentric/conformal plan combination approach.

Inverse (conformal) planning for the CyberKnife is an optimization problem that can be solved using linear programming [Schweikard et al. 1998]. In linear programming, the value of the objective function is minimized or maximized under the condition that a set of linear constraints is fulfilled. The linear constraints can also be weighted according to their relative merit in the clinical situation. The weights define the penalty functions for violating the constraints during the optimization process. A clinical sample set of constraints and their weights is given in Fig. 16.29. The basic formalism of linear programming can be expanded to include 4D planning and potential organ deformation during different phases of the respiratory cycle [Schlaefer et al. 2005].

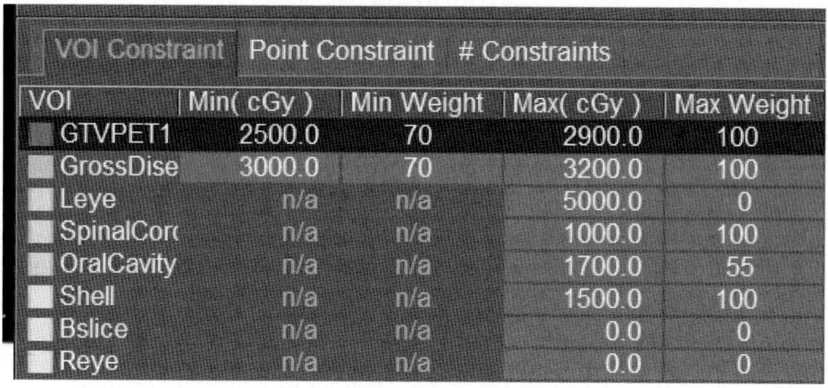

VOI Constraint	Point Constraint	# Constraints		
VOI	Min(cGy)	Min Weight	Max(cGy)	Max Weight
GTVPET1	2500.0	70	2900.0	100
GrossDise	3000.0	70	3200.0	100
Leye	n/a	n/a	5000.0	0
SpinalCorc	n/a	n/a	1000.0	100
OralCavity	n/a	n/a	1700.0	55
Shell	n/a	n/a	1500.0	100
Bslice	n/a	n/a	0.0	0
Reye	n/a	n/a	0.0	0

Fig. 16.29. Example set of linear constraints used in treatment planning

16.4.4   Treatment Delivery

Once the patient is aligned using any of the four tracking modes described earlier, the treatment itself can begin. Before each beam, the system can take an X-ray image to assess the current patient position. The frequency of imaging can be defined by the user before treatment starts, and changed during the treatment. Position changes of the patient during the treatment are automatically corrected by the robot. While this method of image guidance during treatment is not a truly real-time system, residual errors caused by patient motion between images have been shown to be small [Murphy et al. 2003].

16.4.5   Four-Dimensional Real-Time Adaptive Respiratory Tracking (Synchrony) Technology

16.4.5.1 Introduction

Synchrony [Schweikard et al. 2004] is at this time the only FDA approved dynamic SRS device in the US. Its technology is based on the CyberKnife SRS technology [Adler et al. 1997; Kuo et al. 2003; Quinn 2002]. The technology was developed to dynamically track tumor movement with respiration in real-time, without the need for gating. The Synchrony technology is based on a hybrid skin-tumor correlation method for tracking tumor motion in near real-time. It can be applied for all tumors that move with respiration [Dieterich 2005]. The treatment planning process for Synchrony is very similar to regular treatment planning, but has recently been expanded to include 4D treatment planning capabilities.

16.4.5.2 Skin-Tumor Correlation Model

The main challenge for 4D adaptive, real-time techniques is to establish the position of the hidden, moving target. Because of radiation dose, fluoroscopy used for tracking [Kitamura et al. 2002; Berbeco et al. 2005] is feasible only if the treatment times do not exceed a few minutes. Wireless markers [Balter et al. 2005] have been FDA approved for use in the prostate, but have not been tested for use in conjunction with the CyberKnife. Therefore, a hybrid skin-tumor correlation model has been developed for the CyberKnife. This correlation model does not rely on information gathered during simulation, which can be days before treatment, but is established during the treatment in between the initial patient alignment and the start of the radiation delivery.

After the initial patient alignment, several X-ray images of the internal fiducials are taken with the patient breathing freely. These images must be timed so that they are at different phases of the respiratory cycle. At the same instance, the position of the beacons placed on the skin is recorded. A correlation model between the internal and external positions is established. After three images or 40% of the respiratory amplitude is covered, the treatment can begin. With each additional X-ray image during the treatment, the correlation model is updated until the limit of 15 model correlation points is reached. From then on, the model points are updated in a first-in, first-out fashion (Fig. 16.30).

16.4.5.3 Tumor Path Modeling

Three tumor motion path models are available in the current Synchrony release: linear, curvilinear (same inhale and exhale path), and elliptical (different inhale and exhale path). Each of the three models is fitted to the 15 correlation model points. The model with the least root-mean-square error is automatically selected to be the valid tumor motion path model for the following beams until the next image. Because of the nonlinearity of the models, the accuracy of the fiducial tracking has to be carefully monitored. Seemingly small errors such as tracking an adjacent surgical clip instead of a gold fiducial marker may only cause a small error in the determination of translational tumor position, but may cause much larger deviations in the tumor motion path model.

The technical tracking capabilities of Synchrony have been tested with a sophisticated programmable motion platform [Zhou et al. 2004]. If the correlation model is assumed to be known, the technical tracking accuracy can be better than 0.5 mm even for very irregular respiration. However, a patient is not a phantom, and the skin-tumor correlation is complex [Hoisak et al. 2004]. Therefore, an additional residual clinical tracking error [Schweikard et al. 2004] will have to be taken into account.

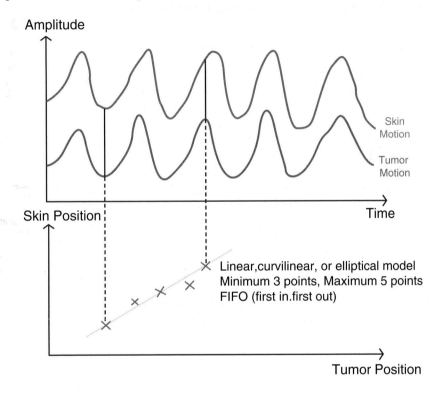

Fig. 16.30. Correlation model between internal and external motion. Several X-ray images at different phases of breathing are taken. The position of the skin marker (beacon) vs. the set of internal fiducials is plotted. Up to 15 model points may be used in the correlation plot and are fitted using the least-squares method. The system automatically fits either a linear, curvilinear, or elliptical model to the data, depending on the best fit

16.4.5.4 Treatment

During the treatment, the robot will correct for tumor motion in real-time. The Synchrony system has an inherent motion lag time of about 250 ms between information on the tumor position as predicted by the beacons and the robot motion. To correct for this, the tumor location is predicted 250 ms ahead using the respiratory motion information from the beacons. Before every beam, an X-ray image can be taken to check the validity of the correlation model and update the tumor motion path model. The user can set software limits on maximum excursions for the beacons and maximum permissible correlation model errors. A typical treatment takes only about 20% longer than a comparable body SRS case with fiducials in soft tissue.

16.5   Future of Image-Guided Radiosurgery

16.5.1   Future Tracking Technologies

As discussed in Sect. 16.4.5, the currently used hybrid tracking technology introduces a residual clinical error caused by the variability of skin-tumor correlation in a patient. An ideal further development would be to directly track the moving tumor. In addition to increasing the precision of treating tumors moving quasi-periodically, nonperiodical motion such as found in the prostate could be followed with less residual error as well.

Currently, external substitute markers are used to predict internal tumor motion. For Synchrony, X-ray images during the treatment verify the accuracy of the correlation model between external and internal motion. Ideally, the tumor motion would be directly tracked continuously throughout the treatment. Because of the long treatment times, nonionizing radiation is the only feasible imaging option.

One method (Aurora, Northern Digital Inc, Ontario, Canada) uses an electromagnetic field generator in a tetrahedron shape to track miniaturized induction coils, which can be placed in the tip of biopsy needles [Seiler et al. 2000]. An AC current excites the six differential coils in the field generator during a measurement cycle. During each cycle, the six induction voltages in the sensor coil are measured and analyzed to determine the position and orientation of the sensor coil. The system was tested in the CyberKnife Suite under treatment conditions (Fig. 16.31) [Mihaescu et al. 2004]. The beam was switched on and pointed in the direction of the sensor coil; the source-to-surface distance (SSD) was about 80 cm. The average error was 1.1–1.2 mm, with a standard deviation of 0.8 mm. There appeared to be no significant effect on the tracking accuracy from turning the CyberKnife beam on. A disadvantage of the current Aurora system is that the sensor coils need to be connected to the readout electronics by a twisted pair of fine wires. While this may be acceptable for single fraction treatments in the liver, pancreas or prostate, it is too invasive for fractionated treatments. For lung tumors, the risk of pneumothorax would be too high. The benefits of continuous electromagnetic tracking may not outweigh the risks, especially since noninvasive alternatives using a combination of internal and external surrogate markers are available [Schweikard et al. 2004].

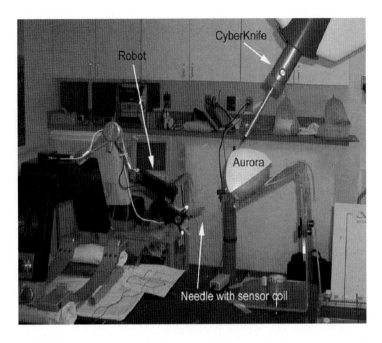

Fig. 16.31. Experimental setup of the Aurora tracking system in the CyberKnife Suite at Georgetown University Hospital. The needle with sensor coil was positioned using a robot platform. The CyberKnife was positioned at about an 80 cm source to needle distance

Implantable, wireless electromagnetic fiducial markers (Calypso Medical Inc., Seattle, WA) are currently under investigation [Balter et al. 2005]. The system consists of an AC magnetic array with four source coils and 32 receiver coils. The position of the array relative to room coordinates can be determined by an integrated optical tracking system (Fig. 16.32).

One or more wireless transponders, which are encapsulated in glass, can be implanted into the tumor using a 14-gauge needle (Fig. 16.33). The transponder location relative to the isocenter is determined by the treatment planning CT. During the treatment, the array is placed over the patient. The transponders are excited sequentially at each transponder's unique frequency by nonionizing AC electromagnetic fields that are generated by the array. Each transponder subsequently responds with a magnetic field at its unique frequency. The process of excitation and sensing is repeated several hundred times for measurement of each transponder. The system software interprets the shape of the AC electromagnetic field to solve for the unknown coordinates for each transponder. The transponder positions are used to register the target to the isocenter in real-time. The system is

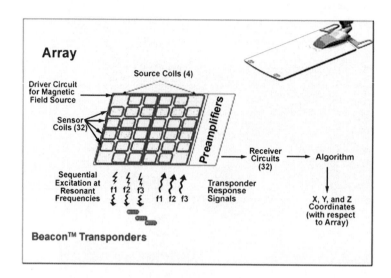

Fig. 16.32. Schematic of source array and detector electronics. Courtesy of Calypso Medical Technologies Inc., Seattle, Washington

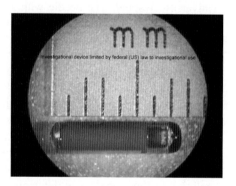

Fig. 16.33. Wireless transponder (beacon). Courtesy of Calypso Medical Technologies Inc., Seattle, Washington

also capable of determining target rotation. It has been tested in an investigational clinical study in a treatment room with a functioning external beam machine. Errors due to cross talk between transponders, conductivity, or motion have been tested and reported to be at the sub-millimeter level. The update frequency is 10 Hz but the product design is capable of variable update rates up to 30 Hz, depending on the clinical application.

16.5.2   Treatment Planning Algorithms

Another important area of ongoing research and clinical improvements are treatment planning algorithms. Current focus areas include Monte-Carlo-based planning and optimization of the linear approach for 4D applications, optimization of beam selection, and variation of collimator sizes [Deng et al. 2003, 2004].

Human beings have complex shapes, and their organs have widely varying characteristics when it comes to attenuation and energy absorption of therapeutic X-ray beams. This is of particular concern in the presence of metallic implants [Ding and Yu 2001; Keall et al. 2003; Laub and Nusslin 2003] or when treating in areas with large inhomogeneities such as the lung [Kavanagh et al. 2006]. A solution to this challenge is to implement Monte-Carlo-based treatment planning for stereotactic radiosurgery applications [Deng et al. 2003, 2004].

16.6   Summary

Image-guided radiosurgery is rapidly being adopted by hospitals to provide accurate, sub-millimeter targeting technologies for treating cancer. Image guidance for setup and during treatment is an integral part of the treatment delivery precision. Technologies for image guidance are developing rapidly, the goal being continuous, real-time tracking for internal targets while minimizing radiation dose due to diagnostic imaging for tracking. Techniques using non-ionizing electromagnetic tracking may be implemented into clinical practice in the near future.

While the technical capabilities of tracking even dynamical targets are at or below 1 mm precision, the target definition itself becomes more and more relevant. Novel diagnostic imaging techniques such as functional imaging or using biological markers as contrast agents, together with automated image registration and target segmentation, may lead to improvements in this area.

References

Adler JR, Jr., Chang SD, Murphy MJ, Doty J, Geis P, and Hancock SL. (1997). The Cyberknife: A frameless robotic system for radiosurgery. *Stereotact Funct Neurosurg*, 69, 124–128

Adler JR, Jr., Colombo F, Heilbrun MP, and Winston K. (2004). Toward an expanded view of radiosurgery. *Neurosurgery*, 55(6), 1374–1376

Balter JM, Wright JN, Newell LN, Friemel B, Dimmer S, Cheng Y, Wong J, Vertatschitsch E, and Mate TP. (2005). Accuracy of a wireless localization system for radiotherapy. *Int J Radiat Oncol Biol Phys*, 61(3), 933–937

Bank MI and Timmerman R. (2002). Superimposition of beams to vary shot size in gamma knife stereotactic radiosurgery. *J Appl Clin Med Phys*, 3(1), 19–25

Berbeco RI, Mostafavi H, Sharp GC, and Jiang SB. (2005). Towards fluoroscopic respiratory gating for lung tumours without radiopaque markers. *Phys Med Biol*, 50(19), 4481–4490

Cheung JY, Yu KN, Yu CP, and Ho RT. (1998). Monte Carlo calculation of single-beam dose profiles used in a gamma knife treatment planning system. *Med Phys*, 25(9), 1673–1675

D'Souza WD, Naqvi SA, and Yu CX. (2005). Real-time intra-fraction-motion tracking using the treatment couch: A feasibility study. *Phys Med Biol*, 50(17), 4021–4033

Deng J, Guerrero T, Ma CM, and Nath R. (2004). Modelling 6 MV photon beams of a stereotactic radiosurgery system for Monte Carlo treatment planning. *Phys Med Biol*, 49(9), 1689–1704

Deng J, Ma CM, Hai J, and Nath R. (2003). Commissioning 6 MV photon beams of a stereotactic radiosurgery system for Monte Carlo treatment planning. *Med Phys*, 30(12), 3124–3134

Dieterich S. (2005). Dynamic tracking of moving tumors in stereotactic radio-surgery. In: *Robotic Radiosurgery*, ed. by Mould RF, (The CyberKnife Society Press, Sunnyvale), pp. 51–63

Ding GX and Yu CW. (2001). A study on beams passing through hip prosthesis for pelvic radiation treatment. *Int J Radiat Oncol Biol Phys*, 51(4), 1167–1175

Fu D and Kuduvalli G. (2006). Enhancing skeletal features in digitally reconstructed radiographs. In: *Medical Imaging 2006: Image Processing*, ed. by Reinhardt JM and Pluim JP, (The International Society for Optical Engineering, San Diego), Abstract 61442M

Fu D, Kuduvalli G, Maurer CJ, Allision J, and Adler J. (2006). 3D target localization using 2D local displacements of skeletal structures in orthogonal X-ray images for image-guided spinal radiosurgery. *Int J CARS*, 1(Suppl 1), 198–200

Gerszten PC, Ozhasoglu C, Burton SA, Vogel W, Atkins B, Kalnicki S, and Welch WC. (2003a). Evaluation of CyberKnife frameless real-time image-guided stereotactic radiosurgery for spinal lesions. *Stereotact Funct Neurosurg*, 81 (1–4), 84–89

Gerszten PC, Ozhasoglu C, Burton SA, Vogel WJ, Atkins BA, Kalnicki S, and Welch WC. (2003b). Cyberknife frameless real-time image-guided stereotactic radiosurgery for the treatment of spinal lesions. *Int J Radiat Oncol Biol Phys*, 57(Suppl. 2), S370–371

Groh BA, Siewerdsen JH, Drake DG, Wong JW, and Jaffray DA. (2002). A performance comparison of flat-panel imager-based mV and kV cone-beam CT. *Med Phys*, 29(6), 967–975

Hoisak JD, Sixel KE, Tirona R, Cheung PC, and Pignol JP. (2004). Correlation of lung tumor motion with external surrogate indicators of respiration. *Int J Radiat Oncol Biol Phys*, 60(4), 1298–1306

Jaffray DA, Siewerdsen JH, Wong JW, and Martinez AA. (2002). Flat-panel cone-beam computed tomography for image-guided radiation therapy. *Int J Radiat Oncol Biol Phys*, 53(5), 1337–1349

Kavanagh BD, Ding M, Schefter TE, Stuhr K, and Newman FA. (2006). The dosimetric effect of inhomogeneity correction in dynamic conformal arc stereotactic body radiation therapy for lung tumors. *J Appl Clin Med Phys*, 7(2), 58–63

Keall PJ, Cattell H, Pokhrel D, Dieterich S, Wong KH, Murphy MJ, Vedam SS, Wijesooriya K, and Mohan R. (2006). Geometric accuracy of a real-time target tracking system with dynamic multileaf collimator tracking system. *Int J Radiat Oncol Biol Phys*, 65(5), 1579–1584

Keall PJ, Siebers JV, Jeraj R, and Mohan R. (2003). Radiotherapy dose calculations in the presence of hip prostheses. *Med Dosim*, 28(2), 107–112

Kitamura K, Shirato H, Shimizu S, Shinohara N, Harabayashi T, Shimizu T, Kodama Y, Endo H, Onimaru R, Nishioka S, Aoyama H, Tsuchiya K, and Miyasaka K. (2002). Registration accuracy and possible migration of internal fiducial gold marker implanted in prostate and liver treated with real-time tumor-tracking radiation therapy (RTRT). *Radiother Oncol*, 62(3), 275–281

Kondziolka D, Maitz AH, Niranjan A, Flickinger JC, and Lunsford LD. (2002). An evaluation of the Model C gamma knife with automatic patient positioning. *Neurosurgery*, 50(2), 429–431

Kuo JS, Yu C, Petrovich Z, and Apuzzo ML. (2003). The cyberknife stereotactic radiosurgery system: Description, installation, and an initial evaluation of use and functionality. *Neurosurgery*, 53(5), 1235–1239

Kupelian PA, Forbes A, Willoughby TR, Wallace K, Manon RR, Meeks SL, Herrera L, Johnston A, and Herran JJ. (2007). Implantation and stability of metallic fiducials within pulmonary lesions. *Int J Radiat Oncol Biol Phys*, 69(3), 777–785

Laub WU and Nusslin F. (2003). Monte Carlo dose calculations in the treatment of a pelvis with implant and comparison with pencil-beam calculations. *Med Dosim*, 28(4), 229–233

Leksell L. (1951). The stereotaxic method and radiosurgery of the brain. *Acta Chir Scand*, 102(4), 316–319

Mihaescu C, Dieterich S, Testa C, Mocanu M, and Cleary K (2004). Electromagnetic marker tracking in the cyberknife suite: A feasibility study. *46th AAPM Annual Meeting*, Pittsburgh, PA, USA, July 25–29

Mu Z, Fu D, and Kuduvally G. (2006). Multiple fiducial identification using the Hidden Markov model in image guided radiosurgery. *Conference on Computer Vision and Pattern Recognition Workshop*, IEEE, June 17–22

Muacevic A, Staehler M, Drexler C, Wowra B, Reiser M, and Tonn JC. (2006). Technical description, phantom accuracy, and clinical feasibility for fiducial-free frameless real-time image-guided spinal radiosurgery. *J Neurosurg Spine*, 5(4), 303–312

Murphy MJ, Chang SD, Gibbs IC, Le QT, Hai J, Kim D, Martin DP, and Adler JR, Jr. (2003). Patterns of patient movement during frameless image-guided radiosurgery. *Int J Radiat Oncol Biol Phys*, 55(5), 1400–1408

Neicu T, Shirato H, Seppenwoolde Y, and Jiang SB. (2003). Synchronized moving aperture radiation therapy (SMART): Average tumour trajectory for lung patients. *Phys Med Biol*, 48(5), 587–598

Pishvaian AC, Collins B, Gagnon G, Ahlawat S, and Haddad NG. (2006). EUS-guided fiducial placement for cyberknife radiotherapy of mediastinal and abdominal malignancies. *Gastrointest Endosc*, 64(3), 412–417

Quinn AM. (2002). CyberKnife: A robotic radiosurgery system. *Clin J Oncol Nurs*, 6(3), 149, 156

Reichner CA, Collins BT, Gagnon GJ, Malik S, Jamis-Dow C, and Anderson ED. (2005). The placement of gold fiducials for cyberknife stereotactic radiosurgery using a modified transbronchial needle aspiration technique. *J Bronchol*, 12(4), 193–195

Ryu SI, Chang SD, Kim DH, Murphy MJ, Le QT, Martin DP, and Adler JR, Jr. (2001). Image-guided hypo-fractionated stereotactic radiosurgery to spinal lesions. *Neurosurgery*, 49(4), 838–846

Schlaefer A, Fisseler J, Dieterich S, Shiomi H, Cleary K, and Schweikard A. (2005). Feasibility of four-dimensional conformal planning for robotic radiosurgery. *Med Phys*, 32(12), 3786–3792

Schweikard A, Bodduluri M, and Adler J. (1998). Planning for camera-guided robotic radiosurgery. *IEEE Trans Rob Autom*, 14(6), 951–962

Schweikard A, Shiomi H, and Adler J. (2004). Respiration tracking in radiosurgery. *Med Phys*, 31(10), 2738–2741

Seiler PG, Blattmann H, Kirsch S, Muench RK, and Schilling C. (2000). A novel tracking technique for the continuous precise measurement of tumour positions in conformal radiotherapy. *Phys Med Biol*, 45(9), N103–110

Shirato H, Harada T, Harabayashi T, Hida K, Endo H, Kitamura K, Onimaru R, Yamazaki K, Kurauchi N, Shimizu T, Shinohara N, Matsushita M, Dosaka-Akita H, and Miyasaka K. (2003). Feasibility of insertion/implantation of 2.0 mm-diameter gold internal fiducial markers for precise setup and real-time tumor tracking in radiotherapy. *Int J Radiat Oncol Biol Phys*, 56(1), 240–247

Willoughby TR, Forbes AR, Buchholz D, Langen KM, Wagner TH, Zeidan OA, Kupelian PA, and Meeks SL. (2006). Evaluation of an infrared camera and X-ray system using implanted fiducials in patients with lung tumors for gated radiation therapy. *Int J Radiat Oncol Biol Phys*, 66(2), 568–575

Wu A, Lindner G, Maitz AH, Kalend AM, Lunsford LD, Flickinger JC, and Bloomer WD. (1990). Physics of gamma knife approach on convergent beams in stereotactic radiosurgery. *Int J Radiat Oncol Biol Phys*, 18(4), 941–949

Yamamoto M. (1999). Gamma Knife radiosurgery: Technology, applications, and future directions. *Neurosurg Clin N Am*, 10(2), 181–202

Yousefi S, Collins BT, Reichner CA, Anderson ED, Jamis-Dow C, Gagnon G, Malik S, Marshall B, Chang T, and Banovac F. (2007). Complications of thoracic computed tomography-guided fiducial placement for the purpose of stereotactic body radiation therapy. *Clin Lung Cancer*, 8(4), 252–256

Yu C, Main W, Taylor D, Kuduvalli G, Apuzzo ML, and Adler JR, Jr. (2004). An anthropomorphic phantom study of the accuracy of cyberknife spinal radiosurgery. *Neurosurgery*, 55(5), 1138–1149

Zhou T, Tang J, Dieterich S, and Cleary K. (2004). A robotic 3D motion simulator for enhanced accuracy in cyberknife stereotactic radiosurgery. In: *Computer Aided Radiology and Surgery*, (Elsevier, London, UK), pp. 323–328

Chapter 17

Radiation Oncology

David Jaffray, Jeffrey Siewerdsen, and Mary Gospodarowicz

Abstract

Radiation and surgical oncology share the common drive for localized intervention and minimal side-effects. These two disciplines are converging in their search for minimally invasive approaches to achieve this objective. New techniques have recently been developed to localize and characterize oncologic targets, and as target localization techniques and treatment approaches have become more precise, the planning and guidance tools for radiation oncology and surgical therapies have converged. Imaging also provides the opportunity to provide feedback relating to the progress of the treatment to the oncologist. This chapter discusses the nature of the cancer intervention philosophy, reviews technological advances in the use of imaging to guide radiation therapy, highlights the potential for fusion of therapies (i.e., surgery and radiation) through the use of image-guidance, and identifies trends for integration of image-guidance approaches in the community.

17.1 Introduction

Oncology is a rapidly evolving field with great promise for both existing and novel forms of localized cancer therapy. At the forefront of this evolution are the development of exquisite characterization of the target *in situ* and the adaptation of imaging technologies to the treatment context.

The advances in diagnostic imaging have increased the sensitivity and specificity for target detection and characterization, which has heightened the interest in conformal targeting of the disease tissues for reduced toxicity. It can be expected that the continued developments in diagnostic imaging will drive this dynamic with growing pressure in the development of minimally invasive approaches to intervention. This chapter reviews the mechanisms and trends for image guidance adoption in the community, after a brief introduction to the nature of the cancer intervention philosophy.

T. Peters and K. Cleary (eds.), *Image-Guided Interventions.*
© Springer Science + Business Media, LLC 2008

17.2   Oncological Targets and the Nature of Disease Management

Successful treatment of localized cancer targets poses a complex and challenging problem. From earliest records, the disease is characterized by its remarkable invasive entanglement in the surrounding normal tissues. The desire to maintain function in the surrounding tissue is often compromised in exchange for confident eradication of the disease from its midst. The aggressive nature of cancer and its capacity to recur, given the slightest of residue, forces the clinician to take an approach of *confident eradication*. Compromising eradication in exchange for reduced toxicity is, in general, a temptation that is not to be taken lightly. More clearly, the concept of a partial intervention is not an approach that applies in such a disease where incomplete resection assures recurrence and leaves the patient with reduced capacity for further intervention.

The invasive nature of the disease has also evolved forms of therapy that can be safely applied under a range of presentations of the disease; from an isolated, accessible target to those intertwined with critical normal tissues. The two major forms of intervention are surgery and radiation therapy. Briefly, surgery involves tissue resection and radiation therapy involves ir- radiation of targets and normal tissues. The latter has the advantage of a preferential cyto-toxicity for cancerous cells relative to normal cells. These two therapies are applied in all varieties of localized cancer therapy and together often provide a complementing pair. No further description of these two interventions is required in this chapter; however, it is important to highlight the differences in the nature of their intervention, as it is relevant to the image guidance context and the ever-present tradeoff between eradi- cation of the tumor and preservation of normal tissue.

In both surgical and radiation intervention, a simplistic but relevant description of the objective is to eliminate cancerous cells. In the surgical context, the cancer cells are physically resected with the removal of tissue. This resection could be considered as a binary intervention – either the cells were removed or not. In the radiation therapy context, each irradiation or fraction has some probability of inducing the death of a cell.

This probabilistic nature of the intervention provides a much more forgiving instrument when geometric uncertainties are present. Furthermore, it allows the therapy to preferentially target cancer cells relative to their normal cells, even when the two cell types are colocalized in space – a situation in which geometric selection of the cancer cells from the normal cells would require a level of precision and accuracy on the scale of a single cell. It is this *selective nature* of the radiation intervention that has made it so attractive to the oncologist, as it allows for some level of selection when geometry does not provide the opportunity. To maximize the potential of this selection process, however, the therapy needs to be broken into a number of repetitive fractions; thereby allowing the differential cancerous cell kill to accumulate to a level of significance [Bernier et al. 2004].

Recent developments in image guidance have begun to shift this radiation therapy practice toward fewer fractions. In the case where the number of fractions is reduced to less than ten, it is referred to as hypofractionation, and often these few numbers of treatments are applied in a stereotactic approach [Leksell 1951]. The broad use of the stereotaxy label is somewhat historical and simply communicates the expectation that these treatments are delivered with a very high level of precision and accuracy, often through *calculated* coordinates of a target.

Recently, image-guided approaches, combined with hypofractionation, have been referred to stereotactic radiosurgery or SRS (in the cranium) and stereotactic body radiation therapy (SBRT). Using different fractionation schedules, radiation intervention has a nature of intervention that ranges from the selective to the ablative, where its mode of use is more akin to surgical intervention. It is of great relevance to this chapter to recognize that this remarkable transformation of radiation intervention was made possible by the development of image guidance methods that offer an appropriate level of precision and accuracy in the geometric targeting of the dose.

Development of more specific imaging techniques in the process of diagnosis will have a synergistic interaction with image guidance technology developments. Conventional radiation oncology practice has targeted the entire volume of the gross disease with uniform dose of a prescribed level. The identification of a subtarget that would represent elevated tumor burden or radiation resistant cells opens the opportunity to apply increased dose to this subregion. Such a dose-sculpting concept [Ling et al. 2000] is exciting, and is only feasible if methods can be developed for assuring the dose is delivered to this region, and not a surrounding normal structure. In this way, the advantages of improved target definition and the advancements in therapy targeting are both required if the full benefit of image-based target characterization is to be exploited for the benefit of the patient.

17.3   Imaging and Feedback in Intervention

17.3.1   Formalisms for Execution of Therapy

The development of image guidance in the context of radiation therapy has been substantially accelerated by the creation of a robust lexicon for communicating the intent of the therapeutic intervention, formalizing the description of the *prescription*. The International Commission of Radiological Units (ICRU) has provided a forum for the generation of standardized methods of prescribing radiation therapy [Measurements 1993, 1999].

The evolution of the ICRU Reports #50 and #62 over the past 20 years has been an important "structural breakthrough" in the development of image guidance as it is currently practiced in radiation oncology. The documents created a nomenclature that allowed the dosimetric and geo-metric objectives of the radiation intervention to be communicated from the clinician to the rest of the treatment team. It also introduced a principle that is central to the image guidance task; geometric constructs or *margins* that explicitly accommodate the technical challenge of colocalizing the radiation dose distribution with respect to the tumor and normal tissues within the human body, over the many fractions of radiation treatment. The formaliza-tion of this margin concept has provided a fulcrum for the advancements of image guidance technologies by clarifying that component of the interven-tion is a by-product of imperfections or incapacity in the fidelity of the delivery scheme. The reduction of these margins has become a focus of the community, as they are directly associated with excess toxicity and, there-fore, constraints on dose escalation of increased cure. Some of the elements of the ICRU formalism employed in radiation oncology are presented in (Fig. 17.1).

The volume of irradiation described by the planning target volume (PTV) can be contrasted against the supporting clinical target volume to illustrate the penalty associated with geometric uncertainties in the delivery of therapy. The methods employed to characterize uncertainty in the sur-gical context have been largely restricted to registration errors related to points in space employed for registration and for targeting [Fitzpatrick et al. 1998]. The development of a formalism in support of surgical intervention is an objective that would assist in the rational deployment of image guidance across the oncology field.

17.3.2   Dimensions of an Image-Guided Solution for Radiation Therapy

The selection or development of an appropriate image guidance solution is a complex process that typically contains compromises between clinical object-tive, availability of technology, efficiency, and manpower [Jaffray et al. 2005]. The simple development of an imaging method falls far short of the successful implementation of improved accuracy and precision in inter-vention. The following list identifies some of the many factors that must be considered in establishing an image guidance solution:

1. Clinical objective (targeting/normal tissue sparing)
2. Structures of interest (target/surrogates, normal structures)
3. Desired level of geometric precision and accuracy
4. Residual uncertainties to be managed (e.g., through the use of margins in RT)
5. Method of intervention (constraints, degrees of freedom)

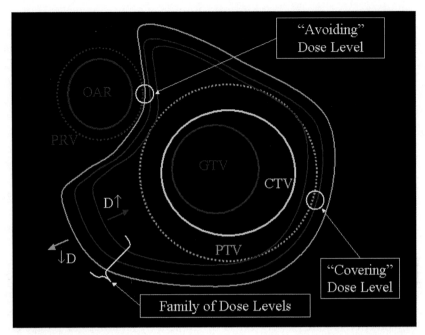

Fig. 17.1. An illustration of the ICRU constructs employed in the prescription and design of radiation therapy. The *gross tumour volume* (GTV) represents the component of the disease wherein imaging methods can be employed to characterize its three-dimensional morphology. The *clinical target volume* (CTV) accommodates the fact that clinical knowledge of the disease supports treating volumes that exceed the "imageable" volume based upon suspicion of microscopic disease extension into the surrounding tissues. It is often the case that GTV and CTV volumes will be prescribed different dose levels (although not reflected in this illustration). In addition to the target volumes, organs at risk (OAR) constrain the placement of dose. These structures are critical to function and have a sensitivity to the radiation. The dotted volumes (*planning target volume* or PTV and *planning risk volume* or PRV) are constructs employed in the design of the therapy. These constructs are generated specifically to accommodate the geometric targeting uncertainties of radiation delivery process. As "volumes" they do not reflect any specific tissues, nor are they related to any volume within the patient. Their purpose is to represent the geometric inaccuracy and imprecision in overall process. The margins between CTV and PTV (or OAR and PRV) are sometimes referred to as "safety margins," as they assure cover and avoidance of the various anatomical volumes. A simple dose distribution has been overlaid (i.e., Family of Dose Levels) to illustrate the selection of the "red" dose level for coverage of the PTV volume and the verification that the "orange" dose level does not reach the OAR. The determination of appropriate safety margins is a challenging element of radiation therapy and it requires an understanding of the sensitivity of the structure to dose variation, the magnitude of the dose gradient at that location, and prior knowledge of the geometric uncertainties in actual CTV and OAR locations over the course of therapy. Typically, this information is generated for a population of patients and a specific treatment technique

6. Gradients in the intervention (dose, ablation)
7. Strength of surrounding surrogates (bone, skin)
8. Consideration of implanted markers as surrogates of target/normal structure
9. The length of the procedure of number of fractions for which guidance is required
10. Available treatment capacity (treatments/hour) on treatment system
11. Application for all or some patients
12. Identification of individuals responsible for development
13. Identification of individuals responsible for commissioning and performance characterization
14. Identification of individuals responsible for performing quality assurance on the system and periodic verification of performance
15. Development of a structure for delegation of responsibility with respect to measurement, analysis, decision, and operation.

These factors highlight the scope of the problem, with issues reaching into the domains of clinical operations, training of staff, and delegation of responsibility. The development of clinical image guidance solutions in oncology practice requires a very broad investment by a number of groups and disciplines. Experience in radiation oncology has demonstrated that effective deployment has even required the development of education programs to bring all the disciplines into the process and to clarify the relative roles these disciplines play in the image guidance paradigm. It is likely that similar investments will be necessary in the surgical context if these advances are to become efficient and broadly applied.

17.3.3 Image Guidance Technologies in Radiation Oncology

The localized nature of the intervention in radiation therapy clearly requires some level of targeting or guidance. Conventional approaches have largely relied on the use of external skin marks for the routine positioning of patients for radiation delivery. Typically, a patient will be imaged using either radiographic or CT methods to determine the location of internal targets. During this process, external reference marks are drawn or tattooed onto the patient's skin. In addition to these marks, anatomical reference points (e.g., sternal notch, scar, umbilicus) will also be documented to reinforce the marks over the course of delivery.

Once the treatment plan is complete, the patient will be positioned for their daily treatment using these reference marks by aligning them to a set of orthogonal lasers located in the treatment room. The lasers beams (typically 5–7) are refracted to generate planes that all intersect at the isocenter of the treatment machine with a tolerance of better than 2 mm [Kutcher et al. 1994]. This isocentre is the point in space at which all treatment beams intersect regardless of the angle of the gantry or couch. It has long been understood that the use of skin-based surrogates for internal target positioning introduces significant geometric inaccuracies in the placement of dose within the body, but imaging methods to resolve this have been slow (decades) in development.

The past 20 years have seen steady improvements in this regard with initial efforts focused on the development of "portal imaging," that is, the use of the radiographic properties of the treatment beam to visualize the internal anatomy and, more recently, a variety of volumetric imaging technologies used in addition to portal imaging to improve visualization and allow 3D assessment of target and normal tissues (Fig. 17.2).

The past 15 years have seen dramatic advances in portal imaging technology. The introduction of the Kodak ECL film system and the development of computed radiography (CR) systems have improved the quality of the images produced with these systems. Munro [1999] provides an excellent review of electronic portal imaging devices in the clinical setting and identifies the current status of the commercially available devices. The quality of images generated with these new devices is satisfactory at clinically acceptable imaging doses (2–8 cGy) and has sufficiently large field-of-view to cover most clinical fields. The images formed with these systems can not only guide the treatment, but can also verify the shape and orientation of the treatment field [Schewe et al. 1998].

Visualizing surrogates of target position and the edge of the treatment field in the same image has made the portal imaging approach extremely robust and relatively easy to integrate into clinical practice. Portal filming can be used as a robust source of data for off-line correction schemes and many of the early feasibility studies on the implementation of off-line correction strategies were tested on portal film based measurements. Electronic portal imaging devices (EPIDs) have spurred the development of online repositioning strategies, as well as provided a wealth of data for support of off-line approaches. The continued development of portal imaging technologies will drive reduced imaging doses and permit more frequent imaging in support of both online and off-line strategies. These technological advances will provide robust systems for monitoring the quality of therapy. However, the inherently low subject contrast in the MV radiographs and restriction associated with imaging through the treatment port has been spurring the development of kilovoltage (kV) imaging systems on the medical linear accelerator. The future of guidance and verification in radiation therapy will most likely be a hybrid of MV and kV technologies.

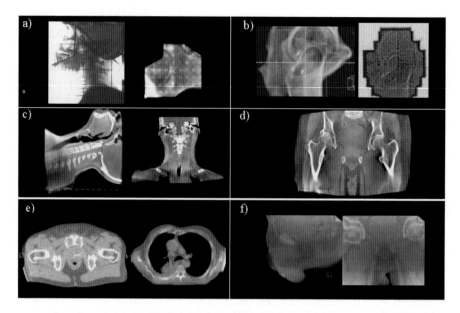

Fig. 17.2. Image guidance methods employed in radiation oncology practice generate a variety of image types. (**a**) Radiographic design of treatment fields using kV radiographs acquired in the planning stages were verified at the time of treatment using portal images. These images were generated with the actual treatment port and provided detection of bony anatomy and air passages. Often the images were reduced in quality by the interference of the treatment table, or trays used to hold the field-shaping blocks in place. (**b**) The development of electronic portal imaging systems allowed images to be detected at the time of treatment and adjustments in patient position could be made before each fraction. This online approach, combined with the implantation of markers, has become a very common method of achieving accurate and precise targeting of the prostate gland. The two images in frame (**b**) would be compared each day to estimate the necessary adjustment to the patient's position. (**c**, **d**) kV volumetric cone-beam CT images acquired on the treatment unit provides soft-tissue visualization without the use of implanted fiducials. The head and neck images shown in (**c**) can be compared with the portal images of the head and neck in the frame directly above. Similarly, the prostate dataset in frame (**d**) can be contrasted with the visualization of prostatic anatomy in the portal image on the right of frame (**b**). Soft-tissue imaging with the megavoltage treatment beam has been progressing well. MV CT from the Tomotherapy platform are shown in frame (**e**) and MV cone-beam CT images from the Siemens MVision system are shown in frame (**f**)

17.3.3.1   Kilovoltage Radiography and Fluoroscopy for Bone and Implanted Surrogates

There have been many embodiments of kV radiography and/or fluoroscopy integrated with the radiation therapy treatment device [Shirato et al. 2000]. Figure 17.3 illustrates direct integration of kV X-ray sources as proposed by multiple investigators. Others have proposed attaching a kV X-ray tube to the gantry and achieving MV and kV source coincidence by a gantry rotation or table translation [Biggs et al. 1985; Drake et al. 2000]. Developments have also proceeded in the construction of room-based kV imaging systems [Raaymakers et al. 2004]. Both approaches are designed to localize the bony anatomy or surrogate structures (markers, etc.) through acquisition of at least two radiographs that are acquired at two distinct and known angles. In the gantry-based approach, a single imaging system is used in conjunction with the gantry rotation to generate the necessary images. Room-based systems typically include a minimum of two complete imaging systems (source and detector) and have been constructed with up to four separate systems. Kurimaya et al. [2003] use four systems to permit continuous stereo monitoring regardless of linear accelerator gantry angle. The types of detectors used in these systems range from conventional radiographic film, to image-intensifiers, to charge-coupled devices/phosphor screen-based systems, to large-area flat-panel detectors. The continued development of large-area, high-performance flat-panel detector technology can be expected to spur this approach in coming years. This is clearly demonstrated in the rapid dissemination of the Elekta Synergy System, the BrainLab Novalis unit, and Varian's OBI Systems as illustrated in Fig. 17.3.

17.3.3.2 Kilovoltage Computed Tomography (kVCT)

Dedicated radiographic imaging systems promise to revolutionize radiation therapy practice by increasing the precision with which the patient's bony anatomy can be positioned with respect to the treatment beam. These systems can also be extended to more mobile targets by implantation of fiducial markers directly in the targeted structures. The generality of this approach is limited, as it does not support visualization of adjacent dose-limiting normal structures. The advancement of a general solution for precision radiation therapy throughout the human body requires the capacity to visualize soft-tissue structures in the treatment context. There have been a number of volumetric imaging modalities proposed for this task, including, ultrasound (US) [Kurimaya et al. 2003], computed tomography (CT) [Court et al. 2003], and magnetic resonance (MR) imaging [Raaymakers et al. 2004].

17.3.3.3 Conventional CT in the Treatment Room

The placement of a conventional CT scanner in the treatment room with a known geometric relationship with respect to the treatment machine offers a feasible and robust approach to implementing CT-guided radiation therapy. Uematsu et al. have been developing this approach over the past 7 years [Simpson et al. 1982].

Currently, multiple manufacturers provide products of this type (e.g., Siemens' Primatom; Mitsubishi's accelerator in combination with a General

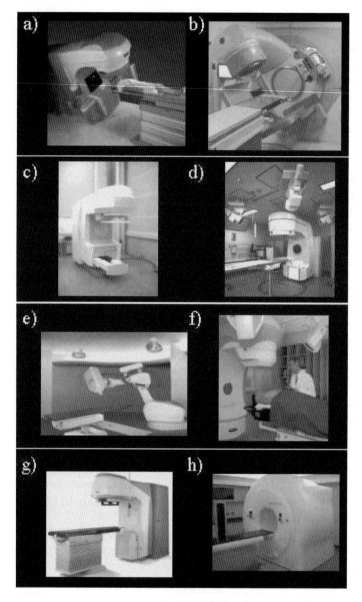

Fig. 17.3. There are numerous forms of image guidance capable treatment machines. The addition of kilovoltage (kV) imaging systems to radiation therapy treatment units has become commonplace. Typically, these systems either integrate the kV system on to the gantry for radiography and cone-beam computed tomography (CBCT) [(**a**) Elekta Synergy, (**b**) Varian Trilogy, (**c**) Siemens Artiste] or employ room-mounted radiographic systems [(**d**) Shirato et al., (**e**) Brainlab Novalis, (**f**) Accuray Cyberknife). Solutions that generate soft-tissue images of the patient using the treatment (MV) beam have also been developed [(**g**) Tomotherapy, (**h**) Siemens MVision]

Electric CT scanner, and Varian's ExaCT targeting system) [Brahme et al. 1987]. All systems are based upon a CT scanner placed in close proximity to the medical linear accelerator, allowing a single couch to be moved from an imaging position to the treatment position. These systems vary in the amount of motion and degrees of freedom required to move the patient from one position to the other. The commercially available systems minimize the amount of couch movement by translating the CT scanner gantry during acquisition. This has the perceived merit of avoiding differences in couch deflection at different couch extensions [Nakagawa et al. 2000].

While the installation of a second costly system in the treatment room is perceived to be somewhat inelegant, it has a clear advantage in that it leverages all the development that has been invested in conventional CT technology over the past 20 years, leading to unquestioned image quality and clinical robustness. Forrest et al. [2004] report a positional accuracy for the Mitsubishi-based system of under 0.5 mm, while Court et al. report an accuracy of 0.7 mm that can be reduced to 0.4 mm when using radio-opaque fiducial markers [Mosleh-Shirazi et al. 1998]. Such accuracy, in combination with excellent image quality, promises excellent management of interfraction setup errors and organ-motion. The issues of motion between imaging and delivery remain and needs to be accommodated through the appropriate selection of PTV margins.

17.3.3.4 Cone-Beam CT on the Medical Linear Accelerator

An alternative approach for CT-based image guidance is to integrate the CT imaging system directly into the mechanics of the medical linear accelerator, providing an integrated approach that echoes the objectives of Uematsu's device. Current medical linear accelerators are limited to approximately 360° of gantry rotation. This would limit a conventional CT approach on such a gantry to one slice per revolution. The IEC limits on gantry rotation rate (~1 rpm) would make imaging with such a platform prohibitive.

Recent advances in large area flat-panel detector technology offer the opportunity to implement cone-beam computed tomography [Groh et al. 2002], permitting a volumetric image to be acquired in a single revolution of the gantry structure. Pouliot et al. [2005] have been exploring this approach over the past 10 years. Figure 17.3 contains a photograph of the cone-beam CT systems offered by Elekta, Varian, and Siemens.

Advantages of such an approach are numerous, provided cone-beam CT image quality is sufficient to visualize soft-tissue structures of interest in the treatment context. This has been examined through numerous investigations [Lattanzi et al. 1998] and current flat-panel technology appears to provide a reasonable level of performance with continued performance enhancements anticipated. The cone-beam CT approach provides volumetric imaging in the treatment position and allows radiographic or fluoroscopic monitoring throughout the treatment procedure. Clinical images generated on the Elekta Synergy system are shown in Fig. 17.2. These images illustrate the system's capacity to visualize soft-tissue structures with substantial detail in all three spatial dimensions. The dose delivered in the imaging process was less than 3 cGy. An integrated imaging system with this level of spatial resolution and soft-tissue visualization capability has a significant potential to alter radiation therapy practice.

17.3.3.5 Megavoltage Computed Tomography (MVCT)

The need for accurate electron density estimates for treatment planning was the initial rationale for developing MVCT imaging systems and their use for patient and target structure localization was secondary. A number of investigators have been exploring the use of MV beams in CT imaging over the past 20 years [Molloy et al. 2004].

The Slice-Based Megavoltage CT

The initial development of a MV CT scanner for radiation therapy is attributed to Simpson et al. [Raaymakers et al. 2004]. Their approach was based upon a 4 mV beam and a single linear array of detectors. Brahme et al. proposed employing a 50 mV treatment beam for CT imaging in 1987 [Mageras 2005]. In their proposal, the high-energy beam would create contrasts comparable to a 300 keV due to the dependence of the pair production X-ray interaction process on atomic number.

Bijhold et al. [1992] were the first group to have reported clinical experience based upon MV CT images, using their single-slice system to treat 15 patients for metastatic and primary lung cancer. In this system, a single linear detector consisting of 75 cadmium tungstate crystals is mounted on the accelerator gantry and can be readily removed. The authors indicate that a spatial resolution of 0.5 mm and contrast resolution of 5% can be resolved with the system. Clinical imaging doses of 2.8 cGy were delivered during patient imaging and sample images are shown in Fig. 17.2. The most recent exploration of MV CT imaging has been in the development of the Tomotherapy™ treatment platform [Van Herk 2004].

MV Cone-Beam CT on the Medical Linear Accelerator

Limitations in gantry rotation have also spurred the development of cone-beam MV CT on a medical linear accelerator. With the exception of Mosleh-Shirazi et al. [Yan et al. 2005], these developments have come as a by-product of advances in commercial portal imaging technology. Groh et al. [Balter and Kessler 2007] have reported on the challenges associated with achieving high signal-to-noise performance at MV energies with low-efficiency flat-panel detector technology. Despite the low efficiency of these systems, the visibility of high contrast structures, such as air and bone, should be reasonable at clinically acceptable doses (~5 cGy). These systems have matured and are becoming commercially available [Kong et al. 2005]. Images acquired with such a system are shown in Fig. 17.2.

17.3.3.6 Ultrasound Approaches in IGRT

The US approach had been proposed for many years [Kong et al. 2006] and became commercially available in the late 1990s with the introduction of the BAT^{TM} system by Nomos Corporation [Blomgren et al. 1995]. Ultrasound has many features that make it a technology well-suited for IGRT applications. It is low-cost, volumetric, has no known side-effects, is interactive in its use, and provides soft-tissue contrast that can challenge more expensive modalities such as CT or MR.

As in any technology, its strengths are also its weaknesses. The contrast-inducing reflections limit the depth of targets to which the modality has been applied and the need for acoustic coupling requires robust physical contact between the probe and the patient's external contour. The ultrasound images are formatted in 3D using an US probe position sensor (either mechanical or optical) and visualization software. The coordinate system of the resulting 3D US dataset is located in treatment reference frame and can be registered to the planning CT dataset through alignment with contours from the planning process. The discrepancy after alignment reflects the appropriate correction to be applied to patient position. The potential of disturbing the target location during imaging has been an area of investigation [Timmerman et al. 2005]. More recent studies provide an excellent review of the relative performance of US-based approaches in targeting of the prostate gland [Purdie et al. 2007]. The low-cost of the technology, its ease of integration, and its ability for real-time monitoring of soft-tissue structures suggest that this technology has a future in radiation therapy for both planning [Keall et al. 2006] and localization.

17.3.3.7 Developments in MR-Guided Radiation Therapy

The high contrast and noninvasive nature of magnetic resonance (MR) imaging has prompted the development of MR-guided radiation therapy systems [Purdie et al. 2006]. These systems seek to exploit the remarkable gains in MR engineering (in particular active shielding) made over the past several years to allow integration of the significant electromechanical elements of a medical linear accelerator into the treatment room. Alternatively, the use of Cobalt-60 sources has been suggested to further reduce the technical challenges.

The merits of these systems are arguably their ability to produce images of the internal anatomy during radiation delivery, and without additional imaging dose associated with X-ray based approaches. The selection of higher field systems would even offer benefits for improved identification of targets at the time of treatment or assessment of therapy induced biological changes. To date, no MR-guided systems have been constructed; however, it is likely that prototypes will be available in the next few years.

17.4   Image-Guided Applications in Radiation Oncology

The growth of image guidance technologies have allowed new treatment approaches to be developed, and existing treatment methods to adopt image-guided approaches. In the following section, methods of oncology intervention that rely on image guidance approaches in the treatment context are described. The intention is not to provide a comprehensive description of these applications, but rather highlight a number of interesting models.

The past 5 years have seen a dramatic increase in the use of formalized, quantitative image guidance approaches in routine radiation therapy practice [Vicini et al. 2005]. While the technologies can be readily applied to various clinical problems, it is most informative to highlight specific clinical applications and comment on the clinical rationale. It is important to note that the advances in image guidance in radiation therapy have been made possible by substantial advances in 3D planning software and the availability of state-of-the-art imaging in the characterization of the target and normal tissues.

17.4.1   Prostate Cancer: Off-Line and Online Models

The past 10 years have seen a sharp increase in image guidance approaches being applied to radiation therapy of prostate cancer. This effort has been part of the broad initiative of dose escalation for increased probability of cure. The dose to the prostate has gone from 66 Gy delivered to simple, nonconformal volumes, to over 80 Gy with highly conformal approaches based upon methods that modulate the intensity of the treatment beam. This dose escalation has heightened the concerns regarding the volume of normal tissues irradiated with particular concern for the dose delivered to the rectal wall. The implementation of image guidance approaches allows confident reduction of the PTV margins and thereby reduction in the volume of normal tissue receiving the therapeutic dose level [Baglan et al. 2003].

Portal imaging approaches allowed bony anatomy to be localized on a routine basis with corrections for systematic errors in treatment setup [White in press; White et al. 2007]. However, the motion of the prostate gland relative to boney anatomy [Islam et al. 2006] is now a recognized and well-documented factor determining the size of the PTV margin [Pisters et al. 2007].

Schemes to accommodate the systematic errors in gland location relative to bony anatomy have been matured using off-line repeat CT imaging with excellent success [Ward et al. 2004]. An alternative to the off-line approach is to image every day and correct for any variations in prostate location by adjustments to the treatment couch. This approach requires visualization of the prostate gland or reasonable soft-tissue surrogate. Such approaches have been effected in many institutions using portal imaging in combination with implanted fiducial (typically gold) markers within the gland prior to the start of therapy [Davis et al. 2005].

This approach allows fairly straightforward interpretation of the marker location and appropriate adjustment in patient position through simple couch translations. Often these approaches are deployed with threshold for adjustment (e.g., no corrections for displacements less than 3 mm) to minimize the number of adjustments, and prevent interventions that are less than the precision of the adjustment. Developments in soft-tissue imaging in the treatment room (e.g., cone-beam CT, Tomotherapy megavoltage CT, and ultrasound) are allowing the soft-tissue anatomy to be targeted directly without the need for fiducials. These approaches have been receiving mixed reviews and there continue to be concerns with regard to consistency of interpretation [Griffin et al. 2007].

Despite these concerns, it can be concluded that growth in the use of these approaches will continue as image quality and confidence in interpretation improves. The merits of soft-tissue guidance approaches include the absence of fiducial placement and the opportunity to track the dose accumulation in surrounding normal tissues. A major challenge in the use of soft-tissue guidance is in the determination of the appropriate intervention under conditions of target or normal tissue deformation. This is currently an area of research and development within the radiation therapy community [O'Sullivan 2007].

17.4.2 Stereotactic Body Radiation Therapy (SBRT) for Cancer of the Lung

Radiation therapy of cancerous lesions in the lung has demonstrated poor outcomes and driven the pursuit of dose escalation. Recent studies are demonstrating the potential clinical gains associated with increasing the applied dose [Bilsky 2005]. However, concerns regarding toxicity continue to constrain dose escalation [Bilsky 2005]. The dependence of lung toxicity on dose and volume makes the lung a clinical site for which increased precision and accuracy would offer further pursuit of dose escalation provided toxicity is limited. However, the technical challenges associated with maintaining high precision and accuracy over the multiple fractions (20+) of conventional dose regimen (~2 Gy/Fx) is forbidding. The past several years have seen significant interest and success in the treatment of early stage lung cancer using stereotactic methods.

As the name implies, the targeting of the radiation dose to the lesion is achieved through 3D localization at the time of treatment. Early pioneers in this approach, such as Kim et al., [2001] have employed a body frame to provide Cartesian referencing of the target within the body at the time of treatment. This frame is to be replaced for each of the few (1–4) fractions delivered. This low number of fractions is the basis for the "hypo"-fractionation label.

Similar hypo-fractionated approaches were developed in Japan during the late 1990s [Siewerdsen et al. 2005] demonstrating the feasibility of these methods using image guidance. The past 5 years have seen maturation of clinical evidence to support these approaches both in terms of benefit and feasibility of applying this approach in the broader community [Wright et al. 2006; Yenice et al. 2003]. The recent completion of the RTOG #0236 clinical trial represented the first multiinstitutional trial of this kind in the North American setting (3 fractions at 20 Gy/Fx). Letourneau et al. [2007] have reported on the employment of cone-beam CT methods in the targeting of these lesions and highlighted inaccuracies in targeting based on boney anatomy alone.

The development of 4D CT methods (Fig. 17.4) have allowed characterization of the respiration-induced movement of these targets in 3D [Ekelman 1988]. This allows development of patient-specific motion profiles and corresponding planning target volumes [Gospodarowicz and O'Sullivan 2003], as well as the development of tracking and gating methodologies [Siker et al. 2006]. The use of SBRT in the lung is likely to increase dramatically over the next few years, given the clinical outcomes and the development of image-guided delivery solutions that are capable of assuring target coverage.

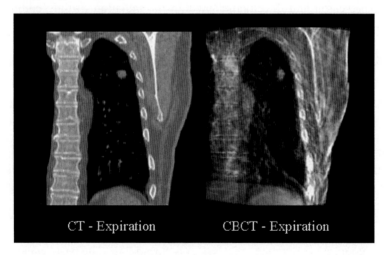

CT - Expiration   CBCT - Expiration

Fig. 17.4. Cone-beam CT guided radiation therapy of lung targets allows soft tissue targeting at the time of treatment. The image on the left illustrates the visibility of the lesion on conventional 4D CT imaging (expiration phase). The image on the right is the same breathing phase, but acquired at the time of treatment using 4D cone-beam CT. The use of images such as these for online guidance is becoming more commonplace

17.4.3   Accelerated Partial Breast Irradiation

The treatment of post-lumpectomy breast cancer has traditionally included uniform coverage of the entire breast and chest wall, as well as a small portion of the underlying lung [Lee et al. 2006]. Recent developments in technological capacity have raised the potential to reduce the volume of irradiation in a selected subset of patients, and furthermore, the fractionation schedule is modified. The rationale for these changes includes convenience, cosmesis, reduced toxicity in surrounding structures, and radiobiological arguments of equivalent control. For example, patients would receive 38.5 Gy in 3.85 Gy/fraction delivered twice daily for 5 consecutive days. The clinical target volume includes the lumpectomy cavity, plus a 10–15 mm margin bounded by 5 mm within the skin surface and the lung–chest wall interface. The planning target volume (PTV) included the clinical target volume plus a 10 mm margin [Von Hippel et al. 1999]. The technical studies to support this level of conformality are maturing. Rosenberg [1999] has reported on the suitability of 10 mm margins in covering the target volume.

In this technique, conventional clinical setup is employed using evaluations performed using portal imaging techniques. These studies examined the mobility of surgical clips relative to bony anatomy to gain confidence in the portal imaging-based assessments. Recent developments in cone-beam CT have allowed evaluation of seroma coverage directly [Nusslin 1995]. This study found that conventional skin mark positioning was able to achieve reasonable levels of targeting accuracy (2–3 mm standard deviation in the mean in the population) and precision (2–3 mm standard deviation in an individual) over the 1 week course of therapy. For the application of online corrections, an action level for correction of errors of 3 mm was demonstrated to be appropriate with more stringent levels producing no further improvements in precision or accuracy.

Overall, these investigations demonstrated that skin-based positioning produced acceptable levels of precision and accuracy for the PTV margins employed (10 mm). The additional benefit of the method may be in the reduction of these volumes, or in the assessment of seroma coverage at the onset of therapy as part of the overall assurance of treatment quality. It should be noted that the imaging doses delivered in these studies are small; however, the benefits of improved geometric targeting needs to be evaluated with respect to the potential risks associated with increased imaging dose to the contralateral breast.

17.5   Image Guidance Approaches that Bridge Therapeutic Modalities

Image guidance approaches are developing across the many forms of oncology intervention with remarkably similar issues and solutions. These approaches share common issues of achieving precision and accuracy in the intervention for the purpose of limiting toxicity while assuring the success of the procedure. If the image-guided approaches are broadly successful, oncology intervention will become a carefully contemplated and meticulously executed series of interventions for the benefit of the patient. This type of execution opens the opportunity for the community to consider a much more coordinated form of cancer care that bridges the disciplines and binds them by the accurate record of intervention performed by their complementary discipline. The evolution of these steps will lead to the creation of intervention planning systems that bridge chemical, cellular, surgical, and radiation-based interventions.

17.5.1   The Optimal Intervention

In the following section, oncology treatment solutions that adopt a combined modality therapy approach with a dependence on image-guided methods are highlighted. The feasibility of these approaches is dependent on the elevated level of precision and accuracy that can be achieved with image guidance.

17.5.1.1   Preoperative Radiation Therapy in the Management of Sarcoma

The management of soft-tissue sarcoma (STS) is a rapidly evolving complex multidis-ciplinary activity. Recent studies have demonstrated the benefits for optimal combination of radiation therapy and surgery in some forms of STS. These investigations have demonstrated that the combination of preoperative radiation therapy followed by surgery permitted improved outcomes, with a penalty of post-surgical wound-healing complication. These observations raised the potential for a more conformal preoperative radiation intervention to minimize damage to normal structures that are supportive of the post-surgical recovery. To this end, a collaboration of surgeons, radiation oncologists, physicists, and therapists have implemented a novel practice for the management of STS that exploit all the elements of modern radiation and surgery (see Fig. 17.5). This approach hinges on a set of assertions:

1.   The anatomy critical to wound healing can be identified and segmented prior to radiation therapy
2.   The precision of therapy delivery allows minimal "safety margins" in the expansion of the CTV to the PTV
3.   The planning process can employ intensity modulated radiation fields to conform the dose to these volumes while simultaneously avoiding the avoidance structures

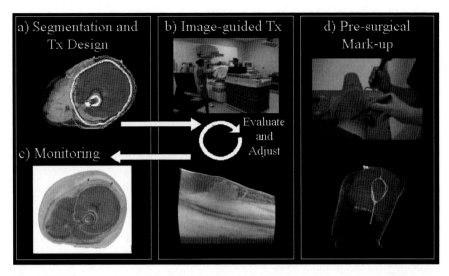

a) Segmentation and Tx Design   b) Image-guided Tx   d) Pre-surgical Mark-up

Evaluate and Adjust

c) Monitoring

Fig. 17.5. The treatment of patients with soft-tissue sarcomas at Princess Margaret Hospital (Toronto, Ontario, Canada) is a multidisciplinary effort with involvement of surgeons, radiation oncologists, therapists, and physicists. (**a**) Disease and normal structures are identified and include volumes of interest in post-surgical wound healing as well as more conventional targets. Avoidance is only feasible if therapy is delivered with sufficient precision and accuracy. (**b**) Online image guidance using cone-beam CT allows assurance of targeting performance while also monitoring the juxtaposition of normal and disease structures over the course of therapy. Following radiation therapy, the regions of elevated dose are marked on the patient prior to surgery using a cross-calibrated optical tracking tool and the dose map used in the treatment design. Future versions of this model will include accurate dose tracking over the course of therapy

4. The surgeon can have knowledge of the regions of applied radiation dose at the time of surgery to appropriately include the viable tissues for postresection wound closure

Each of these steps draws on the latest in technologies to make them possible so that:

1. Target and normal tissues are identified by surgeons and radiation oncologists on multi-modal (CT and MR) datasets
2. Inverse planning methods are employed to design the intensity modulated radiation fields
3. Daily online guidance using cone-beam CT assures target coverage and normal tissue avoidance
4. Preoperative planning using an optical navigation system is employed to map the high dose regions to the skin surface immediately prior to surgical intervention

To date, this has been applied in a population of patients (>20) treated in the sarcoma program at Princess Margaret Hospital, Toronto, Canada.

17.5.1.2 Post-Surgical Radiation Therapy of the Spine

It is estimated that between 5% and 10% of all cancer patients will develop metastatic spinal tumors. Metastasis of cancer to the spine is characterized by both loss in structural integrity of the involved vertebrae and significant pain. The use of radiation therapy in combination with surgical stabilization of the vertebrae is growing in practice.

The developments of MR imaging for characterization of these lesions have allowed optimization of the therapy intervention depending on various parameters. Bilsky [2005] describes a decision-making framework for appropriate combination of surgery and radiation depending on many factors, including mechanical stability and radiation sensitivity (e.g., radiation sensitive lymphoma primary vs. radiation resistant renal cell primary). The surgical techniques applied in these procedures have undergone advancements with the maturation of pedicle screws and the use of polymethyl methacrylate (PMMA) for stabilization of the vertebral body. Image guidance methods have been proposed in these procedures to increase the accuracy of screw placement. These methods use preoperative images in the design of the pedicle placement, and efforts to introduce intraoperative imaging in spine surgery are making progress. Siewerdsen et al. [2005] demonstrated the use of intraoperative cone-beam CT systems for placement of pedicle screws in an application of photodynamic therapy in the treatment of mock metastases in a porcine model.

The application of radiation therapy in the treatment of spinal lesions is dominated by the radiation sensitivity of the spinal cord itself. Conventional radiation therapy used for pain management would irradiate the entire region, lesion, and cord to approximately 30 Gy. If radiation dose to the cord is taken beyond an average 45 Gy or sub-volumes in excess of 50 Gy, radiation myelopathy is likely to develop. These dose thresholds prevented retreatment or even aggressive treatment to adjacent lesions due to the concern of overlap. Image guidance approaches are now allowing cord-avoiding treatments to be applied with confidence and allowing aggressive retreatments to the same or adjacent regions. This technique is illustrated in Fig. 17.6. Recent developments in image guidance technologies may allow these treatments to be delivered in a single fraction that is designed at the treatment unit.

17.6   Opportunities in Image-Guided Therapy: New Information Driving Invention

The growing use of image guidance is evident across all the modalities of cancer management. From the perspective developed over years of involvement of image guidance technologies and processes, there appear to be two important dynamics that will advance these approaches further:

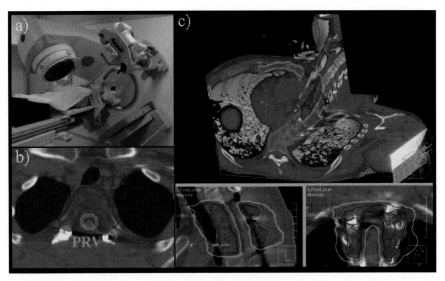

Fig. 17.6. Stereotactic radiation surgery of the spine allows conformality of the target while avoiding the dose-constraining spinal cord. (**a**) The use of image guidance approaches such as cone-beam CT to guide therapy allows use of small PTV margins [see inset (**b**)] and opportunities to spare the cord. (**c**) The use of intensity modulated radiation methods results in highly conformal dose distributions that satisfy the competing objectives of the prescription. While image guidance allows increased conformality, it also provides an accurate record of the treatment to allow for safe retreatment should the need arise

(i) the adaptation dynamic and (ii) the "user as innovator" dynamic as described by W. Lowrance in Ekelman [1988].

17.6.1 Image Guidance, Adaptation, and Innovation by the User

The "adaptation dynamic" is related to the rising availability of information about the patient during the course of intervention. Conventional medical practice is founded on the principles of prognostication [Gospodarowicz and O'Sullivan 2003]. In medical practice, determination of best intervention requires the "freezing" of various prognostic factors to allow timely and appropriate decision making regarding the course of therapy for an individual. Failure to "freeze" the many variables results in endless pursuit of more or "better" information to increase confidence in the predicted outcome, given a specified intervention. Simultaneously, failure to freeze the variables may also result in a loss of opportunity to intervene.

Identification of this fundamental element of medical practice is attributed to Hippocrates wherein he highlighted the importance of honesty in the process of observation and prediction of patient outcome. The development of methods of monitoring or assessing the patient over the course of therapy continues on this philosophy, but the quantity and quality of the information challenges the practice by contributing knowledge that may require *re-prognostication* of an individual patient's outcome during the course of intervention. The risk, of course, is that these modified predictions may be inaccurate. In the context of image guidance, there is nearly a continuous stream of new information being generated for purposes of improved targeting. Whether this information describes the shrinkage in lung tumor volumes during radiation therapy, the realization that complete resection of the tumor is not possible after initiating surgery, or the documented change in MR imaging signatures (e.g., apparent diffusion coefficient) after intervention, inconsistencies between this information and the observations used in the initial prognosis will drive adaptations to the intervention, and put immense pressure on the physicians' capacity to predict outcome for the individual at the onset of therapy. Furthermore, it will make trials-based assessment of the method difficult due to variations in clinical management. Regardless of whether we have the training and tools to deal with this new information, it has begun to arrive through the deployment of image guidance technologies and can be expected to increase. Furthermore, it can be anticipated that the integration of more advanced imaging tools will produce a greater temporal density of this information and significantly stress the traditional prognosis-treat-assess cycle that is at the foundation of modern healthcare.

The second dynamic of interest is that of the "user as innovator." While this concept is mature and highlighted by Lowrance in 1988, its relevance is elevated by the adaptation dynamic described above. Lowrance's comments are in the summary of an interesting and insightful publication entitled *New Medical Devices: Invention, Development, and Use* [Ekelman 1988] This publication arose from a National Academy of Engineering/Institute of Medicine symposium chaired by Robert W. Mann of MIT and Walter L. Robb of the General Electric Company.

In his review of the process of medical device development, Samuel Thier presents a strong case for the central role of the user in development of medical devices, as opposed to industry-initiated developments. Through a review of previous studies, he reinforces that the estimates of 80% of all device developments are instigated by the user. A leader in the identification of this process, E. von Hippel has recently reported commercial successes associated with leveraging this dynamic in a corporate strategy in 3M's medical–surgical division.

Lowrance's synopsis of the entire symposium reduces to a few identified needs and opportunities, wherein, he identifies the "most neglected step in the innovation scheme" as that of the "last long feedback loop: the one from the ultimate user community back to the start of the whole process." Given the importance of the role of the user in this process, what can be done to facilitate this dynamic?

17.6.2 Environments and Conditions that Support Innovations in Image-Guided Therapy

In terms of funding, there are a number of initiatives put forward in the past 10 years to foster health care innovation within the imaging and intervention communities. These include targeted funding opportunities as well as institutional initiatives. The U.S. National Institutes of Health (NIH) have initiated a number of calls for applications in the area of image-guided interventions in cancer. This has been primarily supported by the National Cancer Institute (NCI) with support of the recently formed National Institute of Biomedical Imaging and BioEngineering (NIBIB). The development of the Small Business Innovation Research (SBIR) and Small Business Technology Transfer (STTR) programs recognize the need for the researchers to take their developments to the commercial setting if they are going to have an impact. These are important initiatives that seek to address the need for funding and also provide mechanisms for the maturation of the technologies to product.

Institutional programs that foster the development of the "user" would be consistent with Lowrance's objectives. An approach that has been developed to better integrate the user within the process of innovation is that of the "clinician scientist." There has been over a decade of angst associated with the reduction in the participation of the clinician in scientific research. The past 10 years have seen dramatic increases in the establishment of dedicated clinician scientist support, with an expectation that these individuals contribute to both clinical and research activities. This has been operational in a number of health care systems throughout the world. For example, Singapore's Agency for Science, Technology, and Research works in collaboration with their Ministry of Health to fund 14 clinician scientists for both basic and translational work. In Canada, the Canadian Institute for Health Research (CIHR) has put forth a series of recommendations in a report entitled *The Clinician Scientist: Yesterday, Today, and Tomorrow.* Recommendations such as …develop a national framework (language) for what we mean by clinician-scientist… and …[collect] up-to-date statistics that speak to the composition of the clinician-scientist community… clearly indicate that they seek to maintain a level of clinician involvement in the national biomedical research agenda. It is quite clear from their report that the term "clinician" is not restricted to a physician. They go on to recommend that non-MDs be included in this definition and the development of research activities in this component of the healthcare system also be aggressively pursued. While it is evident that efforts are being made to improve clinician/user involvement in the research agenda, one can still ask "Is medical device development sufficiently supported through these programs?" What is the appropriate training for a clinician scientist if medical device development is to be a successful outcome? Are these clinician scientists providing the "last long feedback loop" for medical device development or are they preferring to focus on the basic science of the disease – an important contribution, but not targeted at device development. Given the multidisciplinary nature of intervention and the complexity of these interventions, it is difficult to imagine the Lowrance's user is actually an individual. Rather, it has become a team that collaborates for healthcare delivery and that this team needs to be fostered and supported in their pursuit of improved health care delivery. One could extend the concept of the clinician scientist to reflect the reality of current health care practice and seek to develop "clinical science teams." In the context of cancer, the relationship between physician and physical scientist (physicist) has been a long-standing and fruitful collaboration. In the context of radiation oncology, this relationship reaches back to the start of technology development in radiation oncology. For example, the collaboration of Henry Kaplan, M.D., and Edward Ginzton, Ph.D., led to the development of the medical linear accelerator at Stanford University and first treatment in 1957, and the development of the Gamma knife unit by the team of Lars Leksell, M.D., and Borje Larsson, Ph.D., in 1968. The changing nature of medical device technology suggests that collaborative relationships with computing and material sciences should be stimulated and fostered.

There have been a number of initiatives to establish infrastructure to foster clinical science teams in image guidance. Examples of which include the Center for Integration of Medicine and Innovative Technology (CIMIT) in Boston, USA (http://www.cimit.org/), the Centre for Surgical Technologies and Advanced Robotics (CSTAR) in London, Canada (http://www.cstar.ca), and the recently initiated Spatio-temporal Targeting and Amplification of Radiation Response (STTARR) program in Toronto, Canada (http://www.sttarr.ca/). Dedicated laboratories that allow the clinician (surgeon, radiation oncologist, physicist, therapist) to test and mature concepts before returning to the clinical environment are critical for the team to progress. Often the technologies employed in these activities are remarkably similar across treatment modalities. The Guided Therapeutics (GTx) Program is a new initiative at the University Health Network and this program seeks to provide a communication channel between disciplines (surgery, radiation, interventional radiology) and among researchers (clinicians, physicists, engineers, computer scientists) to avoid duplication of skill-sets and solutions. This program has harmonized its funding pursuits to develop a common laboratory environment for preclinical work with corresponding clinical facilities that will accept these novel approaches. While the infrastructure is usually perceived to be related to walls, devices, and the like, the greater challenge is in achieving support for these novel approaches in the demanding context of an active hospital with resource constraints. This particular challenge can only be addressed by engaging the senior management of the institution and articulating the value of innovation for the benefit of the patient and the hospital or health system as a whole.

Ultimately, if the initiative is to be successful, the team must reflect all stakeholders (e.g., administration, nursing, biomedical engineering, facilities) and cannot be restricted to the user, the scientist, or the physician.

17.7   Conclusion

The challenge of executing the localized cancer intervention continues to drive innovation in the field of oncology. The development of adaptable imaging systems that can integrate within the interventional setting is allowing these interventions to be applied under guidance for the benefit of both increased probability of cure, as well as the potential for reduced toxicity. The interventions of radiation therapy and surgery are by far the dominant form of local intervention in oncology and these two fields are rapidly adopting image guidance approaches. The "new information" provided in the context of image guidance will not only lead to increased accuracy in intervention, but also create a dynamic course for therapy in which interventions are modified or adapted to the individual patients response. These activities will put immense pressure on the current treatment paradigm and drive the development of devices, like new software tools, and the desire for more robust biological models to guide this adaptation. Despite these concerns, there is genuine potential for the image-guided approaches to become the standard of care. This transition will challenge the traditional educational and operational paradigms of oncology intervention and additional effort must be invested in the development of programs to facilitate the maturation and adoption of image-guided approaches.

Acknowledgments

The authors acknowledge the contributions of individuals who have contributed comments and figures to this chapter. Figure 17.2 contains images provided by Joerg Stein (Siemens Medical Systems), Gustavo Olivera (Tomotherapy, Inc.), and Peter Munro (Varian Medical Systems). The images in Fig. 17.4 have been provided by Drs. D. Moseley, T. Purdie, and A. Bezjak of the Princess Margaret Hospital (PMH). Figure 17.5 is provided by the PMH/Mt. Sinai Sarcoma Program. Figure 17.6 was provided by Drs. B. Millar and D. Letourneau, PMH. The authors thank the contributions of Dr. Jonathan Irish with respect to the discussions on cross-discipline collaboration in cancer intervention.

References

Baglan KL, Sharpe MB, Jaffray D, Frazier RC, Fayad J, Kestin LL, Remouchamps V, Martinez AA, Wong J, Vicini FA, Vicini F, Winter K, Straube W, Pass H, Rabinovitch R, Chafe S, Arthur D, Petersen I, and McCormick B. (2003). Accelerated partial breast irradiation using 3D conformal radiation therapy

(3D-CRT): A phase I/II trial to evaluate three-dimensional conformal radiation therapy confined to the region of the lumpectomy cavity for Stage I/II breast carcinoma. Initial report of feasibility and reproducibility of Radiation Therapy Oncology Group (RTOG) Study 0319. *Int J Radiat Oncol Biol Phys*, 55(2), 302–311

Balter JM and Kessler ML. (2007). Imaging and alignment for image-guided radiation therapy. *J Clin Oncol*, 25(8), 931–937

Bernier J, Hall EJ, and Giaccia A. (2004). Radiation oncology: A century of achievements. *Nat Rev Cancer*, 4(9), 737–747

Biggs PJ, Goitein M, and Russell MD. (1985). A diagnostic X ray field verification device for a 10 mV linear accelerator. *Int J Radiat Oncol Biol Phys*, 11(3), 635–643

Bijhold J, Lebesque JV, Hart AAM, and Vijlbrief RE. (1992). Maximizing setup accuracy using portal images as applied to a conformal boost technique for prostatic cancer. *Radiother Oncol*, 24, 261–271

Bilsky MH. (2005). New therapeutics in spine metastases. *Expert Rev Neurother*, 5(6), 831–840

Blomgren H, Lax I, Naslund I, and Svanstrom R. (1995). Stereotactic high dose fraction radiation therapy of extracranial tumors using an accelerator. Clinical experience of the first thirty-one patients. *Acta Oncol*, 34(6), 861–870

Brahme A, Lind B, and Nafstadius P. (1987). Radiotherapeutic computed tomography with scanned photon beams. *Int J Radiat Oncol Biol Phys*, 13(1), 95–101

Court L, Rosen I, Mohan R, and Dong L. (2003). Evaluation of mechanical precision and alignment uncertainties for an integrated CT/LINAC system. *Med Phys*, 30, 1198–1210

Davis AM, O'Sullivan B, Turcotte R, Bell R, Catton C, Chabot P, Wunder J, Hammond A, Benk V, Kandel R, Goddard K, Freeman C, Sadura A, Zee B, Day A, Tu D, and Pater J. (2005). Late radiation morbidity following randomization to preoperative versus postoperative radiotherapy in extremity soft tissue sarcoma. *Radiother Oncol*, 75(1), 48–53

Drake DG, Jaffray DA, and Wong JW. (2000). Characterization of a fluoroscopic imaging system for kV and MV radiography. *Med Phys* 27(5), 898–905

Ekelman KB. (1988). *New Medical Devices: Invention, Development, and Use*, (National Academy Press, Washington DC)

Fitzpatrick JM, West JB, and Maurer CR, Jr. (1998). Predicting error in rigid-body point-based registration. *IEEE Trans Med Imaging*, 17(5), 694–702

Forrest LJ, Mackie TR, Ruchala K, Turek M, Kapatoes J, Jaradat H, Hui S, Balog J, Vail DM, and Mehta MP. (2004). The utility of megavoltage computed tomography images from a helical tomotherapy system for setup verification purposes. *Int J Radiat Oncol Biol Phys*, 60(5), 1639–1644

Gospodarowicz M and O'Sullivan B. (2003). *Prognostic Factors in Oncology*, (UICC, Geneva, Switzerland)

Griffin AM, Euler CI, Sharpe MB, Ferguson PC, Wunder JS, Bell RS, Chung PW, Catton CN, and O'Sullivan B. (2007). Radiation planning comparison for superficial tissue avoidance in radiotherapy for soft tissue sarcoma of the lower extremity. *Int J Radiat Oncol Biol Phys*, 67(3), 847–856

Groh BA, Siewerdsen JH, Drake DG, Wong JW, and Jaffray DA. (2002). A performance comparison of flat-panel imager-based mV and kV cone-beam CT. *Med Phys*, 29(6), 967–975

Islam MK, Purdie TG, Norrlinger BD, Alasti H, Moseley DJ, Sharpe MB, Siewerdsen JH, and Jaffray DA. (2006). Patient dose from kilovoltage cone beam computed tomography imaging in radiation therapy. *Med Phys*, 33(6), 1573–1582

Jaffray DB, Bissonnette JP, and Craig T. (2005). X-ray imaging for verification and localization in radiation therapy. In: *Modern Technology of Radiation Oncology*, (Medical Physics Publishing, Madison, WI)

Keall PJ, Mageras GS, Balter JM, Emery RS, Forster KM, Jiang SB, Kapatoes JM, Low DA, Murphy MJ, Murray BR, Ramsey CR, Van Herk MB, Vedam SS, Wong JW, and Yorke E. (2006). The management of respiratory motion in radiation oncology report of AAPM Task Group 76. *Med Phys*, 33(10), 3874–3900

Kim KD, Johnson JP, and Babbitz JD. (2001). Image-guided thoracic pedicle screw placement: A technical study in cadavers and preliminary clinical experience. *Neurosurg Focus*, 10(2), E2

Kong FM, Hayman JA, Griffith KA, Kalemkerian GP, Arenberg D, Lyons S, Turrisi A, Lichter A, Fraass B, Eisbruch A, Lawrence TS, and Ten Haken RK. (2006). Final toxicity results of a radiation-dose escalation study in patients with non-small-cell lung cancer (NSCLC): Predictors for radiation pneumonitis and fibrosis. *Int J Radiat Oncol Biol Phys*, 65(4), 1075–1086

Kong FM, Ten Haken RK, Schipper MJ, Sullivan MA, Chen M, Lopez C, Kalemkerian GP, and Hayman JA. (2005). High-dose radiation improved local tumor control and overall survival in patients with inoperable/unresectable non-small-cell lung cancer: Long-term results of a radiation dose escalation study. *Int J Radiat Oncol Biol Phys*, 63(2), 324–333

Kurimaya K, Onishi H, Sano N, Komiyama T, Aikawa Y, Tateda Y, Araki T, and Uematsu M. (2003). A new irradiation unit constructed of self-moving gantry-CT and linac. *Int J Radiat Oncol Biol Phys*, 55, 428–435

Kutcher GJ, Coia L, Gillin M, Hanson WF, Leibel S, Morton RJ, Palta JR, Purdy JA, Reinstein LE, Svenssone GK, Weller M, and Wingfield L. (1994). Comprehensive QA for radiation oncology: Report of the AAPM Radiation Therapy Committee Task Group 40. *Med Phys*, 21, 581–618

Lattanzi J, McNeely S, Hanlon A, Das I, Schultheiss TE, and Hanks GE. (1998). Daily CT localization for correcting portal errors in the treatment of prostate cancer. *Int J Radiat Oncol Biol Phys*, 41(5), 1079–1086

Lee KC, Hall DE, Hoff BA, Moffat BA, Sharma S, Chenevert TL, Meyer CR, Leopold WR, Johnson TD, Mazurchuk RV, Rehemtulla A, and Ross BD. (2006). Dynamic imaging of emerging resistance during cancer therapy. *Cancer Res*, 66(9), 4687–4692

Leksell L. (1951). The stereotaxic method and radiosurgery of the brain. *Acta Chir Scand*, 102(4), 316–319

Letourneau D, Wong R, Moseley D, Sharpe MB, Ansell S, Gospodarowicz M, and Jaffray DA. (2007). Online planning and delivery technique for radiotherapy of spinal metastases using cone-beam CT: Image quality and system performance. *Int J Radiat Oncol Biol Phys*, 67(4), 1229–1237

Ling CC, Humm J, Larson S, Amols H, Fuks Z, Leibel S, and Koutcher JA. (2000). Towards multidimensional radiotherapy (MD-CRT): Biological imaging and biological conformality. *Int J Radiat Oncol Biol Phys*, 47(3), 551–560

Mageras GS. (2005). Introduction: Management of target localization uncertainties in external-beam therapy. *Semin Radiat Oncol*, 15(3), 133–135

Measurements ICoRUa. (1993). ICRU Report 50: Prescribing, recording and reporting photon beam therapy, (Measurements ICoRUa, Bethesda, Maryland, USA)

Measurements ICoRUa. (1999). ICRU Report 62: Prescribing, recording and reporting photon beam therapy, (Measurements ICoRUa, Bethesda, Maryland, USA)

Molloy JA, Srivastava S, and Schneider BF. (2004). A method to compare supra-pubic ultrasound and CT images of the prostate: Technique and early clinical results. *Med Phys*, 31(3), 433–442

Mosleh-Shirazi MA, Evans PM, Swindell W, Webb S, and Partridge M. (1998). A cone-beam megavoltage CT scanner for treatment verification in conformal radiotherapy. *Radiother Oncol*, 48(3), 319–328

Munro P. (1999). Megavoltage radiography for treatment verification. In: *The Modern Technology of Radiation Oncology*, ed. by Dyk JV, (Medical Physics Publishing, Madison, WI), pp. 481–508

Nakagawa K, Aoki Y, Tago M, Terahara A, and Ohtomo K. (2000). Megavoltage CT-assisted stereotactic radiosurgery for thoracic tumors: Original research in the treatment of thoracic neoplasms. *Int J Radiat Oncol Biol Phys*, 48(2), 449–457

Nusslin F. (1995). Relations between physician and physicist. Remarks from the viewpoint of the physicist. *Strahlenther Onkol*, 171(1), 1–4

O'Sullivan B. (2007). Personal Communication

Pisters PW, O'Sullivan B, and Maki RG. (2007). Evidence-based recommendations for local therapy for soft tissue sarcomas. *J Clin Oncol*, 25(8), 1003–1008

Pouliot J, Bani-Hashemi A, Chen J, Svatos M, Ghelmansarai F, Mitschke M, Aubin M, Xia P, Morin O, Bucci K, Roach M, III, Hernandez P, Zheng Z, Hristov D, and Verhey L. (2005). Low-dose megavoltage cone-beam CT for radiation therapy. *Int J Radiat Oncol Biol Phys*, 61(2), 552–560

Purdie TG, Bissonnette JP, Franks K, Bezjak A, Payne D, Sie F, Sharpe MB, and Jaffray DA. (2007). Cone-beam computed tomography for on-line image guidance of lung stereotactic radiotherapy: Localization, verification, and intrafraction tumor position. *Int J Radiat Oncol Biol Phys*, 68(1), 243–252

Purdie TG, Moseley DJ, Bissonnette JP, Sharpe MB, Franks K, Bezjak A, and Jaffray DA. (2006). Respiration correlated cone-beam computed tomography and 4DCT for evaluating target motion in Stereotactic Lung Radiation Therapy. *Acta Oncol*, 45(7), 915–922

Raaymakers BW, Raaijmakers AJ, Kotte AN, Jette D, and Lagendijk JJ. (2004). Integrating a MRI scanner with a 6 MV radiotherapy accelerator: Dose deposition in a transverse magnetic field. *Phys Med Biol*, 49(17), 4109–4118

Rosenberg LE. (1999). The physician-scientist: An essential–and fragile–link in the medical research chain. *J Clin Invest*, 103(12), 1621–1626

Schewe JE, Lam KL, Balter JM, and Ten Haken RK. (1998). A room-based diagnostic imaging system for measurement of patient setup. *Med Phys*, 25(12), 2385–2387

Shirato H, Shimizu S, Kunieda T, Kitamura K, van Herk M, Kagei K, Nishioka T, Hashimoto S, Fujita K, Aoyama H, Tsuchiya K, Kudo K, and Miyasaka K. (2000). Physical aspects of a real-time tumor-tracking system for gated radiotherapy. *Int J Radiat Oncol Biol Phys*, 48(4), 1187–1195

Siewerdsen JH, Moseley DJ, Burch S, Bisland SK, Bogaards A, Wilson BC, and Jaffray DA. (2005). Volume CT with a flat-panel detector on a mobile, isocentric C-arm: Pre-clinical investigation in guidance of minimally invasive surgery. *Med Phys*, 32(1), 241–254

Siker ML, Tome WA, and Mehta MP. (2006). Tumor volume changes on serial imaging with megavoltage CT for non-small-cell lung cancer during intensity-modulated radiotherapy: How reliable, consistent, and meaningful is the effect? *Int J Radiat Oncol Biol Phys*, 66(1), 135–141

Simpson RG, Chen CT, Grubbs EA, and Swindell W. (1982). A 4-MV CT scanner for radiation therapy: The prototype system. Med Phys, 9(4), 574–579

Timmerman RD, Forster KM, and Chinsoo CL. (2005). Extracranial stereotactic radiation delivery. *Semin Radiat Oncol*, 15(3), 202–207

van Herk M. (2004). Errors and margins in radiotherapy. *Semin Radiat Oncol*, 14(1), 52–64

Vicini F, Winter K, Straube W, Wong J, Pass H, Rabinovitch R, Chafe S, Arthur D, Petersen I, and McCormick B. (2005). A phase I/II trial to evaluate three-dimensional conformal radiation therapy confined to the region of the lumpectomy cavity for Stage I/II breast carcinoma: Initial report of feasibility and reproducibility of Radiation Therapy Oncology Group (RTOG) Study 0319. *Int J Radiat Oncol Biol Phys*, 63(5), 1531–1537

von Hippel E, Thomke S, and Sonnack M. (1999). Creating breakthroughs at 3M. *Harv Bus Rev*, 77(5), 47–57

Ward I, Haycocks T, Sharpe M, Griffin A, Catton C, Jaffray D, and O'Sullivan B. (2004). Volume-based radiotherapy targeting in soft tissue sarcoma. *Cancer Treat Res*, 120, 17–42

White E. Volumetric assessment of setup performance in accelerated Partial breast irradiation. *Int J Radiat Oncol Biol Phys*, (in press)

White EA, Cho J, Vallis KA, Sharpe MB, Lee G, Blackburn H, Nageeti T, McGibney C, and Jaffray DA. (2007). Cone beam computed tomography guidance for setup of patients receiving accelerated partial breast irradiation. *Int J Radiat Oncol Biol Phys*, 68(2), 547–554

Wright JL, Lovelock DM, Bilsky MH, Toner S, Zatcky J, and Yamada Y. (2006). Clinical outcomes after reirradiation of paraspinal tumors. *Am J Clin Oncol*, 29(5), 495–502

Yan D, Lockman D, Martinez A, Wong J, Brabbins D, Vicini F, Liang J, and Kestin L. (2005). Computed tomography guided management of interfractional patient variation. *Semin Radiat Oncol*, 15(3), 168–179

Yenice KM, Lovelock DM, Hunt MA, Lutz WR, Fournier-Bidoz N, Hua CH, Yamada J, Bilsky M, Lee H, Pfaff K, Spirou SV, and Amols HI. (2003). CT image-guided intensity-modulated therapy for paraspinal tumors using stereotactic immobilization. *Int J Radiat Oncol Biol Phys*, 55(3), 583–593

Chapter 18

Assessment of Image-Guided Interventions

Pierre Jannin and Werner Korb

Abstract

Assessment of systems and procedures in image-guided interventions (IGI) is crucial but complex, and addresses diverse aspects. This chapter introduces a framework for dealing with this complexity and diversity, and is based on some of the major related concepts in health care. Six assessment levels are distinguished in IGI. The main phases and components of assessment methodology are described with an emphasis on the specification and the reporting phases, and on the clear initial formulation of the assessment objective. The methodology is presented in a systematic order to allow interinstitutional comparison. Finally, we outline the need for standardization in IGI assessment to improve the quality of systems, their acceptance by surgeons, and facilitate their transfer from research to clinical practice.

18.1 Introduction

The use of image-guided interventions (IGI) may have an important influence on the decision and action-making processes before, during, and after surgery. For this reason, it is crucial to assess IGI systems rigorously. Assessment of IGI belongs to the domain of Health Care Technology Assessment (HCTA), which is defined as the "process of examining and reporting properties, effects and/or impacts of a system" [Goodman 2004]. The objective of the assessment is to increase the quality of an IGI system, to reduce risks of malfunctions or misuses, and to enhance customer and user satisfaction. Developers of IGI systems have the responsibility for assessing their systems and to make the results widely available. This chapter aims to provide a framework for the assessment of IGI systems with more focus on the engineering side rather than on the clinical side. The authors have gathered major assessment concepts in health care, according to their current knowledge and vision of the domain. Emphasis has been placed on the correct formulation of the assessment objective, and on the report of the assessment method and results. The latter is crucial in assessment as it provides users with proof of

T. Peters and K. Cleary (eds.), *Image-Guided Interventions.*
© Springer Science + Business Media, LLC 2008

added value, recommendations for optimal use, and an indication of possible risks.

The following statements regarding assessment and their application to IGI directly outline the *complexity and diversity of assessment*.

18.1.1 General Assessment Definitions

In general assessment methodology, it is usual to differentiate the concepts of *Verification*, *Validation*, and *Evaluation* [Balci 2003]. In product engineering, verification and validation are distinguished in the following way: verification is the confirmation, by the provision of objective evidence, that specified requirements have been fulfilled [ISO9000:2000], and it involves assessing that the system is built according to its specifications. Validation is the confirmation, by provision of objective evidence, that requirements for a specific intended use have been fulfilled [ISO9000:2000]. It is the assessment that the system actually fulfils the purpose for which it was intended. In software engineering, it also is usual to differentiate verification and validation from evaluation. Evaluation involves determining that the system is accepted by the end user and that it fulfils its specific purpose.

Efficacy and effectiveness both refer to how well a technology performs to improve patient health, usually measured by changes in one or more pertinent health outcomes. A technology that works under carefully controlled conditions, or with carefully selected patients under the supervision of its developers, does not always work as well in other settings, or as implemented by other practitioners. In HCTA, *efficacy* refers to the benefit of using a technology for a particular problem under ideal conditions, e.g., within the protocol of a carefully managed, randomized controlled trial involving patients, meeting narrowly defined criteria, or conducted at a center of excellence. *Effectiveness* refers to the benefit of using a technology for a particular problem under general or routine conditions, e.g., by a physician in a community hospital for different types of patients [Goodman 2004]. Beside parameters such as efficacy and effectiveness, *efficiency* can also be assessed by HCTA methods to include costs, economic conditions, and other factors.

18.1.2 Complexity of Procedures and Scenarios

IGI is generally used during *complex procedures*, and/or it makes them more complex, because it often integrates various hardware and software components into complex scenarios. Image processing is used intensively for registration, segmentation, and calibration. Each component is a potential source of uncertainties, which may result in errors. Performance of the whole IGI system strongly depends on the performance of each component. Assessment may, therefore, include the whole IGI system or one or more of its components. For example, performance and validity of each component may be studied separately, or the performance and validity of the whole system may be condidered as a single entity. Further uncertainties propagating inside the system also may be investigated.

18.1.3 Direct and Indirect Impact of IGI Systems

Diagnostic technologies have an *indirect* impact on surgery, whereas therapeutic technologies have a *direct* one. The impact of IGI may be both direct and indirect as (1) it can provide surgeons with diagnostic images and further information in the OR, and (2) it directly guides the surgeon during surgical performance by emphasizing areas to be targeted or avoided, and showing the trajectories of instruments. Both direct and indirect impacts should be studied.

18.1.4 Interdisciplinary Collaborations

Technical, clinical, social, economical, and ethical aspects are crucial in IGI assessment, which requires *interdisciplinarity* involving clinicians, computer scientists, natural scientists, ergonomists, and psychologists. The result of this is that different roles, languages, motivations, and methods come into play during assessment studies.

18.1.5 Human–Machine Interaction

Human–machine interaction in IGI is embedded in the surgeon–patient–machine triangle (Fig. 18.1).

In this triangle of the surgeon, the patient, and the IGI system, interactions occur between the three components. The surgeon performs surgery on the patient on the basis of a dedicated surgical procedure. The surgeon communicates with the IGI system through the human/machine

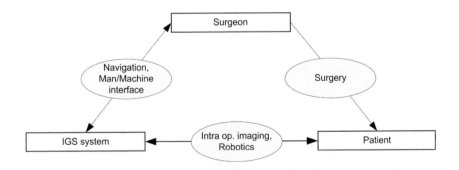

Fig. 18.1. The surgeon–patient–machine triangle in IGI

interface or with the displacement of a surgical tool tracked by a navigation system. In the opposite direction, the IGI system displays images or information to the surgeon. Information about the patient, such as his or her intraoperative images, can be sent to the IGI system. Alternatively, the IGI system may be used to guide a surgical robotic tool.

Table 18.1 The assessment levels for IGI

Levels		Assessed properties	Study conditions	Examples of criteria
Level 1	Technical system properties	Technical parameters	Laboratory	Technical accuracy and precision, latency, noise
Level 2	Diagnostic reliability (indirect assessment)	Reliability in clinical setting	Simulated clinical scenario, laboratory	Sensitivity, specificity, level of quality, level of trust
Level 2	Therapeutic reliability (direct assessment)	Reliability in clinical setting	Simulated clinical scenario, laboratory	Target registration error, safety margins, percentage of resection, cognitive workload
Level 3	Surgical strategy (indirect assessment)	Efficacy	Specific clinical scenario, hospital	Change of strategy, time
Level 3	Surgical performance (direct assessment)	Efficacy	Specific clinical scenario, hospital	Cognitive workload, situational awareness, skill acquisition, time, percentage of resection, histological result, pain, usability
Level 4	Patient outcome	Effectiveness	Routine clinical scenario, multisite clinical trials, meta-analysis	Morbidity (recrudescence), pain, cosmetic results
Level 5	Economic aspects	Efficiency	Multisite clinical trials, Meta-analysis	Cost effectiveness, time saving
Level 6	Social, legal, and ethical aspects	Social, legal, and ethical aspects	Meta-analysis, committees, recognized authorities	Quality of life issues

The degree of complexity of human/machine interaction is particularly high as the operation is often performed under extreme (time) pressure, and physical and physiological stress. In many IGI cases, the information flow is considerable, and the relevant data must be processed and condensed by the surgeon's brain.

18.2 Assessment Methodology

The complexity and diversity in IGI assessment outlines the importance of using a rigorous methodology for (1) specifying requirements and expected outputs of studies, and (2) precisely reporting objectives, methodology, and output of studies as already mentioned by The Global Harmonization Task Force (GHTF) [GHTF 2004]. This leads directly to the three main phases of assessment of an IGI system (Fig. 18.2).

In the **specification phase**, the *assessment objective* is clearly formulated (phase 1a in Fig. 18.2), the *study conditions* are defined (phase 1b), e.g., setting, criteria, data, as well as relevant assessment methodology, which all fulfil the assessment objective. The specification phase should be able to describe *who* is concerned in the assessment, *what* will be assessed, *what* is expected, in *which* domain or context it is to be assessed, *where* it is assessed, and *which* features will be assessed. Such a specification process results in a better and more manageable design of the assessment study. The *assessment method* is chosen according to the assessment objective and the study conditions. Descriptions of each component of the assessment method are fully included in the specification phase (phase 1c in Fig. 18.2). Good specification of the study phase allows proper measuring and computing as well as statistical analysis of data. Describing and specifying all necessary aspects of the assessment protocol before conducting the study enables correct assessment in accordance with the assessment objective.

In the **implementation phase**, the assessment study is performed (phase 2 in Fig. 18.2). The *assessment method* is strictly applied according to the previously defined *study conditions* for verifying the *assessment objective*. The outcome of phase 2 is the assessment results produced according to the previously defined and properly specified method.

The study documentation is written in the **reporting phase** (phase 3 in Fig. 18.2). The report needs to be well structured and describe assessment objective, study conditions, assessment method, and results to facilitate understanding and comparison of the results between different studies. The specification phase is outlined in the following sections.

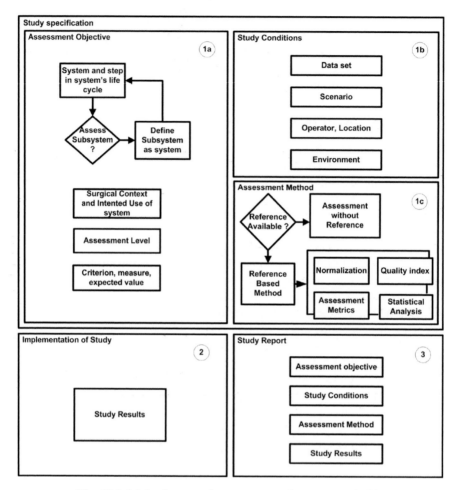

Fig. 18.2. Main phases and components of assessment in IGI

18.2.1 Assessment Objective

Clear and precise design of the *assessment objective* is emphasized as a crucial and required initial step for every assessment study [GHTF 2004; Goodman 2004]. For example, the assessment objective may be formulated as a hypothesis, in which case the assessment study aims to test this hypothesis.

Jannin et al. [2006] proposed a formalization of the assessment objective in medical image processing. Similarly, in IGI, the assessment objective needs to be rigorously formalized and specified before conducting assessment studies. It includes (Fig. 18.2, phase 1a) a precise description of the motivation for assessment, the description of the IGI system to be assessed, the targeted surgical context and intended use of the system, the corresponding assessment level (see later), criteria to be assessed and corresponding measure, and the expected results or performances. The assessment objective usually consists of comparing measured performance with that expected for a specific IGI system in specific study conditions, and with dedicated data sets. Performance of an assessment criterion is measured by the assessment metric applied to information extracted from the assessment data sets. Expected performance may correspond to a value or a model. Comparison may be performed using a statistical hypothesis test.

18.2.1.1 Motivation for Assessment

Starting from a high level, it is important to know the targeted consumer of the study, e.g., the developer of the system, the end-user, the manufacturer, an approval body, or a scientific society. Different needs require different methods. At this initial level, the consumer must have expressed his or her motivations and expectations.

18.2.1.2 Description of the System to be Assessed

It is important to clearly specify and describe the system to be assessed. Not only is the performance of the whole IGI system of interest, but also the performance of its components, such as a module for image to patient registration or tracking cameras as part of a navigation system. Assessment should occur both retrospectively for existing innovative products (e.g., systems or methods), and prospectively during the product life cycle. As mentioned in [GHTF 2004], assessment has to be performed throughout the *product life cycle*. Consequently, the time point along this life cycle and the associated state of the system needs to be described (e.g., whether the system is assessed after specification phase, design phase, or implementation phase).

18.2.1.3 Surgical Context and Intended Use of the System

One essential aspect in the definition of the *assessment objective* is the description of the surgical context in which the IGI system will be used and, therefore, in which the assessment will be performed. The *surgical context* can be considered as a surgical task performed by the surgeon for a targeted population of patients. It is usual to define as many surgical contexts as required and, consequently, to distinguish different corresponding assessment studies. For the chosen surgical context, the system to be assessed is used in a specific manner, which is defined as the *intended use* of the system.

18.2.1.4 Assessment Levels

In HCTA, the complexity and diversity of assessment is usually organised and managed through a hierarchy of levels [Fryback and Thornbury 1991; Goodman 2004; Chow and Liu 2004; Pocock 2004; Korb et al. 2006]. A similar assessment level hierarchy is also relevant and required in IGI (Table 18.1). According to this hierarchy, it is important to decide on the appropriate assessment level during the specification phase of an assessment study.

At **Level 1**, the *technical feasibility and behavior* of the system are checked. Level 1 aims to characterize the intrinsic performance of the system. It is usually the best level at which to verify how technical parameters influence the output of the system. Examples are accuracy or latency investigations, but also may be the impact of noise or the interference of signals or material. It is also the best level for assessing subcomponents of the system independently (e.g., 3D localization, trackers, uninterruptible power supplies, registration components, segmentation modules, or surgical instruments). This level is useful for better understanding possible surgical applications of the system. The clinical realism of the experimental conditions is not crucial, as phantoms and numerical simulations are used for assessment at this level. It often makes sense to perform the technical assessment before doing the assessment studies of Level 2, as Level 1 studies can be considered as verification as defined earlier, and Level 2 studies can be considered as validation as defined earlier.

At **Level 2**, the *diagnostic and therapeutic reliability* is assessed. The technical applicability and reliability of a system for a clinical setting is checked before clinical studies. IGI systems are assessed for their clinical accuracy, patient and user safety, and reliability in a realistic clinical setting context. The methods at Level 2 may include the process of a risk analysis [ISO-14971:2000], as risk analysis is a method to discover the inherent risks of a surgical device or new surgical method. *Diagnostic* and *therapeutic* reliabilities are distinguished, as IGI systems may have indirect and direct impact on surgery as discussed earlier. From this level, the realism is increased from the experimental environment to daily clinical environment at Level 3 and above.

At **Level 3**, the *efficacy* is assessed in clinical trials, including study of the indirect and direct impacts on surgical strategy and performance. Level 3 studies address assessment criteria dedicated to clinical reality, such as patient outcome, surgical time, or the surgeon's cog-nitive workload. Level 3 studies and above can be considered as evaluation, as defined earlier. Design and performance of such clinical trials require inter-disciplinary research groups of surgeons, psychologists, ergonomic scientists, and other related scientists.

It may not be straightforward to measure the outcome or added value of the indirect effects of some IGI systems, such as navigation and intraoperative imaging devices. Indirect effects on the surgical procedure can be assessed either:

1. By performing prospective assessment of therapeutic intent before and after the intervention
2. By asking the surgeons the hypothetical question: "What would you do for the patient, if the information source (navigation or intraoperative imaging) was not available?"
3. By requesting the effect retrospectively from the clinical records
4. By controlled trials in demo-scenarios, i.e., simulations of surgical complications that have to be solved with and without the information provided by the assessed equipment (based on Fryback [1991]).

At **Level 4**, the *effectiveness and comparative effectiveness* are assessed particularly in multisite clinical trials. Facing and addressing clinical assessment of IGI in terms of "large scale multisite randomized clinical trials" (RCT) is difficult for the following reasons: there is a high interpatient and intersurgeon variability that makes large clinical trials difficult; surgical and technological skills are disparate along the population of surgeons; RCTs with randomized assignment of patients mean that some have the opportunity to benefit from a potentially useful technology, which others do not, create a dilemma for surgeons who always want the best possible techniques for all their patients [Paleologos et al. 2000]. Furthermore, IGI technologies are still recent and long-term outcome is usually difficult to study. Therefore, the dedicated methodology of "small clinical trials" could be applied in IGI [Evans and Ildstad 2001].

At **Level 5**, the *economic impact* is assessed, on the basis of criteria like cost-effectiveness [Gibbons et al. 2001; Draaisma et al. 2006]. Such evaluations are mainly done by health organizations or cost bearers, based on political requests. For example, one cost analysis in IGI was performed by Gibbons et al. [2001]. This study included the measurement of the costs and benefit of image-guided surgery with an electromagnetic surgical navigation system in sinus surgery.

At **Level 6**, the *social, legal, and ethical impacts* are assessed. The goal of HCTA is also to advise or inform regulatory agencies, such as the US Food and Drug Administration (FDA) or the European Community about whether to permit the commercial use (e.g., marketing) of a system. HCTA also informs standards-setting organizations for health technology and health care delivery about the manufacture, use, and quality of care [Goodman 2004]. HCTA contributes in many ways to the knowledge base for improving the quality of health care, especially in innovative areas of medicine and surgery, such as image-guided surgery or robot-assisted surgery [Corbillon 2002; OHTAC 2004a,b, National Horizon Scanning Center (NHSC) 2002].

Such reports are usually meta-analyses, based on literature reviews, expert interviews, and local reviews in centers of excellence. These meta-analyses enable governmental organizations to plan future investments, as well as surgeons to consider the use of new technologies in their daily routines.

18.2.1.5 Criteria, Measures, and Expected Values

Surgery with image-guided systems can be seen as a triangle including the surgeon (plus the surgical staff), the patient, and the IGI system (Fig. 18.1). IGI assessment criteria may be characterized along this triangle into six categories:

1. Patient-related criteria, such as clinical scores, functional outcome, pain [Hanssen et al. 2006], cosmetic results [Hanssen et al. 2006], and resection rate
2. Surgeon-related criteria, such as cognitive stress, skill acquisition, and ergonomic working postures [Matern and Waller 1999; van Veelen et al. 2001]
3. IGI system-related criteria, such as technical accuracy and precision of 3D localization, latency, noise, and interference
4. Criteria related to interactions between surgeon and patient, such as time, complexity of procedure, and process-related criteria (e.g., resources, cost effectiveness, complications [Draaisma et al. 2006], reoperation, and change of strategy or planned surgical management [Solomon et al. 1994])
5. Criteria related to the interaction between surgeon and the IGI system, such as human factors [Goossens and van Veelen 2001] (e.g., usability [Martelli et al. 2003], situation awareness [Strauss et al. 2006], hand-eye coordination [Pichler et al. 1996], perception [Crothers et al. 1999; DeLucia et al. 2006], line-of-sight for tracking devices [Langlotz et al. 2006]), and surgical efficiency criteria (e.g., level of trust in a technical system, level of quality, level of reliance, change of strategy) [Strauss et al. 2006]
6. Criteria that express the interaction between the IGI system and the patient, such as clinical accuracy and precision, target registration error [Fitzpatrick et al. 1998; Fitzpatrick and West 2001], and safety margins.

Within each of these six IGI assessment categories, different validation criteria can be used for assessing the various aspects of an IGI system [Jannin et al. 2002], such as *accuracy, precision, robustness, specificity,* and *sensitivity.* For example, the accuracy can be the *spatial accuracy* of a navigation system or the *accuracy of time-synchronization.* Therefore, these terms cannot be included into one specific category only.

Accuracy is defined as the "degree to which a measurement is true or correct" [Goodman 2004]. For each sample of experimental data, local accuracy is defined as the difference between observed values and theoretical ideal expected values. The *precision* of a process is the resolution at which its results are repeatable, i.e., the value of the random fluctuation in the measurement made by the process. Precision is intrinsic to this process. Close to precision, *reliability* is defined as "the extent to which an observation that is repeated in the same, stable population yields the same result" [Goodman 2004]. The *robustness* of a system refers to its performance in the presence of disruptive factors such as intrinsic data variability, data artifacts, pathology, or interindividual anatomic or physiologic variability. *Specificity* and *sensitivity* are also useful for IGI assessment by computation of ratios between true positive, true negative, false-positive, and false-negative values. In IGI, it has to be emphasized that accuracy is not the only impotant criterion: robustness is also highly relevant.

The measures that give values for each criterion are dependent on the targeted categories of assessment criteria and the chosen assessment level. Some criteria and measures may be used for different assessment levels; others are particularly suited for a dedicated assessment level. The evaluation of each criterion needs to be specified and performed separately. Finally, the evaluation of *expected values* includes the definition of what constitutes nonconformance for both measurable and subjective criteria.

18.2.2 Study Conditions and Data Sets

It is crucial to assess the system in experimental conditions that are as close as possible to the surgical context and to the intended use of a system (as outlined earlier). The *Assessment Study Conditions* (i.e. *Assessment Locus*) [Goodman 2004] describe characteristics related to the actual use of the IGI system during assessment studies. Such characteristics include the assessment scenario, location, environment, and data sets. They must be explicitly specified.

18.2.2.1 The Assessment Surgical Scenario

An IGI system is assessed according to a surgical scenario, which mimics its use and includes a list of surgical steps for which the IGI system is assessed. The IGI system can be assessed throughout the whole surgical procedure, or only during single steps of the procedure. Further temporal conditions of the assessment are important. Clinical timing constraints relative to anaesthesia time, for example, are also a crucial characteristic of the surgical procedure and therefore of the assessment surgical scenario.

18.2.2.2 The Assessment Operator, Location, and Environment

Important questions that have to be clarified during the planning phase of the study are as follows:

1. Who will use the IGI system during the assessment study?
2. Where it will be performed?
3. How much of the full clinical environment will be available when performing the study?

18.2.2.3 Assessment Data Sets

The assessment surgical scenario is then applied in an assessment location and environment by an operator using dedicated *assessment data sets*. It is usual to distinguish families of assessment data sets along a continuum between clinical realism and easy control to the parameters to be studied. Along this continuum, three main categories can be identified: numerical simulations, physical phantoms, and clinical data sets (Fig. 18.3). Additional categories are also located along this continuum, such as data acquired from animals or cadavers. Assessment data sets are described by their location along the continuum, by their intrinsic characteristics, such as imaging modalities, spatial resolution or tissue contrast, and by clinical assumptions related to the data sets or to the patient, such as assumptions regarding anatomy, physiology, and pathology.

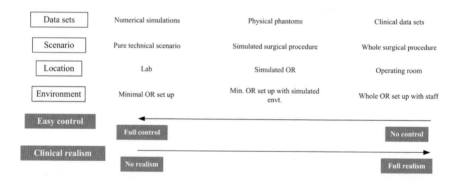

Fig. 18.3. Continuum for assessment data sets, scenario, location, and environment from full control of parameters to full clinical realism

A similar continuum can be used for describing the other study conditions: assessment surgical scenario, location, environment, operator, and temporal conditions. As shown in Fig. 18.3, there is usually a trade-off between control of parameters and clinical realism. Choice of a solution along these continua for all the categories are strongly related to the *assessment levels* as defined above.

18.2.3 Assessment Methods

The main prerequisite of a study is the proper definition of the *assessment objective* and the *study conditions*. This means that for each component as defined earlier (Fig. 18.2), a dedicated *value* (e.g., level, criterion, measure, data sets) is selected. Then a method is chosen to fulfil the assessment objective. The selection of an appropriate method will primarily depend on the assessment objective and secondarily on the study conditions. For some studies, it is possible to choose a reference for assessment (a gold standard), but for others it is impossible. This leads to a categorisation into (1) reference-based assessment and (2) assessment without reference.

18.2.3.1 Reference-Based Assessment

Reference-based assessment compares the direct or indirect results of a system with a reference (also called a *gold standard*)[1] that is assumed to be very close or equal to the ideal expected solution (also called the *ground truth*). Jannin et al. [2006] proposed a model for describing and reporting such reference-based assessment methods for medical image processing. This model is also useful for IGI when assessed criteria require such comparison with a reference (e.g., accuracy).

The main components and the main stages of this model are described as follows. The IGI system to be assessed is used according to the study conditions (surgical scenario, temporal conditions, operator, location, environment, and data sets). Characteristics of the system output are compared with ideal expected results. As ideal expected results are usually not directly available, another method can be used according to the study conditions to provide results that are closer to the ideal expected results than those computed by the system itself. These results are considered to be the *reference* against which results from the system will be compared. Assessment is a comparison of characteristics of both results, with the characteristics being chosen according to the targeted assessed criteria. The reference is generally chosen to be as accurate as possible, but in some situations it may have an error that should be taken into account during the assessment process or at least in the assessment results. The quantitative comparison may require converting those results in a similar format, which may be seen as a *normalization step*.

---

[1] In this chapter, we use the term *reference* rather than *gold standard*. *Reference* can be used in a wider meaning including terms of *gold, bronze,* or *fuzzy* standards.

This normalization aims at transforming the measurements of the assessed criteria in a clinically meaningful format. Normalized results of the system to be assessed, and normalized output of the reference method are comp pared using a *comparison function,* also called the *Assessment Metric.* Statistics of the comparison results distribution may serve as a *quality index,* also called a *figure of merit.* Finally, values of the quality indices are compared with expected values or models using a *statistical hypothesis test.* This consists of testing quality indices computed on comparison results against the assessment hypothesis to provide the assessment result.

To avoid mistakes or bias in reference-based assessment methods, the following aspects have to be carefully checked. The relevance of the data sets used in assessment studies must be verified according to two aspects: the realism of the data sets, and the coherence between the data sets and the assessment objective. The reference usually comes from one of the following methods:

1. It can be an exact and perfect solution computed from numerical simulations
2. It can be an estimated solution from the results of one or several reference methods
3. It can be another estimated solution from the results of the same assessed system but used with different data sets or conditions
4. It can be an expert-based solution relying on assumptions, or on a priori knowledge of the results.

In all cases, the quality of the reference has to be checked according to two aspects: correctness and realism. As the reference is also computed from the reference method, it is only an approximated value of the ideal expected results. A study of the error associated with the reference is crucial.

The comparison function can be considered as an assessment metric, as it quantifies the assessment criteria. This function has to be chosen or defined according to its suitability to fulfil the assessment objective.

Training and testing methods are also usually used for validation, such as the leave-one-out method. They could be considered as reference-based validation methods, since the result of the system when using the training set is compared to the result of the system when using the testing set. These methods can show the independence of the results according to the training set and the coherence of the findings computed with different references.

18.2.3.2 Assessment Without Reference

Some assessment criteria or some assessment objectives do not require any reference. For example, we can mention the consistency criterion for image registration and the Bland and Altman [1986] method for measurements. However, it is hard to define assessment objectives in clinical terms when using such assessment methods, as they mainly characterize intrinsic behavior of a method only. They usually allow evaluation of variability only, as no comparison with ideal expected results is performed. Finally, some assessment without reference methods relies on strong assumptions on the data sets or the assessed methods, which cannot always be verified easily.

18.2.3.3 Statistics

Statistics are crucial in assessment methodology, as assessment is usually performed with multiple studies, multiple data sets, or multiple sites. Finding relevant and appropriate statistical tests is not always straightforward. Statistical hypothesis tests usually rely on strong assumptions about the data that have to be carefully checked. Because of the importance of correct statistical analysis, the assessment team should incorporate statistical skills with knowledgeable partners.

18.3   Discussion

The complexity and diversity of assessment for IGI have been emphasized in this chapter. However, different tools and models are available to deal with this complexity. On the one hand, the effort that is performed in the specification phase of an assessment study, together with a clear and precise definition of the *assessment objective,* also helps to deal with the complexity. The diversity, on the other hand, can be managed with the concept of *assessment levels* in IGI.

The suggested tools, phases, components for each phase, and classifications are not exhaustive. There is no strict sequential structure inside each phase, and there are some dependencies and relationships between components in Fig. 18.2. Also, the assessment levels organization in Table 18.1 may not always be strictly hierarchical.

Obviously, the use of the presented tools does not guarantee the quality of the IGI system; rather it should guarantee the quality of the assessment study and provide a correct understanding and analysis of the assessment results. For the latter, the same rigorous methods that were presented should be used for *assessing* the applied *assessment method* itself. This should include the assessment of its associated components (e.g., criteria, statistical tests). Furthermore, different types of validity [Nelson 1980] (such as face validity, content validity, criterion validity, and construct validity) need to be assessed.

Other aspects close to assessment are not covered in this chapter but are also of great interest for IGI. Risk analysis is the assessment of risk according to a defined methodology. The surgical context and intended use are as important as in assessment studies. On the basis of the specification of these characteristics of an IGI system, the possible hazards are identified and estimated. The estimation is based on the level of severity, occurrence probability, and detection probability. From these estimations, different methods for *risk management* can be performed [Korb et al. 2005].

In this important, diverse, and complex landscape, there is much room for innovation and research. Some directions will now be mentioned. There is still a need for new assessment metrics adapted and relevant to a dedicated surgical context. There is a need for realistic and controllable study conditions, from data sets, surgical scenario, environment, and location. Another important aspect in the assessment methodology for correct dissemination and reproducibility of studies and results is the availability of open source data and tools. Such an open source environment will further facilitate assessment.

Finally, for all assessment aspects, there is a great need for standardization, both for specification, implementation, and reporting assessment. In health care technology assessment, some standards have been recently introduced for reporting of clinical trials, e.g., the *Standard for Reporting of Diagnostic Accuracy* (STARD), The *Grading of Recommendations Assessment, Development and Evaluation* (GRADE) Working Group, and the Current Controlled Trials Ltd. (a part of the Science Navigation Group of companies, which hosts the *International Standard Randomized Controlled Trial Number* (ISRCTN) Register). There is also a standard available for the specification and implementation of clinical patient trials for medical devices [ISO 14155:2003]. Some standards can be directly applied to IGI, some need to be adapted, and some additional ones are required. Standardization in IGI assessment will improve the quality of systems, their acceptance by surgeons, and facilitate their transfer from research to clinic practice.

As mentioned at the beginning of this chapter, each person involved in the development or use of an IGI system should be involved in assessment, at least in a specific assessment level. However, assessment studies can be tedious and difficult, requiring time, energy, and motivation. Results are not always as expected and biases are numerous. Such biases cover the spectrum from the specification of the study to the analysis of the results and can be hidden traps, sometimes requiring restarting the study from the beginning. But rigorous assessment is the only way to develop useful, relevant, and valuable tools for the patient and for society. As we cannot escape assessment, the best way forward is to make it as easy and efficient as possible.

Acknowledgments

The authors thank B. Gibaud, C. Grova, and P. Paul from Visages/INSERM/ University of Rennes and M. Audette, O. Burgert, A. Dietz, E. Dittrich, V. Falk, R. Grunert, M. Hofer, A. Klarmann, S. Jacobs, H. Lemke, J. Meixensberger, E. Nowatius, G. Strauss, and C. Trantakis from ICCAS (The Innovation Center for Computer Assisted Surgery) for fruitful discussions. They also thank participants and speakers of dedicated special sessions and workshops on this topic during the Computer Assisted Radiology and Surgery (CARS) conferences. Finally the authors thank S. Duchesne and M. Melke for their help during the preparation of the manuscript.

References

Balci O (2003). "Verification, validation and certification of modeling and simulation applications". In: *Proceedings of the 35th conference on Winter Simulation: Driving innovation*, New Orleans, Louisiana, 150–158.

Bland JM and Altman DG (1986). "Statistical methods for assessing agreement between two methods of clinical measurement". *Lancet*, 1, 307–310.

Chow S-C and Liu JP (2004). *Design and Analysis of Clinical Trials: Concepts and Methodologies*, Wiley, Hoboken, New Jersey, ISBN 0-471-24985-8.

Corbillon E (2002). "Computer-assisted surgery progress report." *ANAES*, Saint-Denis La Plaine.

Crothers IR, Gallagher AG, McClure N, James DTD, McGuigan (1999). "Experienced laparoscopic surgeons are automated to the "fulcrum effect": An ergonomic demonstration." *Endoscopy*, 31(5), 365–369.

DeLucia PR, Mather RD, Griswold JA, Mitra S (2006). "Toward the improvement of image-guided interventions for minimally invasive surgery: Three factors that affect performance." *Hum Factors*, 48(1), 23–38.

Draaisma WA, Buskens E, Bais JE, Simmermacher RKJ, Rijnhart-de Jong HG, Broeders IAMJ, Gosszen HG (2006). "Randomized clinical trial and follow-up study of cost-effectiveness of laparoscopic versus conventional Nissen fundoplication." *Br J Surg*, 93, 690–697.

Evans CH and Ildstad ST (2001). *Small Clinical Trials: Issues and Challenges*. Institute of Medicine, National Academy Press, Washington DC.

Fitzpatrick JM, West JB, Maurer CR, Jr (1998). "Predicting error in rigid-body, point-based registration." *IEEE Trans Med Imag*, 17, 694–702.

Fitzpatrick JM and West JB (2001). "The distribution of target registration error in rigid-body point-based registration." *IEEE Trans Med Imag* 20(9), 917–927.

Fryback DG and Thornbury JR (1991). "The efficacy of diagnostic imaging." *Med Decis Making*, 11, 88–94.

Gibbons MD, Gunn CG, Niwas S, Sillers MJ (2001). "Cost analysis of computer-aided endoscopic sinus surgery." *Am J Rhinol*, 15(2), 71–75.

Global Harmonization Task Force, Quality Management Systems (2004). "Process validation guidance" *GHTF*/SG3/N99-10: http://www.ghtf.org/sg3/inventorysg3/sg3_fd_n99-10_edition2.pdf [Accessed September 2007].

Goodman CS (2004). "Introduction to health care technology assessment." *Nat. Library of Medicine/NICHSR*: http://www.nlm.nih.gov/nichsr/hta101/ta101_c1.html [Accessed September 2007].

Goossens RHM and van Veelen MA (2001). "Assessment of ergonomics in laparoscopic surgery." *Min Invas Ther Allied Technol*, 10(3), 175–179.

Hanssen WEJ, Kuhry E, Casseres, Herder WW de, Steyerberg EW, Bonjer HJ (2006). "Safety and efficacy of endoscopic retroperitoneal adenalectomy." *Br J Surg*, 93, 715–719.

ISO 14155-1+2 (2003). "Clinical investigation of medical devices for human subjects. Part 1+2."

ISO 14971 (2001). "Medical devices – Application of risk management to medical devices."

ISO 9000 (2000). "Quality management systems – Fundamentals and vocabulary. International organization for standardization."

Jannin P, Fitzpatrick JM, Hawkes DJ, Pennec X, Shahidi R, Vannier MW (2002). "Validation of medical image processing in image-guided therapy." *IEEE Trans Med Imag*, 21(11), 1445–1449.

Jannin P, Grova C, Maurer C (2006). "Model for designing and reporting reference based validation procedures in medical image processing." *Int J Comput Assist Radiol Surg*, 1(2)2, 1001–1115.

Korb W, Kornfeld M, Birkfellner W, Boesecke R, Figl M, Fuerst M, Kettenbach J, Vogler A, Hassfeld S, Kronreif G (2005). "Risk analysis and safety assessment in surgical robotics: A case study on a biopsy robot." *Minim Invasive Ther*, 14(1), 23–31.

Korb W, Grunert R, Burgert O, Dietz A, Jacobs S, Falk V, Meixensberger J, Strauss G, Trantakis C, Lemke HU, Jannin P (2006). "An assessment model of the efficacy of image-guided therapy." *Int J Comp Assist Radiol Surg*, 1, 515–516.

Langlotz F, Kereliuk CM, Anderegg C (2006). "Augmenting the effective field of view of optical tracking cameras – A way to overcome difficulties during intraoperative camera alignment." *Comput Aided Surg*, 11(1), 31–36.

Martelli S, Nofrini L, Vendruscolo P, Visani A (2003). "Criteria of interface evaluation for computer assisted surgery systems." *Int J Med Informat*, 72, 35–45.

Matern U and Waller P (1999). "Instrument for minimally invasive surgery: Principles of ergonomic handles." *Surg Endosc*, 13, 174–182.

Medical Device Directive, Council Directive 93/42/EEC20 of 14 June 1993 concerning medical devices. *European Community, Official Journal* L 169, 1–43.

National Horizon Scanning Centre (NHSC), The University of Birmingham: Surgical Robots.Update (2002) http://www.pcpoh.bham.ac.uk/publichealth/horizon/PDF_files/2002reports/Robots Update.pdf and
http://www.pcpoh.bham.ac.uk/publichealth/horizon/PDF_files/2000reports/Surgical_robots.PDF [Accessed September 2007].

Nelson AA (1980). "Research design: Measurement, reliability and validity." *Am J Hosp Pharm*, 37, 851–857.

OHTAC Recommendation (2004a). "Computer assisted hip and knee arthroplasty: Navigation and robotic systems."http://www.health.gov.on.ca/english/providers/program/mas/tech/reviews/pdf/rev_arthro_020104.pdf [Accessed September 2007].

OHTAC Recommendation (2004b). "Computer assisted surgery using telemanipulators."http://www.health.gov.on.ca/english/providers/program/mas/tech/reviews/pdf/rev_teleman_020104.pdf [Accessed September 2007].

Paleologos TS, Wadley JP, Kitchen ND, Thomas DGT (2000). "Clinical utility and cost-effectiveness of interactive image-guided craniotomy: Clinical comparison between conventional and image-guided meningioma surgery." *Neurosurgery*, 47(1), 40–48.

Pichler C von, Radermacher K, Rau G (1996). "The state of 3D technology and evaluation." *Min Invax Ther Allied Technol*, 5, 419–426.

Pocock SJ (2004). *Clinical Trials: A Practical Approach*, Wiley, New York, ISBN 0-471-90155-5.

Solomon MJ, Stephen MS, Gallinger S, White GH (1994). "Does intraoperative hepatic ultrasonography change surgical decision making during liver resection?". *The Am J Surg*, 168, 307–310.

Strauss G, Koulechov K, Röttger S, Bahner J, Trantakis C, Hofer M, Korb W, Burgert O, Meixensberger J, Manzey D, Dietz A, Lüth T (2006). "Evaluation of a navigation system for ENT with surgical efficiency criteria." *Laryngoscope*, 116(4), 564–572.

Van Veelen MA, Meijer DW, Goossens RHM, Snijders CJ (2001). "New ergonomic design criteria for handles of laparoscopic dissection forceps." *J Laparoendosc Adv Surg Tech*, 11(1), 17–26.

Index

Printed in the United States of America

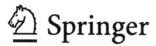